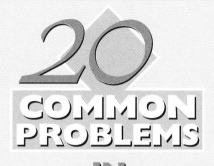

20 COMMON PROBLEMS IN

Preventive Health Care

Notice

Medicine is an ever-changing science. As new research and clinical experience broaden our knowledge, changes in treatment and drug therapy are required. The editor and publisher of this work have checked with sources believed to be reliable in their efforts to provide information that is complete and generally in accord with the standards accepted at the time of publication. However, in view of the possibility of human error or changes in medical sciences, neither the editor nor the publisher nor any other party who has been involved in the preparation or publication of this work warrants that the information contained herein is in every respect accurate or complete, and they are not responsible for any errors or omissions or for the results obtained from use of such information. Readers are encouraged to confirm the information contained herein with other sources. For example and in particular, readers are advised to check the product information sheet included in the package of each drug they plan to administer to be certain that the information contained in this book is accurate and that changes have not been made in the recommended dose or in the contraindications for administration. This recommendation is of particular importance in connection with new or infrequently used drugs.

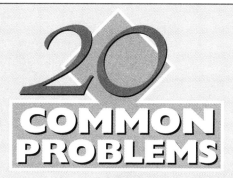

20 COMMON PROBLEMS

IN

Preventive Health Care

EDITOR

DOUGLAS CAMPOS-OUTCALT, M.D., M.P.A.

Medical Director of Preventive Services
Maricopa County Department of Public Health
Phoenix, Arizona

Series Editor

BARRY D. WEISS, M.D.

Professor of Clinical Family and Community Medicine
Univeristy of Arizona College of Medicine
Tucson, Arizona

McGraw-Hill

Health Professions Division

New York   St. Louis   San Francisco   Auckland   Bogotá   Caracas   Lisbon   London   Madrid
Mexico City   Milan   Montreal   New Delhi   San Juan   Singapore   Sydney   Tokyo   Toronto

McGraw-Hill

A Division of The **McGraw·Hill** *Companies*

20 COMMON PROBLEMS IN PREVENTIVE HEALTH CARE

Copyright © 2000 by The McGraw-Hill Companies, Inc. All rights reserved. Printed in the United States of America. Except as permitted under the United States Copyright Act of 1976, no part of this publication may be reproduced or distributed in any form or by any means, or stored in a data base or retrieval system, without prior written permission of the publisher.

1234567890 DOCDOC 09876543210

ISBN 0-07-012044-7

This book was set in Garamond by Better Graphics.
The editors were Martin Wonsowiecz, Susan Noujaim, and Karen G. Edmonson.
The production supervisor was Rick Ruzycka.
The text and cover were designed by Marsha Cohen/Parallelogram.
The indexer was Pat Perrier.

R.R. Donnelley and Sons, Inc., was the printer and binder.

This book was printed on acid-free paper.

Library of Congress Cataloging-in-Publication Data

20 common problems in preventive health care / editor, Douglas Campos-Outcalt.
    p.; cm.
  Includes bibliographical references and index.
  ISBN 0-07-012044-7
    1. Medicine, Preventive--United States. I. Title: Twenty common problems in preventive health care. II. Campos-Outcalt, Douglas.
  [DNLM: 1. Primary Prevention--methods. WA 108 Z999 2000]
RA425 .A15 2000
362.1--dc21   99-089081

This book is dedicated to my parents, Norman and Elizabeth Outcalt, and to my wife, Frances Campos-Outcalt. Words cannot express what I owe to these three.

Contents

Part
3
Adults   203

Contributors

ADULT VACCINATIONS (CHAPTER 19)
Ellen R. Ahwesh, M.A.
Department of Epidemiology
Graduate School of Public Health
University of Pittsburgh
Pittsburgh, Pennsylvania

CARDIOVASCULAR DISEASE (CHAPTER 16)
James L. Arter, M.D.
Greenville Hospital System
Greenville, South Carolina

BREAST CANCER (CHAPTER 13)
Lorne Becker, M.D.
Professor and Chair
Department of Family Medicine
State University of New York
Syracuse, New York

COLON CANCER (CHAPTER 15)
Marvin Moe Bell, M.D., M.P.H.
Associate Director
Scottsdale Healthcare Family Practice Residency
Scottsdale, Arizona

DENTAL DECAY (CHAPTER 4)
Robert J. Berkowitz, D.D.S.
Professor of Dentistry
Chief, Division of Pediatric Dentistry
Eastman Department of Dentistry
University of Rochester Medical Center
Rochester, New York

IMMUNIZATIONS (CHAPTER 1)
Ilene T. Burns M.D., M.P.H.
Assistant Professor
Department of Family Medicine and Clinical Epidemiology
University of Pittsburgh School of Medicine
Pittsburgh, Pennsylvania

CARDIOVASCULAR DISEASE (CHAPTER 16)
Jeffrey L. Bush, M.D.
Greensville Hospital System
Greensville, South Carolina

VISION PROBLEMS (CHAPTER 2)
Lindsay A. Campbell, M.D.
Clinical Assistant Professor
Department of Pediatrics
University of Arizona College of Medicine
Phoenix Children's Hospital
Phoenix, Arizona

PRENATAL CARE/PROSTATE CANCER (CHAPTERS 9 AND 14)
Doug Campos-Outcalt, M.D., M.P.A.
Medical Director, Preventive Services
Maricopa County Department of Public Health
Associate Chair for Phoenix
Department of Family and Community Medicine
University of Arizona College of Medicine
Phoenix, Arizona

CARDIOVASCULAR DISEASE (CHAPTER 16)
James K. Crager, M.D.
Greenville Hospital System
Greenville, South Carolina

NEWBORN METABOLIC SCREENING (CHAPTER 7)
Franklin Desposito, M.D.
Chairman
Department of Pediatrics
New Jersey Medical School
Newark, New Jersey

DENTAL DECAY (CHAPTER 4)
Burton Edelstein, D.D.S., M.P.H.
Clinical Assistant Professor
Harvard School of Dental Medicine
Boston, Massachusetts

SEXUALLY TRANSMITTED DISEASES (CHAPTER 8)
Jonathan M. Ellen, M.D.
Department of Pediatrics
Johns Hopkins Hospital
Baltimore, Maryland

CERVICAL CANCER (CHAPTER 12)
Paul Gordon, M.D.
Associate Professor and Co-Head
Department of Family and Community Medicine
University of Arizona College of Medicine
Tucson, Arizona

IRON DEFICIENCY ANEMIA (CHAPTER 5)
Paul P. Hartlaub, M.D., M.S.P.H.
Associate Professor and Interim Associate Chair
Department of Family Medicine
University of Wisconsin Medical School
Milwaukee, Wisconsin

OSTEOPOROSIS (CHAPTER 18)
Fred E. Heidrich, M.D., M.P.H.
Family Practice Residency Program Director
Group Health Cooperative of Puget Sound
Seattle, Washington

DIABETES (CHAPTER 17)
Lynn Helseth
MD and PhD candidate
University of Nebraska College of Medicine
Omaha, Nebraska

BREAST CANCER (CHAPTER 13)
Pamela Horst, M.D.
Associate Professor
Department of Family Medicine
State University of New York
Syracuse, New York

SMOKING PREVENTION AND CESSATION (CHAPTER 10)
Carlos Roberto, Jaén, M.D., Ph.D.
Associate Professor and Vice Chairman
Department of Family Medicine
Department of Social and Preventive Medicine
State University of New York at Buffalo
Buffalo, New York

THE TRAVELER (CHAPTER 20)
Randa M. Kutob, M.D.
Assistant Professor
Department of Family and Community Medicine
University of Arizona College of Medicine
Tucson, Arizona

IRON DEFICIENCY ANEMIA (CHAPTER 5)
Nuzhat Majid, M.D.
Mora Medical Center
Mora, Minnesota

SEXUALLY TRANSMITTED DISEASES (CHAPTER 8)
Erica B. Monasterio, R.N., M.S., F.N.P.
Associate Clinical Professor
Division of Adolescent Medicine
Department of Pediatrics
University of California, San Francisco
San Francisco, California

PRENATAL CARE (CHAPTER 9)
Elizabeth H. Morrison, M.D., M.S.Ed.
Associate Clinical Professor
Director of Maternity Care Education
Assistant Clinical Professor of Family Medicine
University of California, Irvine
Long Beach, California

THE TRAVELER (CHAPTER 20)
Ron E. Pust, M.D.
Professor
Department of Family and Community Medicine
University of Arizona College of Medicine
Tucson, Arizona

DIABETES (CHAPTER 17)
Jeff Susman, M.D.
Professor and Director
Department of Family Medicine
University of Cincinnati
Cincinnati, Ohio

CARDIOVASCULAR DISEASE (CHAPTER 16)
Randal J. Thomas, M.D., M.S.
Senior Associate Consultant
Division of Cardiovascular Diseases
Department of Internal Medicine
Mayo Clinic
Rochester, Minnesota

Contributors ◆

ALCOHOL AND DRUG ABUSE (CHAPTER 11)
Daniel C. Vinson, M.D., M.S.P.H.
Associate Professor
Department of Family and Community Medicine
University of Missouri-Columbia
Columbia, Missouri

BREAST CANCER (CHAPTER 13)
Pamela Vnenchak
Assistant Professor
Department of Family Medicine
State University of New York
Syracuse, New York

HEARING PROBLEMS (CHAPTER 3)
Jeffrey C. Weiss, M.D.
Chief, Section of General Pediatrics
Phoenix Children's Hospital
Phoenix, Arizona

LEAD POISONING (CHAPTER 6)
Michael Weitzman, M.D.
Professor and Associate Chairman
Department of Pediatrics
University of Rochester School of Medicine and Dentistry
Rochester, New York

DENTAL DECAY (CHAPTER 4)
Dominick Zero, D.D.S., M.S.
Professor of Dentistry
Eastman Department of Dentistry
University of Rochester Medical Center
Rochester, New York

IMMUNIZATIONS/ADULT VACCINATIONS (CHAPTERS 1 AND 19)
Richard Kent Zimmerman, M.D., M.P.H.
Department of Family Medicine and Clinical Epidemiology, School of Medicine
Department of Health Services Administration, Graduate School of Public Health
University of Pittsburgh
Pittsburgh, Pennsylvania

Introduction

Twenty Common Problems in Prevention is an attempt to provide students and clinicians in the health sciences with a firm foundation in the field of clinical preventive medicine. It takes 20 of the most common issues facing clinicians and covers them in depth. The book is organized by topic under three age groups: infants and children, adolescents and young adults, and adults. Mastery and application of the material contained in each section will mean that the clinician and student can competently handle a significant proportion of the prevention challenges faced in primary care practice and will be prepared for the clinical prevention portion of licensing examinations.

The book borrows heavily from several sources that deserve mention. The U.S. Preventive Services Task Force (USPSTF) is a government-sponsored group of experts that reviews screening, counseling, and immunization interventions; evaluates the strength of evidence for or against their effectiveness; and makes recommendations for or against their use. Their methodology is sound, and their work contributes significantly to the field of evidence-based medicine and should be emulated. The Canadian Task Force on the Periodic Health Exam deserves recognition as being the forerunner and model for the USPSTF and for their ongoing work in evaluating prevention interventions. The Centers for Disease Control and Prevention (CDC) regularly produces updated recommendations on vaccines, control of infectious diseases, and other areas of clinical medicine. They are viewed worldwide as a leader in the field of public health and preventive medicine.

Students and clinicians who use this book should be familiar and conversant with certain terms, for example: primary, secondary, and tertiary prevention; sensitivity, specificity, positive predictive value, and negative predictive value; and lead time and length bias. The introductory chapters of the second edition of the *Guide to Clinical Preventive Services* by the USPSTF (1996) can be used as a resource for those unfamiliar with these concepts. Chapter 19, (Preventive Health Examinations) in *Twenty Common Problems in Primary Care* is also recommended to help organize an approach to individual patients and apply the material contained in this text.

Finally, there is a word of caution. As much as we would all like to learn a body of knowledge and then rest content, the rapidly changing knowledge base of medicine does not allow it. Preventive medicine is no different. The USPSTF, at the time of publication of this book, is beginning the process of reviewing and revising their recommendations. The CDC, as previously mentioned, regularly reviews and updates their recommendations. The ready availability of information on the Internet now provides instant updates; we no longer need to wait for books and publications to find their way from the press to our desks. This book represents the authors' interpretation, as well as my own, of the knowledge accumulated on each topic as of the date of publication. The novice would do well to master the material and use it as a foundation but not be tied too tightly to the facts and recommendations; they will change with time. Better to learn the concepts and develop a methodology for remaining current.

Acknowledgments

I thank Barry Weiss, Susan Noujaim, and Ann Dennison for their assistance in preparing this book. I also thank my wife and children for their patience and understanding about the long hours that I spent apart from them while I was working on this project. Most of all, thanks to the authors, who so promptly and competently contributed their chapters. They were a pleasure to work with.

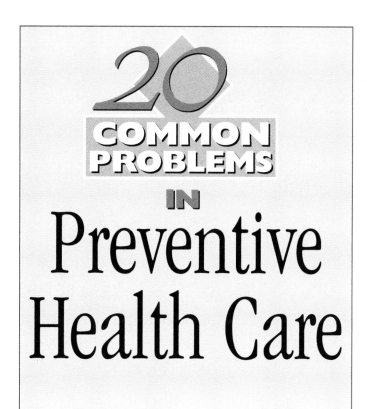

20

COMMON
PROBLEMS

IN

Preventive
Health Care

Part

1

Infants
and Children

Richard Kent Zimmerman
Ilene Timko Burns

Chapter

1

Immunizations

Introduction

The national childhood vaccination program in the United States, including the development of vaccines and guidelines concerning which children should receive vaccination and when, has been tremendously successful in decreasing the incidence of vaccine-preventable diseases in

The bulk of this chapter was modified from a project supported by funding from the Centers for Disease Control and Prevention, National Immunization Program, through Cooperative Agreement U50/CCU300860-10 to the Association of Teachers of Preventive Medicine (ATPM).

The use of trade names and commercial sources is for identification purposes only and does not constitute endorsement by the U.S. Department of Health and Human Services, the U.S. Public Health Service, the Centers for Disease Control and Prevention, or the Association of Teachers of Preventive Medicine.

children. For example, the total number of measles cases among U.S. children dropped from 458,083 in 1964, the year before widespread use of measles vaccine began, to 138 in 1997. Cases of *Haemophilus influenzae* type b (Hib) disease among children in the United States have also dropped dramatically, from an estimated 20,000 annually before introduction of Hib vaccine to fewer than 300 in 1996. Table 1-1 lists the maximum number of cases ever reported of nine vaccine-preventable diseases and compares them with the numbers reported in 1996. The benefits of childhood vaccinations can be further appreciated from Fig. 1-1 through Fig. 1-5, which show the historical incidence rates of selected vaccine-preventable diseases in the United States and the effect of the introduction of vaccine.

As the benefits of each vaccine and guidelines concerning which children should receive it became known, vaccination rates increased dramatically. Nevertheless, childhood vaccina-

Table 1-1

Maximum Number of Cases of Specified Vaccine-preventable Diseases Ever Reported for a Calendar Year Compared with the Number of Cases of Disease in 1996

DISEASE	YEAR(S) MAXIMUM NUMBER REPORTED	MAXIMUM NUMBER OF CASES REPORTED IN PREVACCINE ERA	REPORTED CASES IN 1996	PERCENTAGE CHANGE
Hepatitis B	1989	132,000	10,637	−91%
Diphtheria	1921	206,939	2	−100%
Pertussis	1934	265,269	7,796	−97%
Tetanus	1948	601	36	−94%
Invasive *Haemophilus influenzae*	1984	20,000[a]	1,170	−94%
Poliomyelitis (wild indigenous)	1952	21,269	0	−100%
Measles	1941	894,134	508	−100%
Mumps	1968	152,209	751	−100%
Congenital rubella	1964–1965	20,000[a]	4	−100%

[a] Estimated numbers.

SOURCE: Adapted from Centers for Disease Control and Prevention: Update: vaccine side effects, adverse reactions, contraindications, and precautions—recommendations of the Advisory Committee on Immunization Practices (ACIP). *MMWR* 45(RR-12):2, 1996. Public domain.

Figure 1-1 to 1-5

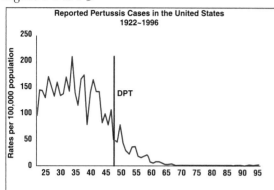

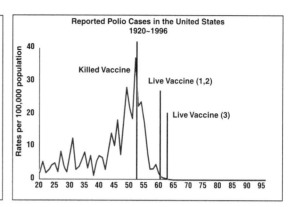

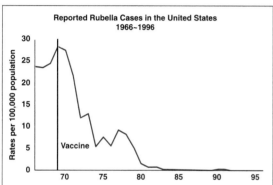

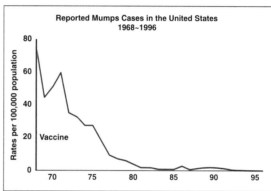

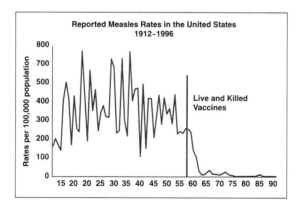

tion rates remain less than optimal. In 1997, among children aged 19 to 35 months, 93% had received three or more doses of Hib vaccine; 81% had received four doses of diphtheria, tetanus toxoids, and pertussis vaccine (DTP) or pediatric diphtheria and tetanus toxoids (DT); and 76% had completed four doses of DTP, three doses of poliovirus vaccine, three doses of Hib, and one dose of measles-containing vaccine. It is important that each primary care clinician understands the benefits of childhood vaccinations, stays well informed about current recommended vaccines and immunization schedules, and stores and uses vaccines properly.

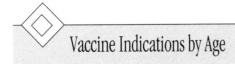

Vaccine Indications by Age

Schedules have been developed for administering doses of vaccine to children based on their age (Fig. 1-6).

Hepatitis B Vaccine

The epidemiology of hepatitis B has changed little over the past 10 years. It is estimated that between 128,000 and 320,000 persons are infected with hepatitis B virus (HBV) annually in the United States, and approximately 6000 persons die annually of HBV-related liver disease. Most of these deaths occur in persons with chronic HBV infection and are due to cirrhosis or primary hepatocellular carcinoma. The number of persons chronically infected with HBV in the United States, each of whom is potentially infectious, is estimated at 1.25 million, and the lifetime risk of acquiring HBV infection has been estimated at 5%. HBV infection is clearly a major health problem in this country.

HBV is transmitted by sexual contact or exposure to contaminated blood. Those at high risk of HBV infection include intravenous drug users, men who have sex with men, health care workers, dialysis patients, staff at institutions for the mentally retarded, and sexual and household contacts of HBV carriers. Immigrants from Asia and sub-Saharan Africa and Alaskan Natives/Pacific Islanders also have higher rates of HBV serologic markers.

The incubation period of HBV averages 120 days, with a range of 45 to 160 days. Clinical symptoms include nausea, vomiting, abdominal pain, malaise, diarrhea, and jaundice, although the disease can cause only minor symptoms or be asymptomatic. Most of those who are infected recover and develop immunity to the disease. Chronic HBV infection results when the infected person does not develop immunity and HBV continues to infect the liver. These individuals continue to test positive for hepatitis B surface antigen (HBsAg) but negative for hepatitis B surface antibody (HBsAb). Any HBV infection lasting longer than 6 months is considered to be chronic. Those with chronic HBV infection are at high risk of cirrhosis, liver failure, and hepatocellular carcinoma.

HBV infection is much more likely to become chronic when it is acquired early in life than when it is contracted during adulthood: chronic HBV infection develops in 90% of those infected as infants, 30% to 60% of those infected before the age of 4 years, and only 5% to 10% of those infected as adults. Although most acute HBV infections in the United States occur in adulthood because of high-risk behaviors, 36% of all persons in the United States with chronic HBV infection contracted the infection during childhood. Up to 25% of individuals infected with HBV as infants will die of HBV-related chronic liver disease as adults.

RATIONALE FOR ROUTINE HEPATITIS B VACCINATION

There are several reasons to recommend routine infant vaccination against HBV. First, there is the concern about morbidity and mortality of HBV infection, especially when contracted in childhood. Moreover, transmission of HBV infection from child to child, although relatively infrequent, has been reported in schools, daycare centers, and families and among playmates. Strategies focusing on immunization of high-risk persons have had little impact, and no risk factor for HBV infection can be identified in at least 30% of infected persons. Those who engage in high-risk forms of behavior (e.g., injection drug use) frequently are not compliant with the needed three-dose vaccination regimen, and many become infected soon after beginning such practices. Finally, routine infant hepatitis B vaccination is as cost-effective as other commonly used preventive measures.

HEPATITIS B VACCINATION POLICY

The prevalence of HBV infection and its associated morbidity and mortality have led to the development of a comprehensive Hepatitis B vaccination policy that includes recommendations for prevention of perinatal HBV infection, routine infant vaccination, catch-up vaccination of adolescents not previously vaccinated, catch-up vaccination of young children at high risk of infection, and preexposure vaccination of adolescents and adults based on lifestyle or environmental, medical, and occupational situations that place them at risk. Hepatitis B vaccination is recommended for all infants and catch-up vaccination for unvaccinated children and adolescents of any age, by the Advisory Committee on Immunization Practices (ACIP), the American Academy of Pediatrics (AAP), and the American Academy of Family Physicians (AAFP).

HEPATITIS B VACCINES AND VACCINATION PROCEDURES

The hepatitis B vaccines currently produced in the United States, Recombivax HB and Engerix-B, are manufactured by recombinant DNA technology using baker's yeast and do not contain human plasma. Preexposure vaccination results in protective antibody levels in almost all infants and children (>95%).

PREVENTION OF PERINATAL HBV INFECTION   According to the ACIP, the American College of Obstetricians and Gynecologists, the AAP, and the U.S. Preventive Services Task Force, all pregnant women should be screened for HBsAg, optimally at an early prenatal visit. According to published calculations, screening all pregnant women in the United States would result in detection of about 22,000 HBsAg-positive women each year and prevent chronic HBV infection in 6000 neonates annually. Women whose initial HBsAg test result is negative but who are at high risk of HBV infection (e.g.,

women who use injection drugs, have a recently diagnosed sexually transmitted disease, have multiple sexual partners, or had hepatitis during pregnancy) should be tested again for HBsAg late in pregnancy.

ROUTINE INFANT VACCINATION   For infants born to mothers with positive or unknown HBsAg status, postexposure prophylaxis, including both hepatitis B immune globulin (HBIG) and hepatitis B vaccine, should be initiated within 12 hours of birth, regardless of gestational age. These infants should receive their second and third doses of vaccine at ages 1 to 2 months and 6 months, respectively. If the mother is chronically infected with HBV, the infant should be tested for HBsAg and anti-HBs at 9 to 15 months of age to determine the success of vaccination.

For infants who weigh less than 2 kg at birth whose mothers are known to be HBsAg negative, the first dose of hepatitis B vaccine should be delayed until the infant weighs 2 kg, because seroconversion rates are lower in infants born prematurely with birth weights less than 2 kg and lower still in those with birth weights less than 1 kg. For newborns weighing more than 2 kg at birth whose mothers are known to be HBsAg negative, the first dose of hepatitis B vaccine can be given at or before the time of hospital discharge.

Table 1-2 lists recommended doses for hepatitis B vaccination by age and vaccine type, and Table 1-3 lists the hepatitis B vaccine schedule based on the patient's age and the indication for vaccination. If the hepatitis B vaccine schedule is interrupted, it should be continued. The second dose can be given as soon as 1 month after the first, and the third dose can be given as soon as 2 months after the second dose, as long as that is at least 4 months after the first dose and the patient is at least 6 months old. COMVAX, a combination of hepatitis B and Hib vaccines, was licensed in October 1996. It is licensed for use only in children born to HBsAg-negative mothers. It should not be used in chil-

Figure 1-6

Vaccine	Birth	1 mo	2 mos	4 mos	6 mos	12 mos	15 mos	18 mos	4–6 yrs	11–12 yrs	14–16 yrs
Hepatitis B[†]	Hep B	Hep B		Hep B						(Hep B)	
Diphtheria and tetanus toxoids and pertussis			DTaP	DTaP	DTaP		DTaP		DTaP	Td	
H. influenzae type b[∥]			Hib	Hib	Hib	Hib					
Poliovirus[**]			IPV	IPV		IPV			IPV		
Measles-mumps-rubella[§§]						MMR			MMR	(MMR)	
Varicella[¶∥]							Var			(Var)	

Age

☐ Range of Acceptable Ages for vaccination

⬭ Vaccines to be Assessed and Administered if Necessary

Recommended childhood immunization schedule.

* This schedule indicates the recommended ages for routine administration of currently licensed childhood vaccines. Any dose not given at the recommended age should be given as a "catch-up" vaccination at any subsequent visit when indicated and feasible. Combination vaccines may be used whenever any components of the combination are indicated and its other components are not contraindicated. Providers should consult the manufacturers' package inserts for detailed recommendations.

† **Infants born to hepatitis B surface antigen (HBsAg)-negative mothers** should receive the second dose of hepatitis B (Hep B) vaccine at least 1 month after the first dose. The third dose should be administered at least 4 months after the first dose and at least 2 months after the second dose, but not before age 6 months. **Infants born to HBsAg-positive mothers** should receive Hep B vaccine and 0.5 mL hepatitis B immune globulin (HBIG) within 12 hours of birth at separate injection sites. The second dose is recommended at age 1–2 months and the third dose at age 6 months. **Infants born to mothers whose HBsAg status is unknown** should receive Hep B vaccine within 12 hours of delivery to determine the mother's HBsAg status; if the HBsAg test is positive, the infant should receive HBIG as soon as possible (no later than age 1 week). All children and adolescents (through age 18 years) who have not been vaccinated against hepatitis B may begin the series during any visit. Special efforts should be made to vaccinate children who were born in or whose parents were born in areas of the world where hepatitis B virus infection is moderately or highly endemic.

§ The fourth dose may be administered as early as age 12 months, provided 6 months have elapsed since the third dose and if the child is unlikely to return at age 15–18 months. Tetanus and diphtheria toxoids (Td) is recommended at age 11–12 years if at least 5 years have elapsed since the last dose of DTP, DTaP, or DT. Subsequent routine Td boosters are recommended every 10 years.

¶ Three *Haemophilus influenzae* type b (Hib) conjugate vaccines are licensed for infant use. If Hib conjugate vaccine (PRP-OMP) (PedvaxHIB® or ComVax® [Merck]) is administered at ages 2 and 4 months, a dose at age 6 months is not required. Because clinical studies in infants have demonstrated that using some combination products may induce a lower immune response to the Hib vaccine component. DTaP/Hib combination products should not be used for primary vaccination in infants at ages 2,4, or 6 months unless approved by the Food and Drug Administration for these ages.

** Two poliovirus vaccines are licensed in the United States: inactivated poliovirus vaccine (IPV) and oral poliovirus vaccine (OPV). The ACIP, AAFP and AAP recommend all IPV series. OPV is no longer recommended and is acceptable only for special circumstances (e.g., use in the sequential schedule when parents do not accept the recommended number of injections, and imminent travel to areas where poliomyelitis is endemic.

§§ The second dose of measles, mumps, and rubella vaccine (MMR) is recommended routinely at age 4–6 years but may be administered during any visit provided at least 4 weeks have elapsed since receipt of the first dose and that both doses are administered beginning at or after age 12 months. Those who have not previously received the second dose should complete the schedule no later than the routine visit to a health-care provider at age 11–12 years.

¶¶ Varicella (Var) vaccine is recommended at any visit on or after the first birthday for susceptible children (i.e., those who lack a reliable history of chickenpox [as judged by a health-care provider] and who have not been vaccinated). Susceptible persons aged ≥13 years should receive two doses given at least 4 weeks apart.

Use of trade names and commercial sources is for identification only and does not imply endorsement by CDC or the U.S. Department of Health and Human Services.

Source: Advisory Committee on Immunization Practices (ACIP), American Academy of Family Physicians (AAFP), and American Academy of Pediatrics (AA).

Table 1-2

Hepatitis B Vaccine Dose by Patient Age and Immune Status and Vaccine Type

| | **EACH DOSE** | | |
PATIENT STATUS	**RECOMBIVAX HB (μG)**	**ENGERIX-B (μG)**	**ADMINISTRATION SITE**
Infant	5	10	Anterolateral thigh
Child or adolescent up to 19 years old	5	10	
Adult 20 years of age or older	10	20	Deltoid muscle
Dialysis patients or immunocompromised patients	40[a]	Total 40[b]	

[a] Special formulation of 40 μg in 1.0 mL.
[b] Four-dose schedule (0, 1, 2, and 6 months) using two 1.0-mL doses (for a total of 40 μg) at one site for each dose.
SOURCE: Modified from Centers for Disease Control and Prevention: Hepatitis B virus infection: A comprehensive immunization strategy to eliminate transmission in the United States—recommendations of the Advisory Committee on Immunization Practices (ACIP). *MMWR* (in press). Public domain.

Table 1-3

Hepatitis B Vaccine Schedule

HEPATITIS B VACCINE DOSE	**VACCINATION OF INFANTS BORN TO HBsAg-POSITIVE MOTHERS AND CATCH-UP VACCINATION AND CHILDREN AND ADOLESCENTS**[a]	**AGE FOR ROUTINE VACCINATION OF INFANTS BORN TO HBsAg-NEGATIVE MOTHERS**	**ALTERNATIVE SCHEDULE FOR CATCH-UP VACCINATION OF CHILDREN AND ADOLESCENTS (1 TO 19 YEARS OLD)**
Dose 1	Start (or within 12 hr of birth if born to HBsAg-positive mother)	Birth to 2 mo	Start
HBIG	Within 12 hr of birth if born to HBsAg-positive mother	N/A	N/A
Dose 2	1–2 mo later	1 to 4 mo of age[b]	2 mo later[c]
Dose 3	6 mo of age (or from first dose)	6 to 18 mo of age	4 mo from first dose

[a] Infants born to mothers who were not screened for HBsAg should receive hepatitis B vaccine within 12 hr of birth at the dose for infants born to HBsAg-positive mothers. Their subsequent treatment depends on their mother's HBsAg status.
[b] The second dose should be administered at least 1 mo after the first dose.
[c] For adolescents 11 to 19 yr old, the second dose may be given 1 to 2 mo after the first.
ABBREVIATIONS: HBsAg, hepatitis B surface antigen; HBIG, hepatitis B immune globulin; NA, not applicable.
SOURCE: Modified from Centers for Disease Control and Prevention: Hepatitis B virus infection: A comprehensive immunization strategy to eliminate transmission in the United States—recommendations of the Advisory Committee on Immunization Practices (ACIP). *MMWR* (in press). Public domain.

dren less than 6 weeks of age. This vaccine is discussed in more detail in the section on Hib vaccines.

Pertussis Vaccine

Before the licensure of pertussis vaccine, pertussis was a major cause of mortality and morbidity in infants and children in the United States. Owing to the widespread use of pertussis vaccines, rates now are only 5% of what they were before the advent of vaccine. In 1996 there were 7796 cases reported. Over the past decade, a higher proportion of cases have been reported in adults; in 1996, 4.5% of cases were in those age 15 and older.

Pertussis (whooping cough) is transmitted by respiratory droplets and occasionally by contact with freshly contaminated objects. Pertussis is highly contagious: from 70% to 100% of susceptible household contacts and 50% to 80% of susceptible school contacts will become infected following exposure to a person who is contagious. (Communicability lasts from 7 days after exposure to 3 weeks after the onset of the symptoms.) Symptoms include a cough that becomes paroxysmal within 1 to 2 weeks with repeated violent coughs followed by a high-pitched whoop on inspiration. Paroxysm can end with vomiting or spitting of clear mucus. Adolescents and adults often do not have paroxysms but instead have a chronic cough that is diagnosed as bronchitis.

Components of *Bordetella pertussis* that are important in the organism's ability to cause disease include tracheal cytotoxin that destroys cilia, making it difficult to clear thickened mucus; pertussis toxin (also called lymphocytosis-promoting factor), which interferes with immune cell function, contributes to ciliary damage, and aids attachment to respiratory epithelium; filamentous hemagglutinin, which helps the bacteria attach to cilia of the respiratory tract; pertactin (also called 69-kd protein), which also aids bacterial attachment to cilia; and agglu-

tinogens, which may aid persistent attachment to cilia.

RATIONALE FOR VACCINATION

Almost half (47%) of reported cases of pertussis occur in infants, and most reported cases (72%) are seen in children younger than 5 years of age. The hospitalization rate is 69% for reported cases of pertussis in infants younger than 12 months of age, and their case fatality rate is 0.6%. Pneumonia is an accompanying feature in about 15% of pertussis cases and is the leading cause of death from pertussis. Seizures occur in 2.2% of cases of pertussis and encephalopathy in 0.7% of cases. Encephalopathy, which may be caused by hypoxia or minute cerebral hemorrhages, is fatal in approximately one-third of cases and causes permanent brain damage in another one-third.

Before routine pertussis vaccination of children, whooping cough incidence peaked approximately every 3 to 4 years, and virtually all children were eventually infected. Between 1925 and 1930, 36,013 persons died in the United States from complications of pertussis. More than one million cases of pertussis were reported in the United States from 1940 through 1945. After pertussis vaccination became widespread in the mid-1940s, the incidence of pertussis dropped by more than 95%.

VACCINE EFFICACY

Two types of vaccines are available for the prevention of pertussis: whole-cell pertussis vaccine (labeled "P" in DTP), which is made from a suspension of killed *Bordetella pertussis*, and acellular pertussis vaccine (labeled "aP" in DTaP), which contains one or more of the antigens of *Bordetella pertussis* that are important to its ability to cause disease. Although adults and adolescents are the primary source of pertussis infection in young infants, their own morbidity from pertussis is low. Furthermore, the incidence of adverse effects after administration of whole-cell pertussis vaccine to older children and adults is relatively high; half of such individuals who receive monovalent or combination whole-cell pertussis vaccine will have induration at the injection site. Therefore, whole-cell pertussis vaccine alone or in combination with other vaccines is not indicated for use in anyone older than 6 years. No acellular vaccines have been licensed for use in persons 7 years of age or older, although there is considerable interest in it.

In studies conducted in the United States, DTP vaccination was found to be between 70% and 90% effective in preventing pertussis disease. In studies conducted in Europe, DTaP vaccines showed efficacies between 59% and 89%, and DTP vaccines had efficacies from 36% to 98%. It is difficult to compare the results of various studies, however, because of differences in study type, degree of blinding, case definition of pertussis, criteria for confirmation of pertussis infection, ethnicity of study population, number of children studied, timing of the vaccine schedule, and manufacturers of whole-cell vaccine used for comparison. The protection afforded by pertussis vaccination wanes with time. For whole-cell (DTP) vaccines, protection against pertussis disease is lost by 12 years after the last dose.

ADVERSE EFFECTS

Although DTP and DTaP vaccines have been found to have similar efficacies, DTaP vaccines have approximately one-fourth to one-half the common adverse effects associated with DTP vaccines. The rates of adverse effects are similar for DTaP and DT. Minor adverse effects associated with DTP vaccination include localized edema at the injection site in 41% of recipients, fever, drowsiness, and fretfulness. Uncommon adverse effects are persistent crying for 3 or more hours after DTP vaccination, an unusual high-pitched cry, seizures, and hypotonic, hyporesponsive episodes. Most seizures that

accompany DTP vaccination are simple febrile seizures that do not have any permanent sequelae. It is generally accepted that on rare occasions a child may have an anaphylactic reaction to DTP, and in these cases further doses of DTP or DTaP are contraindicated. The risk of other serious adverse effects, such as permanent neurologic damage, after a dose of DTP vaccine is the subject of debate and has been discussed in depth. If permanent neurologic damage ever results from vaccination, it does so rarely. Administration of DTaP vaccine has also been associated with seizures, persistent crying, and hypotonic, hyporesponsive episodes, but at lower rates than after administration of a DTP vaccine. Table 1-4 shows the incidence rates of mild or local reactions to DTaP or DTP vaccine administration.

RECOMMENDATIONS

DTaP is recommended for all children because of the lower risk of adverse effects compared with DTP (Fig. 1-6). DTaP is strongly recommended over DTP for children with a family history of seizures. Premature infants should be vaccinated with full doses at the appropriate age. Full doses should be used because fractional doses are not as immunogenic and might not lessen the risk of adverse effects. Completing the recommended series is important for optimal efficacy. For instance, one study found that the efficacy of whole-cell vaccine, based on a case definition of a cough of at least 14 days' duration, with paroxysms, whoop, or vomiting, is 36% after one dose, 49% after two doses, and 83% after three doses. Although five doses of DTP or DTaP vaccine are recommended, persons who receive their fourth dose on or after their fourth birthday do not need the fifth dose.

Diphtheria and Tetanus Toxoids

Diphtheria has become a rare disease in the United States—only 41 cases were reported

Table 1-4

Percentage of Infants with Mild or Local Reactions by the Third Evening After Pertussis Vaccination at Ages 2, 4, and 6 Mo

VACCINE	TEMPERATURE ≥37.8°C (%)	SWELLING >20 MM (%)	SEVERE FUSSINESS (%)[a]
DTaP vaccines			
Connaught/Biken/CB-2/Tripedia	24.5	3.7	3.7
Lederle/Takeda/LPT-4F$_1$/ACEL-IMUNE	19.8	3.2	4.6
SmithKline Beecham/SKB-3P/Infanrix	31.6	5.8	5.0
Overall for 13 DTaP vaccines	24.5	4.2	4.7
DTP vaccines overall	60.4	22.4	12.4

[a] Fussiness was classified as severe when the infant cried persistently and could not be comforted.
ABBREVIATIONS: DTaP, pediatric dose of diphtheria toxoid and tetanus toxoid and acellular pertussis vaccine; DTP, pediatric dose of diphtheria toxoid and tetanus toxoid and whole-cell pertussis vaccine.
SOURCE: Adapted from data in Decker MD, Edwards KM, Steinhoff MC, et al.

between 1980 and 1994. It is believed, however, that mild cases remain unrecognized and that strains of *Corynebacterium* still circulate. Diphtheria has a 10% fatality rate among children who have received no diphtheria immunizations. Recent outbreaks of diphtheria in the newly independent states of the former Soviet Union illustrate how the disease can recur if immunization rates fall. Tetanus has also become a rare disease, with approximately 50 cases reported each year. Because of the widespread use of vaccines containing tetanus toxoid, only a small proportion of cases are seen among infants and children, and these affect children who are inadequately immunized. Children under 7 years of age should receive tetanus and diphtheria toxoids in combination with pertussis vaccine as either DTP or DTaP.

Persons 7 years of age and older should receive adult tetanus and diphtheria toxoids (Td), which contain about the same quantity of tetanus toxoid as the DTP or pediatric DT vaccines but only one-third to one-eleventh as much diphtheria toxoid. Td vaccine should be used for the primary three-dose series in those receiving the first dose at 7 years or older and

for routine booster doses every 10 years. Persons who experience an Arthrus-type hypersensitivity reaction or a fever of more than 39.4°C (103°F) after a dose of tetanus toxoid probably have high serum antitoxin titers and should not be given a dose of Td more often than every 10 years.

Haemophilus Influenzae Type b Vaccines

Hib bacteria are spread by respiratory droplets and nasal or oral discharge and usually infect by way of the nasopharyngeal route.

RATIONALE FOR VACCINATION

In unvaccinated populations, Hib infection is the most common cause of bacterial meningitis in children between 2 months and 5 years of age. Hib infection can also cause epiglottitis, pneumonia, meningitis, septic arthritis, cellulitis, pericarditis, osteomyelitis, empyema, and sepsis. Hib meningitis results in hearing loss or neurological damage in 15% to 30% and has a case fatality rate of 2% to 5%. Since the introduction of Hib vaccines, there has been a dramatic decrease (95%) in the rate of invasive Hib disease in children in the United States, with only 280 cases among children under 5 years reported in 1996.

HIB VACCINES

Starting in 1985, polysaccharide Hib vaccines were introduced in the United States. The human immune system is not able to respond well to the purified polysaccharide antigens in these vaccines until 18 to 24 months of age, however, and 60% to 61% of all cases of invasive Hib disease in unvaccinated populations are found in children younger than 18 months. Consequently, new vaccines were developed by conjugation, that is, chemically bonding polysaccharide vaccine to a protein carrier. These conjugate vaccines are T-dependent, resulting in a good immune response in infancy, in contrast to the T-independent polysaccharide vaccines. Since 1987, four conjugate Hib vaccines have been licensed in the United States:

1. PRP-D (ProHIBit) contains Hib-purified polyribosyribitol phosphate (PRP) conjugated with diphtheria toxoid. Although this conjugated vaccine, the first to achieve Federal Drug Administration approval, seemed to be efficacious in infants in Finnish trials, early results in the United States were disappointing. As a result, PRP-D is approved only for children 12 months of age and older.
2. PRP-OMP (PedvaxHIB) contains Hib PRP conjugated with the outer membrane protein of *Neisseria meningitidis* group b (it is not intended for use against *Neisseria meningitidis*). PRP-OMP is given as a three-dose series, at 2, 4, and 12 months of age.
3. HbOC (HibTITER) contains a subunit of Hib polysaccharide conjugated with a mutant (CRM_{197}) diphtheria protein.
4. PRP-T (OmniHib/ActHIB) contains PRP conjugated with tetanus toxoid. HbOC and PRP-

T are given as a four-dose series at 2, 4, 6, and 12 to 15 months of age.

These last three conjugated vaccines approved for use in infants in the United States have estimated efficacies of 93% to 100% for a completed series.

COMVAX, a vaccine containing both PRP-OMP (PedvaxHIB) and hepatitis B vaccine is available for use in infants. It is licensed for use in children born to mothers who are HBsAg negative. Like any Hib vaccine, it should not be given before 6 weeks of age. COMVAX is licensed for administration at 2, 4, and 12 to 15 months of age. Adverse reactions to conjugate Hib vaccines are generally mild. Fever has been noted infrequently (1% to 4.6% of recipients). Localized erythema, tenderness, or induration at the injection site is relatively common, occurring in about 25% of children.

RECOMMENDATIONS

All children younger than 60 months (after which time the risk of invasive Hib disease is significantly lower) should be vaccinated against Hib according to the recommended schedule shown in Table 1-5 for the particular Hib vaccine chosen. Note that if PRP-OMP (PedvaxHIB) Hib vaccine is administered at 2 and 4 months of age, a dose at 6 months of age is not required. Hib vaccines should not be given before 6 weeks of age because they may induce immune tolerance, preventing adequate antibody response to further doses of Hib vaccine.

Since studies show that administration of Hib conjugate vaccines from different manufacturers results in as good (or better) antibody titers as using the same vaccine throughout the series, interchanging conjugate Hib vaccines is now considered acceptable. HbOC and PRP-T contain diphtheria or tetanus toxoid, and exposure to these agents in DT or DTP/DTaP vaccine may be required for optimal Hib antibody formation. For this reason, PRP-OMP is preferred for chil-

Table 1-5

Detailed Vaccination Schedule for *Haemophilus influenza* Type b Conjugate Vaccines

VACCINE	AGE AT 1ST DOSE (MO)	PRIMARY SERIES	BOOSTER
HbOC or PRP-T	2–6	3 doses, 2 mo apart	12–15 mo
	7–11	2 doses, 2 mo apart	12–18 mo
	12–14	1 dose	2 mo later
	15–59	1 dose	—
PRP-OMP	2–6	2 doses, 2 mo apart	12–15 mo
	7–11	2 doses, 2 mo apart	12–18 mo
	12–14	1 dose	2 mo later
	15–59	1 dose	—
PRP-D (Connaught)	15–59	1 dose	—

ABBREVIATIONS: Hib, *Haemophilus influenzae* type b; HbOC, Hib vaccine conjugated with a pediatric dose of diphtheria toxoid; PRP-T, Hib vaccine conjugated with tetanus toxoid; PRP-OMP, Hib vaccine conjugated with *Neisseria meningitidis* group B; PRP-D, Hib vaccine conjugated with a pediatric dose of diphtheria toxoid.
SOURCE: Modified from *Epidemiology and Prevention of Vaccine-preventable Diseases*, 4th ed. Atlanta, GA, Centers for Disease Control and Prevention, 1997. p. 110. Public domain.

dren in whom DT/DTaP/DTP vaccination is deferred.

Poliovirus Vaccines

Poliovirus is an enterovirus that has three serotypes. The virus is quite infectious, and transmission to susceptible household contacts takes place in 73% to 96% of infections, depending on the contact's age. Transmission is primarily by the fecal–oral route, although oral–oral transmission can occur. After the virus enters the mouth, it multiplies in the pharynx and gastrointestinal tract before invading the bloodstream and, potentially, the central nervous system. The incubation period ranges from 3 to 35 days.

The results of poliovirus infection, in decreasing order of likelihood, are subclinical infection (up to 95% of cases), nonspecific viral illnesses with complete recovery (about 5% of cases), nonparalytic aseptic meningitis (1% to 2% of cases), and paralytic poliomyelitis (less than 2% of cases). The ratio of inapparent to paralytic illness is about 200:1, with a range of 50:1 to

1000:1. The case fatality rate is 2% to 5% in children and 15% to 30% in adults.

RATIONALE FOR VACCINATION

Poliovirus vaccination programs have resulted in dramatic declines in disease incidence. Circulation of indigenous wild polioviruses ceased in the United States in the 1960s, and the last case of wild poliomyelitis contracted in the United States was reported in 1979. The last case of poliomyelitis due to indigenous virus in the New World occurred in 1991 in Peru, and in 1994 the Americas were declared free of indigenous poliomyelitis.

Between 1980 and 1996, 142 confirmed cases of paralytic poliomyelitis (an average of eight cases a year) were reported in the United States. Six of these cases were imported, the last in 1986. (In 1996, only 81% of infants worldwide had received three doses of poliovirus vaccine.) Two were classified as indeterminate in origin, and the remaining 134 were classified as associated with oral poliovirus vaccine (OPV)—due either to receiving OPV or to contact with an OPV recipient.

POLIOVIRUS VACCINES

Two vaccines are available in the United States for use to prevent poliomyelitis—inactivated poliovirus vaccine (IPV) and OPV. *Inactivated poliovirus vaccine*, also known as the Salk vaccine, was licensed in 1955. An enhanced-potency IPV formulation became available in 1988 and is the IPV in use in the United States today. IPV is inactivated, cannot cause poliomyelitis, and thus is safe for immunocompromised persons and contacts of immunocompromised persons. The disadvantages of IPV include administration by injection, less gastrointestinal immunity, and unknown duration of immunity in populations without indigenous poliomyelitis or those that do not use OPV.

A possible consequence of decreased gastrointestinal tract immunity is that wild poliovirus can infect and be shed from the gastrointestinal tract. The IPV-vaccinated person is protected from paralytic poliomyelitis, but he or she could transmit wild virus to other persons. This happened in a 1984 Finnish outbreak in which scattered cases of paralytic poliomyelitis due to wild serotype 3 were seen after almost two decades of freedom from poliomyelitis in Finland; most cases were in persons who had received three to five doses of IPV. The Finnish IPV vaccine then in use appeared to be inferior to that of other manufacturers of serotype 3.

Oral poliovirus vaccine has the advantage of easier administration, induces early intestinal immunity, and confers (probably lifelong) protection from poliomyelitis in more than 95% of those who complete the primary series of three doses of OPV. In one study of inner city children in Detroit and Houston, seropositivity for poliovirus types 1 and 3 ranged from about 80% among 12- to 23-month-old children to more than 90% in children ages 36 to 47 months. In

children unlikely to have been vaccinated, seropositivity rates ranged from 9% to 18% for poliovirus types 1 and 3 and from 29% to 42% for poliovirus type 2; thus, secondary spread of vaccine virus plays a modest role in increasing poliovirus immunity in inner city populations.

The main disadvantage of OPV is that the oral polioviruses can revert to a more virulent form and cause vaccine-associated paralytic poliomyelitis (VAPP). The overall risk of VAPP is quite small: between 1980 and 1994, 303 million doses of OPV were distributed, and 125 cases of VAPP were reported—for a risk of one case per 2.4 million doses of OPV distributed. VAPP developed most often in healthy vaccine recipients (49 cases), followed by healthy contacts of vaccine recipients (40 cases), immunodeficient vaccine recipients (23 cases), and immunodeficient contacts of vaccine recipients (seven cases); in six cases, VAPP was community acquired. In healthy recipients, 82% of cases occur after the first dose of vaccine (one case per 750,000 doses). Among immunodeficient persons, those with B-cell disorders are at highest risk of VAPP; in one series of 20 VAPP cases in immunodeficient persons, 15 arose in persons with hypogammaglobulinemia or agammaglobulinemia (Centers for Disease Control, unpublished data).

VACCINATION SCHEDULES

For the year 2000 and beyond, the all-IPV schedule is recommended although the sequential schedule of two doses of IPV, followed by two doses of OPV, may be used in special circumstances such as when a parent refuses the larger number of injections. The vaccines are given at 2 months, 4 months, 6 to 18 months, and 4 to 6 years. For the sequential schedule, the ACIP recommends that the third dose be given at 12 to 18 months in order to delay administration of OPV until a later age, thereby increasing the likelihood that any immunodeficiencies, if present, would be diagnosed (in which case OPV would be withheld). Advantages and disadvantages of each schedule are listed in Table 1-6.

An all-IPV vaccination schedule results in the lowest risk of VAPP. It adds four injections. The all-OPV regimen is recommended by the World Health Organization for global eradication efforts and provides the earliest mucosal immunity. In terms of the sequential schedule, most studies have shown that two doses of IPV induce protective levels of antibodies in ≥90% of recipients. Thus, administering IPV for the

first two doses of poliovirus vaccine and completing the series with OPV avoids the high risk that VAPP will develop after the first dose of OPV. In Denmark, which has used a six-dose sequential schedule since 1968, the only case of VAPP occurred in 1969 in a child who had only one dose of IPV. The ACIP concluded that use of a four-dose sequential IPV-OPV schedule could reduce the overall risk of VAPP by 50% or more, and among vaccine recipients the sequential schedule should lower the risk of VAPP by 95%.

Table 1-6

Advantages and Disadvantages of Three Poliovirus Vaccination Options

ATTRIBUTE	OPV	IPV	IPV-OPV
Occurrence of VAPP	8–9 cases/year	None	2–5 cases/year (estimated)
Other serious adverse effects	None known	None known	None known
Systemic immunity	High	High	High
Immunity of gastrointestinal musosa	High	Low	High
Secondary transmission of vaccine virus	Yes	No	Some
Extra injections or visits needed	No	Yes	Yes
Compliance with immunization schedule	High	Possibly reduced	Possibly reduced
Future combination vaccines	Unlikely	Likely	Likely (IPV)

ABBREVIATIONS: OPV, oral poliovirus vaccine; IPV, inactivated poliovirus vaccine; IPV-OPV, sequential vaccination with IPV followed by OPV; VAPP, vaccine-associated paralytic poliomyelitis.
SOURCE: Modified from Centers for Disease Control and Prevention: Poliomyelitis prevention in the United States: Introduction of a sequential vaccination schedule of inactivated poliovirus vaccine followed by oral poliovirus vaccine—recommendations of the Advisory Committee on Immunization Practices (ACIP). *MMWR* 46:12, 1997.

In addition to reduction but not elimination of VAPP, other advantages of the sequential schedule are the lack of added injections in the second year of life, the development of eventual mucosal immunity, and postponement of OPV until 12 to 18 months of age, by which time many congenital immunodeficiencies have been diagnosed. The sequential schedule provides better intestinal immunity than does the all-IPV schedule. The percentage of children who shed virus in their stools after being given a challenge dose of OPV was 85% after three doses of IPV, 66% after two doses of IPV and one previous dose of OPV, 25% after two doses of IPV and two previous doses of OPV, and 24% after two doses of IPV and three previous doses of OPV. Thus, the ACIP concluded that two doses of OPV were needed in the sequential schedule. Disadvantages of the sequential schedule include the need for additional injections and the lack of efficacy data from studies conducted within the United States. Although other counties have used the sequential schedule successfully, these countries use more than the four doses recommended in the U.S. schedule.

RECOMMENDATIONS FOR IPV

In 1988, the Institute of Medicine reviewed poliovirus vaccination options for the United States and recommended a sequential schedule if a combination vaccine containing DTP and IPV were to be licensed. For 2000 and beyond the ACIP, the AAP, and the AAFP recommend that the all-IPV schedule be used except in special circumstances such as parental refusal of the larger number of injections. It is expected that OPV will not be available in the US after 2000, except stock piles for emergency use only.

Premature infants vaccinated in the hospital generally should not receive OPV, owing to potential transmission to other high-risk infants. Immunocompromised children and children with immunocompromised household contacts should receive IPV only. When an unvaccinated immunocompetent child is traveling imminently to countries where poliovirus is endemic, OPV may be preferred. For school entry, four doses of vaccine are recommended, and any combination of IPV and OPV by 4 to 6 years of age is acceptable; however, a fourth dose is not required for children receiving an all-IPV or all-OPV series who had the third dose on or after their fourth birthday.

Measles, Mumps, and Rubella Vaccine

Measles, mumps, and rubella (MMR) are viral diseases transmitted person to person by respiratory droplets and direct contact with the saliva of an infected person. Measles, one of the most infectious agents known, can also be spread by smaller aerosolized droplets that pass through ventilation systems within a building and are infective for at least 1 hour. Prodromal symptoms of measles appear 10 to 12 days after exposure, and the characteristic rash appears in 14 days. Infected persons can transmit the disease 4 days before and 4 days after the appearance of the rash. Initial symptoms of the disease are fever, conjunctivitis, coryza, cough, and Koplik spots on the buccal mucosa. The rash appears on the face on the third to seventh day and spreads to the trunk and limbs, lasting 4 to 7 days. Measles is more severe in infants and adults. Complications include diarrhea, middle ear infection, pneumonia, encephalitis (one of every 1000 cases), and death (1 or 2 of every 1000). Case fatality rates in some developing countries are as high as 25%.

Mumps occurs 16 to 18 days after exposure, with symptoms of fever, headache, malaise, myalgia, and parotitis. Orchitis develops in up to 38% of postpubertal men and aseptic meningitis in 4% to 6% of cases. Rubella is a mild, febrile rash illness with an incubation period of 14 to 23 days. The rash is maculopapular and can be mistaken for measles. Other symptoms include postauricular and suboccipital lymphadenopathy and, among young adults, arthralgias. Encephalitis is seen in one of 6000 cases. The most significant complication of rubella affects the fetuses of infected pregnant women, especially in the first trimester. Congenital rubella syndrome (CRS) is associated with deafness, cataracts and other eye anomalies, heart defects, microcephaly, and mental retardation in newborn infants. CRS develops in 20% to 25% of infants whose mothers are infected during the first half of pregnancy and 85% of those whose mothers are infected in the first 4 weeks.

RATIONALE FOR VACCINATION

Measles is highly contagious (the attack rate for unvaccinated household contacts is 90% or higher); before the introduction of vaccine it caused illness in approximately three to four million persons, with 500 reported deaths annually in the United States. Epidemics occurred every 2 to 3 years, and more than 90% of persons contracted measles by age 15. Following the introduction of measles vaccine in 1963, the incidence of measles dropped by more than 98%, although an epidemic during the years 1989 to 1991 led to 55,467 reported cases and 136 deaths.

The introduction of mumps vaccine in 1967 has resulted in a marked decline in reported cases—from over 185,000 in 1968 to 906 in 1995. Still, there were large outbreaks of mumps in 1986 and 1987; 64% of cases occurred in children less than 15 years of age. The introduction of rubella vaccine in 1969 resulted in a decrease of both reported rubella cases and CRS. There were 60,000 rubella cases reported in 1969 and only 567 cases from 1994 to 1996; only 12 cases of CRS were documented in the same time period, down from 20 to 70 cases per year in the 1970s.

MEASLES, RUBELLA, AND MUMPS VACCINES

The measles vaccine used at present in the United States is called the Enders-Edmonston strain, and it contains live, highly attenuated virus. After measles vaccination, seroconver-

sion rates are 95% for children vaccinated at 12 months of age and 98% for children vaccinated at 15 months of age. The vaccine induces both humoral and cellular immunity. Antibody persists for at least 17 years and probably confers lifelong immunity in almost all vaccinated persons who initially seroconvert. Subclinical reinfection may develop after vaccination, but there is no evidence that persons with subclinical disease transmit wild virus to others. Of the few whose antibody level wanes, most are probably still immune because they have secondary immune responses upon revaccination.

The rubella vaccine in use contains the live virus strain RA 27/3. It induces immunity with a single dose in more than 95% of those 12 months of age or older. Immunity lasts at least 15 years and is probably lifelong. Mumps vaccine is also a live virus (Jeryl-Lynn strain). Ninety-seven percent of those vaccinated develop immunity for at least 30 years. Some studies have documented the efficacy of mumps vaccine at 75% to 95%.

RECOMMENDATIONS

The number of doses and recommended ages for administering measles vaccine has changed over time. When the measles vaccine was licensed in 1963, one dose at 9 months of age was recommended. Data showed, however, that seroconversion rates were higher when the vaccine was administered at a later age, because passively acquired maternal antibodies transferred across the placenta persisted beyond 9 months in a number of children and these antibodies interfered with seroconversion. Hence, the recommended age at vaccination was increased to 12 months in 1965 and to 15 months in 1976.

When cases of measles broke out among school-aged children in the United States in the 1980s despite high vaccination levels, measles vaccination guidelines were reassessed. In 1989 the ACIP recommended a second dose of measles-containing vaccine at age 4 to 6 years (entry to kindergarten or first grade) in order to provide protection for most of those who did not respond to the initial measles vaccination.

Two factors may contribute to inadequate protection from the first dose of measles vaccine: lack of initial seroconversion and waning immunity. Lack of initial seroconversion is usually due to the presence of higher initial titers of passively acquired antibody. Mothers whose immunity was acquired actively rather than passively (by vaccination) confer higher initial levels of immunity to their children, and these high titers in turn result in longer periods of protection for the infant. When most mothers had actively acquired immunity to measles infection, they conferred immunity on their children until an average age of 11 months or more, and seroconversion rates were optimal when administration of MMR vaccine was delayed until children were 15 months of age. As the source of maternal immunity to measles shifted to vaccine, the duration of immunity in infants declined, to about 9 months, resulting in a higher proportion of children experiencing a period of inadequate protection from measles. This probably accounts for the fact that in 1990, 26% of measles cases occurred in children ≤16 months of age. In response to these findings, in 1994 the ACIP changed the recommendation for the first dose of MMR from 15 months of age to 12 to 15 months of age. Studies have found that seroconversion fails to occur after the initial dose of measles vaccine at a rate of 2% to 5%. In comparison, the rate of secondary vaccine failure, also known as waning immunity, has been found to be less than 0.2%.

In summary, two doses of MMR vaccine are recommended for children. The first dose should be given at age 12 to 15 months, and the AAFP, the ACIP, and the AAP now advise giving the second dose at 4 to 6 years of age, although it may be administered at any time 1 month or longer after the first dose. Children 7 years of age or older who have not received the second dose of MMR can be given the catch-up dose at any pediatric visit. One study raised concerns about decreased immunogenicity when MMR was administered to children who had a viral illness, but recent studies show no difference in vaccine efficacy when it is given to children with mild illness.

Varicella Vaccine

Varicella in children is typically a self-limited, benign illness. However, complications can arise, and the disease is highly contagious, as indicated by secondary household attack rates as high as 90% in susceptible household contacts. The virus is spread by direct contact, droplet nuclei, and aerosols from vesicles or respiratory tract secretions. Communicability (by the respiratory route) begins 1 to 2 days before the rash develops and lasts until all lesions have formed crusts. Symptoms include mild fever and a skin rash that changes from maculopapular to vesicular in a few hours. The disease is characterized by the simultaneous occurrence of papules, vesicles, and scabs. Lesions also appear in the mouth.

The complications of varicella that most often lead to the need for hospitalization are bacterial skin infections, encephalitis, Reye's syndrome, and dehydration. Pneumonia may also accompany varicella. Most children (81 of 96 in one study) who need hospitalization for varicella are immunologically normal. The overall case fatality rate is 2/100,000. In adults it is 30/100,000. Herpes zoster, or shingles, can develop months to years after varicella infection and is characterized by painful vesicles distributed in one or more dermatomes.

RATIONALE FOR ROUTINE VACCINATION

Varicella is more severe in infants (particularly those with congenitally acquired infection) and adults than in children, as seen by age-specific hospitalization rates of 103, 23, and 65 per 10,000 cases in infants, 1- to 4-year-olds, and 20- to 29-year-olds, respectively. Because the incidence of varicella is so high in young children, however, they have the highest number of hospitalizations. Routine vaccination of children 12 to 18 months of age was determined to be a cost-effective way to minimize the morbidity of varicella in the United States: a study based on an estimated vaccine price of $35 calculated that the cost of routine vaccination in 1990 dollars was $3.21 per case of varicella prevented and that each $1 spent for universal vaccination of children would avoid approximately $5 in costs to care for varicella cases—including indirect costs, such as lost work time.

A concern of some clinicians is that widespread immunization of children against varicella might shift the age of contracting varicella from childhood to adulthood, when disease is more likely to be severe. Mathematical modeling shows that vaccination of children will indeed lead to an increase in the proportion of varicella cases in older patients but that varicella vaccination will result in considerably lower overall numbers of hospitalizations, even if vaccination confers a shorter period of immunity than expected.

VARICELLA VACCINE

The available varicella vaccine contains live, attenuated virus derived from the Oka strain and is highly immunogenic: almost all children 1 to 12 years of age (97%) seroconvert after one dose, and a Japanese study found antibody present in 97% of children for at least 7 years after vaccination. The ACIP concluded that varicella vaccination provides 70% to 90% protection against infection and 95% protection against severe disease for 7 to 10 years after vaccination. Furthermore, when children who have been vaccinated contract varicella, the clinical course is milder than in those who have never been vaccinated.

The long-term duration of varicella immunity in a highly immunized population is unknown. An expert panel estimated that a child receiving one dose of varicella vaccine would have a 15%

likelihood of losing immunity over his or her lifetime. To date, studies of vaccine efficacy have not accounted for the possibility that immunity may have been boosted, and therefore prolonged, by exposure to varicella in the surrounding community. Active surveillance of vaccine-induced immunity is planned by the vaccine manufacturer and public health authorities, to determine the duration of immunity.

The adverse effects of varicella vaccination consist principally of pain and erythema at the injection site. After vaccination, 4% to 6% of recipients report a generalized varicella-like rash consisting of a few (median of five) lesions. Children with leukemia who were immunized and experienced lesions have transmitted the virus to others; however, the virus does not become more virulent through this form of transmission. Administration of varicella vaccine to previously immune individuals does not increase the rate of adverse reactions. The risk of herpes zoster is lower after vaccination than after naturally acquired varicella.

RECOMMENDATIONS

The ACIP, AAFP, and AAP recommend that children receive one dose of varicella vaccine between 12 and 18 months of age. For children with a history of varicella, vaccination is not necessary, although it is not contraindicated. Catch-up varicella vaccination is suggested for children between 18 months and 12 years of age who do *not* have a history of varicella. Varicella vaccine is approved for use in adolescents ($\geq$13 years of age) and adults without a history of chickenpox on a two-dose schedule; the doses should be spaced 4 to 8 weeks apart. If the second dose is late, it can be given without restarting the schedule. The vaccine is heat sensitive and must be stored at $-15°C$ (5°F) or colder. Vaccine not used within 30 minutes after being reconstituted should be discarded. Vaccinees who show signs of a varicelliform rash after vaccination might be contagious; hence, they should avoid contact with individuals at high risk of complications of varicella, such as immunocompromised persons. If there is such contact, however, it is not necessary to give the immunocompromised contact varicella-zoster immune globulin because the virus in the vaccine is attenuated. Varicella vaccine is effective in post-exposure prophylaxis when given within 3–5 days of exposure.

Rotavirus Vaccine

Although rotavirus accounts for only 5% to 16% of all episodes of diarrhea among children younger than 5 years of age, it is the most common cause of severe gastroenteritis in the United States, accounting for 30% to 61% of all hospitalizations for diarrhea in this age group. Published estimates of the annual number of hospitalizations in the United States range from 23,000 to 110,000, with recent data suggesting that the figure is about 50,000. Based on an estimated 3.9 million children in the birth cohort, this means that 1 in 78 children will be hospitalized. Rotavirus results in about 160,000 emergency department visits and about 410,000 physician visits, that is, 10.5% of children will be seen by a clinician in the first 5 years of life for this illness.

Rotavirus infection is spread by the fecal–oral route and may also spread through respiratory secretions and contaminated surfaces. The virus can be passed in the stool for up to 25 days after symptoms resolve. It infects the epithelium of the small intestine, and, after an incubation period of 1 to 3 days, produces vomiting, fever, and watery diarrhea. The major complication is dehydration. In developing countries rotavirus is responsible for an estimated 870,000 deaths per year.

RATIONALE FOR VACCINATION

Since rotavirus is shed in very high concentrations in human feces (i.e., 10^{11} particles per gram) it is highly contagious, but a person also can be infected by a low dose (i.e., about 10 viral particles). It is transmitted primarily by the fecal–oral route; thus, transmission within families of infants (due, in part, to diaper changing) and within day-care institutions is common. The incubation period is less than 48 hours. Rotaviruses are relatively resistant to many disinfectants, and they can remain infectious on inanimate articles for months at ambient temperatures owing to the intense communicability of rotavirus. Environmental approaches such as assuring that water is potable and improving sanitation have limited impact on disease incidence. Natural immunity develops after infection, providing a rationale for vaccine use. The vaccine can prevent 80% of severe rotavirus illness and almost all hospitalizations.

ROTAVIRUS VACCINE

A live, tetravalent (serotypes G1, G2, G3, and G4) rhesus rotavirus vaccine (RRV), RotaShield, was licensed in 1998, based on a modified Jennerian (e.g., smallpox-like) approach to vaccination. In the Jennerian approach, an attenuated virus (e.g., cowpox) from one animal is given to another to prevent infection by a related virus (e.g., smallpox). Since a particular rotavirus serotype replicates in primarily one species of animal host (a property called host restriction), nonhuman strains are usually naturally attenuated when given to humans. RRV is further attenuated by passage 16 times in cell culture.

The efficacy of rotavirus vaccine is moderately good against diarrhea but very good against dehydration and severe diarrhea. In a multicenter, double-blind, placebo-controlled trial conducted in the United States that included infants of multiple races, the efficacy of 4×10^5 plaque forming units (pfu) RRV over one season of observation was 49% for gastroenteritis, 73% for gastroenteritis resulting in clinician intervention, 80% for very severe rotavirus gastroenteritis, and 100% against dehydration. Although most children do not have reactions to RRV, low-grade fever, diarrhea, and irritability sometimes occur. On rare occasions, the fever after the first dose at 2 months of age might lead to precautionary hospitalization. In 1998, the AAP and ACIP recommended routine infant rotavirus vaccination. The AAFP, however, had concerns that rotavirus infection was often mild, that recommendations should not be made before the price was available, and that stronger evidence was required to make a strong recommendation. Consequently, AAFP recommended that the decision should be made by the parent or guardian in consultation with their clinician.

INTUSSUSCEPTION

From licensure through June of 1999, 15 cases of radiographically confirmed intussusception were reported to the Vaccine Adverse Event Reporting System (VAERS); 12 of these 15 cases occurred within one week of RRV. In a Northern California Kaiser Permanente study, the rate of intussusception was 45 per 100,000 infant years among those never vaccinated versus 314 per 100,000 infant years among children who received RRV in the preceding week.

Due to the intussusception reports, use of RRV was postponed from July through October 1999, until after the next meeting of the ACIP in October. In October 1999, the manufacturer voluntarily withdrew rotavirus vaccine from the US market.

At the October 1999 meeting of the ACIP, it was reported that 93 reports of intussusception among confirmed recipients of rotavirus vaccine had been reported to VAERS. One case was fatal. The striking feature was the clustering of intussusception in first 14 days following vaccination. Data from several different sources including a case-control study demonstrate a strong association between rotavirus vaccine and intussusception. The attributable risk is about one case in 5,000 vaccinees. This association appears causal since it is strong, temporally related to rotavirus vaccination, consistently found among the data sources, and plausible as

3–6 days is the time of high viral replication following vaccination. The ACIP recommended *against* further rotavirus vaccination in the United States, although the ACIP noted that the risk-benefit equation might be different in developing countries.

There are several lessons from this situation. First, this is an example of how the VAERS system worked well in giving a signal of a problem to which the National Immunization Program at CDC gave great attention. Second, the AAFP position ended up being wise–the AAFP did not push quickly for mass vaccination given concerns about disease burden, giving approval prior to knowing the price, and the potential for varying parental preferences. Third, all scientific sources of data on adverse effects, particularly for live viral vaccines, should be consulted. Fourth, patient-friendly balance sheets that compare the benefits of vaccination versus the risks may be needed as new vaccines are developed for conditions that are milder and less likely to be fatal.

Preadolescence and Adolescence Checks of Vaccination Status

In 1996, the ACIP, AAFP, AAP, and American Medical Association recommended a well-child office visit at age 11 to 12 years to check vaccination status. Vaccines that might be indicated at this visit include varicella, hepatitis B, the second dose of MMR, and Td (if tetanus toxoid was not given in the past 5 years). Adolescent patients should be screened for high-risk conditions indicating the need for influenza, pneumococcal, or hepatitis A vaccines.

Late Vaccination

If the childhood vaccination schedule is started late or if the child is more than 1 month late receiving a dose of vaccine, then the accelerated vaccination schedule should be used (Table 1-7) until the child catches up. If the vaccination schedule is interrupted, it does not need to be restarted. Instead, the schedule should be resumed using minimal intervals between doses (Table 1-8) to catch up as quickly as possible.

Table 1-7

Recommended Accelerated Immunization Schedule for Infants and Children <7 Yr of Age Who Start the Series Late or Who Are >1 Mo Behind in the Immunization Schedule (i.e., Children Whose Compliance with Scheduled Return Visits Cannot be Assured)[a,b]

TIMING	VACCINE(S)	COMMENT
First visit (≥4 mo of age)	DTaP, IPV, Hib, hepatitis B, MMR, varicella [c,d,e]	Must be ≥12 mo of age to receive MMR and varicella. If ≥5 years of age, Hib is not normally indicated.
Second visit (1 mo after first visit)[f]	DTaP, IPV, Hib, hepatitis B	
Third visit (1 mo after second visit)	DTaP, IPV, Hib	
Fourth visit (≥6 mo after third visit)	DTaP, Hib, hepatitis B	
4–6 yr of age	DTaP, IPV, MMR	Preferably at or before school entry. DTaP is not necessary if fourth dose is given on or after the fourth birthday. IPV is not necessary if third dose of all IPV series is given on or after fourth birthday.
11–12 yr of age	Varicella, MMR, and/or hepatitis B (if not already received); Td if >5 yr since last dose	Repeat Td every 10 yr through-out life.

[a] If immunization is initiated in the first year of life, administer DtaP doses 1, 2, and 3 and IPV doses 1, 2, and 3 according to this schedule; administer MMR and varicella vaccines when the child reaches 12 to 15 mo of age. All vaccines should be administered simultaneously at the appropriate visit.
[b] See individual ACIP recommendations for detailed information on specific vaccines.
[c] DTaP formulation is preferred for all doses of the series. A vaccine containing whole-cell pertussis vaccine is an acceptable alternative.
[d] OPV is no longer recommended and is acceptable only for special circumstances, such as for children whose parents do not accept the recommended number of injections and in cases of imminent travel to polio-endemic areas. If a child has received a mixture of OPV and IPV, then four total doses are recommended even if the third is given after the 4th birthday.
[e] The recommended schedule for Hib vaccination varies by vaccine manufacturer and age of the child when vaccination series is started. If series is begun at <6 mo of age, four doses are needed (only three doses are needed if all doses are PRP-OMP [PedvaxHIB, Merck]). The fourth dose must be ≥2 mo after the third dose and on or after the first birthday. If the series is started between 7 and 11 mo of age, three doses are needed, with the third dose ≥2 mo after the second dose and on or after the first birthday. If the series is started at age 12 to 14 mo, two doses are needed, ≥2 mo apart. If the series is started at age ≥15 mo, one dose of any licensed conjugate Hib vaccine is recommended.
[f] An interval of 28 or more days.
ABBREVIATIONS: DTaP, pediatric dose of diphtheria toxoid and tetanus toxoid and acellular pertussis vaccine; OPV, oral poliovirus vaccine; IPV, inactivated poliovirus vaccine; Hib, *Haemophilus influenzae* type b; MMR, measles, mumps, rubella combination vaccine; Td, adult dose of diphtheria toxoid and tetanus toxoid
SOURCE: General Recommendations on Immunization, Centers for Disease Control and Prevention, Atlanta, GA, 1994, with modifications from subsequent Advisory Committee for Immunization Practices (ACIP) statements and poliovirus recommendations.

Table 1-8

Minimum Age for Initial Vaccination and Minimum Interval Between Vaccine Doses, by Type of Vaccine[a]

VACCINE	MINIMAL AGE FOR DOSE 1	MINIMAL INTERVAL FROM DOSE 1 TO 2	MINIMAL INTERVAL FROM DOSE 2 TO 3	MINIMAL INTERVAL FROM DOSE 3 TO 4
DTP/DTaP (DT)[b]	6 wk	4 wk	4 wk	6 mo
Combined DTP-Hib[c]	6 wk	1 mo	1 mo	6 mo
Hib (primary series)				
HbOC	6 wk	1 mo	1 mo[c]	—
PRP-T	6 wk	1 mo	1 mo[c]	—
PRP-OMP	6 wk	1 mo	—	—
IPV[d]	6 wk	4 wk	4 wk[e,f]	—
MMR	12 mo[g]	1 mo	—	—
Hepatitis B	Birth	1 mo	2 mo[b]	—
Varicella	12 mo	4 wk	—	—

[a] The minimal acceptable ages and intervals may not correspond to the *optimal* recommended ages and intervals for vaccination. For current recommended routine schedules see the annual "Recommended Childhood Immunization Schedule, United States."
[b] The total number of doses of diphtheria and tetanus toxoids should not exceed six each before the seventh birthday.
[c] The booster dose of Hib vaccine that is recommended following the primary vaccination series should be administered no earlier than 12 mo of age *and* at least 2 mo after the previous dose of Hib vaccine (see Table 1-6).
[d] Inactivated poliovirus vaccine (IPV).
[e] For unvaccinated adults at increased risk of exposure to poliovirus with <3 mo but >2 mo available before protection is needed, three doses of IPV should be administered at least 1 mo apart.
[f] If the third dose is given after the third birthday, the fourth (booster) dose is not needed.
[g] Although the age for measles vaccination may be as young as 6 mo in outbreak areas where cases are developing in children <1 yr of age, children initially vaccinated before the first birthday should be revaccinated at 12 to 15 mo of age, and an additional dose of vaccine should be administered at the time of school entry or according to local policy. Doses of MMR or other measles-containing vaccines should be separated by at least 1 mo.
[b] This final dose is recommended at least 4 mo after the first dose and no earlier than 6 mo of age.
ABBREVIATIONS: DTP, pediatric dose of diphtheria toxoid and tetanus toxoid and whole-cell pertussis vaccine; DT, pediatric dose of diphtheria toxoid and tetanus toxoid; Hib, *Haemophilus influenzae* type b vaccine; MMR, measles, mumps, rubella combination vaccine; HbOC, Hib vaccine conjugated with a pediatric dose of diphtheria toxoid; PRP-T, Hib vaccine conjugated with tetanus toxoid; PRP-OMP, Hib vaccine conjugated with *Neisseria meningitidis* group B.

Vaccination Procedures

Health care providers administering vaccinations need to keep in mind the general contraindications to and precautions for vaccination and requirements for record-keeping and informing patients and parents.

Contraindications

There are two absolute contraindications to administering a dose of vaccine: severe allergy to a vaccine component or anaphylactic reaction to a previous dose of the vaccine and, for pertussis vaccine, encephalopathy without a known cause developing within 7 days of a dose of pertussis vaccine. Contact dermatitis from neomycin, however, is a delayed-type (cell-mediated) immune response and is not a contraindication to vaccination. Traces of neomycin are in MMR, OPV, IPV, and varicella vaccine. If the pertussis component is withheld because of a contraindication or precaution, then pediatric DT is administered instead, except in the case of true anaphylaxis, in which the diphtheria and pertussis components are permanently contraindicated. In such cases, referral may be made to an allergist to assess whether tetanus toxoid can be given and for possible desensitization to tetanus toxoid.

Two conditions are temporary contraindications to vaccination in certain situations: immunosuppression and pregnancy. *Immunosuppression* due to an immune-deficiency disease or malignancy or therapy with high-dose corticosteroid drugs, alkylating agents, antimetabolites, or radiation is a contraindication to administration of a live vaccine, although persons infected with HIV who are not severely immunosuppressed should receive MMR vaccine when indicated, based on age. Varicella vaccine should be considered when otherwise indicated in HIV-positive persons whose CD4 percentage is at least 25%. Inactivated vaccines may be given to immunosuppressed individuals because they do not contain live organisms that can replicate; however, immunosuppression may lessen the response to vaccination.

Pregnancy is a contraindication to administration of live-virus vaccines because of the theoretical risk that the live virus could damage the fetus. Furthermore, women should avoid becoming pregnant within 3 months of receiving MMR or rubella vaccine and within 1 month of mumps or varicella vaccination. On the other hand, inadvertent administration of a live-virus vaccine during pregnancy is not an indication for pregnancy termination because there are no data to link live-virus vaccination with increased risk of fetal malformations. Unless otherwise contraindicated, all vaccines may be given to breast-feeding mothers.

Precautions

Precautions for vaccination are conditions that *may* increase the risk of a serious or life-threatening adverse event or compromise the ability of the vaccine to produce immunity. Generally, the vaccine is withheld or postponed in such situations. The decision whether to vaccinate in such cases is made by weighing the individual patient's risk of acquiring the disease against the risk of the adverse event (or inability to produce immunity). Certain uncommon adverse effects of pertussis vaccination are precautions to further doses: temperature of ≥40.5°C (105°F) within 48 hours of a dose (not due to another identifiable cause); collapse or shocklike state (hypotonic, hyporesponsive episode) within 48 hours of a dose; persistent, inconsolable crying lasting ≥3 hours and occurring within 48 hours of a dose; or convulsions within 3 days of a dose. *Severe acute illness* usually warrants postponement of vaccination until the patient has recovered from the acute phase of illness.

Recent administration of blood products can interfere with development of an immune response to a live-virus (but not inactivated-virus) vaccine. Tables have been published that describe when various vaccines can be administered in such cases.

Overly cautious health care providers have misinterpreted a number of other conditions as posing contraindications to vaccination, including local reactions to vaccine administration, low to moderate fevers following previous doses of vaccine, a family history of severe adverse effects related to administration of DTP vaccine, mental retardation, seizures, or allergies.

INFANTS WITH POTENTIAL OR UNDERLYING NEUROLOGIC DISORDERS

DTaP vaccination should be postponed for infants with an evolving neurologic disorder, unevaluated seizures, or a neurologic event between doses of pertussis vaccine. Vaccination should be resumed after evaluation and treatment of the condition.

Vaccine Information Statements for Patients

Patients or their legal guardians should receive information that is easy to understand about the benefits and risks of vaccination. Under the Public Health Service Act, health care providers who administer any vaccine containing diphtheria, tetanus, pertussis, measles, mumps, rubella, poliovirus, varicella, hepatitis B, or Hib antigens are required to provide a copy of the relevant vaccine information statements to the patient before vaccination. These statements are available for most routinely used vaccines. They may be viewed and downloaded from the following World Wide Web site: http://www.cdc.gov/nip/vistable.htm. In the case of vaccines for which such an information statement is not available, the clinician should provide information about the risk of the disease, the protection afforded from vaccination, the risk of vaccine adverse effects, and what to do if a serious adverse event occurs. In cases of vaccine-related injury, there has been successful litigation for failure to provide information statements before vaccination.

Adverse Effect Reporting

Health care providers are required to report certain adverse effects and may report any adverse effects of vaccination to the Vaccine Adverse Event Reporting System. Forms and instructions can be obtained by calling 1–800–822–7967.

Vaccine Injury Compensation Program

The Vaccine Injury Compensation Program (VICP) is a system under which no-fault compensation can be awarded for specified injuries that are temporally related to administration of vaccinations against measles, mumps, rubella, diphtheria, tetanus, pertussis, poliovirus, hepatitis B, varicella, or Hib. For vaccines covered by the VICP, the program has reduced the risk to both providers and vaccine manufacturers of litigation following adverse effects. Information about specific adverse effects that are covered is available from the Health Resources and Services Administration by telephoning (301) 443–6593.

At least two cases have been successfully litigated against providers for failure to administer indicated doses of hepatitis vaccine or hepatitis B immune globulin, and other cases are being brought for failure to vaccinate against hepatitis B, measles, and Hib. Health care providers who administer vaccines covered by the VICP are required to record, either in an office log or the recipient's permanent medical record, the date of vaccine administration, the vaccine's manufacturer and lot number; and the name, address, and title of the person administering the vaccine. The ACIP recommends that providers record these data for all vaccines.

Interchangeability of Vaccines from Different Manufacturers

Vaccines from different manufacturers can be given interchangeably if the disease has a serologic test that shows whether a person is protected. For instance, hepatitis B disease is known to be prevented if vaccination results in at least 10 mIU/ml of HBsAb. Therefore, hepatitis B vaccines from different manufacturers can be substituted for one another. Hib conjugate vaccines from different manufacturers can also be used interchangeably.

No data are yet available on the safety, immunogenicity, or efficacy of acellular pertussis vaccination when different brands are administered for the first three doses of vaccine at 2, 4, and 6 months of age, and very limited data exist on the effects of administering different brands of acellular pertussis vaccine for the fourth and fifth doses in the vaccination series. Thus, when possible, use of the same brand of acellular pertussis vaccine for sequential doses is preferred. When a child who started the vaccination series with one brand of acellular pertussis vaccine is due for another dose and the office or clinic stocks a different brand, any of the licensed acellular pertussis vaccines may be administered rather than miss the opportunity to vaccinate.

Simultaneous Vaccinations and Combination Vaccines

Most vaccines will be efficacious and safe when administered simultaneously with another vaccine. Simultaneous vaccination (e.g., administering MMR and varicella vaccines at the same visit) is preferred when possible, because it may increase compliance with vaccination schedules by limiting the number of visits needed to complete vaccinations. In addition, use of combination vaccine products is generally preferred over separate products, for example, administering MMR instead of separate measles, mumps, and rubella vaccines, to minimize the patient's discomfort from multiple injections and the costs of stocking and administering separate vaccines.

Vaccine Administration Routes

DTaP, Hib, inactivated influenza, hepatitis A, hepatitis B, and Td vaccines are administered intramuscularly. In infants and children 2 years of age or younger, they should be administered intramuscularly in the anterolateral thigh. In older children and adults, they should be administered intramuscularly in the deltoid muscle. Pneumococcal vaccine can be administered either intramuscularly or subcutaneously. MMR, IPV, and varicella vaccine are administered subcutaneously.

Common Errors

Clinician's errors in vaccine administration have potentially serious consequences. Individual patients might receive less than adequate protection against vaccine-preventable diseases, and the community can have less than optimal herd immunity. The most common errors include missing an opportunity for administering a vaccine, not following the recommended vaccine schedules, considering minor illnesses as contraindications to vaccine, and not properly storing vaccines.

Causes of Delayed or Missed Childhood Vaccinations

Causes of delayed or missed vaccinations include limited appreciation of the risks of vaccine-preventable diseases, concerns about the occurrence of and liability for adverse effects of vaccination, and missed opportunities to vaccinate. Another cause of delayed vaccinations is the fact that many children switch clinicians with changes in insurance coverage or after moving to another residence.

FAILURE TO APPRECIATE DISEASE HAZARDS

Appreciation of the communicability and severity of vaccine-preventable diseases in children has diminished with the success of the United States childhood vaccination program. The widespread use of vaccinations has led to the elimination in the United States of indigenous poliomyelitis due to wild virus and dramatically reduced the incidence of diphtheria, pertussis, tetanus, measles, mumps, and rubella. Thus, many parents and some clinicians lack firsthand experience with these diseases, which may lead them to underestimate their communicability and their potential to cause harm.

CONCERNS ABOUT ADVERSE EFFECTS

Concerns about adverse effects associated with vaccine administration have increased as the incidence of the diseases the vaccines prevent has declined. Concerns have been fostered by a wave of anti-vaccine reports in the popular media, which may account for the finding in one national clinician survey that a median of 20% of parents ask clinicians about the safety of pertussis vaccine. Clinicians, however, may also overestimate the risk of serious adverse effects from vaccination. Data from the literature indicate that even the most common serious adverse effects are uncommon: among children administered whole-cell DTP, hypotonic, hyporesponsive episodes and seizures each occurred at a rate of 0.57% (one in 1,750 doses). In a national clinician survey, however, almost one-third (32%) of physicians overestimated the risk of serious adverse effects from pertussis vaccine administration, and 13% overestimated the risks from measles vaccine administration.

This same national survey found that almost one-fifth of responding clinicians had concerns about the possibility of litigation from potential vaccine-related injury. The VICP provides no-fault compensation to patients suffering a permanent injury temporally related to vaccination. Plaintiffs must apply to the VICP for compensation before using the tort system. The VICP affords protection to manufacturers and to vaccine providers and has already substantially reduced the number of cases processed in the tort system.

MISSED OPPORTUNITIES TO VACCINATE

Most children have received their full vaccination series by the time they enter elementary school because prematriculation vaccination is mandated by law, but many are at risk of disease during the preschool years because they do not receive their immunizations according to childhood vaccination guidelines. Some reasons for delays in immunization, such as a family's lack of access to medical care, are too complex to be addressed by individual clinicians. Chart audits show, however, that health care providers contribute significantly to delayed vaccination due to missed opportunities for vaccination and suboptimal rates of simultaneous vaccination of children who access medical care.

A missed opportunity to vaccinate occurs when a child who is a candidate for a dose of vaccine is seen by a health care provider and the child's vaccination status is not assessed or a dose of vaccine is withheld inappropriately. In Rochester, New York, 422 of 515 children (82%) had a missed vaccination opportunity; most missed opportunities (64%) involved withholding vaccination because of the mistaken belief that vaccination was contraindicated by mild acute illness. Another study found that physicians were less likely to recommend vaccination during an acute care visit because they believed vaccination at this time would be associated with a higher risk of adverse effects, the vaccine would be less efficacious, parents would be more likely to object to vaccination at that time, or the procedure would adversely affect practice operations.

Missed opportunities for simultaneous vaccine administration can contribute significantly to vaccine-preventable illnesses in children. In one measles outbreak, for example, 38% of measles cases developed in children who had received OPV and/or DTP at a time when MMR could also have been given. It is encouraging that only 11% of physicians in one study failed to recommend appropriate simultaneous administration of three injectable vaccines to a 2-year-old child who was behind schedule. The reasons cited for not administering vaccines simultaneously included concern about the difficulty of determining which vaccine caused an adverse event (if one were to occur), decreased vaccine efficacy, and parental objection.

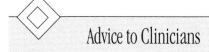

Advice to Clinicians

Strategies for Increasing Vaccination Rates

An office or clinic practice can improve vaccination rates by taking these five steps:

1. Evaluate current vaccination rates.
2. Identify problem areas and plan strategies to address these areas.
3. Set individual clinician goals for vaccination.
4. Implement the strategies to improve vaccination rates.
5. Provide ongoing feedback to individual clinicians about vaccination rates in their patients.

EVALUATING VACCINATION RATES

The first step in improving vaccination rates, a step that is frequently overlooked, is to evaluate the current vaccination rates of the practice. The impact of such evaluations can be large: assessment and feedback is credited with raising childhood vaccination rates in public clinics in Georgia from 53% in 1988 to 89% in 1994. Assessment of vaccination rates can tell clinicians about which barriers to address. For instance, an audit of vaccination practices in one clinic showed the following barriers to vaccination, in descending order: gaps in patient attendance at the clinic, missed opportunities to vaccinate, and overly cautious interpretations of contraindications.

IDENTIFYING PROBLEM AREAS AND PLANNING STRATEGIES

The second step to improving rates of vaccination is identifying the causes of vaccination

problems, such as missed opportunities to vaccinate, and planning strategies to address them. Clinicians and staff may find that a number of the following strategies fit their plan:

1. Have office staff routinely check the vaccination status of patients before the clinician's encounter with the patient, either during registration (perhaps programming electronic reminder notices if registration is computerized) or while nursing personnel obtain vital signs. Colored stickers, checklists, or inked rubber stamps added to the patient's chart are practical ways to communicate the need for vaccinations.
2. Remind parents about needed vaccinations, either by sending postcard reminders or through telephone contact (a telephone autodialing machine may be practical for some practices). A combination of mail and phone reminders may be most cost-effective, since a study of underimmunized children 20 months of age in a large health maintenance organization found that the estimated cost per child immunized was $9.80 using automated telephone messages alone, $10.50 using letters alone, but only $7.00 using both. A recent review of reminder and recall systems for routine childhood vaccines found that six of eight studies had a positive effect and two had no effect.
3. Write standing orders to allow nurses to administer routine vaccines without requiring a new order for each patient.
4. Have nursing personnel, not clinicians, administer the vaccines.
5. Use combination vaccines when available, to limit the number of injections that children receive and thereby decrease discomfort.

COMPLETING THE PROGRAM

The third step in a program to boost vaccination rates is to set measurable goals for vaccination and a time frame for their achievement. For example, the goals may be for each health care provider in the clinic to vaccinate 90% of the 2-year-olds in his or her practice. The fourth step is implementation of the plan. The final step is monitoring vaccination rates and giving feedback to providers. For instance, the percentage of fully vaccinated 2-year-olds can be graphed and displayed, allowing clinicians and teams to compare their records. The clinician or team that vaccinates the highest percentage of patients can be awarded a prize. The impact of evaluation, competition, and feedback should not be underestimated.

KEEPING CURRENT WITH VACCINE RECOMMENDATIONS

The "Recommended Childhood Immunization, United States," is published in January in *American Family Physician*, *Pediatrics*, and *Morbidity and Mortality Weekly Report* (MMWR) (Fig. 1-1). Vaccine information can be accessed at Web sites for the American Academy of Family Physicians (www.aafp.org), the Immunization Action Coalition (www.immunize.org), the National Immunization Program at the Centers for Disease Control (www.cdc.gov/nip/publica.htm), and MMWR (www.cdc.gov/epo/mmwr) and ATPM at (http://www.atpm.org).

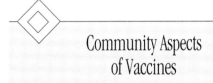

Community Aspects of Vaccines

The prevention potential of vaccines lies not only with individual patients but also with the community. Some of the protection from certain vaccine-preventable diseases comes from achieving and maintaining an adequate level of herd immunity to prevent diseases from spreading. Clinicians can contribute toward this com-

munity goal by ensuring that their patients are immunized according to recommended schedules. Most states have programs that provide free vaccine for clinicians to administer to their patients who do not have medical insurance and who meet eligibility criteria.

States also have school immunization laws that require proof of vaccinations against specified diseases before admission to school is allowed. These laws vary, the strongest ones require adequate documentation before school entry at all levels and allow exceptions only for religious or medical reasons. Universities also have immunization requirements for entry. Clinicians can assist their patients by ensuring that their immunization records are complete and accurate, so they can meet these requirements. Many states have also passed laws initiating statewide immunization registries. This creates a record to which any clinician can refer when a child and parent do not have documentation of past immunization with them. Registries also facilitate accurate records for patients who tend to use several health care providers.

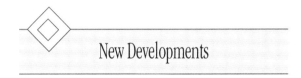

New Developments

Future developments in childhood vaccines are likely to be in three areas; new vaccines, revised vaccine recommendations, and combination vaccines.

New Vaccines and Immunization Recommendations

Research is progressing on vaccines against several important infectious agents, including pneumococcal conjugate vaccine, respiratory syncytial virus vaccine, and live, attenuated influenza vaccine. As new vaccines are developed and introduced, some will become part of the recommendations for routine childhood immunizations. New conjugate vaccines will allow for immunization at younger ages. As experience is gained with newer vaccines, we will learn how long their protection lasts and when boosters are needed. All these developments will lead to periodic changes in the recommendations for routine childhood immunizations. It will be challenging for clinicians to stay abreast of these changes.

Combination Vaccines

As more vaccines are introduced, more injections are required to meet recommendations, leading to problems with acceptance by patients and clinicians alike. There is much interest in vaccine combinations as a way of minimizing the number of needed injections. For example, combination vaccines that include acellular pertussis vaccine are being developed. The first combination licensed, for use in the fourth dose of the series, was TriHIBit, in which the Hib vaccine ActHI is reconstituted with the Tripedia acellular pertussis vaccine.

A combination of effective vaccines and public health efforts has already led to the eradication worldwide of one of the world's scourges, smallpox. It is likely that several other diseases will be eradicated in the next several decades and that vaccines will be a major contributor to these efforts.

Acknowledgments

The authors thank Diana Bosse Mathis, B.S.N., E.L.S., for editorial assistance; Judy Ball, M.S., for preparation of the manuscript; and William Barker, M.D., for project guidance.

Bibliography

Anders J, Jacobson, R, Poland G, et al: Secondary failure rates of measles vaccine: A metaanalysis of published studies. *Pediatr Infect Dis J* 15:62–66, 1996.

Centers for Disease Control: Certification of poliomyelitis eradication—the Americas. *MMWR* 43:720, 1994.

Centers for Disease Control: Prevention of varicella: Recommendations of the Advisory Committee on Immunization Practices (ACIP). *MMWR* 45(RR-11):1–36, 1996.

Centers for Disease Control and Prevention: General recommendations on immunization: Recommendations of the Advisory Committee on Immunization Practices (ACIP). *MMWR* 43(RR-1):1–38, 1994.

Centers for Disease Control and Prevention: Progress toward elimination of *Haemophilus influenzae* type b disease among infants and children—United States, 1987–1995. *MMWR* 45(42):901–906, 1996.

Centers for Disease Control and Prevention: Update: Vaccine side effects, adverse reactions, contraindications, and precautions—recommendations of the Advisory Committee on Immunization Practices (ACIP). *MMWR* 45(RR-12):1–35, 1996.

Centers for Disease Control and Prevention: Pertussis vaccination: Use of acellular pertussis vaccines among infants and young children. *MMWR* 46:1–25, 1997.

Centers for Disease Control and Prevention: Poliomyelitis prevention in the United States: Introduction of a sequential vaccination schedule of inactivated poliovirus vaccine followed by oral poliovirus vaccine—recommendations of the Advisory Committee on Immunization Practices (ACIP). *MMWR* 46(RR-3):1–25, 1997.

Centers for Disease Control and Prevention: Progress toward global eradication of poliomyelitis. *MMWR* 46:579–584, 1997.

Centers for Disease Control and Prevention: Rubella and congenital rubella syndrome—United States, 1994–1997. *MMWR* 46(16):350–354, 1997.

Centers for Disease Control and Prevention: Measles—United States, 1997. *MMWR* 47(14):273–276, 1998.

Centers for Disease Control and Prevention: National, state, and urban area vaccination coverage levels among children aged 19–35 months—United States, 1997. *MMWR* 47(26):547–554, 1998.

Centers for Disease Control and Prevention: Recommended childhood immunization schedule—United States, 1998. *MMWR* 47:8–12, 1998.

Chen RT, Rastogi SC, Mullen JR, et al: The Vaccine Adverse Event Reporting System (VAERS). *Vaccine* 12(6):542–550, 1994.

Decker MD, Edwards KM, Steinhoff MC, et al: Comparison of 13 acellular pertussis vaccines: Adverse reactions. *Pediatrics* 96:557–566, 1995.

Edmonson MB, Davis JP, Hopfensperger DJ, et al: Measles vaccination during the respiratory virus season and risk of vaccine failure. *Pediatrics* 98(5):905–910, 1996.

Freed GL, Katz SL, Clark SJ: Safety of vaccinations: Miss America, the media, and public health. *JAMA* 276(23):1869–1872, 1996.

Gamertsfelder DA, Zimmerman RK, DeSensi EG: Immunization barriers in a family practice residency clinic. *J Am Board Fam Pract* 7(2):100–104, 1994.

Greco D, Salmaso S, Mastrantonio P, et al: A controlled trial of two acellular vaccines and one whole-cell vaccine against pertussis. *N Engl J Med* 334:341–348, 1996.

Halloran ME, Cochi SL, Lieu TA, et al: Theoretical epidemiologic and morbidity effects of routine varicella immunization of preschool children in the United States. *JAMA* 140:81–104, 1994.

Immunization Practices Advisory Committee: Recommendations for use of *Haemophilus* b conjugate vaccines and a combined diphtheria, tetanus, pertusis, and *Haemophilus* b vaccine: Recommendations of the Advisory Committee on Immunization Practices (ACIP). *MMWR* 42(RR-13):1–15, 1993.

Institute of Medicine, Committee to Review the Adverse Consequences of Pertussis and Rubella Vaccines, Howson CP, et al (eds): *Adverse Effects of Pertussis and Rubella Vaccines: A Report of the Committee to Review the Adverse Consequences of Pertussis Vaccines*. Washington, DC; National Academy Press, 1991.

King GE, Markowitz LE, Heath J, et al: Antibody response to measles-mumps-rubella vaccine of children with mild illness during the time of vaccination. *JAMA* 275:704–707, 1996.

LeBaron CW, Chaney M, Baughman AL, et al: Impact of measurement and feedback on vaccination coverage in public clinics, 1988–1994. *JAMA* 277(8):631–635, 1997.

Lieu TA, Capra AM, Makol J, et al: Effectiveness and cost-effectiveness of letters, automated telephone messages, or both for underimmunized children in a health maintenance organization. *Pediatrics* 101(4):1–7, 1998.

Lieu TA, Cochi SL, Black SB, et al: Cost-effectiveness of a routine varicella vaccination program for U.S. children. *JAMA* 271:375–381, 1994.

McConnochie KM, Roghmann KJ: Immunization opportunities missed among urban poor children. *Pediatrics* 89(6 Pt 1):1019–1026, 1992.

Modlin JF, Halsey NA, Thoms ML, et al: Humoral and mucosal immunity in infants induced by three sequential inactivated poliovirus vaccines—live attenuated poliovirus vaccine immunization schedules. *J Infect Dis* 175(suppl 1):S228–S234, 1997.

Moyer LA, Mast EE: Hepatitis B: Virology, epidemiology, disease, and prevention, and an overview of viral hepatitis. *Am J Prev Med* 10(Suppl):45–55, 1994.

Schmitt HJ, von Konig CH, Neiss A, et al: Efficacy of acellular pertussis vaccine in early childhood after household exposure. *JAMA* 275(1):37–41, 1996.

Szilagyi PG, Rodewald LE, Humiston SG, et al: Missed opportunities for childhood vaccinations in office practices and the effect on vaccination status. *Pediatrics* 91:1–7, 1993.

Taylor JA, Darden PM, Slora E, et al: The influence of provider behavior, parental characteristics, and a public policy initiative on the immunization status of children followed by private pediatricians: a study from pediatric research in office settings. *Pediatrics* 99(2):209–215, 1997.

West DJ, Margolis HS: Prevention of hepatitis B virus infection in the United States: a pediatric perspective. *Pediatr Infect Dis* 11:866–874, 1992.

Wood D, Pereyra M, Halfon N, et al: Vaccination levels in Los Angeles public health centers: The contribution of missed opportunities to vaccinate and other factors. *Am J Public Health* 85:850–853, 1995.

Zimmerman RK, Barker WH, Strikas RA, et al: Developing curricula to promote preventive medicine skills: The Teaching Immunization for Medical Education (TIME) Project. *JAMA* 278:705–711, 1997.

Zimmerman RK, Bradford BJ, Janosky JE, et al: Barriers to measles and pertussis immunization: The knowledge and attitudes of Pennsylvania primary care physicians. *Am J Prev Med* 13(2):89–97, 1997.

Zimmerman RK, Schlesselman JJ, Baird AL, et al: A national survey to understand why physicians limit childhood immunizations. *Arch Pediatr Adolesc Med* 151:657–664, 1997.

Zimmerman RK, Schlesselman JJ, Mieczkowski TA, et al: Physician concerns about vaccine adverse effects and potential litigation. *Arch Pediatr Adolesc Med* 152:12–19, 1998.

Chapter

2

Vision Problems

Introduction

Proper vision screening and eye examination are critical for the early detection of conditions that can lead to poor school performance or blindness in children. Vision problems in children occur in as many as 5% to 10% of preschool children and 20% to 30% of school-age children. Primary care clinicians must be aware of the age-appropriate evaluations that will identify infants and children who need early referral to an ophthalmologist for diagnosis and treatment of visual problems to prevent permanent, irreversible blindness. Three major vision-threatening problems that a clinician must recognize are amblyopia, strabismus, and cataracts. Refractive errors should also be recognized.

Amblyopia

Amblyopia, one of the most common physical problems in children, occurs in approximately 2% of the general population. It is defined as loss of vision due to inadequate visual stimulation of the brain during cortical visual development. Anything that interferes with the brain's visual learning process may result in amblyopia. If the retinal image in one eye is distorted or if there is misalignment of the image on the retina (strabismus), the brain will suppress the poorer image from the affected eye to allow for clear vision. Amblyopia is a reversible condition that can be improved if the underlying cause is corrected early enough.

There are many causes of amblyopia (Table 2-1) including strabismus (crossed eyes), hyperopia (farsightedness), astigmatism (unfocused images on the retina), and visual deprivation (i.e., cataract, lid hemangioma, or blepharoptosis). Strabismus, defined as improper alignment of the eyes, is the most common cause of amblyopia. Amblyopia results when the brain ignores the incoming images from the crossed eye to prevent blurry vision. The prefixes *eso* and *exo* signify the direction of the ocular deviation. *Eso* refers to medial deviation and *exo* to lateral deviation. The most common type of strabismus is esodeviation (medial), which accounts for over half of all cases. The suffixes *phoria* and *tropia* indicate that there is a tendency for the eye to drift from the visual axis; this drift may be the result of certain conditions, such as fatigue (*phoria*), or it may always be present (*tropia*) (Figs. 2-1 and 2-2).

Table 2-1

Causes of Amblyopia

Strabismus (Improper Alignment)
Hyperopia (Far Sightedness)
Astigmatism (Unfocused images on the retina due to unequal curvative of the refractive surface)
Cataract
Eye Lid Hemangioma
Blepharoptosis (Drooping eye lid)

Figure 2-1

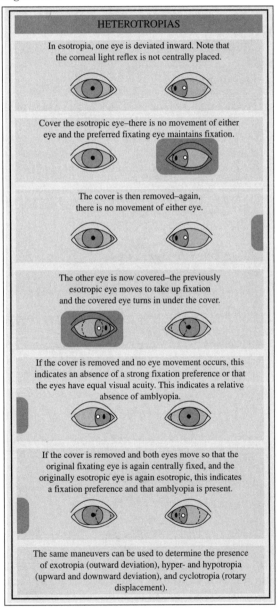

The cover/uncover test for heterotropias. From Chang KB, et al. Ophthalmology. In Zitell BJ and Davis H (eds). *Atlas of Pediatric Diagnosis*, Mosby, 1997. Used with permission.

Figure 2-2

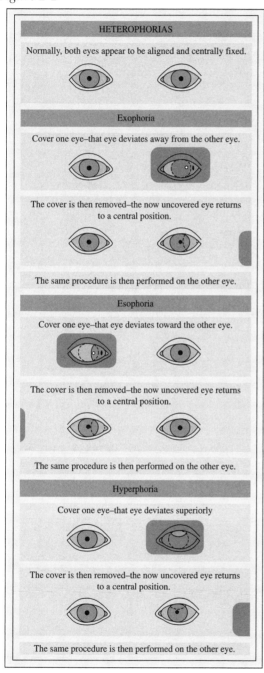

The cover/uncover test for heterophorias. From Chang KB, et al. Ophthalmology. In Zitell BJ and Davis H (eds). *Atlas of Pediatric Diagnosis*, Mosby, 1997. Used with permission.

Strabismus

Infantile strabismus appears before six months of age and is usually associated with a family history of strabismus. There may be alternate fixation, in which either the left eye or, at other times, the right eye turns medially. With this type of strabismus there is less risk of amblyopia, since the deviation alternates, allowing each eye to develop vision. Constant fixation is more likely to result in amblyopia of the eye that is turned inward. This condition may require surgical correction before the age of 2 years.

Accommodative esotropia is usually due to hyperopia (farsightedness). Accommodation allows for the image to be focused on the retinal plane but forces one eye to turn inward to focus. The condition may be intermittent or persistent and is usually hereditary, appearing between the ages of 2 and 3 years. Other causes of esotropia include trauma, prematurity, sixth-nerve palsy, cataract, and congenital syndromes. Exodeviations (turning outward) are often hereditary and usually intermittent, and they appear between infancy and 4 years of age. It is often noticed when the child is tired, ill, or looking into the distance. The prognosis is favorable unless the condition becomes permanent, which may lead to amblyopia. Late-onset, constant exotropia is more worrisome because it may be a sign of ocular or central nervous system disease. Vertical strabismus is often accompanied by a head tilt that allows the eyes to maintain binocularity. Congenital superior oblique muscle palsy is the most common cause.

Cataracts

A cataract is opacity of the lens. Cataracts may be congenital or acquired. One-fourth of cataracts are familial (autosomal dominant), and one-third are related to maternal infection during pregnancy (i.e., rubella). The remainder are sporadic cases, are part of a congenital syndrome (i.e., Down's and Turner's syndrome), or stem from a systemic illness (i.e., metabolic diseases, such as galactosemia). When the cataract diffuses light rays entering the eye, it obstructs the transmission of clear images onto the retina, resulting in abnormal vision. This is a significant cause of deprivation amblyopia.

Refractive Error

Myopia (nearsightedness) is a defect in the ability to see distant objects. Hyperopia (farsightedness) is the inability to see objects at close range and can cause problems with reading. Unilateral hyperopia can lead to amblyopia.

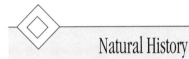

Natural History

Ocular Malalignment and Amblyopia

The human visual system is rudimentary at birth; many anatomical and physiologic changes take place during the first few months of life. By two to three months of age, the infant develops the ability to focus an image on the retina. Development of the visual system depends on stimulation of the visual cortex at an early age. Anything that disrupts this stimulation of the visual cortex will likely result in visual impairment. Morbidity associated with visual defects is significant—if left untreated, amblyopia can lead to irreversible blindness. The duration of amblyopia and the age at onset determine how rapidly normal acuity can be achieved with proper treatment. The cause of amblyopia must also be considered. Amblyopia stemming from a unilateral congenital cataract requires surgery within the first few months of life and is less effectively treated after age 1 to 2 years. In contrast, strabismic amblyopia may be treated effectively up to 4 years of age. Early detection and

treatment improve the likelihood of restoring normal visual acuity.

Infants are often born with benign eso- or exotropia that resolves within two to three months of age. Pseudostrabismus or pseudoesotropia is the appearance of crossed eyes due to a flat nasal bridge, prominent epicanthal folds, or a narrow interpupillary distance. The parents will often comment that one eye turns inward when the child is gazing to either side, but the eyes are actually properly aligned. This is a benign condition that will resolve as the child's nose develops and becomes narrower and more prominent, thus pushing the epicanthal folds away from the eyes. The literature supports that early detection and treatment of visual impairment minimizes morbidity. Unfortunately, preschool children are often not adequately screened for visual problems, resulting in delays in diagnosis. Primary care clinicians must be well informed about vision screening and incorporate it into regular health maintenance visits.

Refractive Error

The issue of refractive error (decreased visual acuity) is more controversial. Refractive error often is first discovered during the early school years. In the range of 7% to 9% of children in grades one to three have prescription glasses, a figure that rises to 20% by the late teenage years. There is disagreement about whether undiscovered refractive error affects academic performance adversely.

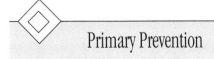

Primary Prevention

Early prenatal care allows screening for treatable maternal infections and the opportunity to counsel mothers about maternal habits or behavior that can affect the fetus (see Chap. 9). Maternal drug use or environmental toxin exposure puts the fetus at risk of congenital malformations. For example, LSD exposure may cause coloboma, a defect in the uveal tract that can affect several structures, including the iris and optic nerve head. Maternal infection during pregnancy can cause many defects of the fetal eye. Cytomegalovirus infection can lead to chorioretinitis, strabismus, optic atrophy, microphthalmia, and cataracts in the newborn. Toxoplasmosis can cause chorioretinitis. Rubella can result in cataracts, pigmentary retinopathy, and microphthalmia. Routine rubella screening of women before pregnancy can identify nonimmune women and permit vaccination before they become pregnant. It is important that pregnant women who contract rubella, cytomegalovirus, or toxoplasmosis during pregnancy be counseled concerning the possible complications in the newborn infant.

Two specific examples of maternal infections that can be transmitted at the time of delivery and lead to eye disease in a newborn infant are those caused by *Chlamydia trachomatis* and *Neisseria gonorrhoeae*. Both can cause ophthalmia neonatorum (neonatal conjunctivitis). Chlamydia is the most common cause of ophthalmia neonatorum, but gonococcal conjunctivitis is the more significant condition, because it can lead to corneal ulceration with scarring and, in severe cases, perforation of the globe. Prevention of gonococcal infection, but not chlamydial disease, is achieved with 1% silver nitrate, 0.5% erythromycin ointment, or 1% tetracycline ointment administered in the immediate postpartum period. Despite topical prophylaxis, eye infection and disseminated disease may still develop in some infants. Identification and treatment of pregnant women are the best ways of preventing chlamydial and gonococcal infection in the newborn infant. The prevention of both congenital and newborn infections that affect the eye is discussed in Chapter 9. It is important that physicians who perform forceps deliveries

be cautious when they are near newborn ocular structures. Forceps trauma may result in lid swelling, corneal opacification and laceration, hemorrhage, and rupture of the globe.

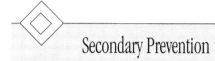

Secondary Prevention

A complete and accurate history is the first tool the primary care clinician should use in vision screening. The clinician should ask the parents if they have any specific concerns about the infant's or child's vision (i.e., the child does not blink at bright light or the infant does not regard the mother's face). Infants whose parents express concern about possible visual problems should have early ophthalmologic examination. Eye examination and vision-screening guidelines have been developed by the American Academy of Pediatrics (AAP) to promote early detection and treatment of conditions that affect visual acuity (Table 2-2). Eye examination should be performed beginning in the newborn period and at each well infant/child visit. The examination should include inspection of the ocular structures for symmetry and function. Pupillary response and the appearance of conjunctiva, cornea, iris, and sclera should be noted. Red reflex should be tested using an ophthalmoscope, from approximately twelve inches away. Asymmetry of the pupils, dark spots within the red reflex, or lack of a red reflex should prompt referral. The presence of a white reflex, known as leukokoria, can indicate retinoblastoma and must be considered an ocular emergency. The following are tests that the practitioner can use in the office to screen vision in infants and children. Formal vision screening should begin at age 3 years, using the most sophisticated test with which the child is capable of cooperating.

Table 2-2
Vision-screening Guidelines[a]

Function	Recommended Tests	Referral Criteria	Comments
Ages 3–5 yr Distance visual acuity	Snellen letters Snellen numbers Tumbling *E* *HOTV* Picture tests Allen figures LH test	1. <4 of 6 correct on 20-ft line with either eye tested at 10 ft monocularly (i.e., <10/20 or 20/40) or 2. Two-line difference between eyes, even within the passing range (i.e., 10/12.5 and 10/20 or 20/25 and 20/40)	1. Tests are listed in decreasing order of cognitive difficulty. The highest test that the child is capable of performing should be used. In general, the tumbling *E* or the *HOTV* test should be used for ages 3–5 yr and Snellen letters or numbers for ages 6 yr and older. 2. Testing distance of 10 ft is recommended for all visual acuity tests. 3. A line of figures is preferred over single figures. 4. The nontested eye should be covered by an occluder held by the examiner or by an adhesive occluder patch applied to eye; the examiner must ensure that it is not possible to peek with the nontested eye.
Ocular alignment	Unilateral cover test at 10 ft or 3 m or Random dot *E* stereogram test at 40 cm (630 s of arc)	Any eye movement ＜4 of 6 correct	

Ages 6 yr and older

Distance visual acuity	Snellen letters Snellen numbers Tumbling *E* *HOTV* Picture tests Allen figures LH test	1. <4 of 6 correct on 15-ft line with either eye tested at 10 ft monocularly (i.e., <10/15 or 20/30) or 2. Two-line difference between eyes, even within the passing range (i.e., 10/10 and 10/15 or 20/20 and 20/30)	1. Tests are listed in decreasing order of cognitive difficulty. The highest test that the child is capable of performing should be used. In general, the tumbling *E* or the *HOTV* test should be used for ages 3–5 yr and Snellen letters or numbers for ages 6 yr and older. 2. Testing distance of 10 ft is recommended for all visual acuity tests. 3. A line of figures is preferred over single figures. 4. The nontested eye should be covered by an occluder held by the examiner or by an adhesive occluder patch applied to the eye; the examiner must ensure that it is not possible to peek with the nontested eye.
Ocular alignment	Unilateral cover test at 3 m or Random dot *E* stereogram test at 40 cm (630 s of arc)	Any eye movement <4 of 6 correct	

*Vision-screening guidelines were developed by the American Academy of Pediatrics Section on Opthalmology Executive Committee, 1991–1992—Robert D. Gross, M.B.A., M.D., Chairman; Walter M. Fierson, M.D.; Jane D. Kivlin, M.D.; I. Matthew Rabinowicz, M.D.; David R. Stager, M.D.; Mark S. Ruttum, M.D., A.A.P.O.S.; and Earl R. Crouch, Jr, M.D., A.A.O. Used with permission of the American Academy of Pediatrics from *Pediatrics* 98:156; 1996.

Screening Tests

CORNEAL LIGHT REFLEX (HIRSCHBERG TEST)

A child looks directly into a penlight. The examiner checks that the light reflected off the corneas is positioned in the center of the pupil and is symmetrical in location. This test will give normal results in the case of pseudostrabismus. Asymmetry may indicate ocular malalignment that requires follow-up by a pediatric ophthalmologist (Fig. 2-3).

COVER/UNCOVER TEST

This test requires that the child focus on an object at a distance with both eyes open. The examiner occludes one eye while he or she looks for movement in the uncovered eye. The occlusion device is removed to allow binocular viewing to return. The examiner then occludes the alternate eye while again observing the uncovered eye. This process is repeated over and over to obtain reproducible results. Movement of the nonoccluded eye indicates that a tropia exists. Any movement that occurs when the eyes are covered and uncovered is considered a positive test result and requires evaluation by a pediatric ophthalmologist (Figs. 2-1 and 2-2).

ALTERNATE COVER TEST

This test is performed by alternating the cover from one eye to the other without allowing adjustment to binocular vision. If any eye movement is noted, it is considered an abnormal test result that requires referral to an ophthalmologist.

EYE CHARTS FOR VISUAL ACUITY

Allen cards use simple pictures and are appropriate for children 2 to 3 years old. It is important to be sure that the child is able to identify the figures before conducting the actual vision testing. The tumbling *E* chart consists of several capital letter *E*'s oriented in different

Figure 2-3

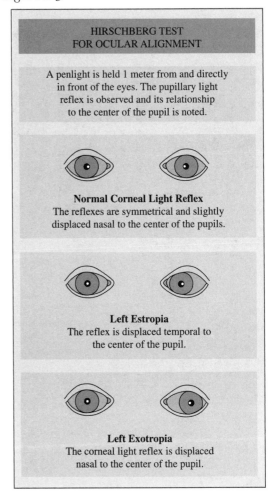

The Hirschberg test for ocular alignment. From Chang KB, et al. Ophthalmology. In Zitell BJ and Davis H (eds). *Atlas of Pediatric Diagnosis*, Mosby, 1997. Used with permission.

directions. The examiner points to a specific *E*, and the child must indicate the direction of the arms by using his or her fingers. This is an appropriate tool for a 4- to 5-year-old child. An alternative to the *E* chart is the *HOTV* chart, which consists of a combination of differently sized letters *H, O, T,* and *V.* When the examiner points to a letter, the child is asked to match the letter on a card that the child holds. This is a useful test for 3- to 5-year-olds. The Snellen acuity chart consists of letters and numbers. The child must know his or her numbers and letters, so this test is best used with school-aged children.

The distance for all vision testing using a chart is at 10 to 20 feet, except the Allen cards, which are placed at 10 feet. A well-lit area and proper occlusion of the untested eye are important. If a child wears corrective lenses, they should be worn during testing. The area should have a limited number of distractions to maximize cooperation. Screening devices, such as the Optec Vision Testing System, are available to evaluate near and far visual acuity, phorias, and color and contrast vision. The child looks into the viewer, and the examiner selects the test to be administered. There is less peripheral distraction with the viewer than with the wall chart. The cost of the system is about $2000. In interpreting results of vision screening, acuity of 20/40 is normal for 3-year-olds, 20/30 for 4-year-olds, and 20/20 for 5- to 6-year-olds. A difference of more than one line between the two eyes is abnormal and may indicate amblyopia or a refractive error, which requires referral to an ophthalmologist.

STEREOSCOPIC TESTING

Stereoscopic tests detect amblyopia and strabismus. Binocular vision develops by four months of age and should be included in early vision screening. The AAP recommends the unilateral cover test or the random dot *E* stereogram to test for ocular alignment. In the random dot *E* test, the stereogram appears to be a page of dots until the child puts on three-dimensional glasses that enable him or her to see geometric figures, such as an *E*. Children with amblyopia will not see these shapes. The test is easy to administer and takes only a few minutes.

PHOTOREFRACTION

Standard refraction testing involves determining the proper eyeglass lens to correct vision. Photorefraction is a photographic technique designed to detect ocular anomalies by using a light reflex that is generated by placing a flash source slightly above or below a camera lens. In this way it is possible to determine refractive error, ocular alignment, and clarity of the lens. Benefits of using this screening method are that it is compact and easy to use and does not require a response from the child. The limitations of photorefraction include the expense and the delay in obtaining results, because the film must be sent out for processing and analysis.

Accuracy of Screening Tests

Despite the common use of the Hirschberg test and the cover/uncover test, there is no information available on their sensitivity and specificity.

Follow-up and Treatment

A child who fails any of the vision-screening tests should be referred to an ophthalmologist for evaluation and treatment of the underlying disorder (see Table 2-2 for referral criteria). Amblyopia is treated by eliminating the cause of the inadequate stimuli to the brain. If there is a refractive error, glasses can be used to correct it. Patching the stronger eye with an occlusive, adhesive eye patch will help normalize visual acuity in the weaker, amblyopic eye. A detailed patching schedule should be developed and carefully monitored by the ophthalmologist, working closely with the family. It is important to avoid development of occlusion amblyopia, which can occur if the patch is left in place too long. Successful treatment depends on the age at onset of amblyopia and the length of time before diagnosis and treatment is initiated. Strabismus is treated by realigning the eyes to eliminate amblyopia. Nonsurgical treatments include occlusion patches or prescription glasses. If nonsurgical methods fail to correct the problem, surgery is indicated. The primary care clinician should emphasize to families that the operation is a short procedure and rarely has complications.

School-based Screening

Most states have adopted some form of required school-based vision screening, usually school-entry screening and screening two to three times during the elementary and middle-school years. This has proved to be an important way to identify problems that have gone undetected or have recently developed. School-entry screening programs detect some form of vision deficit in 10% to 13% of children tested, the majority being a form of refractive error. A significant number of ocular alignment problems are also detected. Snellen chart testing screens for myopia and is the most common tool used for school screening. Some programs have adopted multiple screening methods, including a test for visual acuity, stereo-acuity, and ocular alignment.

The sensitivity of school-based vision-screening programs has been reported to be 60% to 70% and the specificity, 70% to 80%. This means that 20% to 30% of children with normal vision will have abnormal test results and that the positive predictive value of an abnormal test will be 25% to 33%. Any child referred to a primary care clinician for failing a school vision test should undergo an eye examination and office vision screening and be referred to an ophthalmologist if a deficit is confirmed. School nurses or teachers frequently refer children with headaches, blurry vision, difficulty in reading, or poor school performance to primary care clinicians. These children should have a thorough evaluation, including a complete medical history, neurological examination, and vision screening. The majority of them do not have primary visual problems and should not be automatically referred to an ophthalmologist.

Evidence That Screening and Treatment Are Effective

There is good evidence that early detection and treatment of amblyopia and strabismus in infants and children improve outcomes. There is also evidence that early detection and correction of refractive errors lead to less visual impairment. There is very little evidence that screening for refractive errors in school-age children, compared with evaluating those complaining of symptoms or those referred because of parents' concerns, results in improved school performance.

Recommendations

The AAP recommendations for vision screening are listed in Table 2-2; they include tests for visual acuity and ocular alignment starting at age three. The U.S. Preventive Services Task Force (USPSTF) recommends screening for ocular alignment between ages three and four. The AAP advocates testing for visual acuity and ocular alignment for school-age children every 1 to 2 years through adolescence. The USPSTF does not sanction routine screening in this age group. Recommendations from other groups, such as the American Academy of Ophthalmology and the American Optometric Association, are in agreement with those of the AAP.

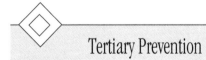

Tertiary Prevention

It is important for the primary care clinician to work closely with the pediatric ophthalmologist and the family of a visually impaired child. With proper treatment, some vision problems will result in full recovery of vision, whereas other conditions will leave the child permanently visually impaired. Even children who are legally blind, however, may have a degree of useful vision that will allow for normal schooling. The visually impaired child is often developmentally delayed, especially in gross motor skills. Parents can help minimize these delays by enriching the child's environment with sensory stimuli. For example, blind infants and children should have toys that are tactilely stimulating and make interesting sounds. The child with partial vision should have an environment with bright colors or toys.

The visually impaired child should be encouraged to develop socialization skills. Until the age of 4 or 5 years, visually impaired children may not realize that they are different from other children. Developing play and cooperative skills is important, but the socialization process will also make a visually impaired child aware of the abilities he or she lacks. Parents should be honest with the child about the visual impairment and encourage the child to participate in nursery school or kindergarten programs. Most children can attend a non-handicapped school if the class sizes are limited and the teacher is caring and willing to deal with the visually impaired child.

Once the child is of school age, there are a variety of programs available through the public school system. For example, classes may be limited in the number of students and taught by special education teachers certified to teach visually impaired students. Some programs allow the child to spend a portion of the school day in a traditional classroom setting and part of the day with individualized instruction in a resource room. In such a room, the special education instructor may use special lighting effects and innovative computer equipment to enhance learning. The educational placement of the child is a decision that should be made by the parents in conjunction with school educators. Children's

books in Braille are available to help minimize disability. Before school entry, the parents should arrange with the local school officials for an evaluation of their child. Often a psychological assessment, individualized for the visually impaired child, is performed to help the school determine specific educational goals and objectives for the child's school program. Parents are encouraged to take an active part in the process.

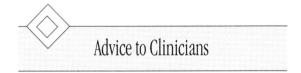

Advice to Clinicians

Routine Screening Practices

Primary care clinicians should incorporate eye and vision screening into newborn, infant, and childhood wellness exams. Many tests can be performed on children when they are being examined for other illnesses and complaints. For infants and children through age 3 to 4 years, concentrate on looking for fixation problems, malalignment, and presence of disease. Ask parents and caregivers about any observed or suspected problems with the child's vision. Inspect the eye, as previously described, and perform tests for ocular alignment. Having children sit on their parents' laps during the exam can help put them at ease.

Vision testing should begin at age three or as soon thereafter as the child can cooperate. If a child wears glasses, conduct the tests with the glasses on, unless the glasses are for reading. Have a selection of visual acuity tests available and use the one of highest cognitive difficulty for the particular child. Vision testing wall charts can be ordered from medical supply houses. Most are available for testing at either a 10 or a 20 foot distance. It is important to test at the correct distance and to conduct the testing in a location free of distraction. Primary care clinicians should have a working relationship with a pediatric ophthalmologist and an optometrist who has experience with children.

The Visually Impaired Child

The primary care clinician plays an important role in advising the parents of the visually impaired child and must be well informed and have a positive attitude to be able to help the parents accept their child's impairment. The age at which the child lost his or her vision as well as the level of impairment affect how the parents and child will cope with the impairment. Professional counseling for the entire family is often valuable in easing the adjustment and preventing depression. Clinicians should also be familiar with local support groups, so that they can help the family network with other families who have had similar problems. For example, the National Association of Parents of the Visually Impaired has local chapters throughout the country. The clinician should advise families that through the Internet, they can visit Web sites for the visually impaired that offer information about a multitude of currently available resources and technology.

Clinicians should also be familiar with problems that can arise during development, so that they can provide quality anticipatory guidance for the visually impaired child. These children may develop strange mannerisms, including rocking, eye gouging, and other socially unacceptable forms of behavior. Parents should be advised to deal with these the way they would any other objectionable behavior, by not dwelling on them but by using behavioral modification techniques. When examining a child with a serious visual impairment, the clinician should not touch the child before explaining what will be done and should allow the child to

touch the instruments that will be used. Always speak softly and be gentle, because the child has no visual clues to help him or her anticipate actions. It is important not to focus on the child's visual impairment but to help the family foster the development of the child's talents and skills to maximize his or her potential.

Common Errors

Not Providing Screening

In spite of evidence that screening for ocular malalignment and early intervention can minimize the adverse consequences of strabismus and other causes of amblyopia, many primary care clinicians do not conduct screening.

Lack of Follow-up

Many parents of children who have positive results on vision-screening tests at school are unaware of the results, and referral appointments with specialists for eye evaluations are frequently not made or kept. Primary care clinicians need to emphasize the importance of following up with an eye specialist whenever there is a suspicion of vision problems. School screening programs should inform parents and primary care clinicians of results, make referrals, and follow-up on referral results.

Performing Tests Improperly

Visual acuity tests can result in false-positive results if the child is not capable of following instructions for the testing procedure. It is important to use a test with a cognitive difficulty that matches the child's ability. False-negative tests can result from not occluding the opposite eye completely and from the nonverbal and other unintentional clues of the tester.

Referrals for Pseudostrabismus

Pseudostrabismus can be mistaken for esotropia if the clinician is unfamiliar with this normal condition. Pinching the bridge of the nose to make it narrow can demonstrate the normal eye alignment. Along with normal Hirschberg test results, this should help the clinician distinguish pseudo- from true strabismus.

Emerging Trends

Screening

New software for personal computers is being developed and tested for mass screening in preschool programs. Automated vision-testing equipment for clinicians' offices is also being developed and will likely become more widely available. Technological improvements and decreases in the cost of photorefraction for diagnosing vision problems are also in the offing. An easy-to-use camera will allow clinicians to download images onto a computer that will immediately perform analysis, eliminating delay and expediting referral.

Assistance for the Visually Impaired Child

The expanding role of technology offers sophisticated devices for the education of visually impaired children. For example, a camera can project enlarged newsprint onto a screen, thus allowing the visually impaired child to read the daily newspaper. Web sites designed specifically for visually impaired children offer information about newsletters, libraries, and books on tape, Braille transcription services, and more.

Validation of Current Screening Tests and Their Benefits

Studies are needed to document the sensitivity and specificity of commonly used screening tests. This accuracy can then be compared with that of new automated screening devices. Studies are also needed to validate the cost-effectiveness of universal, periodic visual acuity screening in schools. School health resources are not sufficient to continue to support mass interventions of no value or unproven benefit. It is hoped that the relationship of asymptomatic refractive errors to school performance and outcomes will be explored more fully.

Bibliography

Broderick P: Pediatric vision screening for the family physician. *Am Fam Physician* 58:3, 691–700, 1998.

Brown MS: Vision screening of preschool children. *Clin Pediatr* 14:10, 968–973, 1975.

Committee on Practice and Ambulatory Medicine, Section on Ophthalmology: Eye examination and vision screening in infants, children, and young adults. *Pediatrics* 98:1, 153–157, 1996.

Committee on School Health, American Academy of Pediatrics, Nader PR: School Health Services: *School Health: Policy and Practice.* American Academy of Pediatrics, 1993.

Ehrlich MI, Reinecke RD, Simons K: Preschool vision screening for amblyopia and strabismus: Programs, methods, guidelines. *Surv Ophthalmol* 28:145–163, 1983.

King RA: Common ocular signs and symptoms in childhood. *Pediatr Clin North Am Pediatr Ophthalmol* 40(4):753–766, 1993.

Magramm I: Amblyopia: Etiology, detection, and treatment. *Pediatr Rev* 13(1):7–14, 1992.

Moller MA: Working with visually impaired children and their families. *Pediatr Clin North Am Pediatr Ophthalmol* 40(4):881–891, 1993.

Nelson LB: *Pediatric Ophthalmology*. Philadelphia, WB Saunders, 1984.

Robinson B, Bobier WR, Martin E, Bryant L: Measurement of the validity of a pre-school vision screening program. *Am J Public Health* 89:193, 1999.

Stager DR: Amblyopia and the pediatrician. *Pediatr Ann* reprint, 1977.

Traboulsi EI, Maumenee IH: Eye problems, in Oski FA, DeAngelis CD, Feigin RD, McMillan JA, Warshaw JB (eds): *Principles and Practice of Pediatrics*, 2d ed. Philadelphia, Lippincott, 1994, p 878.

Jeffrey C. Weiss

Hearing Problems

Introduction

Definition

Hearing loss in children can be categorized in several ways. It may be congenital or acquired, static or progressive, unilateral or bilateral. The condition may or may not be inherited and can be either an isolated finding or part of a recognized syndrome. The severity can be mild, moderate, severe, or profound. Some patients have hearing loss that occurs at all frequencies, whereas others have losses only at certain specific frequencies, such as with high-frequency hearing loss. Finally, the hearing loss may be categorized as conductive, sensorineural, or mixed, depending on the underlying pathophysiologic condition.

A conductive hearing loss results from interference with sound transmission through the external auditory canal, tympanic membrane, middle ear, or ossicular chain. A conductive loss is most commonly the result of severe cerumen impaction, eustachian tube dysfunction, or otitis media and its complications. Conductive losses may also result from trauma or be due to inherited or congenital anatomic anomalies of the ear canal or middle ear apparatus.

Sensorineural hearing loss is caused by abnormalities in the cochlea and the neural auditory pathways. Sensorineural loss may be due to genetic factors (50%) or environmental causes (20% to 25%) such as infection, noise, drugs, anoxia, and hyperbilirubinemia. Unknown causes account for about 25% of cases, but this percentage is likely to decrease as more genes are discovered that are associated with non-syndrome-related hereditary hearing loss.

The severity of hearing loss is generally expressed in decibels (dB), a measure of sound intensity. The decibel is a logarithmic unit, so a 10-dB increase is a tenfold increase in energy intensity, 20 dB is a 100-fold increase, 30 dB is a 1000-fold increase, and so forth. A child who can hear sounds at a threshold of 0 to 15 dB has hearing that is considered normal. "Slight" hearing loss is associated with thresholds of 16 to 25 dB, "mild" with thresholds of 26 to 40 dB, "moderate" with thresholds of 41 to 65 dB, and "severe" hearing loss with thresholds of 66 to 95 dB. A threshold of more than 95 dB is called "profound" hearing loss.

Prevalence

NEWBORN AND INFANT HEARING LOSS

The prevalence of newborn and infant hearing loss is estimated to range from 1 to 5 per 1000 live births. The prevalence is determined to some degree by the definition of hearing loss, with higher rates resulting if mild and/or unilateral cases are included. Several authors indicate that severe or profound bilateral sensorineural hearing loss occurs in 1 per 1000 births.

Approximately half of the newborns with hearing loss have risk factors that can be identified at or near the time of birth. These risks are listed in Table 3-1. Additional risk factors in older children include head trauma with associated loss of consciousness or skull fracture, recurrent or persistent otitis media with effusion for longer than three months, and neurodegenerative disorders. Any parental concern regarding

Table 3-1

Risks Associated with Sensorineural and/or Conductive Hearing Loss in Newborns

Family history of hereditary childhood sensorineural hearing loss
In utero infection with cytomegalovirus, rubella, syphilis, herpes virus, toxoplasmosis
Craniofacial anomalies, including abnormalities of the pinna and ear canal and preauricular tags and pits
Birth weight less than 1500 grams
Hyperbilirubinemia requiring exchange transfusion
Ototoxic medications, such as aminoglycosides, used in multiple courses or in combination with loop
    diuretics
Bacterial meningitis
Apgar scores of ≤4 at 1 min or ≤6 at 5 min
Mechanical ventilation lasting 5 days or longer
Signs or other findings associated with a syndrome known to include hearing loss

SOURCE: From American Academy of Pediatric Joint Committee on Infant Hearing 1994 position paper.

hearing, speech, language, and/or developmental delay should always be considered a risk factor for hearing loss and taken seriously.

The prevalence of hearing loss in children 6 to 19 years of age was studied in the third National Health and Nutrition Examination Survey between 1988 and 1994. Close to 15% of all children tested had hearing loss in one or both ears of at least 16 dB; 7.1% had low-frequency hearing loss (generally conductive hearing loss), and 12.7% had high-frequency loss (generally sensorineural hearing loss). Most of the hearing deficits documented were slight, but 4.7% had mild loss or worse in one or both ears. Mexican American children had higher rates of high-frequency hearing loss, as did children from the lowest socioeconomic groups. It is unknown what proportion of the hearing loss detected was temporary or transient.

OTITIS MEDIA

Children under 15 years old make 20 million office visits each year for treatment of acute otitis media. Between 1975 and 1990, the number of office visits for acute otitis media among children increased by 150%. While many of these infections resolve spontaneously or with antibiotic treatment, otitis media with effusion (OME) develops in many children. Some children get OME without having had an acute infection, possibly as the result of respiratory allergy or a viral upper respiratory infection.

A diagnosis of OME suggests that there is eustachian tube malfunction with associated negative middle ear pressure, a retracted tympanic membrane, middle ear effusion, and hearing loss. OME can be a transient condition that resolves over time without treatment, or it can become a chronic problem requiring medical or surgical treatment. At any point, up to 7% of children age 5 to 8 years experience mild temporary hearing loss due to otitis media.

Risk factors that are associated with recurrent and chronic OME include day-care attendance, lack of breast feeding, regular exposure to tobacco smoke, young age at time of first infection, craniofacial abnormality (e.g., cleft palate and Down's, Turner's, and Pierre Robin syndromes), and immunodeficiency. OME is 15 times more likely to develop in Native American children than white or black children.

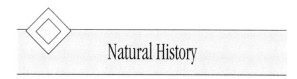

Natural History

Profoundly hearing-impaired newborns can look and act like any normal baby. Initially, they may even coo and babble normally. Before initiation of newborn screening programs, the average age at which a hearing-impaired child was diagnosed was between 2 and 3 years. A National Institutes of Health consensus statement (1993) indicates that "reduced hearing ability during infancy and early childhood interferes with the development of speech and normal verbal language skills." It goes on to say that "reduced auditory input affects the developing auditory nervous system and can have harmful effects on social, emotional, cognitive and academic development, as well as on a person's vocational and economic potential."

By age 8 years, children with severe bilateral hearing loss are already 1 to 2 years behind their peers in reading comprehension. The gap widens with time, so that at the completion of high school, reading levels are usually between the third and seventh grade levels. Children with mild or moderate bilateral hearing loss generally perform at grade level if they receive proper educational support; however, children with unilateral loss of more than 45 dB were shown to lag substantially behind their peers in reading. In fact, in one study 35% of children with unilateral hearing loss failed a grade in school. Hearing-impaired children have been shown to have a greater incidence of problems with self-esteem and social adjustment. They are often described as impulsive and physically aggressive. These findings may be due in part to family stress and parenting style, which is sometimes intrusive and overly controlling.

Benefits of Early Detection

NEWBORNS AND INFANTS

Because we have not been able to identify severe hearing loss at an early age until recently, no large prospective, long-term, randomized study proves that early identification and early intervention clearly have a beneficial effect. There are, however, solid studies that do suggest that significant benefits may result. Apuzzo and Yoshinaga-Itano (1995) have found that children with severe bilateral hearing loss diagnosed before 6 months of age had significantly better language comprehension, expressive language, and vocabulary than those children whose hearing loss was identified after age 6 months. Children whose severe hearing loss was discovered by 2 months of age were functioning almost at grade level. In another study, children who received 9 months of early home-based intervention before age 30 months did better than control children on measures of reading, arithmetic, vocabulary, articulation, social adjustment, and behavior (Watkins, 1987).

OTITIS MEDIA WITH EFFUSION

In 1994, the United States Public Health Service published a clinical practice guideline, entitled *Otitis Media with Effusion in Young Children*. The report states that "OME can produce mild to moderate conductive hearing impairment, which can fluctuate, remain stable, or alternate with periods of normal hearing. It is not known how many days of effusion or reduced hearing are required before development is adversely affected." A detailed review of the medical literature "failed to find rigorous, methodologically sound research to support the theory that untreated OME results in speech/language delays or deficits." The review did sug-

gest a "weak association between early OME and delay in expressive language development in children over age 4 years."

Despite the lack of hard evidence that OME results in language delay and the reality that OME-associated hearing loss is usually temporary, it is common practice for primary care clinicians to refer young children with chronic and recurrent middle ear disease for audiologic testing. Furthermore, speech and language development should be carefully monitored at least until school entry in all children with a history of chronic OME.

Primary Prevention

Intrauterine Infections

Infectious teratogenic agents most commonly associated with congenital hearing loss include rubella, cytomegalovirus, syphilis, toxoplasmosis, herpes simplex, and varicella. Since the development of rubella vaccine, the incidence of congenital infection with this virus has fallen dramatically, to about 50 children per year. Varicella vaccine has recently been released for general use, but effective vaccines for the other common organisms responsible for congenital hearing loss are not currently available.

Pregnant women are routinely screened for their rubella titer, to check for previous infection. Nonimmune individuals are advised to report any rash or illness to their clinicians, so that a follow-up rubella titer can be obtained 3 to 4 weeks after the illness. If a follow-up titer is positive, infection is assumed to have occurred, and counseling regarding congenital rubella syndrome and possible termination of the pregnancy may be warranted.

Pregnant women are also generally screened for the presence of syphilis infection. There is some evidence that prompt treatment of an active infection can prevent the sequelae of intrauterine infection in the neonate. For other congenital infections, however, primary prevention consists of minimizing exposure of the pregnant woman to the infectious organism. For example, pregnant women should be advised to limit their exposure to toxoplasmosis by refraining from eating raw meat or eggs and avoiding exposure to cat feces. Chapter 9 contains a more complete discussion concerning the primary and secondary prevention of infections during pregnancy.

Intrauterine Medication Exposure

There are a few drugs and chemical agents that have been proved to cause hearing loss in the infants of mothers who take them during pregnancy. Thalidomide, which caused an epidemic of severe congenital malformations and sensorineural hearing loss in the 1960s, is no longer being prescribed except in rare circumstances.

The aminoglycoside antibiotic streptomycin has been shown to be teratogenic to the developing fetal auditory system. While the evidence is less well established, kanamycin and gentamicin have also been reported to cause newborn hearing loss when used during pregnancy, particularly taken in conjunction with diuretics, such as furosemide or ethacrynic acid. The antimalarial drug chloroquine may cause deafness, but it seems to be of little risk when used in standard doses during pregnancy.

Ethyl alcohol exposure in pregnancy remains a major problem, with an estimated incidence of fetal alcohol syndrome (FAS) of between 1:550 and 1:2500 live births. Children with FAS have dysmorphic craniofacial features that are commonly associated with bilateral recurrent OME and conductive hearing problems. For this reason, and because permanent sensorineural hearing loss has also been reported with FAS, pregnant women should avoid the use of alcohol.

Noise

Exposure to very loud noise can cause high-frequency hearing loss. While there is no evidence regarding the benefit of noise avoidance in children, it is probably wise to advise children to avoid constant, high-level noise exposure from headsets. Any child with a documented high-frequency hearing deficit should use earplugs when exposed to loud noise, such as in shop class or at a noisy concert.

Otitis Media with Effusion

Otitis media has been associated with two modifiable risk factors: lack of breast feeding and exposure to second-hand tobacco smoke. In spite of a lack of evidence of efficacy, it is reasonable to encourage mothers to breast-feed and to avoid exposing children to cigarette smoke.

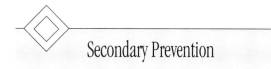

Secondary Prevention

Newborn Screening

In the past, only newborns with certain risk factors were screened for hearing loss. In 1993, the National Institutes of Health Consensus Development Conference on Early Identification of Hearing Impairment in Infants and Young Children concluded, "All infants should be screened for hearing impairment." This recommendation for universal newborn screening was based on several facts, among them, that 50% of children with hearing loss do not have any high-risk factors that would trigger an evaluation; the average age for detection of hearing loss is between 2 and 3 years; and delay in diagnosis causes permanent speech and language problems, with associated harmful effects on social, emotional, cognitive, and academic development. Moreover, early intervention can prevent many of these problems, and new technology has made screening more cost-effective and feasible.

Initial resistance toward universal screening came from individuals and organizations that felt, first, that a high number of false-positive test results would result in parental anxiety and unacceptable costs for unnecessary referrals for detailed, diagnostic follow-up studies and, second, that no solid evidence exists to support the benefit of early versus later treatment. In the past few years, because of improved screening accuracy, resistance to universal screening has declined, and several states have passed laws requiring such screening.

The ideal hearing screening test should be simple to perform and interpret, inexpensive, fast, reliable, and valid. Because the incidence of hearing loss is low, universal screening is relatively new, the testing equipment is rapidly evolving, and good studies of sensitivity and specificity of screening tests are very limited at this time. Often, newborn screening tests are compared with gold standard diagnostic tests rather than a child's confirmed hearing status at an older age. Furthermore, debates among audiologists about the most appropriate cutoff levels for various screening tests make comparison of sensitivity and specificity difficult.

Brainstem Auditory-evoked Response

Historically, newborns who were thought to have hearing loss and those with specific risk factors for hearing loss were evaluated with brainstem auditory evoked-response audiometry (BAER). This test is often the gold standard against which other diagnostic and screening tests are compared. In a BAER, a multifrequency click and/or frequency-specific tone bursts are delivered to the ear by way of an earphone or through a bone conduction device. Electrodes are applied to the surface of the head, often on the mastoids and forehead, in order to detect electrical signals in the cochlea, auditory nerve,

and brainstem auditory nucleii. Each ear is tested separately, and threshold response levels are determined over a range of frequencies. The BAER can be used at any age, but young infants and children require sedation with an agent such as chloral hydrate. Because of the time required (about 1 hour), the high cost, and the need for expert interpretation, the BAER is not suitable for any type of universal mass screening program. Since the BAER is often scheduled for a time after the baby is discharged from the nursery, broken appointments and incomplete follow-up are frequent problems.

In comparing the results of the newborn BAER to the hearing status of children at 4 years old, Hyde et al. (1990) found that the sensitivity of the test was 98%, and the specificity was 96%, using a screening threshold level of 40 dB. As with any diagnostic test, the sensitivity and specificity of the BAER depend on the definition of a positive test result. When the screening threshold is lowered to 30 dB, even those children with mild hearing loss are identified, but the number of false-positive test results is also increased.

Automated Brainstem Response

New technology has become available that can be used to screen large numbers of infants in an efficient and cost-effective way. The automated brainstem response (ABR) is faster (about 15 minutes per test) than the BAER and does not require interpretation by an audiologist. After the stimulus clicks are delivered at the screening intensity (usually between 30 and 40 dB), brain wave activity is recorded from three scalp electrodes and processed by a computer. The computer software compares the results with a template developed with data from normal infants. Results are reported as "pass" or "refer." The equipment costs about $16,000, and the cost of disposables for each test is about $10. Compared with the conventional BAER, the sensitivity and specificity of the screening ABR are 98% and 96%, respectively.

OTOACOUSTIC EMISSIONS

The transient evoked otoacoustic emissions (TEOAE) test makes use of the principle that cochlear hair cells produce measurable sounds when they are stimulated. After a sound probe is placed into the ear canal, the computerized system presents a series of clicks and then records the sounds generated by the cochlear hair cells. The test requires relative quiet and is difficult to administer in a noisy nursery. Furthermore, the test requires interpretation by an audiologist, and it often has a false-positive rate of more than 10%, especially when it is performed in the first 24 hours of life. Since the TEOAE is not actually a test of hearing, it may not detect "auditory neuropathy," defined as hearing loss due to such nervous system diseases as meningitis, congenital cytomegalovirus infection, intraventricular hemorrhage, hyperbilirubinemia, and degenerative diseases. Taken together, the causes of auditory neuropathy probably represent only 1% of all the cases of hearing loss in children, so this is not a major limitation of the TEOAE screen.

Another version of the otoacoustic emissions (OAE) test, called distortion product otoacoustic emissions (DPOAE), presents two tones of different frequency to the ear. The emissions from the cochlear outer hair cells give information about hearing deficits at various frequencies. The equipment, which costs about $5000, is handheld, fast (less than 5 minutes), can be used in a busy nursery, and generates a pass/refer response that does not require interpretation by an audiologist. No large studies with long term follow-up are available to determine the sensitivity of the DPOAE. In a study of 105 high-risk infants, Salata (1998) found that DPOAE sensitivity was 67% and specificity was 68% compared with ABR. The National Center for Hearing Assessment and Management reports an average false-positive rate of about 8% for DPOAE, but since this test is usually part of a two-stage screen, only about 1% of children require referral for diagnostic testing.

RECOMMENDATIONS

Unfortunately, there is currently no protocol for newborn hearing screening that is accepted by all audiologists and screening programs. Some favor the use of ABR, and others favor OAE as the initial test. The advantages of the ABR are that it has a lower false-positive rate and that it is capable of detecting hearing loss from auditory neuropathy, whereas the main advantages of the OAE are its faster speed and much lower cost. Many programs are now using the OAE as a first step and then performing an ABR or BAER on those infants who get a "refer" result. Infants with clinical conditions known to be associated with auditory neuropathy should not be screened with OAE alone. At this time, there is little information that compares the efficacy of the various two-stage screening protocols currently in use. The primary care clinician should be aware that rapid improvements in the accuracy, ease of use, and costs of testing equipment are likely to alter screening strategies in the future.

While universal screening is gaining acceptance, it is not without controversy. In its last review, published in 1996, the U.S. Preventive Services Task Force (USPSTF) did not find sufficient evidence to recommend for or against universal screening. There is consensus that those neonates with any of the risk factors listed in Table 3-1 should be screened, preferably before leaving the hospital but at least by the age of 3 months.

Screening Older Children

HIGH RISK

If universal newborn screening is not available in the hospital nursery, the Joint Committee on Infant Hearing (JCIH) suggests that infants be screened at some time before 3 months of age if any of the newborn indicators mentioned in Table 3-1 are present. Health conditions that require rescreening of children up to age 2 years (even if the child has passed a newborn screen) include parents' concern regarding speech or hearing, bacterial meningitis infection, head trauma with loss of consciousness, signs of a syndrome associated with hearing loss, previous use of ototoxic medications, and recurrent or persistent OME that lasts for at least 3 months (Table 3-2). To detect delayed-onset sensorineural or conductive hearing loss, JCIH also recommends that certain children with the risk factors shown in Table 3-3 be screened every 6 months until age 3.

At present, accurate hearing evaluation of children less than 3 years of age cannot generally be accomplished in the office of a primary care clinician. The new handheld equipment for performing OAE tests may be within a price range that is feasible for office practice, but this technology is not in widespread use in such settings at this time. Young children with the appropriate risk factors should be referred to a trained pediatric audiologist. Older children diagnosed with bacterial meningitis should have hearing evaluations once they have recovered well enough to tolerate the testing. Recent studies suggest that most cases of hearing loss due to meningitis result from cochlear lesions, rather than from lesions located in the auditory nerves or higher centers. In a British study, the OAE was found to be a feasible method to diagnose most hearing loss after meningitis; however,

Table 3-3

Detection of Delayed-onset Hearing Loss: JCIH Indications for Performing a Hearing Evaluation Every 6 mos Until Age 3 yrs

Family history of hereditary childhood hearing loss
In utero infection (e.g., rubella, CMV, syphilis)
Neurofibromatosis type 2 and neurodegenerative disorders
Recurrent or persistent otitis media with effusion
Anatomic deformities and other disorders that affect eustachian tube function

ABBREVIATIONS: JCIH, Joint Committee on Infant Hearing; CMV, cytomegalovirus.
SOURCE: From American Academy of Pediatrics Joint Committee on Infant Hearing 1994 position paper.

routine follow-up is needed in order to detect retrocochlear or late-onset hearing loss (Richardson et al., 1998).

NON HIGH RISK

The American Academy of Pediatrics recommends that parents be questioned about their child's hearing at every routine health maintenance visit and that a standard audiogram be

Table 3-2

Conditions in Infants 1 mo to 2 yrs Old That Are Associated with Hearing Loss

Parent or caregiver concern regarding hearing, speech, language, or developmental delay
Bacterial meningitis
Head trauma with loss of consciousness or skull fracture
Signs or other findings associated with a syndrome known to include hearing loss
Ototoxic medications, such as chemotherapeutic agents or aminoglycosides, used in multiple courses or in combination with loop diuretics
Recurrent or persistent otitis media with effusion for at least 3 mo

SOURCE: From American Academy of Pediatrics Joint Committee on Infant Hearing 1994 position paper.

performed at ages 3, 4, 5, 10, 12, 15, and 18 years of age. Audiometry is reported to have a sensitivity of 92% and a specificity of 94% when screening for sensorineural loss. The audiogram should be performed in a quiet room, and the child should be asked to indicate when he or she hears a tone by raising a hand. Pure tones of various frequencies (usually 500, 1000, 2000, 4000, 6000, and 8000 Hz) are presented through earphones at a 20-dB intensity, one ear at a time. If the child is unable to hear the tone at this volume, the operator raises the intensity and presents the stimulus repeatedly, until the child indicates that the sound is heard.

Normally, children should be able to hear all of the frequencies at the 20-dB screening level. If the child fails to hear the 20-dB tone at two of the test frequencies in one ear, referral to an audiologist should be considered. Because the transient presence of fluid in the middle ear often causes temporary hearing loss, children unable to hear the stimulus sounds can be retested after approximately 2 weeks. In the absence of middle ear disease, another failure is ground for referral.

For young children who cannot cooperate with the standard audiogram instructions, audiotape equipment is available that instructs the child to point at a series of pictures. With each instruction, the voice on the audiotape becomes progressively softer, each instruction corresponding to an approximate decibel level. The operator can determine the child's hearing threshold by noting the last instruction that the child performs properly.

The audiogram conducted by an audiologist provides significantly more information than the screening exam done in the primary care clinician's office. In addition to measuring thresholds for air conduction, the audiologist will determine bone conduction (a measure of sensorineural function), speech reception thresholds, and a speech discrimination score. The speech-associated tests measure the child's ability to recognize and differentiate specific words that are presented at various levels of sound inten-

sity. The audiogram in Fig. 3-1 shows a mild sensorineural hearing loss evidenced by a 30-dB threshold for bone conduction. An additional 20-dB deficit, called the air-bone gap, is due to conductive hearing loss, as is verified by the air conduction measurements.

Many organizations, including the American Academy of Pediatrics and the American Speech–Language–Hearing Association, recommend periodic audiometry screening. The USP-STF, however, does not recommend routine screening beyond age 3 and states that if screening is conducted, abnormal results should be confirmed by retesting before referral.

Evaluation of Middle Ear Disease

Children with middle ear disease frequently have a blocked eustachian tube, which prevents normal ventilation of the middle ear cavity. When the surrounding tissues absorb the air in the middle ear, a vacuum develops. This negative pressure retracts the tympanic membrane and causes fluid to be drawn into the middle ear cavity, a condition known as otitis media with effusion. OME is often associated with various degrees of conductive hearing loss. Although there is no proof that treatment of OME prevents long-term language delay, most primary care clinicians treat or follow this condition until it resolves. Middle ear diseases such as OME are most often diagnosed clinically by examination of the tympanic membrane with an otoscope. Additional diagnostic accuracy can be obtained by pneumatic otoscopy, in which a small rubber bulb attached to the otoscope is used to apply pressure or suction to the tympanic membrane. Rubber-tipped specula help maintain an airtight system. The presence of middle ear fluid or a high negative middle ear pressure will dampen the mobility of the eardrum. The positive predictive value of a distinctly immobile tympanic membrane to detect a middle ear effusion has been shown by Karma et al. (1991) to be between 78% and 94%.

Figure 3-1

Date: ____________________

Audiometer: ________ Serial No.: ________ Calibration Checked: ________ Examined By: ____________

AUDIOGRAM KEY		RIGHT EAR	LEFT EAR
Air Conduction	Unmasked	O	X
	Masked	Δ	□
Bone Conduction	Unmasked	<	>
	Masked	[	]

(ANSI-1969)

☒ Pure Tone Audiometry
☒ Play Audiometry
☐ Minimal Response Levels

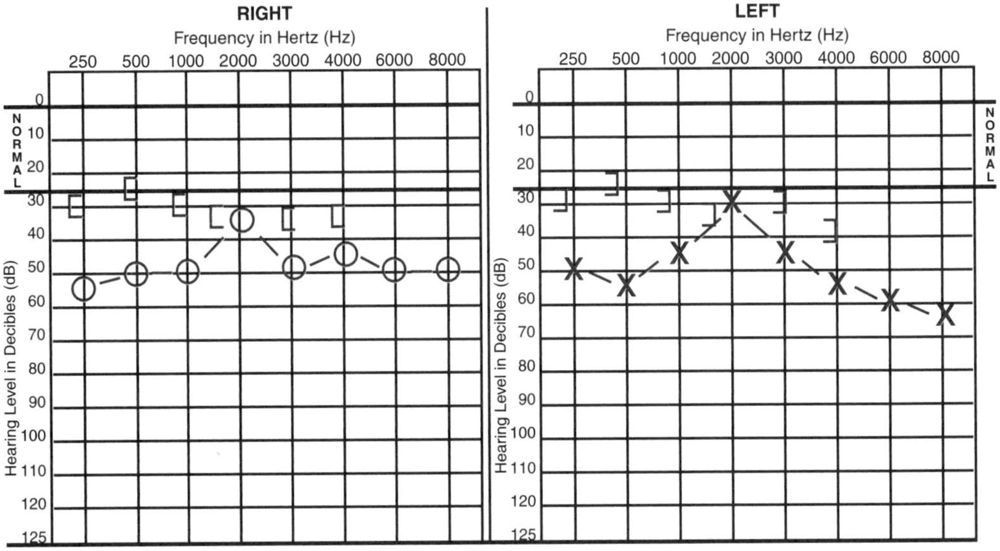
RIGHT
Frequency in Hertz (Hz)
250 500 1000 2000 3000 4000 6000 8000
0 10 20 30 40 50 60 70 80 90 100 110 120 125
NORMAL
Hearing Level in Decibles (dB)
LEFT
Frequency in Hertz (Hz)
250 500 1000 2000 3000 4000 6000 8000
0 10 20 30 40 50 60 70 80 90 100 110 120 125
NORMAL
Hearing Level in Decibles (dB)

Speech Audiometry

Speech Audiometry ☒ Pictures		Right		Left		Through Loudspeakers
Threshold (SRT)	(HL)	45	dB	45	dB	dB
Opposite Ear Masked			dB		dB	
Discrimination (SDS) * ☒ MLV ☐ Recorded		96	%	96	%	%
WIPI ☐			%		%	%
Opposite Ear Masked ☐						
Hearing Level	(HL)	75	dB	75	dB	dB
Comfort	(HL)		dB		dB	dB
Discomfort Level	(HL)		dB		dB	dB

* Monitored Live Voice Presentation

Overall Reliability ☒ **Good** ☐ **Fair** ☐ **Poor**

AUDIOLOGICAL REPORT FORM

OVER

00-3545 Rev 6/95

This audiogram report shows a mixed hearing loss. The 30- to 40-dB bone conduction thresholds indicate the presence of a sensorineural hearing loss. An additional deficit, demonstrated by the 35- to 55-dB air conduction thresholds, is evidence of a conductive hearing loss as well.

TYMPANOMETRY

While it is not actually a test of hearing, tympanometry is used by many primary care clinicians to help with decision-making in children with chronic or recurrent middle ear infections and effusions. The tympanometer indirectly measures the pressure in the middle ear and gives some information about the presence or absence of an effusion. This equipment is designed to gauge the acoustic admittance, a measure of the ease with which sound energy is transmitted from one medium to another.

The tympanometer consists of a probe that fits into the ear canal tightly enough to prevent an air leak, a sound generator, a microphone to detect sound in the external ear canal, and a vacuum pump capable of altering the pressure (measured in deca-pascal units) in the ear canal. When the stimulus tone (266 Hz) is introduced, some of the acoustic energy enters the middle ear (admittance), and some is reflected off the tympanic membrane and measured by the microphone in the ear canal. This process is repeated rapidly many times while the ear canal pressure is varied over a range of positive and negative pressures. The resultant tympanogram is a graph of ear canal pressure on the x-axis and admittance on the y-axis (Fig. 3-2).

Maximum admittance occurs when the air pressure in the ear canal is equal to the air pressure in the middle ear. The pressure at which this admittance peak is highest, called the tympanic peak pressure (TPP), is an approximation of the middle ear pressure. The TPP provides clinically useful information about eustachian tube function, but it does not indicate whether a middle ear effusion is present. The tympanic width (TW), defined by the sides of the tympanogram tracing at 50% of the peak admittance, is a measure of the sharpness of the tympanic peak. A rounded peak and a wider than normal tympanic width are indicators of middle ear effusion.

Most tympanometer equipment can also measure the volume of the ear canal and the acoustic reflex. In the presence of a perforation of the tympanic membrane or patent tympanostomy tubes, the volume of air measured is increased over normal ear canal values because the air in the middle ear is included. The acoustic reflex makes use of a 105-dB tone to stimulate contraction of the stapedius muscle, which causes stiffening of the ossicular chain and decreased admittance. Lack of an acoustic reflex can indicate the presence of a hearing loss, but this is not a particularly accurate or valuable screening test in most clinical situations.

Although more elaborate classifications have been developed, it is clinically useful for the primary care clinician to determine if the tympanogram pattern falls into the type A, type B, or type C category. The type A pattern has a sharp peak that is located along the x-axis at a pressure between −100 and +100 daPa. This is considered normal. The type B pattern has a low admittance over the entire pressure range and has no clear peak. Most ears (88%) with a type B pattern have a middle ear effusion. The type C tympanogram pattern is defined by a negative TPP of less than −100 daPa, with or without an abnormally large TW. This type of pattern indicates eustachian tube obstruction with negative middle ear pressure.

Nozza et al. (1994) compared tympanogram results with the presence or absence of middle ear effusion on myringotomy. TW was the single best variable for differentiating the ear with an effusion from an effusion-free middle ear. The TW upper limit of normal for children is 150 daPa, but using that value as a screening cutoff would result in a very high number of false-positive results (positive predictive value {PPV} of 61%). Using a TW of more than 275 daPa was found to have a sensitivity of 81%, a specificity of 82%, a positive predictive value of 85%, and a negative predictive value of 78%.

Figure 3-2

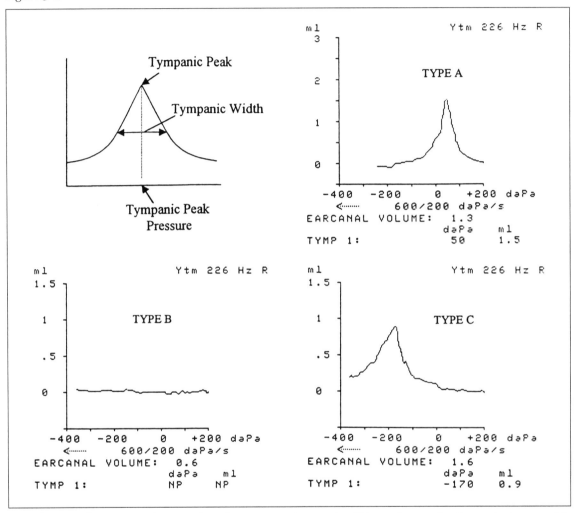

The definitions of tympanic peak, tympanic peak pressure, and tympanic width are given on the diagram in the upper left. Examples of the major types of tympanogram are shown.

Some office tympanometers can analyze the TPP and the TW measurements to provide an interpretation of whether the tympanogram has a normal configuration.

ACOUSTIC REFLECTOMETRY

Acoustic reflectometry is another office technique to determine whether an effusion is present in the middle ear. This test does not measure middle ear pressure, and, like tympanometry, it does not measure hearing. The instrument, which is handheld and light in weight, and does not require an airtight system, emits a chirp consisting of several tone frequencies (from 1.8 to 4.4 Hz) into the ear canal. By plotting the reflected acoustic energy over a range of frequencies, a microprocessor calculates the spectral gradient angle, which correlates with the likelihood of an effusion. Barnett has shown that angles of less than 49° are associated with ear effusions 88% of the time. As the spectral gradient angle increases, the likelihood of effusion decreases such that an angle of 49° to 69° is associated with effusion in 70% of cases, an angle of 70° to 95° has a 44% chance of effusion, and an angle of larger than 95° is associated with effusion only 17% of the time.

MANAGEMENT OF OME

The combination of clinical examination (with pneumatic otoscopy), tympanometry, and acoustic reflectometry allows the primary care clinician to make a diagnosis of OME. Children with OME can simply be observed for spontaneous resolution. Initial management should not include myringotomy with insertion of tympanostomy tubes at this stage. Although a trial of oral antibiotics is considered acceptable, many experts suggest that antibiotic use be minimized, to avoid the growing problem of bacterial antibiotic resistance.

The Agency for Health Care Policy and Research clinical practice guideline recommends a hearing evaluation for a child with a history of middle ear effusion for 3 or more months. The results of this hearing evaluation determine whether surgical tympanostomy tube insertion is a reasonable option. If the audiogram shows hearing thresholds of more than 20 dB, referral for tube placement is acceptable. Even with an abnormal audiogram result, some experts would use oral antibiotics and/or oral corticosteroids before referral for surgery.

School-based Screening

The American Academy of Pediatrics recommends that at school entry, a child whose hearing has not been tested during a recent medical evaluation should be screened with pure-tone audiometry at 25 dB over at least three frequencies. Those who fail should be retested 6 to 12 weeks later, and those who fail again should have a third screening in another 6 weeks. Children who fail two or more tests should be referred to a primary care clinician for examination of the ears and appropriate treatment and further testing.

Some schools also use tympanometry for detection of middle ear fluid, which can be associated with hearing loss. Most children who have abnormal tympanogram results actually have normal hearing. Furthermore, children with upper respiratory infections or nasal allergy will often have transient middle ear fluid that clears spontaneously. For these reasons, tympanometry is not appropriate for mass screening and should not be used as a substitute for pure-tone audiometry. Tympanometry can be useful, however, when used in conjunction with a pure-tone audiogram. There is no reason to delay medical referral for an abnormal audiogram if middle ear disease is ruled out by a normal tympanogram result.

Tertiary Prevention

Children with severe unilateral hearing loss have difficulty hearing speech clearly in noisy environments. For this reason, when they are in school they should be seated as close to the teacher as possible, with the better ear directed toward the teacher. Since these children also have trouble localizing sounds, they need to be given special instructions regarding pedestrian and bicycle safety. Conventional hearing aids provide little benefit to the child with unilateral deafness, but every effort should be made to conserve hearing in the better ear. Parents and the child should be counseled about avoiding loud noises and loud music and about the need to seek prompt medical attention for ear infections and middle ear effusions.

For the child with severe bilateral sensorineural deafness, early use of hearing aids for amplification is critical. Speech and language skills, as well as some aspects of cognitive and emotional development, are maximized if the hearing aids are put in place before 6 months of age. There are a variety of aids available, but air conduction models with an ear mold that fits comfortably into the external ear canal are most commonly used. The ear mold must provide a good acoustic seal or else a high-pitched whistle will be heard when sound escapes and is reamplified. Since children grow rapidly, it is important to refit ear molds often. Bone conduction hearing aids are available for children who have congenital anatomical ear deformities of the pinna or external auditory canal.

A hearing aid should be selected to provide adequate amplification at the proper frequencies. The volume should be loud enough to be helpful but not so loud as to be uncomfortable. Unfortunately, conventional hearing aids are not effective at separating speech from background noise. To rectify this problem, systems that use FM radio signals transmitted to the child's personal hearing aid are used in schools for hearing-impaired children.

Deaf children generally require special education. While some experts believe that children should be taught in schools for the deaf, others think that "mainstreaming" them has advantages. There is still controversy regarding whether deaf children should be taught sign language, and debate about which type of sign language is best for stimulation of the child's overall development is ongoing.

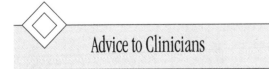

Advice to Clinicians

The primary care clinician who cares for children must always take parental concerns about

hearing seriously and arrange for proper hearing evaluation. Clapping or jingling keys to see if the child turns toward the sound or grimaces is not an adequate measure of hearing. As the technology for hearing testing of newborns improves, with lower costs and fewer false-positive tests, clinicians would be wise to become advocates for universal screening in the hospitals where they care for newborns. For the older child, hearing testing is a part of routine care, and an office audiogram should be undertaken, with results recorded on a regular schedule.

Parents of children with hearing problems have many questions regarding the cause of the problem and the best types of treatments, and the clinician should address these concerns and other parenting and educational issues. Referral to a multidisciplinary team consisting of an otolaryngologist, speech therapist, and audiologist is often available through the state agency responsible for handicapped or hearing-impaired children. Fortunately, there are many sources of good information for parents. The National Information Center on Deafness at Gallaudet University maintains an extensive site on the Internet (http://www.gallaudet.edu/~nicd/index.html), with on-line publications, catalogues of educational materials, instructions about how to find a parent support group, lists of relevant state agencies, and links to many organizations that focus on the interests of people with hearing impairment.

Common Errors

Not Screening High-risk Neonates

While universal screening is still somewhat controversial and not yet universally accepted or implemented, there is no disagreement that those with any of the risk factors listed in Table 3-1 should be screened before age 3 months. These risk factors are often not inquired about, and newborns who fall into these categories are frequently not screened.

Inaccurate Audiograms

Audiogram accuracy is affected by improper techniques and background noise. The test is frequently not performed properly, leading to false-positive results.

Using Tympanometry as a Screening Tool

Tympanometry is a useful diagnostic tool, but it is not recommended as a technique for universal screening. It is, however, often used for this purpose, leading to inappropriate referrals.

Emerging Concepts in Screening and Treatment

Screening Technology

The technology for hearing testing has been rapidly advancing, so that universal screening for newborns is now less expensive, faster, and more accurate. As the resistance to newborn screening diminishes, more and more hospitals are performing screening with either OAEs or the ABR test. The new technology, such as a handheld device to measure OAEs, may soon become standard equipment for the primary care clinician's office, allowing for hearing screening at a much younger age than with a pure-tone audiogram.

Hearing Aid Technology

Great technological improvements are also being made with hearing aids, which are becoming smaller and better able to filter out background noise. Educational improvements using closed-caption television and computer games for deaf children, as well as special telephone systems, are becoming available to larger numbers of children.

Cochlear Implants

A small percentage of children with profound hearing loss who are not adequately helped by conventional hearing aids may benefit from a cochlear implant. When a transmitter sends electrical signals to electrodes that have been surgically implanted into the cochlea, auditory neurons are stimulated, creating the sensation of hearing. As the hardware and software for speech processing continue to improve, cochlear implantation has the capability to make a major positive impact on the lives of severely hearing impaired children.

Research on Efficacy of Screening and Treatment

As described in this chapter, much of what is recommended for hearing screening and treatment is not based on solid evidence. While it may not be possible for ethical reasons to conduct controlled trials in some situations, more research will be conducted on the validity of existing and new screening tools and on the efficacy of early diagnosis and treatment of different forms of hearing loss.

Bibliography

Agency for Health Care Policy and Research: *Otitis Media with Effusion in Young Children: Clinical Practice Guideline.* AHCRP Publication 94-0622. Rockville, MD, US Department of Health and Human Services, Public Health Service, Agency for Health Care Policy and Research, 1994.

American Academy of Pediatrics: *School Health: Policy and Practice.* Elk Grove Village, IL, 1993.

American Academy of Pediatrics: Joint Committee on Infant Hearing 1994 position statement. *Pediatrics* 95:152–156, 1995.

Apuzzo ML, Yoshinaga-Itano C: Early identification of infants with significant hearing loss and the Minnesota Child Development Inventory. *Semin Hear* 16:124–137, 1995.

Barnett ED, Klein JO, Hawkins KA: Comparison of spectral gradient acoustic reflectometry and other diagnostic techniques for detection of middle ear effusion in children with middle ear disease. *Pediatr Infect Dis J* 17:556–559, 1998.

Bess FH, Paradise JL: Universal screening for infant hearing impairment: not simple, not risk free, not necessarily beneficial, not presently justified. *Pediatrics* 93:330–334, 1994.

Guidelines for Health Supervision 3. Elk Grove Village, IL, American Academy of Pediatrics, 1997. http://www.usu.edu/~ncham/publications/equipment.html

Hyde ML, Riko K, Malizia K: Audiometric accuracy of the click ABR in infants at risk for hearing loss. *J Am Acad Audiol* 1:59–66, 1990.

Karma PH, Sipila MM, Kataja MJ: Pneumatic otoscopy and otitis media: Value of different tympanic membrane findings and their combinations, in *Recent Advances in Otitis Media, Proceedings of the Fifth International Symposium*, 1991, p 41–45.

National Center for Hearing Assessment and Management: Selecting equipment

National Institutes of Health Consensus Development Conference: Early Identification of Hearing Impairment in Infants and Young Children. March 1–3, 1993.

Niskar AS, Kiezak SM, Holmes A, Esteban E, et al: Prevalence of hearing loss among children 6 to 19 years of age. The Third National Health and Nutrition Examination Survey. *JAMA*; 279:1071–1075, 1998.

Nozza RJ, Bluestone CD, Kardatzke D: Identification of middle ear effusion by aural acoustic admittance and otoscopy. *Ear Hear* 15:310–323, 1994

Richardson MP, Williamson TJ, Reid A: Otoacoustic emissions as a screening test for hearing impairment in children recovering from acute bacterial meningitis. *Pediatrics* 102:1364–1368, 1998.

Salata JA, Jacobson JT, Strasnick B: Distortion-product otoacoustic emissions hearing screening in high-risk newborns. *Otolaryngol Head Neck Surg* 118:37–43, 1998.

Schuman AJ: Universal newborn hearing screening: The time is right. *Contemp Pediatr* 15:49–60, 1998.

Strasnick B, Jacobson JT: Teratogenic hearing loss. *J Am Acad Audiol* 6:28–38, 1995.

Watkins S: Long term effects of home intervention with hearing-impaired children. *Am Ann Deaf* 132:267–271, 1987.

Robert J. Berkowitz
Dominick Zero
Burton Edelstein

Dental Caries

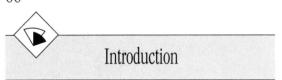

Introduction

Anatomy of a Tooth

A tooth comprises three calcified tissues—enamel, dentin, and cementum—that encase the dental pulp. The pulp is composed of cells, intercellular substance, fiber elements, vessels, and nerves. The anatomic relationship of these tissues to one another and to the periodontium is illustrated in Fig. 4-1.

Development and Names of Teeth

The primary dentition is made up of 20 teeth, whereas the permanent dentition is composed of 32 teeth. The names of these teeth and the chronology of human dental development is summarized in Table 4-1.

Figure 4-1

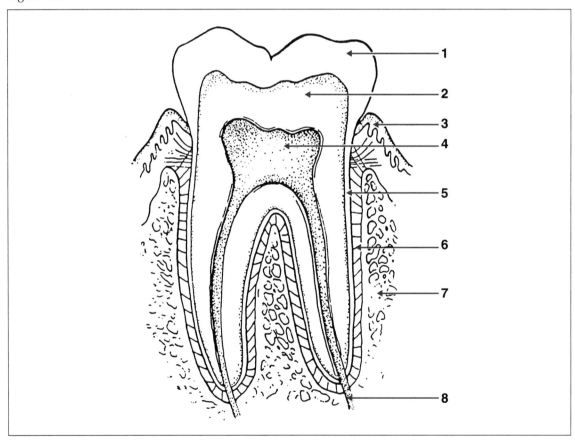

Diagram showing anatomy of the tooth and adjacent structures: enamel (1), dentin (2), gingival margin (3), pulp (4), cementum (5), periodontal ligament (6), alveolar bone (7), and neurovascular bundle (8).

Table 4-1

Chronology of the Human Dentition

			PRIMARY DENTITION			
TOOTH	HARD TISSUE FORMATION BEGINS	AMOUNT OF ENAMEL AT BIRTH	ENAMEL COMPLETED	ERUPTION	ROOT COMPLETED	EXFOLIATION
Maxillary						
Central	3½ mo in utero	Five-sixths	1½ mo	7½ mo	1½ yr	6–7 yr
Lateral	4 mo in utero	Two-thirds	2½ mo	9 mo	2 yr	7–8 yr
Cuspid	4½ mo in utero	One-third	9 mo	18 mo	3½ yr	10–12 yr
1st molar	4 mo in utero	Cusps united	6 mo	14 mo	2½ yr	9–11 yr
2nd molar	4½ mo in utero	Cusp tips still isolated	11 mo	24 mo	3 yr	10–12 yr
Mandibular						
Central	3½ mo in utero	Three-fifths	2½ mo	6 mo	1½ yr	6–7 yr
Lateral	4 mo in utero	Three-fifths	3 mo	7 mo	1½ yr	7–8 yr
Cuspid	4½ mo in utero	One-third	9 mo	16 mo	3½ yr	9–12 yr
1st molar	4 mo in utero	Cusps united	5½ mo	12 mo	1½ yr	9–11 yr
2nd molar	4½ mo in utero	Cusp tips still isolated	10 mo	20 mo	3 yr	10–12 yr
		PERMANENT DENTITION				
Maxillary						
Central	3–4 mo		4–5 yr	7–8 yr	10 yr	
Lateral	10–12 mo		4–5 yr	8–9 yr	11 yr	
Cuspid	4–5 mo		6–7 yr	11–12 yr	13–15 yr	
1st bicuspid	1½–1¾ yr		5–6 yr	10–11 yr	12–13 yr	
2nd bicuspid	2–2¼ yr		6–7 yr	10–12 yr	12–14 yr	
1st molar	At birth	Sometimes a trace	2½–3 yr	6–7 yr	9–10 yr	
2nd molar	2½–3 yr		7–8 yr	12–13 yr	14–16 yr	
3rd molar	7–9 yr		12–16 yr	17–21 yr	18–25 yr	
Mandibular						
Central	3–4 mo		4–5 yr	6–7 yr	9 yr	
Lateral	3–4 mo		4–5 yr	7–8 yr	10 yr	
Cuspid	4–5 mo		6–7 yr	9–10 yr	12–14 yr	
1st bicuspid	1¾–2 yr		5–6 yr	10–12 yr	12–13 yr	
2nd bicuspid	2¼–2½ yr		6–7 yr	11–12 yr	13–14 yr	
1st molar	At birth	Sometimes a trace	2½–3 yr	6–7 yr	9–10 yr	
2nd molar	2½–3 yr		7–8 yr	11–13 yr	14–15 yr	
3rd molar	8–10 yr		12–16 yr	17–21 yr	18–25 yr	

SOURCE: From Logan and Kronfeld, slightly modified by McCall and Schour, and revised by Kraus.

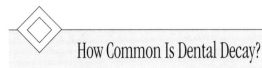

How Common Is Dental Decay?

Prevalence of Caries

EARLY CHILDHOOD CARIES

During the first few years of life, dental caries (also called nursing caries) is usually a rampant process. Stated differently, babies and toddlers either have rampant caries or are caries-free. Excessive dental caries in babies and toddlers is routinely associated with prolonged and frequent oral exposure to cariogenic substrates, including chronic ingestion of sucrose-sweetened liquid medications, use of sweetened pacifiers, ad libitum breast feeding, and, more commonly, use of a nap-time and/or bedtime nursing bottle that contains a cariogenic substrate. This type of dental caries is characterized by a distinctive pattern. The primary maxillary incisors are routinely affected, but the primary mandibular incisors are rarely involved. The involvement of other primary teeth varies.

A recent and comprehensive review regarding the epidemiology of early childhood caries indicates that it has a global occurrence (Milnes, 1996). Its prevalence varies with different populations; disadvantaged children, regardless of ethnicity, race, or culture, are most vulnerable. High-risk populations in the United States include immigrant eastern European children, immigrant Hispanic children, American Indian children, inner city African-American children, and children enrolled in Head Start programs. Disease prevalence rates for these high-risk U.S. populations range from approximately 5% to 70%.

EPIDEMIOLOGY OF CARIES OF PRIMARY AND PERMANENT TEETH

Li et al. (1993) conducted an in-depth comparison of the caries attack patterns in U.S.

schoolchildren using data from the 1979 to 1980 and the 1986 to 1987 National Institute of Dental Research surveys. Previous reports based on these data had indicated that there was a dramatic decline in caries prevalence for both the permanent and primary dentition. When combining all surfaces of the primary teeth, the average attack rates were 76 per thousand surfaces in 1979 to 1980 and 54 per thousand surfaces in 1986 to 1987, representing an overall 28% reduction in the caries attack rate for primary teeth. For the permanent teeth the average attack rates were 47 surfaces per thousand in 1979 to 1980 and 31 surfaces per thousand in 1986 to 1987, representing an overall 35% reduction in the caries attack rate for permanent teeth. The pit and fissures of molars of both primary and permanent teeth were found to have the greatest susceptibility to caries.

Based on a recent review of caries prevalence among children in North America, it appears that caries prevalence and severity are continuing to decline in terms of the permanent dentition in the general population of Canada and the United States but that caries experience in the primary dentition has stabilized since the years 1986 to 1987 (Burt, 1994). It was suggested that fluoride effects may now have been maximized in the primary dentition. The North American findings are similar to the European data. Downer (1994) reported that between 1973 and 1993 there was a caries decline of 55% in primary teeth of 5-year-old children and 75% in the permanent teeth of 12-year-old children in the United Kingdom; however, the data for younger children suggest that the decline in caries experience has ceased and may even have started to rise. Marthaler et al. (1996) amassed an extensive compilation of caries prevalence data from countries throughout Europe. One of the conclusions in their report was that in countries with low caries prevalence in the primary teeth, there does not appear to be a further decline.

Risk Factors: Causes of Tooth Decay

The development of dental caries is dependent on critical interrelationships between the tooth, dietary carbohydrate, saliva, and specific oral bacteria. The decay process is initiated by demineralization of the outer tooth surface as a result of organic acids formed during bacterial fermentation of dietary carbohydrates. Simultaneously, saliva functions as a remineralizing and buffering solution to counter the effect of demineralization. Should bacteria-derived demineralization exceed saliva's remineralization and buffering capacity, caries lesions form. Incipient lesions first appear as opaque white spots; as loss of mineral progresses, cavitation occurs. Accordingly, major risk factors for dental caries are categorized as microbial, salivary, and dietary.

MICROBIAL RISK FACTOR

Current knowledge of oral microbial ecology indicates that human dental caries is initiated by a group of oral streptococci collectively designated as mutans streptococci. Children with dense oral populations of mutans streptococci are at higher risk of dental caries relative to children with low or negligible oral levels of these organisms. In addition, children who are colonized by these organisms early in life (12 to 24 months of age) are at greater risk of future dental caries relative to children who are not.

SALIVARY RISK FACTOR

Saliva is the primary host defense against dental caries. First, the physical flow of saliva, augmented by the activity of the oral musculature, removes a large number of bacteria and food particles from the teeth. Second, saliva possesses numerous antibacterial systems. Finally, saliva has properties that directly protect the tooth surface from demineralization. Salivary bicarbonate, phosphate, and histidine-rich peptides diffuse into plaque and act directly as buffers. Besides helping to counter plaque acidity, saliva helps protect the teeth from demineralization through a mechanism called remineralization, which is defined as the deposition of salivary minerals into incipient enamel defects.

The presence of fluoride in trace quantities is critical to the inhibition of demineralization and enhancement of remineralization. Fluoride enhances enamel crystal growth and hence makes remineralization more rapid and effective. Because remineralization is promoted by the frequent introduction of a low concentration of fluoride into the mouth, the small amount of fluoride in fluoridated drinking water is sufficient to promote remineralization (Mandel, 1987).

Salivary hypofunction can be a consequence of a variety of factors, such as radiotherapy, when the salivary glands are within the radiation ports; long-term administration of anticholinergic or parasympatholytic drugs; and salivary gland disease (e.g., Sjögren's syndrome). In this regard, salivary hypofunction represents an important, although uncommon, risk factor for the development of dental caries.

DIETARY RISK FACTOR

All fermentable carbohydrates (sugars and breakdown products of starches) are readily metabolized to organic acids by mutans streptococci. Thus, such dietary substances are called *cariogenic substrates*. Numerous investigations in humans and laboratory animals demonstrate that frequent, prolonged oral exposure to cariogenic substrates facilitates dental caries activity. Stated differently, it's not how much sugar you eat but the form of sugar and frequency with which you eat it that determines its relative cariogenic potential. For example, the cariogenic potential of apple juice in a nursing bottle that is sampled throughout the night or during nap times or both is quite different from that of the same volume of apple juice consumed at a single meal. Similarly, the sugars in food products retained orally for a long time (e.g., caramel candies) are more cariogenic than those in food products retained for a short time (e.g., ice cream).

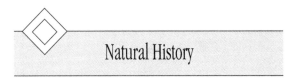

Natural History

Definition of Dental Caries

Dental caries is a localized area of decay that starts with demineralization of the tooth enamel caused by organic acids.

Untreated

Dental caries will usually destroy most of the tooth if it is not treated. Bacterial invasion of the dental pulp (Fig. 4-1) initiates an inflammatory response (pulpitis) that can result in significant pain. Pulpitis, in turn, can progress to pulp necrosis with bacterial invasion of the alveolar bone (periapical infection). Periapical infection is a well-known cause of sepsis and facial cellulitis. In addition, periapical infection of a primary tooth can disrupt normal development of the succeeding permanent teeth.

Treated

Modern dental therapeutics can salvage most carious teeth. When extraction is indicated, treatment must also focus on the problem that teeth surrounding the extraction site will change position in the dental arch. This is of particular importance when a primary tooth is extracted. One of the functions of the primary teeth is to maintain space for the permanent teeth. Accordingly, premature loss of a primary tooth can

result in impaction or ectopic eruption of permanent teeth.

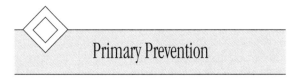

Primary Prevention

There are many proven methods of preventing tooth decay, including fluoride, oral hygiene, sealants, and diet. All should be used concurrently.

Fluoride

WATER FLUORIDATION

The relationships between natural water fluoride concentrations, caries prevalence, and enamel fluorosis were determined in classic epidemiological studies by H. Trendley Dean in the 1930s and 1940s. It was through these studies as well as subsequent community trials with artificial water fluoridation that the level of 1 ppm fluoride in drinking water was determined as optimal for caries prevention, with a minimal risk of fluorosis. Later, the recommendation for an optimal level of water fluoridation was refined to a range of 0.7 to 1.2 ppm fluoride, depending on the amount of water intake as a function of the annual average maximum daily air temperature in a community. Since these early studies, fluoridation of public water supplies has proved to be the most effective, convenient, and economical measure available to reduce dental caries prevalence. The average cost per child is less than one dollar per year.

Not only is water fluoridation one of the most cost-effective preventive measures, it also has proved to cause no adverse effects. Organized efforts against water fluoridation are often vocal and too often are successful. Claims that fluoride, at recommended levels, causes cancer or any other disease have been found to be baseless. Nevertheless, today only 62% of the population has the benefit of optimally fluoridated water.

FLUORIDE SUPPLEMENTS

The dramatic reduction in caries susceptibility in populations drinking fluoridated water led to recommendations to administer fluoride as a dietary supplement to those who do not receive it in their drinking water. Fluoride was assumed to have a systemic mode of action resulting in the formation of a more caries-resistant enamel structure, which led to the conclusion that fluoride supplements should mimic previous estimates of dietary fluoride intake. Fluoride supplements were therefore proposed for the period of time during which teeth are developing.

Newer research has shown that the most important mechanism by which fluoride results in caries prevention is the topical effect. Accordingly, children should slowly dissolve fluoride supplements in their mouth to enhance this topical effect. Fluoride promotes salivary remineralization of demineralized enamel. This effect is enhanced by exposing the teeth frequently to relatively low levels of fluoride, as occurs with drinking fluoridated water. The realization that systemic fluoride ingestion is not the major mechanism of action of fluoride in caries prevention, along with reports on increased dental fluorosis, has led to a reassessment of fluoride supplementation recommendations.

Dental fluorosis is a hypomineralization of enamel that takes place when higher than optimal levels of fluoride are ingested during the period of enamel formation. Fluorosis may vary from very mild to severe. Very mild to mild cases appear as chalky whitening of the enamel, whereas severe fluorosis takes the form of mottled enamel that is pitted and brown in color. Reports have shown a trend toward a higher prevalence of dental fluorosis relative to historical data from earlier studies. This increase in the prevalence of fluorosis was found to correlate with the ingestion of fluoride from sources other than drinking water, including fluoride supplements and fluoridated toothpaste. Accordingly, since fluoride's major mechanism of caries prevention is topical, the Council on Scientific Affairs of the American Dental Association has endorsed a new fluoride supplementation schedule (Table 4-2). In this regard, fluoride supplements are not recommended for mothers during pregnancy or for infants in the first 6 months of life. In addition, breast-fed infants residing in optimally fluoridated communities should not receive fluoride supplements.

As indicated in Table 4-2, dosage is based on the patient's age and the fluoride content of the water supply. The fluoride level of a water supply can usually be obtained by calling the local water board. Should the patient use a private water supply, a fluoride analysis is indicated. The patient's parent should be instructed to use

Table 4-2

Fluoride Supplement Dosage Schedule[a]

	CONCENTRATION OF FLUORIDE IN DRINKING WATER (PPM)		
AGE	<0.3	0.3–0.6	>0.6
Birth to 6 mo	0	0	0
6 mo–3 yr	0.25	0	0
3 yr–6 yr	0.5	0.25	0
6 yr–16 yr	1.0	0.5	0

[a] Fluoride dosage regimen accepted by the American Academy of Pediatrics, American Academy of Pediatric Dentistry, and the American Dental Association (1994).

a plastic container for the water specimen (a glass container can impair the accuracy of the fluoride assay). No fluoride prescription should be written for more than 120 mg of fluoride. Even if a child ingested the entire supply, probably only mild gastric upset would ensue. Nonetheless, in such an event, a poison control center should be contacted immediately.

FLUORIDE TOOTHPASTE

Fluoride-containing dentifrices are highly effective in preventing dental decay. Before the age of 6 years, children tend to swallow rather than expectorate toothpaste, and nearly all of the ingested fluoride is absorbed, primarily from the small intestine. Furthermore, fluoride toothpaste constitutes over 95% of all toothpastes sold.

The ingestion of fluoride-containing toothpaste is responsible for the strong association between early use of fluoride dentifrice and increased risk of dental fluorosis. To lower the risk of dental fluorosis from toothpaste ingestion, a small (pea-sized) amount of toothpaste should be used in brushing a young child's teeth. In this regard, toothpaste should be stored in a childproof area and dispensed by parents or guardians.

FLUORIDE RINSES

Fluoride rinses containing 0.05% fluoride have been shown to be highly effective in limiting dental decay. These products are available without a prescription and should be recommended for children more than 6 years of age who are at risk of dental decay owing to such conditions as compromised salivary flow rates, orthodontic therapy, and a strong susceptibility to caries. They are not recommended for children less than 6 years of age because of their inability to properly expectorate, resulting in excessive fluoride ingestion.

Oral Hygiene

Thorough daily brushing and flossing of the teeth helps prevent dental caries and periodontal disease. Ideally, teeth should be brushed after every meal. Parents should receive professional instruction regarding oral hygiene techniques for children. Clinical studies show that most children 8 years of age and younger do not have the hand–eye coordination required for adequate oral hygiene; accordingly, parents must assume responsibility for oral hygiene. The degree of parental involvement should reflect the child's level of competency.

Sealants

Epidemiological data indicate that caries of pits and fissures accounts for more than 90% of dental caries. Excellent oral hygiene and optimal fluoride exposure have a limited effect in preventing dental caries in the pits and fissures on the occlusal (biting) surfaces of the posterior teeth. The use of sealants has been shown to be effective in the prevention of pit and fissure caries. Sealants are plastic coatings that are professionally applied to the occlusal surfaces of the posterior teeth. Unfortunately, irrespective of proven clinical efficacy, the use of sealants is not routine in prevention of dental caries. A survey conducted by the National Institute of Dental Research indicated that relatively few U.S. schoolchildren have sealants on their teeth.

Diet

Limiting the frequency of cariogenic substrate ingestion prevents dental caries. Parents and children should be encouraged to avoid between-meal snacks that contain cariogenic substrates. The use of gum, candy, and soft drinks containing sugar substitutes (mannitol, sorbitol, xylitol, and aspartame—with precautions, since these agents can cause osmotic diarrhea in small children) is an effective approach for the child with a "sweet tooth." Chewing sugarless gum has been clinically established to enhance the salivary flow rate and in turn neutralize plaque pH.

Infants should be weaned from a bottle by 1 year of age to eliminate their risk of early childhood caries. Otherwise, bedtime and nap-time nursing bottles should contain only water. Finally, sweetened elixirs of medications used on a long-term basis result in an increase in oral exposure to cariogenic substrates, thereby increasing caries risk. Drug manufacturers need to be encouraged to formulate noncariogenic elixirs. Patients who require such medication should be referred for aggressive caries preventive measures.

Controversy

Current oral health policy of the American Academy of Pediatric Dentistry states that infants should be weaned from the bottle at 12 to 14 months of age. Most clinicians support this recommendation and will accept water as a reasonable alternative. Compelling data from new animal model studies and clinical studies indicate, however, that cow's milk is not cariogenic. Accordingly, allowing babies to feed with nursing bottles containing only cow's milk or water past 12 to 14 months of age does not appear to be a caries risk factor.

Secondary Prevention: Professional Intervention

Timing of Visits to the Dentist

AGE AT FIRST VISIT

Current American Academy of Pediatrics policy calls for referral of children to the dentist at age 3 unless the clinician notes dental or oral pathologic symptoms for which earlier referral is indicated. The tacit assumptions underlying this policy are that oral disease is rarely present before age 3, that it is readily discernible to the clinician, and that the clinician's oral health supervision expertise is sufficient to counsel parents regarding oral disease risk and prevention.

A call for a dental visit at age 1 implicitly challenges these assumptions. Such visits are recommended by the American Academy of Pediatric Dentistry (AAPD, 1997). Issues regarding fluoride supplementation, oral hygiene, feeding habits, dental development, injury prevention, and periodontal health need to be addressed by 1 year of age. Consequently, clinicians who don't provide these services should refer their patients to dentists at age 1.

HOW FREQUENTLY SHOULD CHILDREN SEE A DENTIST?

The traditional biannual dentist visit is under scrutiny at present. There is little evidence to support one recommendation over another. Children who are caries-free and who practice good oral hygiene and consume optimally fluoridated water probably need annual dental evaluation. On the other hand, children with a history of extensive dental caries most likely should be evaluated every 3 months.

Examination of the Dentition

The child's dentition should be examined at every visit to the clinician's office for routine preventive care. The required equipment consists of an intraoral light and pediatric tongue blade. The examiner should begin with the most distal maxillary molar and continue with the inspection of each tooth, proceeding from right to left. The procedure should be repeated, proceeding from the patient's left to right side in the mandibular arch.

Dental decay usually begins in the pits and fissures on the occlusal (biting) surfaces of the molar teeth. The second most common sites for caries development are the contact surfaces between the molar teeth. These areas are difficult to examine, even by the dentist, who usually depends on intraoral radiographs. Carious lesions are least frequently detected on the necks (cervical areas) of the teeth near the gingiva. It is usually necessary to retract the lips and cheeks to adequately inspect the latter sites.

When cavitation is detected, the clinician is obliged to inform the parents that dental treatment must be instituted. The advice to go see the dentist does not constitute an appropriate referral. Many parents never seek dental care, while others encounter dentists who prefer not to treat children. The clinician should therefore become familiar with general dentists and/or pediatric dentists who are capable of treating, and willing to treat, pediatric patients. The referral should be as formal and precise as a referral to any other member of a comprehensive health care team.

Tertiary Prevention

Treatment of Dental Caries

Caries lesions are generally managed by mechanical debridement of the infected tooth tissue using rotary and/or hand instruments, followed by placement of dental material to restore form and function. Dental amalgam has historically been the material of choice for intracoronal restorations, owing to its relative ease of use and longevity. Because of the high mercury content of amalgam, however, concerns have been raised over its safety and environmental impact. Composite resins and other materials, such as glass ionomer cements, are now coming into

more common use owing to their aesthetic attributes, the ability to bond them to the tooth, and improvements in their wear characteristics. When decay is extensive, intracoronal restorations are not indicated. Extensive loss of tooth tissue necessitates restoration with a crown. In the permanent dentition, crowns are custom-fabricated, whereas in the primary dentition, preformed stainless steel crowns are used.

There has been a change in treatment philosophy to a more conservative approach in the management of caries lesions. The practice of minimum intervention dentistry is now advocated. Several factors have influenced this change:

1. It is now recognized that traditional restorative dentistry has its limitations in preserving teeth. Placing conventional amalgam restorations can predispose teeth to a cascade of events that can ultimately lead to tooth loss. Restorations have a limited life expectancy, and their replacement usually involves the loss of additional tooth structure. The cusps of the teeth can become undermined, resulting in cracking of the tooth and fracture of the cusp. Repeated restorative intervention and bacterial invasion of the pulp tissue can result in irreversible pulpitis requiring endodontic therapy or extraction. This leads to removal of more tooth structure and may require the placement of crowns.

2. The widespread use of fluoride products and introduction of water fluoridation have slowed the rate of caries progression. This has provided dentists with a greater safety margin to observe incipient caries lesions before intervention becomes prudent.

3. The introduction of adhesive dentistry and the development of improved restorative materials are revolutionizing dentistry. Preventive resin restorations (PRRs) are now indicated in many cases, instead of traditional amalgam restorations. This approach

involves minimal exploratory opening of the enamel, removal of carious tooth tissue without extension into surrounding healthy tooth tissue, obturating the cavity with a filled resin restorative material, and sealing the remainder of the occlusal surface with pit and fissure sealant.

PRRs have several advantages over traditional amalgam restorations in that tooth tissue is conserved and other caries-susceptible surfaces of the tooth are protected. While this technique can be highly recommended, there is the need for careful monitoring during recall visits, because the filling may not be retained in all cases. This technique is also more operator sensitive, and care must be taken to ensure that the tooth surface is free of contamination when placing this type of filling material.

Treatment of Complications of Caries

Clinical management of the pain and infection associated with dental caries varies with the extent of involvement and the medical status of the patient. In general, dental infection localized to the dentoalveolar unit can be treated by local measures (e.g., extraction, pulpectomy). Antibiotics are usually not indicated except in those patients with compromised host defenses, impaired wound healing, or risk of endocarditis.

In contrast, antibiotics are routinely indicated for dental infections that have spread to structures outside the dentoalveolar unit. The oral route can usually be used for patients with unremarkable medical histories if the infection does not involve a nonvital area (such as the buccal space). If the infection involves a vital area, however (e.g., submandibular space, which can lead to Ludwig angina; facial triangle, which can lead to cavernous sinus thrombosis, or periorbital space, which can lead to orbital involvement), parenteral routes are indicated.

Parenteral routes are also indicated for patients with compromised host defenses or

impaired wound healing or for those at risk of endocarditis. Blood cultures should be obtained before initiating parenteral antibiotic therapy. Areas of fluctuance should be incised and drained. Penicillin is the antibiotic of choice, except in patients with a history of allergy to this agent; clindamycin is a suitable alternative for such patients. Finally, the offending tooth must be identified and local treatment instituted to ensure resolution of the infection. Measures for control of pain are adjusted to the need of the patient. Combinations of acetaminophen with codeine or ibuprofen given orally are usually adequate.

Elimination of periapical infection is dependent on removing the necrotic pulp focus. The small opening at the apex of the root (Fig. 4-1) coupled with the destruction of the pulpal vasculature, limits host defenses from accessing the pulp focus. In addition, these anatomic constraints prevent intrapulpal delivery of systemic antibiotics. For this reason, surgical removal of the necrotic pulp (via extraction or root canal therapy) is a mandatory component of treatment for periapical infection.

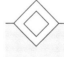

Recommendations to Clinicians

Clinicians who provide preventive care for infants and children should include the prevention of tooth decay in their list of priorities. Diet and oral hygiene should be discussed with parents and guardians and the prevention of bottle caries emphasized. Clinicians should encourage the optimum use of fluoride, including fluoride supplementation based on the water fluoride content in their area. Children should have regular dental examinations, and referral dentists should have training and experience in treating pediatric patients and should use sealants as a routine practice.

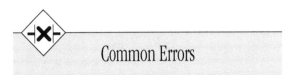

Common Errors

Waiting Too Long to Consider Preventive Dentistry

Depending upon the magnitude of the mother's salivary mutans reservoir and frequency of mutans transmissions, the child can acquire cariogenic flora as soon as a hard surface (usually the first tooth) appears in the mouth. Examination of the teeth should be part of all well-child examinations. Children of mothers who have had serious tooth decay or children whose siblings suffered early caries are at highest risk of early mutans acquisition and consequently an early caries experience. Since cariogenic flora can be acquired as soon as the first tooth erupts and decay can be devastating by the second birthday, high-risk children should receive dental intervention by their first birthdays.

Inappropriate Fluoride Management

A variety of common errors related to prescribing systemic and topical fluorides have been long documented in the medical and dental literature. These include inappropriate prescribing, over- and underprescribing, and inconsistent prescribing of systemic fluorides and inappropriate use of topicals. Inappropriate prescription of supplemental fluoride occurs when a child's fluoride exposure is not assessed before supplementation. For example, a child who resides in a fluoridated area but whose home environment rigorously constrains use of tap water will nonetheless require supplementation, and a child from a nonfluoridated area

who regularly ingests fluoridated water at an alternative site may not require supplementation. As with all prescriptions, a benefit/risk analysis will tend toward errors of commission for children at high risk of decay and errors of omission for children at low risk of decay.

Under- and overprescribing can be markedly limited by fully adhering to the recognized American Academy of Pediatrics, American Academy of Pediatric Dentistry, and American Dental Association accepted dosage schedule. Inconsistent prescribing only adds to the confusion over a child's fluoride ingestion. In short, the supplemental fluoride prescription should be tailored to take into account the ambient fluoride in a particular child's environment. Use of fluoride rinse should be based on the caries activity level and risk of caries of each child.

Failure to Manage the Impact of Systemic Illness or Medication

Any disease or intervention that disrupts the balance between decalcification and recalcification can cause rapid dental destruction. The most common situations encountered by primary care clinicians pertain to medications. Some cause decreased salivary flow (Imipramine); others affect the gums (Dilantin). The issue of long-term medications in sugar-based liquids was discussed earlier. Less common disorders, such as chronic graft versus host disease and head and neck radiation, are also associated with impaired salivary flow.

Disregard for oral care of patients in these situations can readily tip the scales toward both decalcification and acute gingival inflammation, with resultant inducement of dental caries activity and bacteremia. Thus, aggressive preventive care is needed, and these patients may require daily topical fluoride therapy to prevent dental caries. Those with xerostomia may need additional supplementation with oral wetting agents (e.g., synthetic saliva substitutes).

Failure to Use Sealants

As stated previously, sealants are underused. Some clinicians recommend the use of sealants in all children; others endorse the use of sealants only once the process of decay has begun. Clinicians should communicate with their referral dentists to ensure that sealants are part of their patients' routine care.

Emerging Approaches to Diagnosis, Treatment, and Primary and Secondary Prevention

Caries Diagnosis

With technological advances, many of the current approaches used in the practice of dentistry are expected to change over the next 10 years. There is a high level of interest in new approaches to the diagnosis of caries. At present, most dentists use visual and tactile methods assisted by a mirror and dental exploration in combination with conventional dental radiography. Newer approaches involve the use of digital radiography in combination with image processing to aid the dentist in detecting caries lesions. Emerging technologies for detecting caries include the use of electrical detection methods, qualitative light-induced fluorescence methods, and fiber-optic transillumination combined with digital imaging and computer processing. Many of these methods are being developed in response to the need for better methods of detecting caries at an early stage, especially occlusal caries, and also to provide the dentist with a means of measuring changes in the mineral status of teeth so that they can accurately determine caries activity and monitor the effectiveness of preventive interventions.

Treatment

New methods of treating caries lesions are also being evaluated, to replace the dental drill. Lasers and microabrasion devices are being used to remove caries and tooth structure in preparation for placement of restorations. These methods may minimize the need for local anesthesia. There has been an explosion of new restorative materials that involve enamel and dentin bonding technology that allow the placement of aesthetic tooth-colored materials with minimal removal of tooth tissue. New fluoride-releasing materials also have been developed, which have the added benefit of resisting formation of secondary caries around the margins of restorations.

Prevention

New approaches for caries prevention are actively being sought to improve and enhance the anticaries benefits of fluoride products, including better fluoride delivery vehicles and new formulations. Fluoride varnishes that can be painted on the teeth are now available in the United States. Toothpastes with mineral additives intended to improve the remineralizing ability of fluoride are being evaluated. Antimicrobial agents, such as chlorohexidine, are being used alone and in combination with fluoride. Laser treatments for tooth enamel are being tested for their ability to increase caries resistance alone and in combination with fluoride. There is also work being done to formulate a vaccine against oral streptococci, which, if it is effective, could revolutionize the prevention of tooth decay.

Bibliography

ADA Council on Access, Prevention and Interprofessional Relations: Caries diagnosis and risk assessment. *J Am Dent Assoc* 1S–24S, 1995.

American Academy of Pediatric Dentistry: Oral health policies: Baby bottle tooth decay/early childhood caries. *Pediatr Dent* 19(7):24–27, 1997.

Beltran ED, Burt BA: The pre- and posteruptive effects of fluoride in the caries decline. *J Public Health Dent* 48:233–240, 1988.

Bibby B: Influence of diet on the bacterial composition of plaques, in Stiles HM, Loesche WJ, O'Brien TC (eds): *Microbiologic Aspects of Dental Caries*, vol 2, London, Information Retrieval, 1976, pp 477–490.

Bowen WH, Pearson SK, Rosalen PL, et al. Assessing the cariogenic potential of some infant formulas, milk and sugar solutions. *J Am Dent Assoc* 128:865–871, 1997.

Burt BA: Trends in caries prevalence in North American children. *Int Dent J* 44:403–413, 1994.

Downer MC: Caries prevalence in the United Kingdom. *Int Den J* 44:365–370, 1994.

Kraus BS: Calcification of the human deciduous teeth. *J Am Dent Assoc* 59:1128, 1959.

Li SH, Kingman A, Forthofer R, Swango P: Comparison of tooth surface–specific dental caries attack patterns in US schoolchildren from two national surveys. *J Dent Res* 72:1398–1405, 1993.

Loesche WJ: Role of *Streptococcus mutans* in human dental decay. *Microbiol Rev* 50:353–380, 1986.

Logan WHG, Kronfield R: Development of the human jaw and surrounding structures from birth to age fifteen years. *J Am Dent Assoc* 20:379, 1933.

Lopez L, Berkowitz R, Zlotnik H, et al.: Topical antimicrobial therapy in the prevention of early childhood caries. *Pediatr Dent* 21:9–11, 1999.

Mandel ID: The functions of saliva. *J Dent Res* 66(special issue):623–627, 1987.

Marthaler TM, Brunelle J, Downer MC, et al: The prevalence of dental caries in Europe 1990–1995. *Caries Res* 30:237–255, 1996.

Milnes AR: Description and epidemiology of nursing caries. *J Public Health Dent* 56:38–50, 1996.

Newbrun E: Effectiveness of water fluoridation. *J Public Health Dent* 49(special issue):279–289, 1989.

Pendrys DG: Dental fluorosis in perspective. *J Am Dent Assoc* 122:63–66, 1991.

Ripa LW: The current status of pit and fissure sealants: A review. *J Can Dent Assoc* 51:367–375, 377–380, 1985.

Ripa LW: Nursing caries: A comprehensive review. *Pediatr Dent* 10:268–282, 1988.

Van Houte J: Bacterial specificity in the etiology of dental caries. *Int Dent J* 30:305–326, 1980.

Paul P. Hartlaub
Nuzhat Majid

Chapter 5

Iron-deficiency Anemia in Children

Introduction

Anemia is defined as any condition in which the number of red blood cells, the amount of hemoglobin (Hb), or the volume of packed red blood cells, that is, the hematocrit (Hct), is less than normal. In practice, this abnormality can be characterized as a level of these markers less than the 5th percentile of a healthy reference population. The term *anemia* must be distinguished from the terms *iron-deficiency anemia*, which is anemia caused by iron deficiency, and *iron deficiency*, which may be present without associated anemia. Eighty-five percent of the anemias worldwide, or 500 to 600 million cases, are due to iron deficiency. The third National Health and Nutrition Examination Survey (NHANES III) data indicate that there are about 700,000 toddlers in the United States with iron deficiency; 240,000 of them have iron-deficiency anemia.

Other common causes of anemia include the thalassemias, found chiefly in populations living around the Mediterranean Sea and in Burma, Democratic Kampuchea (Cambodia), Thailand, and Vietnam. Malaria is also a major cause of anemia in young children in developing countries, and sickle-cell disease is a major cause in black children in Africa and America. Less common sources of anemia include drug effects, aplastic anemias, transient erythroblastopenia of childhood, pure red blood cell aplasia, alloimmune hemolytic disease of the newborn, autoimmune hemolytic anemia, hereditary spherocytosis, such enzymatic defects as glucose-6-phosphate dehydrogenase (G6PD) deficiency, folic acid and vitamin B_{12} deficiencies, severe lead toxicity, malignancies, and such chronic diseases as tuberculosis, juvenile rheumatoid arthritis, and liver, renal, and thyroid disease (Table 5-1). Because iron deficiency is the most preventable as well as the most common cause of anemia in children, the remainder of the chapter will focus on this entity.

Prevalence of Iron-deficiency Anemia

The prevalence of iron-deficiency anemia in young children has declined over recent years in the United States in association with higher iron intake during infancy. For example, in the states consistently monitored by the Pediatric Nutrition Surveillance System of the Centers for Disease Control and Prevention (CDC), the overall prevalence of iron-deficiency anemia decreased from 7.8% in 1975 to 2.9% in 1985. Data from NHANES II, conducted during the years 1976–1980, and NHANES III, conducted

Table 5-1

Causes of Anemia in Children

Iron deficiency
Thalassemia
Sickle cell disease
Lead toxicity
Drug effects
Chronic diseases
Tuberculosis
Juvenile rheumatoid arthritis
Liver disease
Kidney disease
Thyroid disease
Aplastic anemia
Transient erythroblastopenia
Red blood cell aplasia
Alloimmune hemolytic disease of the newborn
Autoimmune hemolytic anemia
Hereditary spherocytosis
Glucose-6-phosphate dehydrogenase deficiency
Folic acid and vitamin B_{12} deficiencies
Malignancy

during 1988–1994, indicate that the prevalence of iron-deficiency anemia in children age 12 to 36 months in the United States has leveled off at about 3% (Table 5-2). The prevalence of iron deficiency is about threefold higher than iron-deficiency anemia.

Young children and women of reproductive age have a relatively high prevalence of iron-deficiency anemia, with the highest risk group being children age 9 to 18 months. This high risk in young children is related to a rapid rate of growth and an intake of dietary iron that is often inadequate. The reason that full-term infants do not become iron deficient sooner than about 9 months of age is that they are born with enough iron stores to last until about 6 months. In contrast, preterm and low birth weight babies are born with smaller iron stores

Table 5-2

Prevalence (%) of Iron Deficiency and Iron-Deficiency Anemia, United States, Third
National Health and Nutrition Examination Survey, 1988–1994

SEX AND AGE (YR)	IRON DEFICIENCY	IRON-DEFICIENCY ANEMIA
Both sexes		
1–2	9	3^a
3–5	3	<1
6–11	2	<1
Nonpregnant females		
12–15	9	2^a
16–19	11^a	3^a
Males		
12–15	1	<1
16–19	<1	<1

^{a} Prevalence in nonblacks is one percentage point lower than prevalence in all races.
SOURCE: From Centers for Disease Control and Prevention: Recommendation to prevent and control
iron deficiency in the United States. *MMWR* 47:RR-3, 1998.

and grow faster during infancy, making them vulnerable to iron deficiency by 2 to 3 months of age.

Beyond 2 or 3 years of age, iron deficiency is less common because of more varied, iron-rich diets and slower growth. When it is present in children older than 3 years of age, iron deficiency generally results from bleeding disorders, inflammatory disorders, or inadequate intake because of special diets or decreased nutritional consumption. Older children once again become at risk for iron deficiency as adolescents, which is related to pregnancy and menstruation in girls and the relatively rapid growth during puberty for both genders.

According to NHANES III, Mexican American children have a higher prevalence of iron deficiency than African American children, who in turn have a higher prevalence than Caucasian children, even after controlling for poverty. Children living below the poverty level have a higher rate of iron deficiency than those living above the poverty level. Other groups at high risk include preterm and low-birth-weight

infants, Native Americans, Alaska Natives, immigrants from developing countries, and infants whose principal dietary intake is unfortified cow's milk (Table 5-3). In 1980, the World Health Organization compiled prevalence data on anemia of all causes in children. Prevalence data specific to iron deficiency was not separated out, and it is difficult to tell just how many of the anemias resulted from this nutritional deficit. Nevertheless, it is estimated that the highest prevalence rates of iron-deficiency ane-

Table 5-3

Risk Factors for Iron Deficiency in Infants and Children

Race (higher in Mexican American, African American, Native American, Alaska Natives)
Poverty
Premature birth
Recent immigration from developing countries
Unfortified cow's milk as principal dietary constituent

mia are in Africa and southern Asia, followed by Latin America, eastern Asia, Oceania, and North America, respectively.

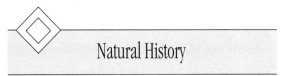

Natural History

Iron Metabolism

The amount of iron needed in the human diet is about 1 mg/kg/day up to a maximum of about 15 mg/day. Some variation in the physiologic demand for iron occurs as the result of rapid growth, for example, in low birth-weight infants, premature infants, adolescents and pregnant women, and in any condition associated with physiologic (e.g., menstrual) or abnormal blood loss.

IRON STORES

Infants have about 75 mg/kg of total body iron on average, which is relatively high compared with about 50 mg/kg in adult men and 42 mg/kg in adult women. Most of the iron in the body is in a "functional" state, incorporated into hemoglobin, myoglobin, and respiratory enzymes. About one-third takes the form of storage or transport iron. Iron is stored in the liver, bone marrow, spleen, and skeletal muscles. This storage is primarily in the form of the soluble protein complex ferritin and, to a lesser degree, the insoluble protein complex hemosiderin.

DIETARY IRON

The total amount of body iron represents the balance between intake and loss. In an adult, most of the iron required for the production of red blood cells comes from recycled old red blood cells. In adult men, for example, only about 5% comes from dietary sources, such as meat, poultry, fish, whole grains, enriched bread

and cereal, dark green vegetables, and legumes, including nuts. In the infant, by contrast, about 30% of the required iron needs to come from dietary sources, and 70% is derived from red blood cell turnover. Unfortunately, many infants and children do not consume the recommended daily allowance of iron in their diets (Table 5-4).

IRON ABSORPTION

Dietary intake is modified significantly in the gastrointestinal tract, where absorption can vary widely, from less than 1% to more than 50%. This variation in absorption, or bioavailability, is affected by many factors, including the amount of iron in the body, the amount and kind of iron ingested, and the presence of absorption enhancers or inhibitors (Table 5-5) in the diet. One of the most powerful of these absorption factors is the amount of iron already in the body, which leads to increased absorption when the body stores are low and decreased absorption when the stores are high.

Other enhancers of iron absorption include the heme form of iron (in poultry, fish, or other meat) and vitamin C. The heme iron sources mentioned earlier have generally two to three times more bioavailability than non-heme sources, such as plant-based foods and iron-fortified foods. Inhibitors of iron absorption include calcium, phytates (in bran), tannins (in tea), and polyphenols found in some vegetables. The bioavailability of iron from breast milk or bottled formula varies greatly (Table 5-6). In fact, an infant will absorb five times more iron from breast milk than cow's milk owing to increased bioavailability, even though these sources have the same concentration of iron. Vegetarian diets are very low in heme iron. Careful planning can maximize iron absorption with these diets, however, by including enhancers of iron absorption (Table 5-5). Vitamin A deficiency has been associated with iron deficiency, most likely related to this vitamin's ability to mobilize or reutilize iron from storage sites for

Table 5-4

1989 Recommended Dietary Allowance (RDA) for Iron and the Proportion of Americans Having Diets Meeting 100% of the RDA for Iron, 1994–1996

SEX AND AGE (YR)	RDA (MG/DAY)[a]	PROPORTION OF AMERICANS MEETING 100% OF THE 1989 RDA for Iron (%)[b]
Both sexes		
<1	6–10	87.9[c]
1–2	10	43.9
3–5	10	61.7
Females		
6–11	10	60.9
12–19	15	27.7
Males		
6–11	10	79.8
12–19	12	83.1

[a] National Research Council (1989). The age groups designated by the council are slightly different from those presented in this table.

[b] Two-day average dietary intakes, from the U.S. Department of Agriculture Continuing Survey of Food Intakes by Individuals, 1994–1996.

[c] Excludes breast-fed infants.

SOURCE: From Centers for Disease Control and Prevention: Recommendation to prevent and control iron deficiency in the United States. *MMWR* 47:RR-3, 1998.

hematopoiesis. Vitamin A deficiency is primarily a problem in developing countries.

NORMAL IRON LOSSES

The loss of iron occurs primarily through feces and desquamated mucosal and skin cells at a rate of about a milligram per day in adults. Menstruating women lose an additional 0.3 to 0.5 mg daily on average.

Morbidity

In addition to being important for hemoglobin production, iron is an essential component in the physiologic processes of brain growth. It is necessary for cell differentiation, protein synthesis, hormone production, and fundamental

Table 5-5

Enhancers and Inhibitors of Iron Absorption

ENHANCERS	INHIBITORS
Low body iron	Calcium
Vitamin C	Phytates (in bran)
Heme iron (in fish, poultry, or other meat)	Tannins (in tea) Polyphenols (in some vegetables)

SOURCE: From Centers for Disease Control and Prevention: Recommendation to prevent and control iron deficiency in the United States. *MMWR* 47:RR-3, 1998.

aspects of cellular energy metabolism and functioning. Brain cells need iron for many cellular oxidative and synthetic processes. Iron is also

Table 5-6

Iron Absorption by Infants Fed Formula or Milk

SUBSTANCE	IRON CONTENT (MG/L)	BIOAVAILABLE IRON (%)	ABSORBED IRON (MG/L)
Nonfortified formula	1.5–4.8[a]	~10	0.15–0.48
Iron-fortified formula[b]	10.0–12.8[a]	~4	0.40–0.51
Whole cow's milk	0.5	~10	0.05
Breast milk	0.5	~50	0.25

[a] Values are given for commonly marketed infant formulas.
[b] Iron-fortified formula contains ≥1.0 mg iron/100 kcal formula. Most iron-fortified formulas contain approximately 680 kcal/L, which is equivalent to ≥6.8 mg iron/L.
SOURCE: From Centers for Disease Control and Prevention: Recommendation to prevent and control iron deficiency in the United States. *MMWR* 47:RR-3, 1998.

essential for the production and catabolism of several neurotransmitters. Based on this information, it is easy to understand how a lack of iron, especially during the first year or two of life, when biological development of the brain is very rapid, could lead to a variety of psychological, developmental, and behavioral adverse effects.

Despite the biological plausibility of the neural effects noted, the literature is varied and inconclusive as to whether iron deficiency in the absence of anemia or other nutritional or socioeconomic factors causes adverse effects. When adverse outcomes have been associated with iron deficiency, they have included abnormal growth and development and behavioral effects, such as decreased motor activity, social interaction, and attention to tasks. On the other hand, iron-deficiency anemias, defined as a Hb less than 10.5 g/dL, have been repeatedly associated with multiple physiological abnormalities, such as blue sclerae, koilonychia, impaired exercise capacity, functional alterations in the small bowel, glossitis, cheilosis, and abnormal growth and development. Whether milder iron-deficiency anemias are associated with harmful effects is not known.

Iron-deficiency anemia contributes to lead poisoning in children by increasing the gastrointestinal tract's ability to absorb heavy metals, including iron and lead. Iron-deficiency anemia has also been associated with conditions that may in turn affect infant and child development, such as low birth weight, generalized undernutrition, and poverty.

Evidence That Treatment Improves Outcomes

The studies that have tried to answer the question of whether treatment of iron-deficiency anemia with iron therapy improves outcomes have had mixed results. Good studies showing a benefit are somewhat limited. Out of four large, well-conducted, randomized, controlled trials of infants in developing countries, for example, only one found a benefit. The largest and most recent of these four trials reported sizable, statistically significant improvements in both mental and motor development after 4 months of oral therapy (Goyer, 1995). Studies of older children in developing countries who were malnourished and anemic have consistently shown growth and weight gain attributable to iron supplementation.

It is not clear why there are mixed results in these outcome studies, although some researchers believe that the adequacy or duration of therapy might explain the differences. It is also not clear whether similar results would be seen if these studies were repeated in the United States, where children are likely to be healthy and otherwise adequately nourished.

Primary Prevention

Primary prevention of iron-deficiency anemia refers to measures that will maintain adequate stores of iron so that anemia does not occur. There is good evidence to recommend primary prevention measures for infants and young children. Infants are at risk of inadequate iron stores by about 9 months of age, and therefore effective primary prevention measures must be considered at an early age. The primary prevention measures available include breast feeding, iron-fortified formulas, iron-fortified cereal, avoidance of cow's milk before age 12 months, and limiting cow's milk after age 12 months.

Breast Feeding and Iron-fortified Formula and Cereal

One of the most powerful measures available to avoid depletion of iron stores in the newborn is breast feeding. Breast milk has the highest percentage of bioavailable iron of all milks and formulas (Table 5-6) and is therefore the preferred nutritional source of iron for at least the first 4 to 6 months of life. When breast feeding is not chosen by the parents or is discontinued before 12 months of age, iron-fortified formula should be substituted for the milk-based part of the diet. Infants breast-fed or fed with iron-fortified formula (at least 1.0 mg iron/100 kcal formula) are not likely to become iron deficient. The iron fortification of cereals also aids the primary prevention of iron deficiency. One study showed

that breast-fed infants who were randomized to receive iron-fortified cereal at 4 months of age had iron-deficiency anemia at 8 months of age about one-fifth as often as those randomized to receive non-iron-fortified cereal (Walter et al., 1993).

Avoiding Cow's Milk

Avoiding cow's milk before 12 months of age and limiting it after 12 months of age to less than about 24 ounces per day will also reduce the risk of iron deficiency. Whole milk causes occult bleeding from the gastrointestinal tract and has relatively low iron bioavailability. Furthermore, if cow's milk is consumed in large amounts, it may serve to replace milks, formulas, or other foods with more bioavailable iron.

Nutrition Programs

Several social programs contribute to the primary prevention of iron-deficiency anemia through nutritional education and support with obtaining or purchasing foods. The Women, Infants and Children (WIC) program, funded by the U.S. Department of Agriculture, helps supply food to pregnant women, women who are breast-feeding, and their infants and children who are at nutritional risk, up to age 5.

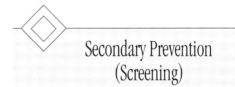

Secondary Prevention (Screening)

Iron-deficiency anemia can be detected by such signs and symptoms as fatigue, tachycardia, heart murmur, or poor appetite. With mild anemias, however, such signs and symptoms may be subtle or not present at all. Secondary prevention of anemia refers to the detection and treatment of asymptomatic anemia.

Hematocrit and Hemoglobin Concentrations

The principal screening tests for anemia are the Hct and the Hb concentrations. Hb samples are obtained by venipuncture, and Hct samples are obtained by either venipuncture or capillary sampling, usually by finger puncture. Age- and gender-specific cutoff values to define anemia using Hb and Hct are listed in Table 5-7. Capillary samples for Hct determinations are inexpensive and relatively easy to obtain in ambulatory practices and are particularly convenient with infant populations. Capillary samples are less reliable than venous samples, however. The sensitivity and specificity of capillary Hct determinations have been estimated to be 90% and 44%, respectively, when compared with venous blood determinations with an automated cell counter.

The sensitivity and specificity of Hb concentrations for detecting iron-deficiency anemia are also variable. Estimates of the sensitivity and specificity of this test are 8% to 90% and 65% to 99%, respectively, depending on the cutoff used. These test characteristics vary with the race of the population studied. For example, in one national sample, a Hb of less than 12 g/dL had a sensitivity and specificity for iron deficiency of 90% and 78%, respectively, in African American

Table 5-7

Maximum Hemoglobin Concentration and Hematocrit Values for Anemia [a]

	HEMOGLOBIN CONCENTRATION ($<$G/DL)	HEMATOCRIT (%)
Children (age, in yr)		
1–<2[b]	11.0	32.9
2–<5	11.1	33.0
5–<8	11.5	34.5
8–<12	11.9	35.4
Men (age, in yr)		
12–<15	12.5	37.3
15–<18	13.3	39.7
≥18	13.5	39.9
Nonpregnant women and lactating women (age, in yr)		
12–<15	11.8	35.7
15–<18	12.0	35.9
≥18	12.0	35.7

[a] Age- and sex-specific cutoff values for anemia are based on the 5th percentile from the third National Health and Nutrition Examination Survey (NHANES III), which excluded persons who had a high likelihood of iron deficiency by using the same methods described by Looker et al. (1997).
[b] Although no data are available from NHANES III to determine the maximum hemoglobin concentration and hematocrit values for anemia among infants, the values listed for children ages 1–<2 years can be used for infants ages 6–12 months.
SOURCE: From Centers for Disease Control and Prevention: Recommendation to prevent and control iron deficiency in the United States. *MMWR* 47:RR-3, 1998.

women, and 36% and 95%, respectively, in Caucasian women (Johnson-Spear and Yip, 1994).

Predictive values for Hct and Hb screening tests, representing true iron-deficiency anemia, vary by the sensitivity and specificity as well as the prevalence of iron-deficiency anemia in the reference population. As noted, the 1975 U.S. prevalence of iron-deficiency anemia was 7.8% in young children. Assuming sensitivity for Hct screening of 90% and specificity of 44% for anemia, as reported, the positive predictive value of Hct screening for iron-deficiency anemia would be only 12%. The Public Health Service goal for the year 2000 is a prevalence of anemia of 3%. With a 3% prevalence and the same sensitivity and specificity, the positive predictive value would be 4.7%. This example demonstrates the decreasing utility of iron-deficiency anemia screening with decreasing prevalence. It is somewhat ironic that the value of screening declines proportionately to our prevention successes. The negative predictive value increases with decreasing prevalence, but the change is of marginal clinical significance. In the example just given, the negative predictive value would increase from 98.1% (7.8% prevalence) to 99.3% (3% prevalence).

Other Screening Tests

There are five other tests that are available to screen for iron deficiency. None have proved superior to Hb or Hct. These tests are described briefly and are listed in Table 5-8, along with the cutoff values generally used.

MEAN CELL VOLUME

The mean cell volume (MCV) is the average red blood cell volume measured in femtoliters (10^{-15} liters). Iron-deficiency anemia results in a low MCV, which indicates microcytic red blood cells. Other causes of microcytosis include chronic infection, lead toxicity, and thalassemia.

Table 5-8

Cutoff Values for Laboratory Tests to Detect Iron Deficiency

LABORATORY TEST	AGE	CUTOFF VALUE
Mean cell volume (microcytic anemia)	1–2 yr	<77 fL
	3–5 yr	<79 fL
	6–11 yr	<80 fL
	12–15 yr	<82 fL
	>15 yr	<85 fL
Red blood cell distribution width (iron-deficiency anemia)[a]	—	>14.0%
Erythrocyte protoporphyrin concentration (iron deficiency)	Adults	>30 μg/dL of whole blood or >70 μg/dL of red blood cells
	Children aged 1–2 yrs	>80 μg/dL of red blood cells
Serum ferritin concentration (iron deficiency)	>6 mo	≤15 mg/L
Transferrin saturation (iron deficiency)	—	<16%

[a] The cutoff is instrument specific and may not apply in all laboratories.

SOURCE: From Centers for Disease Control and Prevention: Recommendation to prevent and control iron deficiency in the United States. *MMWR* 47:RR-3, 1998.

RED BLOOD CELL DISTRIBUTION WIDTH

The red blood cell distribution width (RDW) is a measurement of the variation in red blood cell size. It is calculated by dividing the standard deviation of red cell volume by the MCV and multiplying by 100 to give a percentage. Although it is useful in characterizing and diagnosing the cause of anemia, the RDW has not proved to be a useful screening test.

ERYTHROCYTE PROTOPORPHYRIN CONCENTRATION

As iron availability declines, erythrocyte protoporphyrin concentration increases. The erythrocyte protoporphyrin concentration increases before the Hb and Hct decline. The sensitivity for detecting iron deficiency has been estimated at 42%, with a specificity of 61%. Other causes of elevated erythrocyte protoporphyrin include infection and lead poisoning. At present, inexpensive methods for measuring erythrocyte protoporphyrin are available, but they are not sufficiently standardized to use for population screening.

SERUM FERRITIN

There is a direct correlation between the serum ferritin concentration and the total amount of iron stored in the body. It is the most specific test to detect iron deficiency and the test that detects iron deficiency the earliest. It is currently not used as a screening test because of cost and lack of standardization between laboratories. It is mainly used as a method to confirm iron deficiency in those with low Hb or Hct values.

TRANSFERRIN SATURATION

Transferrin saturation measures the availability of iron-binding sites on transferrin. It is calculated by dividing the serum iron concentration by the total iron-binding capacity (TIBC) and multiplying by 100. As iron stores are depleted, the serum iron concentration decreases, the TIBC increases, and the transferrin saturation decreases. Transferrin saturation is also affected by other conditions, such as chronic infection, cancer, liver disease, and malnutrition. The costs involved with measuring it make it unsuitable as a screening test.

Screening Recommendations

The United States Preventive Services Taskforce (USPSTF) recommends that high-risk infants (as defined in Table 5-3) be screened for iron-deficiency anemia with Hb or Hct testing, preferably between 6 and 12 months of age. The USPSTF does not state whether a capillary sample, which is easier to obtain in infants, is preferable to the more accurate and reliable venous sample. The USPSTF has found insufficient evidence to recommend for or against periodic screening of high-risk infants not found to be anemic at the initial screening or of older, asymptomatic children. The American Academy of Family Physicians (AAFP) agrees with the USPSTF. The American Academy of Pediatrics suggests that all infants undergo Hb or Hct testing once at or before 9 months of age. The Canadian Task Force on the Periodic Health Examination, Bright Futures, and the Institute of Medicine agree with the USPSTF in advocating screening of high-risk infants between 6 or 9 and 12 months of age. The CDC recommends universal screening for high-risk populations between the ages of 9 and 12 months, again 6 months later, and annually between ages 2 to 5 years. In populations not at high risk, they endorse the selective screening approach described in Table 5-9 for infants and preschool children. The CDC also recommends screening of adolescent girls every 5 to 10 years and annual screening of those at high risk of iron deficiency (e.g., those with heavy menses, low iron intake, or a history of iron deficiency).

Table 5-9

CDC Recommendations for Selective Screening in Infants and Preschool Children Not at High Risk for Iron Deficiency

Consider anemia screening before age 6 mo for preterm infants and low-birth-weight infants who are not fed iron-fortified infant formula.

Annually assess children ages 2–5 yr for risk factors for iron-deficiency anemia (e.g., a low-iron diet, limited access to food because of poverty or neglect, or special health care needs). Screen these children if they have any of these risk factors.

At ages 9–12 mo and 6 mo later (at ages 15–18 mo), assess infants and young children for risk factors for anemia. Screen the following children:

Preterm or low-birth-weight infants

Infants fed a diet of non-iron-fortified infant formula for >2 mo

Infants introduced to cow's milk before age 12 mo

Breast-fed infants who do not consume a diet adequate in iron after age 6 mo (i.e., those who receive insufficient iron from supplementary foods)

Children who consume >24 oz daily of cow's milk

Children who have special health care needs (e.g., children who use medications that interfere with iron absorption and children who have chronic infection, inflammatory disorders, restricted diets, or extensive blood loss from a wound, an accident, or surgery).

ABBREVIATIONS: CDC, Centers for Disease Control.

SOURCE: From Centers for Disease Control and Prevention: Recommendations to prevent and control iron deficiency in the United States. *MMWR* 47:RR-3, 1998.

Follow-up of Positive Screening Tests

Appropriate hematologic confirmation of iron deficiency and nutrition counseling or supplementation should be used when infants are found to be anemic. If a screening capillary Hct or Hb level is determined to be low, clinical judgment and the patient's (or caretaker's) preference will determine further management strategies. Options include immediate confirmation of iron deficiency before treatment or empiric supplementation with diet or iron formulations and retesting of Hb or Hct after 4 weeks to confirm therapeutic benefit (as described in Table 5-10). If immediate confirmation of iron deficiency is chosen, a second capillary Hct or Hb, venous Hct or Hb, or serum ferritin level may be used. Of the laboratory options, the serum ferritin level has the best sensitivity and specificity for detecting iron deficiency. A serum ferritin value of 15 μg/L or less confirms iron deficiency, and a higher level indicates the need for further diagnostic workup to rule out other causes of anemia, such as thalassemia, sickle cell disease, or other conditions.

TREATMENT CONSIDERATIONS

There are important considerations when deciding whether to treat anemia empirically, as if it were an iron-deficiency anemia. First is the relative proportion of iron deficiency in the screened populations. The lower the prevalence, the less the likelihood that a positive result on screening will actually be associated with iron-deficiency anemia. As noted, a prevalence of iron-deficiency anemia of 3% and a screening test sensitivity of 90%, with a speci-

Table 5-10

Empiric Approach to Diagnosis and Treatment of Presumed Iron-deficiency Anemia

Check a positive anemia screening result by performing another Hb concentration or Hct test. If the tests agree and the child is not ill, a presumptive diagnosis of iron-deficiency anemia can be made and treatment begun.

Treat presumptive iron-deficiency anemia by prescribing 3 mg/kg per day of iron drops to be administered between meals. Counsel the parents or guardians about adequate diet to correct the underlying problem of low iron intake.

Repeat the anemia screening in 4 wk. An increase in Hb concentration of ≥1 g/dL or in Hct of ≥3% confirms the diagnosis of iron-deficiency anemia. If iron-deficiency anemia is confirmed, reinforce dietary counseling, continue iron treatment for 2 more mo, then recheck Hb concentration or Hct. Reassess Hb concentration or Hct approximately 6 mo after successful treatment is completed.

If after 4 wk, the anemia does not respond to iron treatment despite compliance with the iron supplementation regimen and the absence of acute illness, further evaluate anemia by using other laboratory tests, including MCV, RDW, and serum ferritin concentration. For example, a serum ferritin concentration of ≤15 μg/L confirms iron deficiency, and a concentration of >15 μg/L suggests that iron deficiency is not the cause of the anemia.

ABBREVIATIONS: Hb, hemoglobin; Hct, hematocrit; MCV, mean cell volume; RDW, red blood cell distribution width.
SOURCE: From Centers for Disease Control and Prevention: Recommendations to prevent and control iron deficiency in the United States. *MMWR* 47:RR-3, 1998.

ficity of 44%, would lead to a positive predictive value of 4.7%. This would mean that more than 95% of the positive screening results would represent false-positives. In other words, only one in 20 positive screens would represent an iron-deficiency anemia.

Another important consideration in deciding whether to treat someone with a positive Hb or Hct screen is that iron therapy carries a small, but real risk. Chronic iron overload has been reported to result in such morbid conditions as cirrhosis, hepatoma, diabetes, cardiomyopathy, arthritis, arthropathy, and hypopituitarism. In extreme cases, overdoses can be fatal.

TREATMENT REGIMENS

When iron supplementation is indicated for an infant, give 3 mg/kg of elemental iron per day between meals for a period of 4 weeks.

Age-appropriate dietary instruction is also indicated. A minimal rise of Hb of 1 g/dL or Hct of 3% confirms a therapeutic benefit. Where such a benefit is not shown, further diagnostic testing should be performed to elucidate the cause of anemia. If a therapeutic benefit is confirmed, continue iron therapy for 2 more months to replenish iron stores, and recheck the Hb or Hct level. If the Hb or Hct is still low, continue therapy as indicated. If this retest shows that the Hb or Hct is back to normal levels, stop therapy and screen for recurrence in about 6 months.

IRON PREPARATIONS

There are a variety of iron preparations available for infants and children. They come as drops, syrups, or elixir and as either ferrous sulfate or ferrous gluconate (Table 5-11).

Table 5-11

Liquid Iron Preparations

TYPE OF IRON	TRADE NAME	STRENGTH	IRON CONTENT (MG FE/ML)
Ferrous sulfate			
Syrup	Fer-in-Sol	18 mg/cc	3.6
Elixir	Feosol	44 mg/cc	8.8
Drops	Fer-in-Sol	125 mg/cc	25.0
Ferrous gluconate			
Elixir	Fergon	60 mg/cc	7

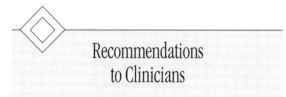

Recommendations to Clinicians

There have been few observational data that have shown adverse effects from iron-deficiency anemia in healthy, low-risk populations. Many observational studies, however, have found an association between iron-deficiency anemia and abnormal growth and development in high-risk infants. One randomized trial, as noted earlier, has shown a beneficial effect on this abnormal development by correcting the iron deficiency. Breast feeding and ensuring an adequate iron intake in the diets of all infants are safe interventions, often associated with additional benefits. Therefore, primary prevention of iron-deficiency anemia in infants and screening of high-risk infants for iron-deficiency are supported in the literature, and the following interventions are recommended.

Primary Prevention

- *Breast-feeding should be encouraged in all infants for at least the first 6 months after birth.* In addition to preventing iron-deficiency anemia and the potential adverse

outcomes previously noted, evidence suggests that breast feeding during this period may reduce the risk of otitis media, lower respiratory tract illness, meningitis, allergic illnesses, diarrhea, hospital admissions, and abnormal cognitive development.

- *When formulas and other foods are introduced, parents should be encouraged to include iron-enriched products in the diets of infants and young children.* Two or more servings per day of iron-fortified infant cereal can meet the iron requirements at this age. When it is age appropriate, good dietary sources of iron can be used, such as meat, poultry, and fish, with their well-absorbed heme iron, and plant-based foods, such as whole grains, enriched bread and cereal, dark green vegetables, and legumes, including nuts. Consider adding the enhancers of iron absorption listed in Table 5-5 to diets low in sources of heme iron.

- The use of low-iron milk products, such as cow's, goat's, and soy milk, should be discouraged during the first 12 months of life, and the intake of these forms of milk in children ages 1 to 5 years should be limited to 24 oz/day.

- When supplemental formulas and foods are being given to infants and they do not provide about 1 mg/kg/day of iron, supplementation with iron drops to reach this goal should be recommended.

- When solid foods are being used, some foods rich in vitamin C (e.g., fruits, vegetables, or juice) should be added to the diet, preferably with meals, to increase the absorption of iron.
- High-risk infants and children should be referred to WIC for assistance with nutrition counseling and purchasing of foods.

A CDC-recommended source for dietary information regarding iron is *Nutrition and Your Health: Dietary Guidelines for Americans* (U.S. Department of Agriculture, 1995).

Secondary Prevention

- Primary care clinicians should assess their communities and patient populations and decide, based on the prevalence of iron deficiency, if they want to implement a universal or selective screening policy for infants.
- In addition, consideration should be given to annual screening of young children, ages 1 to 5 years, for risk factors for iron-deficiency anemia, such as dietary insufficiency or relevant health care needs. Relevant health care needs include chronic infectious or inflammatory disorders or the use of medications that decrease the absorption of iron. When risk factors are identified, screen for anemia.

Errors to Avoid

Improper Collection of Capillary Blood

When capillary blood is used to measure Hb concentration or Hct, a false-positive screen can result from excessive squeezing at the puncture site. This causes tissue fluid to dilute the blood

sample, leading to a false-positive (low) test result.

Failure to Address the Root Cause of Iron Deficiency

If iron deficiency is detected, it is common for it to be treated by iron supplementation. The root cause of the problem, however, is inadequate dietary intake of iron. This problem needs to be addressed by dietary education of parents and caregivers.

Screening Older Children

For school-age children and male adolescents, universal screening for iron deficiency anemia is not recommended. The CDC currently advocates the most aggressive screening policies, and their recommendations include screening school-age children and male adolescents only if they have a history of iron deficiency, special health care needs, or inadequate iron intake.

Emerging Trends

Much remains to be learned about the extent of the morbidity and mortality caused by iron deficiency and iron-deficiency anemia. Future studies will look at this question and provide more evidence for or against the effectiveness of early detection and treatment in preventing cognitive, behavioral, and psychological adverse effects. As more experience is gained with alternative screening tests and they become standardized, more universally available, and more affordable, alternatives to the Hb concentration and Hct for screening will be proposed and tested.

Bibliography

American Academy of Family Physicians: *Age Charts for Periodic Health Examination*. Kansas City, MO, American Academy of Family Physicians, 1996.

American Academy of Pediatrics, Committee on Practice and Ambulatory Medicine: Recommendations for preventive pediatric health care. *Pediatrics* 96(2 Pt 1):373–374, 1995.

Barness LA (ed): *Pediatric Nutrition Handbook*, 3rd ed. Elk Grove Village, IL, American Academy of Pediatrics, 1993.

Beard J: One person's view of iron deficiency, development, and cognitive function. *Am J Clin Nutr* 62;709–710,1995.

Centers for Disease Control and Prevention. Recommendations to prevent and control iron deficiency in the U.S. *MMWR* 47:(RR-3):23. 1998.

Goyer RA: Nutrition and metal toxicity. *Am J Clin Nutr* 61(suppl):646S–650S, 1995.

Guyatt GH, Oxman AD, Ali M, et al: Laboratory diagnosis of iron-deficiency anemia: An overview. *J Gen Intern Med* 7(1):145–153, 1992. Published erratum appears in *J Gen Intern Med* 7(4):423, 1992.

Johnson-Spear MA, Yip R: Hemoglobin difference between black and white women with comparable iron status: Justification for race-specific anemia criteria. *Am J Clin Nutr* 60:117–121, 1994.

Koeller JM, Van Den Berg C: Anemia, in Young LJ, Koda-Kimble MA (eds): *Applied Therapeutics: The Clinical Use of Drugs*, 6th ed. Vancouver, Applied Therapeutics, 1995.

Looker AC, Dallman PR, Carroll MD, et al: Prevalence of iron deficiency in the United States. *JAMA* 277: 973–979, 1997.

Lukens JN: Iron metabolism and iron deficiency, in Miller DR, Baehner RL, Miller LP (eds): *Blood Diseases of Infancy and Childhood*. St. Louis, MO, Mosby, 1995, pp 193–219.

National Research Council: *Recommended Dietary Allowances*, 10th ed. Washington, DC, National Academy Press, 1989.

Oski FA: Iron deficiency in infancy and childhood. *N Engl J Med* 329:190–193, 1993.

Public Health Service: *Healthy People 2000: National Health Promotion and Disease Prevention Objectives*. Washington, DC, US Department of Health and Human Services, Public Health Service, 1991, p 94.

Swain RA, Kaplan B, Montgomery E: Iron deficiency anemia: When is parenteral therapy warranted? *Postgrad Med* 100(5):181–193, 1996.

US Department of Agriculture, Agriculture Research Service. *Data Tables: Results from USDA's 1994–96 Continuing Survey of Food Intakes by Individuals and 1994-96 Diet and Health Knowledge Survey* (online). Riverdale, MD, USDA, Agriculture Research Service, Beltsville Human Nutrition Center, 1997.

US Department of Agriculture and US Department of Health and Human Services: *Nutrition and Your Health: Dietary Guidelines for Americans*, 4th ed, Home and Garden Bulletin no. 232. Washington, DC, US Department of Agriculture and US Department of Health and Human Services, 1995.

US Preventive Services Task Force: *Guide to Clinical Preventive Services*, 2nd ed. Alexandria, Virginia, International Medical Publishing, 1996.

Underwood BA, Arthur P: The contribution of vitamin A to public health. *FASEB J* 10:1044–1045, 1996.

Viteri FE: Iron supplementation for the control of iron deficiency in populations at risk. *Nutr Rev* 55(6): 195, 1997.

Walter T, Dallman PR, Pizarro F, et al: Effectiveness of iron-fortified infant cereal in prevention of iron-deficiency anemia. *Pediatrics* 91(5):976, 1993.

Young PC, Hamill B, Wasserman RC, et al: Evaluation of the capillary microhematocrit as a screening test for anemia in pediatric office practice. *Pediatrics* 78(2):206–209, 1986.

Michael Weitzman

Chapter 6

Lead Poisoning

Introduction

Childhood lead poisoning has attracted a great deal of attention and controversy among clinicians, public health practitioners, policymakers and the public at large. It also represents one of the great pediatric public health success stories in the United States, with major reductions in children's mean blood lead levels and in the number of children with elevated blood lead levels. These changes have been so profound that it is now very rare for a child to suffer from acute lead encephalopathy. Virtually no children in the United States now die of this disease, and the vast majority of clinicians caring for children have never seen a child who has overt symptoms of lead poisoning. The changes also have been accompanied by marked gains in our understanding of lead's untoward effects on children's health and the means by which children are exposed.

Despite these successes, however, environmental lead continues to be a significant child health problem. Large numbers of children still have levels of exposure that negatively affect their health. Substantial amounts of lead remain in our environment, posing an ongoing hazard for children. The ways in which to attain further reductions in children's exposure in a practical and effective manner are not apparent at this time. Many controversies and unanswered questions remain, and those in the medical or public health fields have not universally adopted much of what we know is effective.

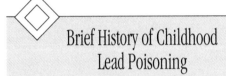

Brief History of Childhood Lead Poisoning

Humankind has used lead for several thousand years. In the times of the pharaohs, the Egyptians used lead in cosmetics. The Romans lined their extensive system of aqueducts with lead and made goblets with lead, from which the aristocracy drank wine. Some historians have suggested that the rapid decline of the Roman Empire was due, at least in part, to the Romans' widespread use of lead.

With the Industrial Revolution, the use of lead increased exponentially. When added to paint, lead has two properties that contribute to its almost ubiquitous dispersion in our environment: it enhances the brilliance of primary colors, and it tends to make paint chalk, rather than chip. While increasing the longevity of a coat of paint, the latter property also amplifies the insidious exposure of children to lead, as described later in this chapter. In the early twentieth century, lead was introduced into our environment in unprecedented quantities, in the form of tetraethyl lead in gasoline.

Whereas lead's adverse effects on adults have been known since antiquity, knowledge about

lead's deleterious effects on children have begun to be recognized only during this past century. Hippocrates wrote about the "abdominal gripes," that is, crampy abdominal pain and constipation that can occur with high levels of exposure. In the eighteenth century, Benjamin Franklin wrote about the folly of continuing to use lead when its negative health consequences were so well known. In the nineteenth century, as women entered the urban workforce, working in factories, decreased fertility and increased pregnancy loss due to lead exposure became prevalent.

It was not until the 1890s, however, that the first description of childhood lead poisoning appeared, when, in 1894, Gibson and associates used rudimentary epidemiologic techniques to tie several cases of childhood lead poisoning to peeling and chipping paint on verandas in the outback of Australia. The pediatric community in the United States remained skeptical for another 20 years. Then in the late 1940s, Byers and Lord published their landmark study showing that a large percentage of children who survived acute lead encephalopathy had serious and permanent neurological and developmental problems. This opened the field to the extensive series of epidemiologic investigations that commenced in the 1970s and that continue today, showing long-term subtle, but serious neurodevelopmental problems among seemingly asymptomatic children with levels of lead exposure previously believed to be safe.

New Knowledge and Approaches

A related field of investigation has been directed toward identifying the sources of children's exposure and ways to prevent poisoning. These advances in understanding have transformed the way we think about this disease, the ways in which children are exposed, its consequences, and our approaches to prevention and treatment. For example, it was long believed that children got lead poisoning by ingesting lead-contaminated paint chips, whereas today we recognize that children most often are exposed as a consequence of developmentally normal hand-to-mouth activity, resulting in the ingestion of lead-contaminated house dust. Just several decades ago lead poisoning was conceptualized as a disease only when a child had acute encephalopathy, which either killed the child or left a very high percentage of children disabled. Today we view it as a disease affecting substantially larger percentages of children, the majority of whom have no symptoms immediately referable to their lead exposure.

Increased knowledge and awareness have led to major changes in public policies and public health and medical management practices. From the 1950s through the 1970s paint manufacturers voluntarily lowered the content of lead in interior household paint. The Consumer Product Safety Commission limited the content of household lead to 0.7% in 1977. In the late 1970s the Centers for Disease Control and Prevention (CDC) began to fund state and local health department childhood lead poisoning prevention programs, a practice that continues to this day. As shown in Table 6-1, the CDC has continually lowered the level of children's blood lead that is defined as poisonous or elevated. These moves have been accompanied by the development in many communities of regional lead-treatment centers, some funded in part by state health department funds and many affili-

ated with hospital-based pediatric training programs.

Centers for Disease Control's Plan of Action

The concern with lower levels of lead exposure has led to new strategies aimed at preventing this condition, new approaches to identifying children with elevated lead levels or those who are at risk of having elevated levels, and new methods of treatment. In 1991 the CDC issued a strategic plan for the elimination of childhood lead poisoning in the United States by the year 2010. This plan acknowledged that public education and screening practices, which had previously been the cornerstones of our preventive strategies, were insufficient. The plan calls for an extensive campaign of increased support for prevention programs, increased abatement of lead-contaminated paint and dust in high-risk housing stock, reductions in lead in other sources and pathways of exposure, the development of lead-poisoning prevention advisory groups at state and local levels, and a broadened research agenda on the prevention of childhood lead poisoning. The cost of such an agenda is estimated at $164 million per year for 20 years, with estimated savings of $64 billion dollars over that same period.

The CDC supported its proposal with the proposition that finding and treating children with lead poisoning is critical, but not sufficient, and that removing the sources of lead before children are poisoned is the prudent approach to this problem. This recommendation firmly redirected our approach away from secondary to primary prevention strategies. The plan was supported by cost-benefit data suggesting that $4600 is saved in medical and special education costs for each child who is prevented from having a blood lead level in excess of 24 μg/dL. Recognizing the hodgepodge of abatement strategies and the paucity of rigorous data on the cost and effectiveness of various abatement activities, the CDC, the Environmental Protection

Table 6-1

The Centers for Disease Control's Action Level for Childhood Lead

1960s	60 μg/dL
1975	30 μg/dL
1985	25 μg/dL
1991	10 μg/dL
1997	10 μg/dL

Agency, the federal Department of Housing and Urban Development, and the National Center for Lead Safe Housing embarked on an ambitious program of targeted abatement and scientific projects aimed at identifying effective approaches to lead-based paint abatement and household dust control. These projects are currently under way.

Role of Deleading Gasoline

Ironically, the most positive influence in reducing children's exposure to lead to date has not been public education campaigns, screening programs, or new abatement or treatment methods, but rather the deleading of gasoline. Gasoline was deleaded not as a consequence of public policy aimed at protecting children from this potent toxin, however; it was the direct result of the development of catalytic converters for automobiles that are incompatible with lead-containing gasoline. It was more than a decade after gasoline was deleaded that the temporal relationship of this action to the profound decrease in blood lead levels was recognized. Despite these declines, large numbers of children continue to have unacceptably high levels of lead in their blood, requiring continued vigilance and efforts in the areas of screening, public education, and removal of sources of lead from children's environments.

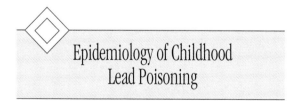

Epidemiology of Childhood Lead Poisoning

Why Children Are at Risk

Although individuals of all ages can get lead poisoning, most of our concern is directed toward infants and preschool children. This is a consequence of the fact that children's lead levels are highest between 1 and 3 years of age and that most of our efforts are aimed at protecting the developing brain from the effects of clinically asymptomatic lead exposure. As much as 90% of brain growth and synaptic sculpting occur in the first several years of life. Thus, the vast majority of studies of lead's neurocognitive effects have focused on preschool children.

Children's lead levels are highest between 1 and 3 years as the result of four factors. First, this is an age of exploration, during which infants and toddlers have achieved new mobility and avidly investigate their environments, often crawling and touching the floors, woodwork, and windowsills of their homes. Second, hand-to-mouth activity of many children peaks at this age, that is, they mouth many objects with which they come in contact as part of their normal development. Third, the efficiency of absorption of gastrointestinal lead is greater in children than it is in older individuals (adults absorb approximately 10% of lead in the gastrointestinal tract, whereas children with normal iron status absorb 40% to 50%). And, fourth, the prevalence of iron deficiency and iron-deficiency anemia also peak at this age, and in the context of iron deficiency the efficiency of gastrointestinal absorption of lead approaches 90%.

At this age, some children also have a condition known as pica, which refers to an abnormal tendency to eat large amounts of nonfood products, such as dirt. This condition, which exacerbates children's potential exposure to lead, should be distinguished from normal hand-to-mouth activity. Virtually all children of this age engage in some hand-to mouth activity. It is generally agreed that the most common way in which children with low (10 to 20 µg/dL) to moderate (21 to 44 µg/dL) elevations of blood lead levels have been exposed to lead is through household dust that they get on their hands and then ingest by hand-to-mouth exposure.

Prevalence and Distribution

There has been a remarkable reduction in the mean blood lead levels of children in the United States and the numbers and percentages of children with elevated blood lead levels. Whereas the mean blood lead level of children 1 to 5 years was 15 μg/dL in 1976 through 1980, from 1991 to 1994 it was 2.7. These data are derived from the National Health and Nutrition Examination Surveys II (1976 to 1980) and III (1988 to 1994). Data from these two national surveys also show that the prevalence of children with blood lead levels of 10 μg/dL or more declined from 88.2% to 8.9% and that the prevalence of blood lead levels above 25 μg/dL declined from 9.3% to 0.5%.

Despite these declines, an estimated 890,000 children still have blood lead levels of 10 μg/dL or higher, a level high enough to lead to adverse neurocognitive effects. Moreover, the racial, social, and economic disparities in occurrence that have long been recognized have increased. Among all children, 21% of those living in cities with more than one million people have blood lead levels of 10 μg/dL or more, compared with 16% of children in smaller cities and 6% of children not living in cities. In large cities, 37% of African-American and 6% of Caucasian children have levels above 10 μg/dL, whereas the rates for African-American and Caucasian children living in non-city settings are 11% and 5%, respectively.

Similarly, blood lead levels vary inversely with family income: 28% of African-American children with low family incomes have blood lead levels of 10 μg/dL or higher compared with 6% of those living in homes with high incomes. On the other hand, 10% of Caucasian children from low-income homes compared with 4% of Caucasian children from high-income homes have blood lead levels of 10 μg/dL or more. These numbers refer to national averages, and there is a great deal of local variation. For example, in New York State in 1994, 1% of children screened still had blood lead levels greater than 20 μg/dL. Within Monroe County, New York, where the city of Rochester is located, 35% of children had blood lead levels of 10 μg/dL or higher in 1993, and 10% had blood lead levels of 20 μg/dL or higher. Because of uneven screening rates in local areas, data based on findings among children screened are not directly comparable to nationally representative survey results, but these numbers highlight the geographic variation in this problem and the fact that in many communities very large numbers of children are still being exposed.

Seasonal Variation

Several other aspects of the epidemiology of childhood lead poisoning are worthy of mention. First, it has long been recognized that there are seasonal variations in the occurrence of lead poisoning—children's blood lead levels increase during the summer. Although the reasons behind this well-observed phenomenon are unknown, it is believed to be due to the effects of ultraviolet light on the absorption of lead; children's extended time outdoors during the summer, increasing their exposure to lead in soil and to peeling paint on porches; and the inclusion of topsoil in the house dust in the homes of children at this time of year.

Cultural Factors

Immigrant children may be at heightened risk because of exposure in their country of origin, the use of folk medicines containing lead, and the use of ceramics with lead glazes. Still another epidemiologic phenomenon deserving mention is "Yuppie Plumbism." In many urban areas, young, middle-class families are moving into neighborhoods that went through a period of being occupied by more impoverished families.

These new families frequently renovate older homes in these communities, and the renovations themselves can result in the exposure of their children to large amounts of lead in the form of paint chips and lead-contaminated house dust unless the job is performed properly and the lead cleaned up.

Causes and Determinants

In the language of environmental health, lead is what is called a multimedia exposure problem, meaning that children are exposed by many routes. As noted in Table 6-2, children may be exposed to lead in water, food, soil, toys, ceramics, and many other sources. For most children in the United States, lead-contaminated interior and exterior household paint remains the most common and the most concentrated source of their exposure by far. Moreover, lead-contaminated paint is the origin of much of the lead in lead-contaminated house dust and residential soil, so that in circumstances where house dust or residential soil is the vector, the original source of the lead often is paint that has chipped, peeled, or become chalky.

Eighty-three percent of all homes built in the United States before 1978 contain at least some lead-based paint at a concentration of at least 1 mg/cm^2. The older the house, the more likely it is to contain lead-based paint, and the less affluent the family, the more likely this paint is to be in disrepair. Housing built before 1950 poses the greatest danger of exposure, and 27% of all housing in the United States was built before 1950. Moreover, there are enormous regional variations in the age of housing stock.

Numerous studies underscore the dangers of improperly performed lead-based paint abatements and of having children present in the home during abatements. As mentioned earlier, this problem has been exacerbated by the reclaiming of many rundown urban residences by young professionals, who then undertake to renovate their houses themselves. This sometimes results in disruptions of intact paint surfaces, releasing lead that then becomes available

Table 6-2
Sources of Children's Lead Exposure

Common sources
  Lead-contaminated household dust and paint
  Lead-contaminated paint on porches and the exterior of homes
  Lead-contaminated residential soil
Less common sources
  Certain home remedies
  Certain toys or household goods imported from abroad
  Household water supply
Industries, work sites, occupations, and associated materials
  Secondary smelting and refining of nonferrous metals
  Brass/copper foundries
  Firing ranges
  Automotive repair shops
  Bridge, tunnel, and elevated highway construction
  Primary and storage batteries
  Valve and pipe fittings
  Plumbing
  Pottery
Hobbies and home activities
  Recreational use of firing ranges
  Home repairs, repainting, and remodeling
  Furniture refinishing
  Stained glass making
  Casting ammunition
  Making fishing weights or sinkers or toy soldiers
  Using lead solder
  Using lead-containing artists' paints or ceramic glazes
  Burning lead-painted wood
  Car or boat repair

SOURCE: Adapted, in part, from the Centers for Disease Control, 1997.

to children in the home in the form of paint chips or lead-contaminated house dust.

It is essential that children not be present when lead-based paint abatements or major renovations to homes with significant amounts of lead-based paint are undertaken. Meticulous cleanup must be done after abatements or significant renovations, preferably by professional housecleaners, before children move back into the home. Some states have developed lead paint abatement standards and certification programs for those who clean up lead. The federal Department of Housing and Urban Development, in concert with the Environmental Protection Agency, has advanced standards for post-abatement dust lead levels that are aimed at protecting children from undue exposures as a consequence of abatements resulting in increases in lead-contaminated house dust available to children. The standard has been set at 200 $\mu g/ft^2$ for floors, 500 $\mu g/ft^2$ for windowsills, and 800 $\mu g/ft^2$ for window wells. While it may be impractical to achieve levels of lead in house dust below these standards, little empirical data show that these levels are safe, and recent studies suggest that the recommended levels still pose a threat that could result in low-level lead poisoning.

Food and Water

The amount of lead in food or food containers has been greatly reduced by the Food and Drug Administration, so that foods produced in the United States pose a minimal risk of significant exposure to lead. Similarly, the Consumer Product Safety Commission limits the amount of lead in children's toys and many household products. Nevertheless, children at times are placed at risk because of the importation of products from abroad, such as was recently the case with crayons and miniblinds from China.

Household water levels also are regulated—these regulations have no benefit, however, in protecting children from lead that leaches from

solder or old piping within one's home or from well water. It also is true that although each of these sources probably contributes only modestly to exposure, together they may add up to an unacceptable level of exposure. Knowing the lead level in drinking water at a community level is somewhat useful, and, in most cases of elevated blood lead levels in children, there is little utility in testing the home's water lead level. This truism does not apply (a) when children have prolonged periods of elevated blood lead levels and the source of their exposure is not readily apparent or (b) when infants who are formula-fed become poisoned, since lead poisoning in infants is unusual and has been shown to be due in many cases to lead-contaminated water used in their formula.

Soil

Lead in soil has received a great deal of attention as a potential source of significant exposure. This is based on cross-sectional studies that have shown that rates of childhood lead poisoning are higher in communities with higher soil lead levels and generalizations from situations where there have been industrial or similar types of contamination of soil. In cases where there have been industrial sources of lead contamination of soil, such as near lead smelters, battery plants, or garages where batteries are discarded in the soil, soil lead levels may be very high and may serve as serious sources of exposure for children.

Urban residential soil may also be contaminated with lead, but usually to a lesser degree. In urban settings, properties closer to highways or busy roads often have higher soil lead levels than those with lesser degrees of exposure to gasoline emissions before 1977, when gasoline was deleaded. Similarly, in urban areas, soil that is closer to the road and soil in proximity to the house tend to have the highest lead levels. Proximity to the road results in higher soil lead levels from gas emissions, and soil close to the house may be contaminated by peeling or chipping external paint.

A randomized, controlled study of lead-contaminated soil removal as a way to reduce children's blood lead levels (among children with lead levels in the range of 10 to 24 μg/dL) showed that while the lead in urban soil is bioavailable to children, it is usually only a modest contributor to their blood lead levels. That is, the reduction in blood lead levels independently associated with the removal of the top three inches of soil, contaminated with lead to a level of 2000 parts per million, was approximately 1.5 μg/dL at 1 year and 2.5 μg/dL at 2 years after abatement. This finding suggests that when urban soil is contaminated to this extent, it is unlikely to be a significant contributor to children's blood lead levels in most cases.

In cases where the level of soil lead is significantly higher, soil may be a very serious source of exposure for children. Examples of such potentially hazardous places are where there have been industrial exposures, on farms where gasoline-powered vehicles and tools are used extensively (gasoline for farm vehicles is not lead-free, in contrast to gasoline for other vehicles), or where soil has been contaminated with lead from paint on bridges. Similarly, children with pica who ingest soil may be at significant risk of exposure to lead.

Other Sources

There are many other potential sources of children's exposure to lead. Parents whose clothing becomes contaminated with lead at work may inadvertently bring lead home on their clothing. Occupations at high risk of "take home exposures" include those involving battery production or repair, pottery making, work in a smelter or brass foundry, demolition and renovation of outdoor structures, printing, work on a firing range, or paint contracting. There also are a number of hobbies that place children at risk of lead poisoning, such as making lead fishing sinkers or bullets, collecting lead figurines, spending time in indoor firing ranges, and ceramic pottery making.

In certain cultures, such as several from Latin America and Southeast Asia, a number of home remedies, such as azarcon or greta, can serve as sources of lead poisoning. Lead-glazed ceramics brought home from numerous developing countries also can lead to lead poisoning, especially if acidic foods, such as salad dressings or citric acid juices, are eaten off them or stored in them. These sources should be sought when children who are recent immigrants, or whose parents have traveled abroad or who work in relevant jobs, are poisoned or whenever more common sources are not found. In most cases, children are exposed in their primary residences or in relatives', babysitters', or day-care providers' homes. The most common source, as noted, is lead-contaminated house dust, which has become contaminated from peeling or chipping paint, often on windowsills, in window wells, or from baseboards and wooden doors.

Adverse Health Effects

Lead has numerous adverse health consequences, including increased rates of fetal loss; decreased birth weight; long-term effects on blood pressure, contributing to adult hypertension; and alterations in vitamin D metabolism. Most of our concern for children's exposure, however, has to do with lead's adverse neurocognitive effects. An impressive array of studies has identified a series of subtle, but potentially serious alterations of children's neurocognitive functioning associated with lead exposure at levels previously believed to be innocuous (Table 6-3).

As noted previously, lead encephalopathy resulting in death or long-term developmental

Table 6-3

Threshold Blood Lead Levels Above Which Adverse Effects
May Occur

BLOOD LEAD LEVEL	TOXIC EFFECT
≥10 µg/dL	Decreased IQ
	Decreased hearing acuity
	Decreased growth
≥20 µg/dL	Decreased nerve conduction velocity
≥30 µg/dL	Decreased vitamin D metabolism
≥40 µg/dL	Decreased hemoglobin synthesis
≥90 µg/dL	Nephropathy
	Encephalopathy

SOURCE: Adapted from the Centers for Disease Control, 1991.

disability has been recognized for most of this century and, until 20 years ago, defined our approach to the problem. The past 20 years have witnessed numerous cross-sectional and longitudinal studies, meta-analyses of series of studies, and reviews by such prestigious scientific bodies as the National Research Council that identify untoward effects of lead at levels as low as 10 µg/dL. *It is important to note that there is no evidence of a threshold for the toxic effects of lead—that is, negative effects are seen at all levels of exposure.* The adverse effects on cognition of blood lead levels as low as 10 µg/dL have been well documented, and the findings of the literature are remarkably consistent. The magnitude of the effect of blood lead on IQ is estimated to be in the range of a loss of two to three IQ points for each 10 µg/dL increase in blood lead. These data are based on large series of children, and the effect of lead on individual children may be greater or lesser than the effect estimated for a population of children. In addition to effects on IQ, many studies have identified adverse effects on other aspects of children's functioning, including attention, vigilance, language development, the transfer of

information from short-term to long-term memory, aggression, and antisocial or delinquent behaviors. The facts in Table 6-4 are central to our current understanding of lead's adverse effects on the neurocognitive functioning of children.

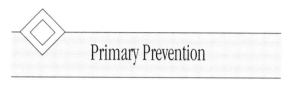

Primary Prevention

Three broad categories have been employed to attempt to achieve primary prevention of childhood lead poisoning. The first involves parent education in the form of public awareness announcements, anticipatory guidance provided by public health or medical care providers, or written materials, all aimed at helping parents limit their children's exposure to environmental sources of lead.

Table 6-4

Current State of Knowledge Regarding Effects of Lead
on Development

There is no evidence that lead's adverse neurocognitive effects are reversible.

It is unclear whether the peak blood lead level or some as yet undetermined length of time with elevated blood lead levels results in these adverse effects.

A critical age for exposure that results in neurocognitive damage has not been identified.

No specific behavioral signals of lead's negative effects have been identified.

While it is clear that the consequences of lead exposure exert negative effects on a population basis, it is unclear whether an individual child is adversely affected, and whether such effects are clinically meaningful for the individual child.

The second has involved the control of environmental sources of lead via regulatory mechanisms. Examples of the latter include reductions in interior household paint lead levels; control of the lead in water, food, food containers, and toys; and, most important to date, deleading gasoline.

A potential third category, which has largely been used thus far as a means of secondary prevention, involves abatement of lead-contaminated properties before children become poisoned and relocating children to lead-safe housing. Many critics of our approach to childhood lead poisoning liken children to the canaries that were used earlier this century to alert coal miners to the presence of dangerous gases in coal mines. It is thought that we use our children to identify environmental dangers rather than taking proactive steps to prevent lead poisoning before children are injured.

A number of studies demonstrate the clear geographic dimensions of the childhood lead-poisoning problem in the United States. That is, children living in older homes in poor condition are those at greatest risk. While paint produced between 1950 and 1977 had varying degrees of lead that could pose a danger, pre-1950 housing usually contains paint with dangerous levels of lead. Lead in paint in these homes poses a limited danger to children unless the paint is in disrepair, which is more often true in poorer neighborhoods and most often in rented properties.

Virtually all lead-poisoning treatment centers and state or local health departments with lead-poisoning-prevention programs recognize that the children who become poisoned tend to come from the same neighborhoods or blocks within small geographic areas. To date, the expense of taking the initiative to abate properties before children become poisoned has led to the policy decision to rely on the regulations listed earlier, parent education, and screening efforts as the major preventive strategies for childhood lead poisoning.

As part of the secondary prevention-related case management recommended for children with elevated blood lead levels, Table 6-5 lists the sorts of things that parents can do that are likely to reduce children's exposure to lead. Table 6-6 outlines recommendations for preventing "Yuppie Plumbism." Although many of these recommendations are contained in the CDC's guide *Preventing Childhood Lead Poisoning* (1991) and represent the consensus of many lead-prevention experts, there are little data to show that these recommendations are effective as secondary prevention strategies. There are no data to show that they work as primary prevention strategies. Nevertheless, it appears reasonable to offer these guidelines as suggestions to parents in an effort to accomplish primary prevention.

Table 6-5

Avoiding Lead Hazards in the Home

Stabilize or cover leaded paint that is chipping or peeling.

Move cribs, playpens, furniture, and play areas away from peeling paint.

Wet mop floors and wet clean windowsills and window wells with high-phosphate detergent.

Avoid dry dusting or sweeping.

Regularly wash children's hands, toys, and pacifiers.

Use cold water for cooking; run tap water for two to three min in the morning before using.

Repair deteriorated paint in home and on porch.

Replace old windows.

Relocate family to lead-safe housing.

Table 6-6

Preventing Yuppie Plumbism

> Inform families that all preschoolers are at risk
>   of lead poisoning, especially if they live in or
>   regularly visit pre-1950 homes.
> Renovations and paint removal in old homes
>   should be done only by trained contractors.
> Families must be out of their homes during
>   remodeling of homes with paint containing
>   lead.
> Post abatement cleanup, preferably by profes-
>   sional housecleaners, is essential.

Secondary Prevention

Screening is an essential component of a comprehensive approach to preventing childhood
lead poisoning. The goal of screening is to identify children who need individual interventions
to reduce their blood lead levels.

Until the past decade, the cornerstone of preventive efforts relied on screening programs for
the secondary prevention of childhood lead poisoning. With the CDC's *Lead Guidelines* and
Strategic Plan to End Lead Poisoning (1991),
much more of the focus has been redirected to
the primary prevention of lead poisoning, but
screening programs and the screening efforts of
primary care providers remain essential in minimizing the disease burden of excessive lead
exposure.

Screening Tests

Children's blood lead levels are a very imperfect
measure of their exposure because the half-life
of lead in blood is only about 28 days. After this
period of time, most of the lead re-equilibrates
to soft tissues, bones (which become the main
reservoir), and the brain. Lead shifts from one
compartment to another over the course of an
individual's life. Thus, blood lead levels are a
composite of recent and long-term exposures,
and there is no way to tell, using only blood
lead levels, how much of the blood lead reflects
recent versus past exposure. This has led many
researchers to try to identify biochemical or
other measures that reflect cumulative exposures. Screening tests that have been tried and
proved to be of no value include basophilic
stippling of red blood cells, bone lead lines
(these actually are growth-arrest plates), and
abdominal flat plates.

For much of the 1980s many clinicians relied
on free erythrocyte protoporphyrin (FEP) levels
as a screening tool. Unfortunately, FEP is very
insensitive with blood lead levels below
35 μg/dL and no longer is recommended as a
screening test for elevated blood lead levels. For
clinicians caring for children with blood lead
levels of 35 μg/dL or higher, however, FEP levels continue to be quite useful in helping distinguish recent from long-term elevations. FEP
levels do not rise with short-term unusual exposures, and it takes 1 to 3 months of elevated
blood lead levels before the FEP begins to rise.
FEP levels also are useful in monitoring the
effects of chelation therapy or environmental
efforts to diminish ongoing exposure, since they
will begin to decline within 1 to 3 months after
body stores decrease.

It is now recommended that lead screening
be conducted by measuring a blood lead level
collected by venipuncture. A capillary blood
sample collected by finger stick is an acceptable
alternative if it is collected properly. Table 6-7
lists the steps needed to perform this test correctly and to avoid surface lead contamination.
Because of the potential for contamination, capillary specimens with lead values of >10 μg/dL
should be confirmed with a venous sample.

Table 6-7

Proper Technique for Collecting a Capillary (Fingerstick) Sample for Lead Testing

Preparing for blood collection
  Use well-trained personnel.
  Clean work environment; use appropriate waste containers.
  All equipment should be within reach.
Preparing the finger for puncture
  Personnel should wear examination gloves throughout the procedure.
  Thoroughly clean the child's finger with soap and water.
  Briefly massage the fleshy portion of the finger gently.
  Clean the finger pad to be punctured with an alcohol swab; dry with sterile gauze or a cotton ball.
Puncturing the finger
  Grasp the finger and quickly puncture it with a sterile lancet.
  Wipe off the first droplet of blood with the sterile gauze or cotton ball.
  Let a well-beaded drop of blood form at the puncture site.
  Do not let blood run down the finger or onto the fingernail.
Specimen collection
  Continue to grasp the finger and touch the tip of the collection container to the beaded drop of blood.
  When the container is full, cap or seal it.
  Agitate the specimen to mix the anticoagulant through the blood.
  Label and store the specimen properly.

Screening Recommendations

UNIVERSAL SCREENING

In 1991 the CDC issued new lead screening guidelines for the first time since 1985. These guidelines contained important and controversial changes to the previous approach to secondary prevention, including the following suggestions.

1. Children were to be considered to have elevated blood lead levels if their levels were 10 μg/dL or higher, rather than 25 μg/dL.
2. Screening was to be accomplished using blood lead levels rather than FEP levels because of the insensitivity of FEP values in the blood lead range of 10 to 25 μg/dL.
3. Universal screening was recommended for all children 12 to 36 months of age, irrespective of social class or geographic location.
4. The risk of lead poisoning was to be assessed using lead-screening questionnaires, which would guide decisions about the age to begin screening and the frequency of screening.
5. Environmental assessment and intervention were to be considered at blood lead levels of 20 μg/dL or higher, rather than at 25 μg/dL, as was previously the case.

The medical community met these recommendations with mixed reviews. The most controversial recommendation was the one calling for universal screening. Numerous articles and commentaries appeared in medical journals contesting this recommendation. These articles argued that children were needlessly being subjected to painful finger sticks and venipunctures.

They also claimed that physicians' time and the public's money were being wasted by screening in many communities where it was unusual for a child to be found with a blood lead level above 10 μg/dL and where it was rare for children to have levels warranting chelation therapy. Moreover, many began to describe anecdotal experiences with what was called "lead hysteria," which was the supposed phenomenon of excessive parental anxiety about subsequent cognitive functioning among children with mild elevations in blood lead levels. It was questioned whether this anxiety was warranted, and ill effects of such parental anxiety were proposed. There were no empirical data to guide clinicians in ways to reduce parental anxiety or their children's lead burdens.

Not surprisingly, almost one-half of all pediatricians in the United States reported not universally screening all children in their practices in 1995, and marked regional variations in screening practices were noted. Even more disturbing, Medicaid children are three times as likely as non-Medicaid children to have elevated lead levels, and even though Congress passed a law in 1989 requiring lead screening as part of Medicaid's special preventive health program for children, a report from the United States General Accounting Office in February 1998 indicated that 81% of Medicaid children were not screened at all for lead toxicity. This report also found that 65% of Medicaid children with elevated blood lead levels had not been properly screened. Thus, despite a national policy aimed at screening all children, even the majority of high-risk children are not being screened.

HIGH-RISK SCREENING

Since the 1991 CDC lead-screening guidelines were published, a number of studies have evaluated the utility of the proposed questionnaire aimed at identifying high-risk children. These studies showed that such questionnaires had reasonably good screening characteristics in terms of sensitivity, specificity, and negative predictive values. They also were better at identifying children with blood lead levels >15 to 20 μg/dL than children with levels >10 μg/dL, adding further support to the notion of targeted screening.

As a consequence of concerns about universal screening, the documentation of markedly diminishing rates of elevated blood lead levels among children in the United States, and evidence that high-risk children could be identified before screening, the CDC issued new guidelines for screening in 1997. These guidelines advise state health officials to devise systems to facilitate targeted screening. Within the state or locale for which recommendations are made, it is advised that child health care providers use blood lead tests to screen children 1 and 2 years old and children 36 to 72 months of age who have not previously been screened and found to have low levels of exposure, if they meet one of the criteria in Table 6-8. It has been estimated that just screening all children who live in zip codes or census tracts in which 27% or more of the houses were built before 1950 would identify 92% to 93% of all children with blood lead levels of 10 μg/dL or more.

In addition, health care providers are encouraged to identify children who should be screened because of their increased risk of being exposed to less usual sources, such as those associated with various parental occupations or hobbies or other sources listed in the section of this chapter on causes and determinants. In the absence of a statewide plan or other formal guidelines from public health officials, universal screening for virtually all young children, as was called for in the 1991 CDC guidelines was again encouraged. *Similarly, whenever a parent or health care provider suspects that a child may be at risk of lead exposure, the child should be screened with a blood lead test, irrespective of health department recommendations or positive responses to questionnaires.*

Table 6-8

Recommendations for Lead Screening in Those at Risk

Child resides in a zip code where ≥27% of housing stock was built before 1950 or ≥12% of children have blood lead levels of ≥10 μg/dL.

Child receives services from public assistance programs for the poor, such as Medicaid or the Supplemental Food Program for Women, Infants, and Children (WIC).

Child's parent or guardian answers "yes" or "don't know" to any of the following three questions:

Does your child live in or regularly visit a house that was built before 1950? This question could apply to a facility such as a home day-care center or the home of a babysitter or relative.

Does your child live in or regularly visit a house built before 1978 with recent or ongoing renovations or remodeling (within the past 6 months)?

Does your child have a sibling or playmate who has or has had lead poisoning?

Follow-up of Positive Screens

Children whose blood lead screening test is <10 μg/dL at 1 year of age should be screened again at 2 years of age. If there is a change in the child's potential exposures or if the parent or primary care provider is concerned that the child is at heightened risk, the child should be screened again before 2 years of age. If, at the 2-year screen, the blood lead level is again <10 μg/dL and the child's potential exposures have not increased, the child need no longer be screened. Children with blood lead levels of ≥10 μg/dL should undergo a confirmatory diagnostic test using a venous sample. Table 6-9 lists the recommended time frames for confirmation, based on the screening test results.

CHILDREN WITH BLOOD LEAD VALUES OF 10–19 μG/DL

If the venous blood lead test confirms that the child has an elevated blood lead level, then the parents are counseled on ways to minimize ongoing exposure (Table 6-4). To date, there is no evidence to show that those recommendations to parents whose children have blood lead

levels in this range are effective in reducing blood lead levels. Recommended activities, however, are believed to be innocuous and relatively easy to accomplish and seem likely to have a beneficial effect on children's blood lead levels. Children with blood lead levels between 10 and 14 μg/dL should be retested every 3 months; those with levels between 15 and 19 μg/dL should be retested every 2 months.

Table 6-9

Schedule for Diagnostic Testing of Children with Elevated Blood Lead Levels on Screening Tests

SCREENING TEST RESULT (μG/DL)	PERFORM DIAGNOSTIC TEST ON VENOUS BLOOD WITHIN
10–19	3 mo
20–44	1 mo to 1 wk[a]
45–59	48 hr
60–69	24 hr
>69	Immediately as an emergency laboratory test

[a] The higher the screening blood lead level, the more urgent the need for a diagnostic test.

SOURCE: From the Centers for Disease Control, 1997.

CHILDREN WITH BLOOD LEAD VALUES OF 20 TO 44 µG/DL

Children with blood lead levels in this range are described as having moderately elevated blood lead levels. Children with blood lead levels of 20 µg/dL or higher require both medical and environmental intervention. If the confirmatory venous lead level is 20 µg/dL or more, the following interventions are indicated: a medical evaluation, consisting of a detailed medical, nutritional, developmental, and environmental history and a physical examination; a laboratory evaluation of the child's iron status, including hematocrit and mean corpuscular volume (MCV) and either ferritin or iron and iron-binding capacity; an environmental inspection and, where indicated, environmental intervention to diminish or curtail further environmental exposure to lead; and case management to assure that the needed counseling and medical, nutritional, and environmental interventions are provided in a timely and effective fashion.

The medical evaluation is done to identify signs or symptoms of lead poisoning, which would be very unusual at this level. The developmental assessment is conducted to see if the child is developmentally delayed and in need of early intervention services, although it is very unlikely that blood lead levels in this range would result in demonstrable delays using regularly employed developmental screening tests. Which developmental tests are best remains unclear. Delays or concerns about inattention and hyperactivity should result in referral for early intervention services. Nutritional assessment is conducted to identify eating patterns that may result in increased absorption of lead from the gastrointestinal tract, such as iron deficiency, low calcium intake, or infrequent meals. Many children with blood lead levels in this range will be found to be eligible for the Supplemental Food Program for Women, Infants, and Children (WIC) and should be referred for help. If the child is iron deficient, he or she should receive iron supplements.

Such children require home inspections, usually performed by local public health departments, to identify sources of a child's lead exposure. The primary care clinician also should ask about the child's primary residence and other places where the child spends significant amounts of time; hobbies and occupations of family members that might result in exposure; and other sources of potential exposure, such as glazed pottery, folk remedies, or cosmetics. *Abatement of lead-based hazards and subsequent dust control are the cornerstones of treatment for children with blood lead levels in this range.* As noted elsewhere in this chapter, parents should be counseled to have lead-based paint abatements performed by a properly licensed contractor and, if possible, with supervision of the local health department; to relocate children and pregnant women to another site while abatement is being done; and to thoroughly clean up dust before allowing children to reinhabit the home.

Medical treatment of children with blood lead levels in this range with chelating agents continues to be the subject of controversy. *The use of chelating agents for children with blood lead levels <25 µg/dL is not indicated.* For children with blood lead levels in the range of 25 to 44 µg/dL, the 1991 CDC guidelines suggested using the $CaNa_2EDTA$ challenge test to determine whether chelation therapy is indicated. This test is performed by administering a single dose of 500 mg/m^2 $CaNa_2EDTA$ intramuscularly or intravenously and collecting the child's urine over the next 8 hours. The test result is considered positive if the ratio of the child's urine lead (in micrograms) to $CaNa_2EDTA$ (in milligrams) is ≥0.6.

The 1997 CDC guidelines do not mention the challenge test, and some authorities have raised concerns that a single dose of this drug might actually increase brain lead levels. Others have questioned this concern because it is based on one study using rats who received a much higher dose of $CaNa_2EDTA$ than is used with children in the challenge test. Children with positive challenge test results who have blood lead levels in this range can be treated with any of the four chelating agents described in the next section. Primary care clinicians should seek consultation with clinicians experienced in lead-toxicity treatment when considering a $CaNa_2EDTA$ challenge test or chelation therapy. Children with blood lead levels in this range should have blood lead tests every month to week (the higher the blood lead level, the more frequently the child should be tested).

CHILDREN WITH BLOOD LEAD VALUES OF 45 μG/DL AND HIGHER

The clearest management strategies exist for children in this category. Children with blood lead screens of 45 to 59 μg/dL should have venous blood retested within 48 hours, those with levels of 60 to 69 μg/dL should be retested within 24 hours, and those with blood lead levels of >70 μg/dL should have venous blood lead level screening on an emergency basis. *There is broad consensus that such children must be removed from sources of lead in their environments and receive chelation therapy.*

Chelation therapy consists of the administration of one of four medications that join to lead in the child's body. The resultant compound is then excreted, either via urine or bile, thereby reducing the child's body burden of lead. Each of the four chelating agents has certain advantages and disadvantages, side effects, and many unanswered questions associated with them. The following limitations of chelation therapy should be noted:

- Chelation cannot repair or reverse neurologic damage.
- Chelation does not reduce brain lead levels and may actually increase them.

- Chelation is expensive and potentially dangerous.
- Chelation is not effective if the child returns to a lead-infested environment.

The most widely used chelating agent is $CaNa_2EDTA$, which must be given intramuscularly or intravenously. $CaNa_2EDTA$ does not cross the blood-brain barrier and works largely by attaching to lead that is in the intravascular space. It usually is given in 5-day courses, either as twice-daily intramuscular injections or continuously via the intravenous route, with regular checks on the child's urine and some other measure of kidney function (since this therapy can be nephrotoxic). Most clinicians are reluctant to use it continuously for more than 5 days because of concern about its nephrotoxicity. Intramuscular injections of this medication are very painful, and so the medication is mixed with lidocaine to minimize pain.

At the end of the 5-day course, there are a number of approaches available to the clinician to determine whether the child needs additional chelation. In some centers the final 8 to 12 hours of urine production during the 5-day chelation cycle are collected and analyzed, similarly to the way in which $CaNa_2EDTA$ provocative tests are analyzed, as described earlier. If the results of these analyses suggest that the child still has elevated body stores of lead, the clinician may decide to give another 5-day course of chelation with $CaNa_2EDTA$ or to place the child on an oral chelating agent, described later herein.

An alternative strategy is to follow the child's blood lead level closely over the next 6 months to 1 year. If it rises above 45 μg/dL again, the child receives another course of $CaNa_2EDTA$. In situations where children have had blood lead levels in excess of 45 μg/dL, serial evaluations of the FEP were found to be very useful. If the child continues to be exposed to environmental sources of lead, the FEP will remain elevated or continue to rise. In contrast, if the environmental exposures have been greatly reduced, the FEP will gradually decline over a course of many months. FEP testing is an especially useful clinical adjunct, since $CaNa_2EDTA$ does not cross the blood-brain barrier and largely leaches lead in blood. Thus, 1 to 3 weeks after chelation with this agent, many children will experience a rebound in their blood lead levels, often due to reequilibration of lead that results from some lead moving from the boney compartment to the blood.

The other parenteral chelating agent is British Anti-Lewisite (BAL), which is reserved for children with evidence of acute encephalopathy or venous blood lead levels of 70 μg/dL or more. Oral chelators consist of penicillamine and dimercaptosuccinic acid (DMSA). These agents are relatively new, and much information is still needed about them. In general, they appear to reduce blood lead levels initially by about 70%. Blood lead levels then bounce back up, so that within 2 weeks of stopping treatment, children's blood lead levels are approximately 70% of pre-treatment values.

Recommendations for Primary Care Clinicians

Recommendations for primary care clinicians are contained in Table 6-10. Pediatric clinicians should incorporate lead screening into their practice routines based upon the epidemiology of lead poisoning in their communities. Clinicians can consult state and local health departments for epidemiologic information and screening recommendations. In low-prevalence areas, screening can consist of a short questionnaire, with blood lead sampling restricted to those children whose parents respond "yes" or "not sure" to any question. In areas with a higher prevalence of older housing or where 12% or more of children have blood lead levels of 10 μg/dL or higher, universal screening at ages 1 and 2 years is recommended. Clinicians should be familiar with follow-up and intervention recommendations for children with elevated

Table 6-10

Role of Child Health Care Providers in Childhood Lead Poisoning Prevention

Use and disseminate information from state and local public health agencies.
Give anticipatory guidance.
Perform routine blood lead screening, as recommended.
Interpret blood lead values for parents.
Provide diagnostic and follow-up testing for children with elevated blood lead levels.
Provide family education regarding nutritional and environmental ways to reduce children's blood lead levels.
Provide medical treatment when indicated.
Refer child and family to local health department when environmental evaluation and management are indicated.
Participate in a follow-up team.
Collaborate with public health agencies.

SOURCE: Adapted in part from the Centers for Disease Control and Prevention, 1997.

lead levels. They should also know the available public and private resources in the community for case management and lead abatement.

The primary care clinician is often the only source of information for high-risk families, and he or she needs to be able to provide information on nutritional and environmental ways to reduce children's lead levels. In many areas elevated lead levels are a condition reportable to the local health department. Clinicians should comply with this requirement, since it helps in delineating high-risk areas and situations and can avail families of resources to assist them. It is essential for the primary care clinician to recognize the social and environmental aspects of lead poisoning and not think of it or its management exclusively in medical terms. This requires collaboration with many community agencies, including health departments, social services, housing authorities, WIC, and early intervention services. Attention to screening and family counseling, coupled with collaboration with nonmedical child health experts and medical subspecialists will provide children and families with the comprehensive array of services that this problem demands.

Common Errors to Avoid

The most common error made by clinicians is not screening for lead poisoning. As mentioned earlier, many high-risk children are not being screened for their lead levels. A second common error is to perform a finger-stick sampling incorrectly, leading to falsely elevated results from surface lead contamination. Common causes of contamination include not using gloves when collecting the specimen, using alcohol wipes with lead-based ink, inadequate cleansing of the child's finger, and failure to wipe off the first drops of blood.

Other errors made frequently include not confirming an elevated capillary lead level with a venous sample, not providing advice to fami-

lies on how to minimize the risks of lead exposure, and not utilizing local resources for environmental evaluation and management.

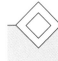

Emerging Approaches to Screening, Diagnosis, Treatment, and Prevention

There are a number of strategies currently being tested for utility in the screening, diagnosis, treatment, and prevention of childhood lead poisoning.

Screening

Many states will soon implement targeted screening programs, which should provide useful information about the effectiveness of such an approach. Portable machines may allow for rapid and accurate testing in clinicians' offices and in the community.

Diagnosis

X-ray fluorimeter machines that measure bone lead content are available for research purposes. They give a good estimation of total body lead stores but are far too expensive for clinical use at present. This technology should advance and become more widely available.

Treatment

A large multicenter study of the effects of oral chelators on cognitive development is under way and will provide needed information about the utility of such agents.

Primary Prevention

The Department of Housing and Urban Development and the Environmental Protection Agency are evaluating a variety of environmental approaches to the primary prevention of childhood lead poisoning and improved abatement methods.

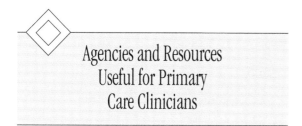

Agencies and Resources
Useful for Primary
Care Clinicians

Many federal agencies have lead-related responsibilities, including the Environmental Protection Agency, the Department of Housing and Urban Development, and the Consumer Product Safety Commission. The CDC, however, offers guidance for state and local public health officials on lead-related activities and is likely to be the federal agency with the most useful information for primary care clinicians. Most clinicians will benefit by referring to CDC publications but will not need to directly contact the CDC. In contrast, state and county health departments often have lead-prevention programs and offer substantial expertise in preventing and managing childhood lead poisoning. If a clinician's state or local health department does not have such a program, the respective department's Maternal and Child Health or Environmental Health divisions are likely places to find useful expertise. Within medical centers, academic generalists or hematologists or metabolic specialists within departments of pediatrics usually have expertise in childhood lead poisoning. *It is not recommended that primary care clinicians attempt to treat children with chelating agents without consultation from experts in childhood lead poisoning.*

Bibliography

Agency for Toxic Substances and Disease Registry: *The Nature and Extent of Lead Poisoning in Children in the United States: A Report to Congress, 1988.* Atlanta, GA, US Department of Health and Human Services, 1988.

American Academy of Pediatrics, Committee on Environmental Health. Lead poisoning: From screening to primary prevention. *Pediatrics* 92:76–183, 1993.

American Academy of Pediatrics, Committee on Drugs: Treatment guidelines for lead exposure in children. *Pediatrics* 96:155–160, 1995.

American Academy of Pediatrics, Committee on Environmental Health: Screening for elevated blood lead levels. *Pediatrics* 101:1072–1078, 1998.

Aschengrau A, Beiser A, Bellinger D, Copenhafer D, Weitzman M: The impact of soil lead abatement on urban children's blood lead levels: Phase II results from the Boston Lead-In-Soil Study. *Environ Res* 67:125–148, 1994.

Aschengrau A, Beiser A, Bellinger D, Copenhafen D, Weitzman M: The impact of residential lead-based paint hazard remediation and soil lead abatement among children with mildly elevated blood lead levels. *Am J Public Health* 87:1698–1702, 1997.

Bellinger D, Dietrich KN: Low-level lead exposure and cognitive function in children. *Pediatr Ann* 23:600–605, 1994.

Campbell J, McConnochie K, Weitzman M: Lead screening among high risk urban children: Are the 1991 CDC guidelines feasible? *Arch Pediatr Adolesc Med* 148:688–693, 1994.

Campbell JR, Schaffer SJ, Szilagyi P, O'Connor KG, Briss P, Weitzman M: Screening for elevated blood lead practices among United States' pediatricians. *Pediatrics* 98:372–377, 1996.

Centers for Disease Control and Prevention: *Preventing Lead Poisoning in Young Children: A Statement by the Centers for Disease Control.* Atlanta, GA, US Department of Health and Human Services, 1991.

Centers for Disease Control and Prevention: *Screening Young Children for Lead Poisoning: Guidance for State and Local Public Health Officials.* Atlanta, GA, US Department of Health and Human Services, Public Health Service, 1997.

Glotzer D, Weitzman M: Commonly asked questions about childhood lead poisoning. *Pediatr Ann* 24: 630–639, 1995.

Harvey B. Should blood lead screening recommendations be revised? *Pediatrics* 93:201–204, 1994.

Lanphear BP, Byrd RS, Auinger P, Schaffer SJ: Community characteristics associated with elevated blood lead levels in children. *Pediatrics* 101:264–271, 1998.

Lanphear BP, Weitzman, M, Eberly S: Racial differences in environmental exposures to lead. *Am J Public Health* 86:1460–1463, 1996.

Lanphear BP, Weitzman M, Yakir B, et al: The relation of lead-contaminated house dust and blood lead levels among urban children. *Am J Public Health* 86:1416–1421, 1996.

Lanphear BP, Winter NL, Apetz LJ, Eberly S, Weitzman M: A randomized trial of the effect of dust control on children's blood lead levels. *Pediatrics* 98:35–40, 1996.

National Research Council: *Measuring Lead Exposure in Infants, Children, and Other Sensitive Populations.* Washington, DC, National Academy Press, 1993.

Needleman HL, Gatsonis CA: Low-level lead exposure and the IQ of children. *JAMA* 263:673–678, 1990.

Schaffer SJ, Kincaid MS, Endres N, Weitzman M: Lead poisoning risk determination in a rural setting. *Pediatrics* 97:84–90, 1996.

Schaffer SJ, Szilagyi PG, Weitzman M: Lead poisoning risk determination through the use of a standardized questionnaire. *Pediatrics* 93:159–163, 1994.

Schwartz J: Low-level lead exposure and children's IQ: A meta-analysis and search for a threshold. *Environ Res* 65:42–55, 1994.

United States General Accounting Office: *Medicaid: Elevated Blood Lead Levels in Children.* Washington, DC, General Accounting Office/Health, Education and Human Services Division-98-78, 1998.

Weitzman M, Aschengrau A, Bellinger D, Jones R, Hamlin JA, Beiser A: Lead contaminated soil abatement and urban children's blood lead levels: Results of a randomized environmental trial. *JAMA* 269:1647–1654, 1993.

Weitzman M, Glotzer D: Lead poisoning. *Pediatr Rev* 13:461–468, 1992.

Franklin Desposito

Newborn Screening

Introduction

Newborn screening for metabolic and other diseases is now mandated in some form by every state in the United States. While there is some variation state to state in the specific conditions for which screening is performed, the universal acceptance of newborn screening attests to the benefits that result from newborn testing and preventive therapy. The purpose of newborn screening programs is to identify disorders in which early recognition and intervention can eliminate or reduce the morbidity and mortality that would otherwise result. Newborn screening systems have been established to facilitate specimen collection, laboratory analysis, follow-up contact, and treatment. Primary care clinicians need to be familiar with these programs to explain these tests to their patients' parents or caretakers, encourage participation in the program, interpret abnormal results, and facilitate treatment and referral of newborns who are discovered to have one of these conditions.

Scope of Newborn Screening

The system of universal newborn screening has five components: screening tests, follow-up and referral of newborns with positive results, diagnosis, disease management, and program evaluation. It is designed to respond to general federal and state mandates to give all children with special needs, particularly those in traditionally underserved populations, access to effective treatment and appropriate care in a timely and cost-effective manner. Newborn screening systems vary from program to program, depending upon state statutory and regulatory structures. All states, as well as Puerto Rico, the U.S. Virgin Islands, and the District of Columbia, now screen newborns for phenylketonuria (PKU) and congenital hypothyroidism. More than 40 programs screen for hemoglo-

binopathies and galactosemia. Still other programs include congenital adrenal hyperplasia, homocystinuria, maple syrup urine disease (MSUD), biotinidase deficiency, tyrosinemia, cystic fibrosis, and toxoplasmosis. (See Table 7-1 on page 118–119, for a listing of state screening requirements as of fall 1998.)

Newborn screening is a preventive public health procedure that should be available to all neonates. There are approximately four million births per year in the United States and approximately 370,000 per year in Canada. Because the numbers to be screened are so large, even if a relatively small percentage of babies are excluded, a significant number of infants will be missed. For example, if 5% of the neonatal population in Canada and the United States were not screened during a 1-year period, there would be 14 or more children with undetected PKU (13 in the United States and one in Canada) and some 43 with undetected congenital hypothyroidism (40 in the United States and three in Canada).

Limitations of Newborn Screening Programs

Confirmation of positive newborn screen test results is always necessary. A positive test does not always mean that a particular disorder is present. The necessary confirmatory tests are discussed in the following sections.

Moreover, newborn screening programs should not preclude the primary care clinician's assessment of clinical symptoms at any age. False-negative test results can crop up for a variety of reasons. Some disorders (e.g., galactosemia and MSUD) might become symptomatic before the availability of the results of newborn screening and could warrant specific testing when they are clinically suspected. Some infants with disorders included in the newborn screening battery will be missed, even when properly screened, owing to individual or biological variations. Although the primary care clinician cannot be held responsible for these problems, he or she must recognize that any child with a negative newborn screening test result can still be affected by one of these disorders. The primary care clinician should trust his or her clinical judgment, even in the face of a normal newborn screening report, and should carry out appropriate diagnostic testing when indicated by clinical signs and symptoms.

In addition, some infants may not be screened or may be inadequately screened. Clinicians should be knowledgeable about the procedures used in their state programs and need to be aware of inadequately screened infants (i.e., those born prematurely, those who have received blood transfusions, those who were born out of state or out of the country, and those who underwent testing too early). Under such circumstances, follow-up testing might be required for certain infants even if the newborn screening results are negative.

It is recommended that the screening status of all patients be entered into the medical record (e.g., on a flowchart such as that used for recording immunization status). Unfortunately, some states do not report negative results directly to the primary care clinician, particularly if he or she is not the clinician of record during the infant's neonatal stay. Instead, reports are sent to the hospital of birth and not necessarily to the clinician, making transfer of such information highly variable from state to state and institution to institution. Many states have developed or are in the process of developing a direct electronic system or telephone call-in system, whereby these results can be obtained easily. In many instances, however, a direct and easily accessible system is not in place and may require time-consuming efforts on the part of the office staff to obtain a hard copy of the newborn screening results.

Even so, clinicians should still recognize the need for careful documentation of newborn screening results on each patient entering the practice for the purpose of comprehensive care. This documentation on patients who transfer between practices should be easily accessible in the records sent to the new practice. Newborn screening is a standard procedure that should be performed on each patient in the practice. It is analogous to immunizations, and the results should be recorded in a similar fashion, perhaps on the well-baby flowcharts along with immunization status. Documentation in this manner will assure that patients are not missed because of administrative oversights.

General Recommendations

The American Academy of Pediatrics has suggested four goals and 18 recommendations regarding newborn screening.

Goal 1: The primary care clinician should be recognized as a key but certainly not the only component in the newborn screening system.

- An adequate neonatal screening program involves not only the laboratory but also education of clinicians, health care providers, families, and the lay public.
- The primary care provider is an important component of the five-part system of disease prevention (Table 7-2, page 120).
- The clinician should inform the parents or caretakers of abnormal results, rapidly initiate and facilitate follow-up testing until a definitive diagnosis is established (either confirmed or ruled out), recommend expert consultation and long-term management, and enhance communication between the newborn screening program, the expert consultants, and the family.
- The responsibility for transmission of screening test results should rest with the authority (state agency) that performed the test.
- When a patient enters a practice for comprehensive care by birth or transfer, the clinician should evaluate clinical signs and symptoms

Table 7-1
Newborn Screening by States as of October 1998

STATE	PHENYLKE- TONURIA	HYPOTHY- ROIDISM	GALAC- TOSEMIA	MAPLE SYRUP URINE DISEASE	HOMO- CYSTIN- URIA	BIO- TINIDASE DEFICIENCY	CYSTIC FIBROSIS	ADRENAL HYPER- PLASIA	TYROSIN- EMIA	TOXO- PLAS- MOSIS	HEMO- GLOBIN- OPATHY
Alabama	X	X	X					X			X
Alaska	X	X	X					X			X
Arizona	X	X	X	X	X	X					X
Arkansas	X	X	X								X
California	X	X	X								X
Colorado	X	X	X			X	X				X
Connecticut	X	X	X	X	X	X		X			X
Delaware	X	X	X	X		X					X
District of Columbia	X	X	X	X	X						X
Florida	X	X	X					X			X
Georgia	X	X	X	X	X	X		X	X		X
Hawaii	X	X	X	X		X		X			X
Idaho	X	X	X	X		X			X		
Illinois	X	X	X	X		X		X			X
Indiana	X	X	X		X						X
Iowa	X	X	X					X			X
Kansas	X	X	X								X
Kentucky	X	X	X								X
Louisiana	X	X	X								X
Maine	X	X	X	X	X						A
Maryland	X	X	X	X	B	X			B		X
Massachusetts	X	X	X	X	X	X		X		X	X
Michigan	X	X	X	X		X		X			X
Minnesota	X	X	X			X		X			X
Mississippi	X	X	X								X
Missouri	X	X	X				A				
Montana	X	X	X								
Nebraska	X	X	X			X					X

State											
Nevada	X	X	X			X					X
New Hampshire	X	X	X	X	X					X	A
New Jersey	X	X	X								X
New Mexico	X	X	X	X		X					X
New York	X	X	X	X	X	X					X
North Carolina	X	X	X					X			X
North Dakota	X	X	X					X			X
Ohio	X	X	X		X						X
Oklahoma	X	X	X								X
Oregon	X	X	X	X		X					X
Pennsylvania	X	X	X	X							X
Rhode Island	X	X	X	X	X	X		X			X
South Carolina	X	X	X					X			X
South Dakota	X	X	X								A
Tennessee	X	X	X					X			X
Texas	X	X	X					X			X
Utah	X	X	X								
Vermont	X	X	X	X	X	X		X			X
Virginia	X	X	X	X	X	X					X
Washington	X	X	X					X			X
West Virginia	X	X	X								A
Wisconsin	X	X	X			X	X	X			X
Wyoming	X	X	X			X	X				X
Puerto Rico	X	X	X	X	X	X					X
Virgin Islands	X	X	X			X					X
Total Count	53	53	49	21	15	22	4	19	3	2	49

A, by specific physician request—selected population; B, performed only on second screen at 2 wk of age.

Table 7-2

Five-Part System of Disease Prevention Through Newborn Screening

Screening:	Universal testing of neonates
Follow-up:	Rapid retrieval and referral of screen-positive neonates for confirmatory testing
Diagnosis;	Confirmation or denial of a positive screening test result
Management:	Rapid implementation and long-term planning of therapy
Evaluation:	Validation of testing procedures, efficiency of follow-up and intervention, and benefit to the patient, family, and society

and, if indicated, carry out appropriate diagnostic testing regardless of the initial test results or whether the results of such initial screening can be ascertained.

- The screening status (both positive and negative) should be entered into the patient's record and preferably documented by a hard copy of the results.

Goal 2: There should be total participation of all newborns in the screening program.

- A blood specimen should be obtained from every neonate before the baby is discharged or transferred from the nursery, regardless of the nature or status of the infant's feeding or age.
- Younger siblings of children previously diagnosed with one of the disorders on the screening panel have an increased risk of that disorder and, therefore, deserve special attention so that the appropriate diagnostic test can rapidly determine whether or not the newborn is affected. A specimen should also be sent for the complete routine screening battery, since this infant is at the same risk as the general population for one of the other screened disorders.
- A specimen should be obtained for screening of any premature infant, any infant receiving parenteral feeding, or any neonate being treated for illness, at or near the seventh day of age if a specimen has not been obtained before that time (preferably 48 to 72 hours

after feeding started), regardless of feeding status.

- The clinician should recognize those patients who are at substantial risk of not being screened and take particular care to document that appropriate screening is performed. Examples of the latter include infants born at home, children of transient or homeless families, infants transferred within or between hospitals, and those undergoing adoption. If screening cannot be documented, then the clinician should obtain a specimen for screening, even if the infant is beyond the neonatal period.

Goal 3: An adequate specimen should be provided to the designated laboratory for analysis.

- The specimen should be obtained as close as possible to the time of discharge from the full-term well neonate and in no case later than 7 days of age.
- Cord blood is not adequate for detection of PKU or other disorders with metabolite accumulation after birth.
- If an infant requires transfusion or dialysis before the routine time for acquisition of the newborn screening specimen, and if the clinical status of the newborn permits, it is optimal to obtain the sample for screening before transfusion or dialysis. If a sample cannot be obtained before dialysis or transfusion, the clinician should then ensure that an adequate second specimen is obtained at the appropri-

ate time, when the plasma and/or red blood cells will again reflect the child's own metabolic process or phenotype. In instances of blood transfusion, this may be as long as 6 to 8 weeks for red blood cell analytes (e.g., homoglobinopathies and galactosemia).

- If the initial specimen is obtained before 24 hours (see note on early discharge), a second specimen should be obtained at 1 to 2 weeks of age to minimize the probability that PKU and other disorders with metabolite accumulation will be missed as a consequence of testing on the first day of life. Data also indicate that 6% to 12% of patients with congenital hypothyroidism show normal results on the initial screening test and abnormal results on a second test.

Goal 4: Systematic follow-up and treatment should be a part of the comprehensive newborn screening program.

- Confirmatory testing is a mandatory step in the laboratory follow-up and diagnosis of disorders detected through newborn screening. With rare exceptions (galactosemia and MSUD), patients should not be started on treatment until a diagnostic specimen has been obtained. Prompt physical examination is a part of newborn screening and takes particular priority in the case of such life-threatening disorders as galactosemia, MSUD, and congenital adrenal hyperplasia.
- The primary care clinician should be aware of the local resources, including expert consultation and comprehensive programs available for both the initial and long-range management of these complex disorders. Primary care providers should consider referral to a comprehensive metabolic center, pediatric endocrinologist, or pediatric hematologist to aid in establishing the diagnosis and providing long-term specialty care. It remains important that all infants have a medical "home" for general health maintenance, able to provide continuing patient and family con-

tact and educational information even when treatment is being administered through a metabolic center or by an expert specialist.
- The evaluation of the efficacy of detection and treatment of these disorders requires routine follow-up and good communication at regular intervals between the state screening laboratory, the newborn screening follow-up personnel, and the expert consultants and comprehensive centers. Clinicians should assist health authorities in the acquisition of data necessary for systematic program and outcome evaluation.
- The primary care provider's role and position of trust with the family gives this clinician a unique ability to educate the family regarding the disorder and to assist the family in obtaining needed services (e.g., dietary foods, registration with state programs, access to support groups and other families, genetic counseling services) and in assuring and monitoring compliance with recommended and ongoing therapies.

Practical Considerations

Collecting the Specimen

Newborn screening blood samples are generally collected by capillary heel stick. Care should be taken to collect the specimen properly to prevent contamination and to ensure a specimen adequate for testing. Recommendations for specimen collection are listed in Table 7-3.

Laboratory Methods

Historically, newborn screening systems in the United States have relied mainly on the use of the Guthrie spot (bacterial inhibition assay) for sample collection and analysis. Such procedures

Table 7-3

Instructions for Capillary Heel-stick Specimen Collection

The infant's leg and foot should be placed lower than the heart in order to increase the blood supply to the foot.

To increase blood flow further, the heel can be covered by a warm, moist towel. Use a temperature no greater than 42°C to avoid burning the skin.

Clean the puncture side with 70% isopropanol alcohol. Wipe away excess alcohol with sterile gauze. Allow the skin to dry.

The puncture site should be the medial or lateral one-third of the plantar surface of the heel.

Use a sterile lancet with a point no longer than 2.4 mm.

Wipe away the first drop of blood with sterile gauze. Allow a second large drop to form.

With the blotter below the foot, touch the filter paper gently against the blood drop, allowing it to soak and fill one preprinted circle.

Avoid pressing the paper against the foot.

Avoid squeezing the puncture site.

Avoid applying layering (applying successive drops to the same circle).

Fill all required circles.

Apply pressure to the puncture site until bleeding stops.

depend on identification of the accumulation of a marker metabolite (e.g., phenylalanine) for a positive screening test result. Several manufacturers now supply automated methods for screening for the disorders previously tested by the Guthrie bacterial inhibition assay. Such techniques involve automated fluorimetric testing, enzymatic methodologies, and multiplex methods that make it possible to determine many analytes in a single procedure using the filter paper blood spot. Some new tests are based on a nonradioactive immunoassay that allows for the diagnosis of hypothyroidism, congenital adrenal hyperplasia, and cystic fibrosis. The use of tandem mass spectrometry, currently available in several state and other diagnostic laboratories, permits the rapid quantitation of amino acids and organic acids, which can enlarge the number of metabolic disorders recognized by this methodology.

Early Hospital Discharge

With the trend toward early hospital discharge and the collection of specimens for screening when the newborn is younger than 24 hours, concerns have arisen regarding the reliability of the assay results in pinpointing all infants with these disorders. Many newborn screening tests rely on time-dependent changes in the concentration of an analyte in blood to identify the congenital condition. The conference Early Hospital Discharge: Impact on Newborn Screening came to several conclusions, reflected in the following consensus recommendations. First, the initial newborn screening specimen should be collected from all infants as close as possible to the time of discharge from the nursery and in no case later than 7 days of age. If the initial specimen for newborn screening is collected before 24 hours of age, a second specimen should be collected before 2 weeks of age. Finally, all newborns should have a primary care provider designated before discharge, to ensure prompt and appropriate follow-up of newborn screening results. Additional monitoring of the true incidence of false-positive and false-negative test results in samples obtained before 24 hours of age and the development and assessment of technical strategies to increase sensitivity of testing were also recommended. Clinicians should be aware of current practices in their community and state with regard to discharge before 24 hours of age, timeliness of obtaining second specimens, and follow-up of test results.

Mandatory Second Screens

Nine states (Alabama, Delaware, District of Columbia, Maryland, Nevada, New Mexico, Oregon, Texas, and Utah) require that newborn screening specimens be taken a second time. These states report a second-screen compliance rate of about 80% to 90%. The time at which the second test is required varies from 1 to 4 weeks. Data from the 1994 National Newborn Screening Report (the latest national report available) indicate that of approximately one million infants who underwent a second screening, eight with classic PKU (representing 4% of the total confirmed PKU cases for that year), 83 (or 7%) with primary congenital hypothyroidism, one with classic galactosemia, and 26 with variant forms of galactosemia (11.5%) were detected. At present, many programs are weighing the cost and health benefit ratios involved in mandatory second screens.

Informed Consent

Our knowledge base regarding newborn screening is expanding rapidly, and there are numerous areas of controversy. The Committee on Assessing Genetic Risks of the Institute of Medicine has recommended that ongoing newborn

screening programs be reviewed periodically, preferably by an independent body that is authorized to add, eliminate, or modify existing programs. Furthermore, the committee advocated that all programs assure that necessary treatment and follow-up services be provided to affected children identified through newborn screening, without regard to ability to pay.

Although no clear consensus of the committee was forthcoming regarding informed consent for newborn screening, such consent was strongly endorsed as an integral part of newborn screening, including disclosure of the benefits and risks of the test and treatments. It was also advocated that information unrelated to the health of the individual (e.g., carrier status and paternity) might be disclosed by such testing. For established tests in which patients would clearly benefit from early diagnosis and treatment (e.g., PKU, congenital hypothyroidism), it was thought appropriate for state departments of health to mandate the offering of such testing. A minority view, expressed by several committee members, was that all testing be universally mandated. In accordance with state and institutional guidelines, a consent form, along with an educational brochure, is usually provided by most hospitals to the parents at the time of delivery; ideally, this could be supplied before the delivery of the infant in a prenatal setting.

Almost all states mandate newborn screening, with provisions for informed refusal by parents. Unfortunately, the information provided to the parents about the risks and benefits of newborn screening is often minimal. Most states are in the process of upgrading and reevaluating their educational parental material. In some states special procedures and forms are required if the parents refuse testing. Primary care clinicians should ensure that parents understand in full the risks of not screening their infants. It is recommended that clinicians have parents who decide against screening sign a document that indicates they understand these risks. The waiver document should be placed in the infant's medical record.

Cost

Newborn screening entails substantial costs, some of which are inherent in the screening process. All abnormal test results trigger a cascade of diagnostic and sometimes therapeutic interventions, with associated economic costs, parental anxiety, and potential for iatrogenic side effects. As more conditions are considered for universal newborn screening, psychologic and economic costs loom large, even given an acceptable 1% to 3% false-positive level for each screening test performed. This is a particular concern when the benefit of early detection of affected children may not be clear. Nevertheless, the conclusion that newborn screening for a selected group of treatable devastating disorders has a favorable cost-benefit ratio compared with long-term treatment of persons not identified and treated seems reasonable. On the other hand, such a cost-benefit analysis completely ignores the cost in human terms of not identifying and treating these conditions.

The costs for newborn screening vary and are generally cited as the initial fees for neonatal testing in a state or regional laboratory. Historically, program costs of $1 to $2 for specimen handling, administration, and overhead have been ascribed to PKU alone. Charges for patients range from no fee to $50. These charges may not cover the total system cost for repeated and confirmatory testing (additional in some states), education, patient and clinician notification and contact, follow-up of affected patients, and treatment (e.g., the cost of special dietary supplements). Neither are the charges necessarily related to the number of disorders included in the screening program.

Disorders Identified Through Newborn Screening Programs

Information is provided in some detail for the following five conditions: PKU, congenital hypothyroidism, galactosemia, hemoglobinopathies, and MSUD. Less detailed information is provided on six disorders that are screened for in less than half of the state programs; homocystinuria, biotinidase deficiency, congenital adrenal hyperplasia, tyrosinemia, cystic fibrosis, and congenital toxoplasmosis. A summary of the information on each disorder is listed in Table 7-4.

Phenylketonuria

PKU is an autosomal recessive disorder of phenylalanine hydroxylation leading to the accumulation in the blood of the amino acid phenylalanine. Phenylalanine is an essential amino acid that is present in dietary protein. It is normally converted to tyrosine by the enzyme phenylalanine hydoxylase and the cofactor tetrahydrobiopterin. Classic PKU results in blood phenylalanine levels of more than 20 mg/dL. Other causes of hyperphenylalanemia (blood levels of 4 to 20 mg/dL) include liver damage, mutation of the phenylalanine hydroxylase gene, cofactor disorders, and transient conditions of prematurity.

NATURAL HISTORY WITHOUT SCREENING

While classic PKU is not lethal, without treatment 95% of those affected will have severe mental retardation and other symptoms, including hyperactivity, spasticity, seizures, eczema, a

Table 7-4

The Most Common Disorders Identified Through Newborn Screening Programs

CONDITION	ANALYTE TESTED	INCIDENCE	OUTCOME IF NOT TREATED	TREATMENT
Phenylketonuria	Phenylalanine	1:10,000–1:25,000	Severe mental retardation	Low phenylalanine diet
Congenital hypothyroidism	T₄ with TSH confirmation	1:3600–1:5000	Mental retardation, other brain damage, growth delay	Thyroid hormone (L-thyroxine)
Galactosemia	GALT, total galactose	1:60,000–1:80,000	Death	Galactose-free diet
Sickle cell disease and hemoglobinopathies	Hemoglobin types	Varies among ethnic groups; sickle cell disease, 1:375 in blacks	For sickle cell disease, lifelong hemolytic anemia and a variety of complications stemming from increased propensity to infection and vasoocclusive episodes	Early comprehensive care, prophylactic penicillin, aggressive diagnosis and treatment of infections, other treatments (see text)
Maple syrup urine disease	Leucine	1:250,000	Death	Diet low in branched-chain amino acids

ABBREVIATIONS: TSH, thyroid stimulating hormone; GALT, galactose-1-phosphate uridyltransferase.

peculiar mousey odor, and autistic-like behavior. Some milder forms of hyperphenylalanemia may not adversely affect intelligence. The disease is rarely diagnosed before 6 months of age and usually only after mental retardation becomes obvious. Because of universal newborn screening, PKU may not be considered in the differential diagnosis of an infant with progressive developmental delay.

OUTCOME WITH SCREENING AND TREATMENT

The treatment of PKU is dietary restriction of phenylalanine. A special formula of amino acids, excluding phenylalanine, with supplemental tyrosine is necessary, along with a carefully planned diet to prevent other nutritional disorders. Frequent laboratory monitoring is needed to ensure that phenylalanine is maintained at a safe level. Specialized teams of nutritionists and specially trained physicians are necessary for optimal treatment. A treatment and follow-up guideline used at our PKU center is given in Table 7-5. Treatment should be started as soon as the diagnosis is made and needs to be maintained indefinitely. Late treatment will not reverse mental retardation but may lead to some improvement in behavior control. Cofactor disorders need to be identified early, because dietary restriction alone will not prevent progressive neurological deficits. These infants need additional therapy.

INCIDENCE

The incidence of PKU is 1:10,000 to 1:25,000 in the United States; 1:20,000 for classic PKU, and 1:16,000 for clinically significant hyperphenylalanemia. There is considerable racial and ethnic variability. Rates that have been documented include 1:6000 in Ireland and Scotland, 1:10,000 in Germany, 1:16,000 in Italy, 1:20,000 in U.S. Hispanics, 1:6000 among Yemenite Jews, 1:60,000 in Ashkenazi Jews, 1:60,000 in native Chinese and Japanese, and 1:90,000 in African Americans.

Table 7-5

Classic Phenylketonuria Treatment Guidelines

Management by experienced physician, metabolic or clinical geneticist, nutritionist, genetic counselor, and psychoeducationalist
Immediate dietary therapy and supplemental tyrosine
Monitoring of plasma amino acids, growth development, and diet with adjustment of changing Phe/Tyr needs
First year follow-up
  Regular visits to treatment centers
  Weekly Phe and Tyr levels for the first month
  Biweekly to triweekly levels for the first 2 yr of life, trying to maintain Phe at <6 mg/dL
Ages 2–7 yr
  Monthly Phe and Tyr levels
  Regular nutritional evaluations
Ages 7–10 yr
  Quarterly Phe and Tyr levels
  Nutritional evaluations
10 yr and older
  Biannual Phe and Tyr levels
  Nutritional evaluations
  Transition of dietary responsibilities to patient as adulthood approaches

ABBREVIATIONS: phe, phenylalanine; Tyr, tyrosine.

SCREENING TEST

PKU is screened by measuring the blood phenylalanine level using a dried blood spot. The cutoff level in most states for an abnormal test is 4 mg/dL. Some states use a cutoff level of 2 to 3 mg/dL. The test should be performed 24 hours after birth and before 5 days. Infants screened before 24 hours should be rescreened by 2 weeks of age. Some experts believe retesting is indicated if the first test is performed before 48 hours. The test is 90% sensitive using a cutoff of 4 mg/dL, if performed at 24 to 48 hours, and 99.85% sensitive after 48 hours. False-positive rates are 1:3300 using a 4 mg/dL cutoff and 1:1000 using a 2 mg/dL cutoff. If the disease incidence is 1:15,000, the positive predictive value would be 17% with the 4 mg/dL cutoff and 6% with the 2 mg/dL cutoff. Workup of abnormal tests should include serum phenylalanine to confirm the elevated level, serum tyrosine to rule out hepatic causes of hyperphenylalaninemia, and urine and serum pterins to diagnose cofactor disorders.

Congenital Hypothyroidism

Congenital hypothyroidism results from inadequate production of thyroid hormone, which may be due to a number of factors: agenesis or ectopic thyroid gland (85% of congenital hypothroidism), genetic disorders of thyroid hormonogenesis (10% to 15% of cases), or defects of the pituitary or hypothalamus (called secondary or tertiary hypothyroidism, <5% of cases). Infants who are not identified and treated promptly have mental retardation and variable degrees of growth failure, deafness, and neurologic abnormalities as well as classic hypometabolic symptoms of hypothyroidism. Inheritance is sporadic. Disorders of thyroid hormonogenesis may be inherited as autosomal recessive traits. Thyroid hormone transport defects may be X-linked, with a male/female ratio of 3:1.

NATURAL HISTORY WITHOUT SCREENING

The fetal hypothalamic-pituitary-thyroid axis begins to function by midgestation and is mature in the full-term infant. If fetal hypothyroidism develops, untoward effects may be noted in the central nervous system and skeleton. Most infants with congenital hypothyroidism appear normal at birth, however. The hypothyroid fetus is partially protected by placental transfer of maternal thyroid hormone; the T_4 levels in cord blood of an athyroid fetus are approximately one-third of maternal levels. Undetected hypothyroidism results in mental retardation and other neuropsychological problems. The mean IQ is 80, and 20% of children have an IQ less than 55. Other findings include poor growth, delayed bone age, goiter, low metabolic rate, constipation, poor peripheral circulation, bradycardia, and myxedema. More than 95% of infants with sporadic hypothyroidism show such minimal signs at birth that the diagnosis is missed.

OUTCOME WITH SCREENING AND TREATMENT

Treatment involves administration of levothyroxine at a dose to produce a T_4 concentration in the upper half of the normal range. It should be started in the first few weeks of life to prevent retardation of intellectual function and bone growth. Growth and development must be monitored at monthly intervals, with frequent laboratory evaluations of thyroid hormone levels to prevent poor achievement associated with low levels (e.g., inadequate dosage and noncompliance) and behavioral problems associated with high levels. Consultation and follow-up with a pediatric endocrinologist is advisable.

Results from studies of treatment have been contradictory. The New England Congenital Hypothyroidism Collaborative Study showed normal IQ, visual motor integration, and neuropsychological profiles when compared with controls. A Quebec study showed normal developmental quotients, but the test scores were significantly lower than for sibling controls; no growth or physical abnormalities were noted. An Ontario study also showed intelligence within the normal range, but the children had cognitive and neuromuscular impairment that seemed to reflect the severity and time of onset of thyroid hormone deficiency. An initial T_4 screening level of less than 50 μmol/L was predictive of a lower IQ score in a Netherlands study. There appears to be good correlation between outcome and time of treatment,

treatment adequacy, and compliance with treatment. Some studies have suggested that low thyroid hormone levels, agenesis of the thyroid gland, and evidence of fetal hypothyroidism are associated with poor outcome in some cognitive areas because of in utero effects.

INCIDENCE

Congenital hypothyroidism in the United States has an incidence of 1:3600 to 1:5000. The incidence is lower in African American populations (1:17,000 in Georgia and 1:10,000 in Texas) and most prevalent among Hispanics (1:2700) and American Indians (1:700). In Japan the incidence is 1:5700, and in Sweden it is 1:7000. Thyroxine-binding globulin deficiency occurs at a rate of 1:10,000 and hypothalamic pituitary hypothyroidism at a rate of 1:50,000.

SCREENING TEST

The screening test for congenital hypothyroidism is assessment of the serum T_4 level; this is followed by evaluation of the thyroid-stimulating hormone (TSH) levels among those with the lowest 5% to 10% of T_4 test results. Both tests are conducted from dried blood spot specimens on filter paper. This method detects both primary hypothyroidism (low or low normal T_4 with high TSH) and thyroxine-binding globulin deficiency or hypothalamic-pituitary hypothyroidism (low to low normal T_4 with normal TSH). The sensitivity of this method depends on the T_4 level used as a cutoff. Testing the bottom 20% of T_4 levels results in a sensitivity of better than 90%. Ten percent of cases of congenital hypothyroidism, however, are detected at a second screening at 2 to 6 weeks or because of symptoms. This may be due to errors in screening methods, a later appearance of some forms of the disease, or both. False-positive rates also vary by test and cutoff used, with an average of four to eight false-positive results for every true positive (positive predictive value of 11% to 20%). False-positive tests are more likely in the

first 24 to 48 hours of life, when TSH levels are higher. Workup of positive screens should consist of a complete history (including mother's thyroid status and medications) and physical examination and a serum measurement of TSH and T_4. Once hypothyroidism is confirmed, consultation with or referral to a pediatric endocrinologist is recommended. Immediate evaluation and treatment are needed. There is controversy concerning the role and value of thyroid scanning. Table 7-6 lists a clinical guideline used by some specialists.

Table 7-6

Guidelines for Workup and Treatment of Confirmed Hypothyroidism

History, physical, lab evaluation of thyroid-binding globulin, thyroid antibodies
Iodine 123 or technetium 99 thyroid scans to evaluate the presence or absence and location of thyroid tissue
Perchorate washout—rapid washout suggests an organification defect
Thyroid ultrasonography to look for nodules
Bone age to assess severity of intrauterine hypothyroidism
Discuss initial developmental, psychological, and educational issues with family
Begin treatment with crushed tablet of L-thyroxine in liquid, 12.5 mcg/kg/day by mouth (not less than 37.5 mcg/day for term infants).
Repeat assessment and T_4 level at 2 wk.
Assessments at 3-mo intervals during the first 2 yr of life, 6-mo intervals from 2 to 10 yr, and yearly in adolescents, with adjustment of T_4 dose to achieve a level in the upper quartile for age and suppression of TSH
Bones ages at 12 and 24 mo and 2-yr intervals thereafter
Formal development assessments at 12 and 24 mo, at preschool age, and periodically thereafter while in school

Galactosemia

Galactosemia is an autosomal recessive disorder that results in elevated levels of blood galactose. It can be caused by a deficiency in any of three enzymes in the galactose catabolic pathway. Deficiency of galactose-1-phosphate uridyltransferase (GALT) is the cause of classic galactosemia. Some variants, such as the Duarte variant, which has 50% of normal erythrocyte transferase activity, have higher enzyme activity and less severe clinical symptoms.

NATURAL HISTORY WITHOUT SCREENING

The disease is usually fatal if it is unrecognized. Symptoms appear in the first 2 weeks of life and include jaundice, vomiting, lethargy, hepatosplenomegaly, cataracts, and failure to thrive and positive non-glucose urine reducing substances. Death is the result of liver failure, sepsis, or bleeding. Survivors suffer cognitive and developmental disabilities.

OUTCOME WITH SCREENING AND TREATMENT

Some infants die of the disease before screening results are available, because of a susceptibility to *Escherichia coli* sepsis. The treatment is a galactose-free diet started as soon as possible and continued through life. Galactose is a product of lactose metabolism, and for this reason lactose must also be avoided. Some variants require a less restrictive diet. Even with early treatment, the mean IQ of those affected is at the low end of the normal range; the intellectual range is wide, however, and includes normal levels. The IQ seems to be dependent on the time of treatment, with best results obtained when treatment is started before 10 days of age. Visual-perceptual, speech, and other learning disabilities are common. The majority of treated females have ovarian failure, with hypergonadotropic hypogonadism and primary and secondary amenorrhea.

INCIDENCE

Galactosemia occurs in 1:60,000 to 1:80,000 newborns and in 1:16,000 for variant forms. There has not been any racial or ethnic variability in these rates

SCREENING TEST

Two tests are available. Some states screen for total galactose (looking for high levels); others test for GALT enzyme activity (looking for low levels). GALT enzyme can be measured at any time, but galactose needs to be measured after milk ingestion. Newborns who have had transfusions may have a false-negative GALT enzyme tests for 2 to 3 months. False-positive test results can stem from improper specimen handling because of the instability of GALT in heat. Abnormal galactose test results can also be caused by a large milk feeding immediately before specimen collection.

The sensitivity and specificity of these tests are not fully known. False-negative results appear to be rare in classic galactosemia and more common in variant forms; they occur more frequently in hot summer months. With a disease as rare as galactosemia, even extremely low false-positive rates will result in far more false positives than true positives. Owing to the short time frame in which to act, however, positive tests should be treated as an emergency, with immediate consultation with a metabolic center for diagnostic testing and treatment. Workup of positive screens should include quantitative measurement of galactose and galactose-1-phospate and electrophoresis for transferase activity. Results of these tests are interpreted in Table 7-7. Nonlactose formula should be substituted during the workup.

Sickle Cell Diseases and Hemoglobinopathies

These are a group of genetic disorders of red blood cells that involve inherited defects of the ß-globin chain of adult hemoglobin. Most are

Table 7-7

Test Results for Confirmation of Galactosemia

	CLASSIC GALACTOSEMIA	VARIANT GALACTOSEMIA	*Not* GALACTOSEMIA
GALT enzyme activity	0% to 5% of control	5% to 20%	>25%
RBC Galactose-1-Phosphate Transferase	>10 μg/dL	1.5–10 μg/dL	<1μg/dL
Genotype	G/G	G/? or G/D	D or unknown, with one normal allele
Diet	Restrict	Restrict	Reinstitute normal diet and repeat lab tests 2–4 wk after normal diet; reassure if normal.

ABBREVIATIONS: GALT, galactose-1-phosphate uridyltransferase; RBC, red blood cell; G, galactosemia; D, Duarte variant.

autosomal recessive disorders that result in single amino acid substitutions. Those with one abnormal gene (heterozygotes) have a hemoglobin trait and are carriers. Those with two abnormal genes (homozygotes or compound heterozygotes) have the disease. Sickle cell disease is caused by two sickle genes (Hbss or sickle cell anemia), or one gene for sickle hemoglobin and one for hemoglobin C (hemoglobin SC), or one gene for sickle hemoglobin and one for β thalassemia (sickle β thalassemia). Sickling disease can also be caused by hemoglobin S in combination with other abnormal hemoglobin (C$_{harlem}$, D, E, O). Thalassemias result from impaired synthesis of globin chains. Newborns with ∂ thalassemia and with β thalassemia major are not detected by most screening.

NATURAL HISTORY WITHOUT SCREENING

Affected individuals with sickle cell diseases (SS, SC, or Sβ thalassemia) have lifelong hemolytic anemia with acute and chronic tissue damage stemming from the blockage of blood flow produced by the abnormally shaped red cells. Additional clinical manifestations include episodic vasoocclusive crises, functional asplenia, sepsis, infections, splenic sequestration, and bone marrow aplasia. Symptoms become evident at about 6 months of age as fetal hemoglobin is replaced by adult hemoglobin. Sickle cell disease can be lethal, especially in early infancy or childhood, as the result of overwhelming sepsis or splenic sequestration (10% mortality rate). Previous indications of reduced life span in adults are being reevaluated in light of more aggressive and careful management; current predictions indicate an 85% chance that infants with HbSS will survive to 20 years of age.

Cerebrovascular accidents (stroke) or side effects of meningitis can lead to neurologic deficits. Aseptic necrosis of bones, leg ulcers, priapism, neuroproliferative retinopathy, serious infections, cerebral thrombosis, renal concentrating defects, and delayed growth and sexual maturation are common. Clinical symptoms of other hemoglobin diseases vary. Homozygous hemoglobin C and E cause mild anemia. Homozygous hemoglobin E produces microcytosis. Thalassemia causes microcytic, hypochromic anemia. Those who are heterozygote carriers of abnormal hemoglobin usually have no clinical problems.

OUTCOME WITH SCREENING AND TREATMENT

Treatment for sickle cell diseases includes penicillin prophylaxis, 125 mg PO bid, started by 2 months of age for children with sickle cell anemia and sickle β thalassemia; prompt medical evaluation, including appropriate cultures and parenteral antibiotics (e.g., ceftriaxone), for all significant febrile illnesses (>101°F); prompt medical evaluation for signs and symptoms of splenetic sequestration; and routine immunizations plus pneumococcal vaccine at 2 and 5 years of age. Other treatments, including red cell transfusion, are based on clinical course and need. Education and genetic counseling should be provided to parents, and overall medical treatment should be undertaken in consultation with a comprehensive sickle cell center or a pediatric hematologist.

Guidelines for specific management of sickle cell events (e.g., painful crisis, infants with fever, stroke prevention) and newer therapies (e.g., hydroxyurea, long-term transfusion with its attendant iron overload, cord blood or stem cell transfusions, and bone marrow transplantation) are under evaluation. There is evidence that

with screening, penicillin prophylaxis, and heightened vigilance, early death and morbidity from overwhelming sepsis can be significantly decreased. Death from acute splenetic sequestration and aplastic crises can be prevented or minimized. Disability can be diminished by aggressive treatment of infection, dehydration, and stroke. Long-term clinical outcomes of patients identified by newborn screening programs are unclear. Since carriers are asymptomatic, there is no clear benefit to detecting them by screening other than to provide potentially useful genetic information to parents to use for planning subsequent pregnancies and to pass on to the child as she or he grows into adulthood. Potential harm from carrier identification includes stigmatization, loss of confidentiality, discrimination in the workplace, problems with insurability, and potential identification of nonpaternity.

INCIDENCE

In the United States, live-born African American infants have the following rates of sickle cell disease: HbSS, 1:375; HbSC, 1:835; and HbSβ thalassemia 1:1667. Among newborns who are not African American in California, New York, and Texas, HbSS has an incidence of 1:40,000 to 1:60,000. While sickle cell diseases are most commonly found in persons of African ancestry, it is also seen in persons of Mediterranean, Caribbean, Central and South American, Arabian, and East Indian ancestry. The incidence of sickle cell diseases in Hispanic populations from eastern states is 1:1100, in Hispanics from western states is 1:32,000, in Asians is 1:11,500, and in American Indians is 1:2700.

SCREENING TEST

Screening is performed on cord blood or a dried heel-stick blood spot. The specimen can be obtained at any time after birth. The test is isoelectric focusing, which involves identifying individual hemoglobin bands by their migration in an electrophoretic field. It is highly accurate, with a sensitivity of 100% and a false-positive rate of 1:3000. Specificity has been 100% in some programs. Confirmation of abnormal screens is required to adequately diagnose hemoglobinopathy. This calls for repeated electrophoresis. Several laboratory methods are available. Common electrophoresis results are listed in Table 7-8, along with suggested actions for primary care clinicians.

Maple Syrup Urine Disease

MSUD is a rare autosomal recessive disorder with several phenotypes ranging from mild to severe. It is characterized by decreased or absent activity of branched-chain ketoacid decarboxylation, resulting in high levels of leucine, isoleucine, and valine in blood, urine, and spinal fluid. Several different allelic variants have been described, which vary in clinical severity, age at onset, clinical symptoms, and thiamine responsiveness. The classic form has

Table 7-8

Results of Hemoglobin Electrophoresis and Suggested Actions

COMMON LAB RESULTS[a]	LIKELY CAUSES	PRIMARY CARE CLINICIAN SUGGESTED ACTIONS
FA	Normal	None
FS	Sickle cell anemia or sickle β thalassemia	Immediate confirmatory test by at least 2 mo of age
FSC	Sickle hemoglobin C disease	Immediate confirmatory test by at least 2 mo of age
FSA	Sickle β thalassemia or sickle cell anemia after blood transfusion	Immediate confirmatory test by at least 2 mo of age
FC	Homozygous hemoglobin C	Confirmatory test at 2 mo of age
FU (no A)	Possibilities include homozygous hemoglobin E or hemoglobin E-β thalassemia	Confirmatory test at 2–4 mo of age
FAS	Sickle cell trait (rarely, sickle β thalassemia or sickle cell[b] anemia after blood transfusion)	Confirmatory test at 2–4 mo of age
FAC	Hemoglobin C trait	Confirmatory test at 2–4 mo of age
F only	Premature infant or β thalassemia major	Confirmatory test at 2 mo of age
AF (predominantly A)	Transfused infant or normal infant	If transfused[b], repeat test 3–4 mo after last transfusion; if not transfused, result is normal.

[a] Hemoglobins are reported in order of quantity (e.g., FSA = F>S>A).
[b] DNA testing for the S mutation will be helpful.
ABBREVIATIONS: F, fetal hemoglobin; U, unidentified; C, hemoglobin C; S, sickle hemoglobin; A, adult hemoglobin.
SOURCE: Adapted from *Newborn Screening Practitioner's Manual*, 2d ed. Davidson A, Chair Newborn Screening Committee of the Mountain States Regional Genetic Service Network, Mountain States Regional Genetic Services Network, 1996, Denver, CO.

severe early onset, continuous branched-chain amino acid urinary excretion, and 0% to 2% of normal substrate oxidation. One intermittent form is triggered by protein stress (high protein intake) and intermittent branched-chain amino acid excretion, with 2% to 40% of normal substrate oxidation. Another intermediate form is associated with ataxia and mental retardation but not ketoacidosis, mild constant urinary branched-chain amino acid excretion, and 5% to 25% of normal substrate oxidation. The thiamine-responsive form is usually milder and of later onset and is characterized by recurrent ataxia and, occasionally, developmental delay. Such patients show constant branched-chain amino acid excretion, no ketoacidosis, and about 40% of normal substrate oxidation.

NATURAL HISTORY WITHOUT SCREENING

Symptoms develop shortly after birth with the ingestion of protein and include poor feeding, irritability, vomiting, and acidosis. The odor of the urine is characteristic. Symptoms progress to include lethargy and coma, and the classic form of disease is fatal within the first month.

OUTCOME WITH SCREENING AND TREATMENT

All deaths cannot be prevented. Death within the first 2 weeks is not uncommon, and about one-third of infants die before dietary intervention can be instituted. Reported deaths have occurred at older ages despite therapy. The age and presence of neurologic symptoms at the time of diagnosis or institution of therapy, as well as adequacy of continued control, affect outcome. Sadly, treated patients frequently have irreversible retardation. Although approximately 30% of more recently reported treated patients have IQs higher than 90, the outcome is related to the time between the onset of symptoms and therapy. The best outcomes have been achieved in second affected newborns in identified families when treatment is initiated promptly after birth.

The outcomes of treated patients are available only for the classic form. Additional data are needed to evaluate the outcomes of other genetic variants detected by newborn screening programs. Screening programs require immediate retrieval of positive test results and rapid diagnosis and treatment of affected infants. Treatment involves restriction of branched-chain amino acids and requires frequent monitoring that must be continued indefinitely, with individual titration of protein intake. A metabolic nutritionist and specially trained physician must coordinate care, and immediate referral is indicated.

INCIDENCE

In mixed populations MSUD occurs in 1:250,000 newborns. The highest incidence documented has been in the Mennonite population, at 1:760. It appears to be more common in African and Asian populations.

SCREENING TEST

Screening involves measuring blood leucine levels from a dried blood spot. Normal levels are <4 mg/dL. Prematurity and receipt of IV amino acid preparations can cause false-positive results. The test can be performed at any time, since elevated leucine levels are present within 4 hours regardless of diet. To improve the outcome, the test must be performed early, and results must be available within 2 weeks. Sensitivity appears to be close to 100%, although it is not known if milder variant forms are detected. There is limited information on the rates of false-positive results. Any positive or borderline test result is a neonatal emergency. Immediate referral to a specialized center is indicated. A decision tree for borderline and high screening results is described in Figure 7-1.

Other Conditions

The following six conditions are part of newborn screening programs in less than half of all

Figure 7-1

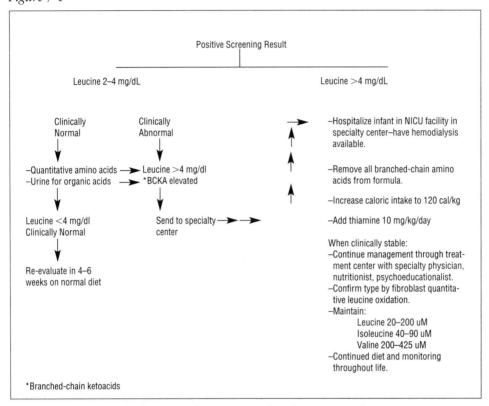

Example of decision tree for diagnosis and management of maple syrup urine disease.

states. A brief summary of these disorders and their screening characteristics is provided in Table 7-9.

HOMOCYSTINURIA

This is an autosomal recessive disorder of methionine metabolism, leading to elevated blood levels of methionine and urine levels of homocysteine. The incidence is 1:80,000 to 1:150,000. The screening test involves measuring blood methionine levels. The false negative rate is higher in the newborn period, and the test is preferably performed at 2 to 4 weeks. False-positive results occur in approximately 1:5000 infants who have transient elevations in methionine levels. The disease causes developmental delay, marfanoid features, optic lens displacement, arterial and venous thrombosis, seizures, and psychiatric disorders in childhood. Treatment calls for large doses of vitamin B_6 in pyridine-responsive cases and methionine-restricted, cystine-supplemented diet in others. Aspirin is used to prevent thromboembolic disease. The value of early detection by screening is unclear, but early treatment appears to lower the risk of thromboembolism.

BIOTINIDASE DEFICIENCY

Biotinidase deficiency is another autosomal recessive disorder. It results in a shortage of biotin, an essential cofactor in several enzyme systems. The incidence is approximately 1:100,000 in the United States. The onset of symptoms varies from 2 weeks to 3 years, and symptoms include seizures, skin rash, hair loss, optic atrophy, ataxia, hearing loss, developmental delay, and metabolic acidosis, which can result in coma and death. The screening test detects low levels of biotinidase activity. The optimal timing of the test is unknown, but test sensitivity appears to be good right after birth. The treatment is oral biotin, which, if given early enough, results in normal growth and development. If treatment is instituted after neurological damage, further harm can be prevented, but mental retardation, hearing loss, and optic atrophy will not be reversed.

CONGENITAL ADRENAL HYPERPLASIA

This is a family of defects in the enzymes of the adrenal cortex needed in the synthesis of corticosteroids. The most common form, accounting for more than 90% of defects, is 21-hydroxylase deficiency. The incidence is 1:12,000, and inheritance is autosomal recessive. Congenital adrenal hyperplasia causes masculinization of female genitalia, early virilization in boys, early-accelerated growth, and premature fusion of epiphyses. Of major concern are those newborns who have a defect in their ability to synthesize aldosterone, who can die in the neonatal period from shock caused by salt wasting. The screening test is immunoassay measurement of 17-hydroxyprogesterone. Test sensitivity is high after 24 hours, but testing will miss 3% of cases if performed earlier. False-positive results range from 0.29% to 0.5%, depending on the cutoff level chosen. Treatment is corticosteroids and mineralocorticoids, which diminish mortality and morbidity.

TYROSINEMIA

Neonatal tyrosinemia results from elevated blood levels of tyrosine. It is an autosomal disorder with two types; type 1, or tyrosinosis, and type II. Type I clinical features range from mild retardation to acute failure to thrive, vomiting, diarrhea, liver disease, and death from liver failure. Chronic type I is characterized by chronic liver disease, renal dysfunction, and rickets. In type II, liver and renal functions are normal. This form of the disease results in corneal lesions and hyperkeratosis. These are autosomal recessive disorders that to date have been detected mainly in Caucasian populations at rates of 1:12,000 (French-Canadians) to 1:100,000 (Scandinavians). It is not clear whether early detection with newborn screening affects outcomes. Treatment is dietary restriction of protein.

TOXOPLASMOSIS

Congenital toxoplasmosis is a protozoan infection that can result in blindness and mental retardation. Most infected newborn infants have no symptoms at birth, but by 20 years of age, as many as 85% of affected individuals have chorioretinitis, including many who were free of symptoms at birth. The incidence is 1:8000 to 1:12,000 births. Fetal infection occurs only when pregnant women contract an acute infection. In the first trimester there is a 17% transmission rate to the fetus, with more severe resulting disease. If infection is acquired in the last two trimesters, the transmission rate is 65%, but the disease is mild or unapparent at birth. The screening test is an IGM-specific enzyme-linked immunosorbent assay from filter paper specimens. Sensitivity is 75%; there are two false-positives for every one true positive. Treatment includes pyrimethamine, sulfadiazine, and spiramycin. The effectiveness of early detection and screening is not firmly established; early results suggest improved outcomes.

Table 7-9
Other Disorders That Are Part of Newborn Screening Programs

Disorder	Incidence in the United States	Disease Characteristics	Expected Benefits of Newborn Screening (i.e., Presymptomatic Diagnosis)	Screening Test	Confirmation	Interventions
Homocystinuria	1:80,000–150,000	65% developmental delay/mental retardation Marfanoid habitus Optic lens displacement Arterial/venous thrombosis Psychiatric disturbances	Clinical variability despite treatment Reduction in mental neurologic, eye changes and thromboembolic phenomena have been cited.	Methionine levels >2 mg/dL	Quantitative serum amino acids Methionine >100 μM Homocysteine >15 μM Absence of urinary methylmalonic acid	Requires a metabolic center 50% are pyridoxine responsive Methione-restricted cystine-supplemented diet Aspirin to prevent thromboembolic disease
Biotinidase deficiency	1:100,000	Profound deficiency (<10% activity) Myoclonic seizures Hypotonia Developmental delay Organic acidemia Seborrhea, atopic dermatitis, alopecia Acute metabolic decompensation	Limited follow-up. All treated patients have remained asymptomatic.	Biotinidase <10% = affected; 10% to 30% = partial deficiency	Colorometric or radioimmune assay	Biotin 10–20 mg/day
Congenital adrenal hyperplasia	1:12,000	Increased androgen production with adrenocortical insufficiency Masculinization of female genitalia 75% with salt-losing syndrome Somatic and sexual precocity	Avoid shock from salt wasting Correct sex identification Eliminate problems of masculinization, precocious puberty, accelerated growth, and decreased fertility in affected girls	17-hydroxy-progesterone	Quantitative measurement of 17 hydroxy-progesterone >100 μg/ml, >40 μg/ml with presence of virilization of genitalia in a female	Pediatric endocrine consultation Glucocorticoids Mineralocorticoid therapy for salt wasting

Tyrosinemia Type I—Tyrosinosis	1:100,000	Ranges from mild retardation and speech delay to acute failure to thrive and death from liver failure, hepatocarcinoma, renal tubular acidosis with hypophosphatemic rickets	Tyrosine >6 mg/dL	Insufficient data Decrease in early mortality and liver failure Long-term developmental outcomes less clear	Ion exchange chromatography tyrosine >200 μm Urine succinyl-acetone >1,000 IU/ml	Requires metabolic center Dietary restriction of protein Liver transplantation for type I
Toxoplasmosis	1:8,000–1:12,000	Most infants considered normal in newborn period; over time in those with clinically apparent disease before age 1 yr. 90% chorioretinitis 50% convulsions 85% mental retardation 60% neurologic complication: cerebral calcification, hydrocephaly or microcephaly, spasticity 15% deafness	IgM-specific enzyme-linked immuno-sorbent assay test	Prematurity and stillbirths will not be prevented. Preliminary studies suggest reduction in neurologic sequelae and eye findings to less than 10% with treatment.	Serologic testing of mother and infant	Treatment regimens include combinations of pyrimethamine, sulfonamides, and spiramycin
Cystic Fibrosis	Caucasians, 1:3300 Hispanics, 1:9000 African Americans, 1:15,000 Asian Americans, 1:32,000	Pancreatic insufficiency Chronic obstructive lung disease Recurrent pulmonary infections Failure to thrive Mean life span of about 30 yr	Immunoreactive trypsinogen (IRT) >140 μg/mL	Earlier recognition may provide better nutrition and growth. more aggressive treatment of pulmonary disease.	IRT elevation *plus* DNA testing *plus* sweat test	Pancreatic enzyme replacement Fat-soluble vitamins Pulmonary and antibiotic therapy Management in a cystic fibrosis center

CYSTIC FIBROSIS

Cystic fibrosis is an autosomal recessive disorder of exocrine function that can first appear in the neonatal period in the form of meconium ileus or later as growth retardation, malabsorption, and pulmonary disease. The severity varies, with death occurring, on average, between ages 20 and 40 as a result of lung disease and infection. There is a 13% mortality rate among neonates and infants. The incidence varies by ethnic groups, with about 1:3300 Caucasians, 1:9000 Hispanics, and 1:15,000 African Americans affected. The screening test uses a dried blood spot to measure for elevated immunoreactive trypsinogen. The test is performed in the neonatal period and has 95% to 97% sensitivity. There are 12 false-positives for every one true positive in some populations. Treatment is a predigested formula, vitamin supplements, pancreatic enzyme replacement, bronchodilator therapy, and aggressive treatment of lung infections. Benefit from early detection through screening has not been proved, although improved nutritional status and lessened pulmonary complications have been reported. There is some concern that children whose test results are false-positive and their families may be harmed and that false-negative test results may cause clinicians to dismiss consideration of cystic fibrosis later in symptomatic children.

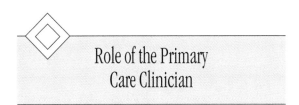

Role of the Primary Care Clinician

The role of the primary care clinician is to ensure that all neonates are tested, inform parents of abnormal results and explain the applications, initiate follow-up testing of abnormal results, refer to experts as needed, and order diagnostic tests on newborns and infants, regardless of screening test results, if evaluation indicates a possible abnormality.

Common Errors

The most common errors committed by primary care clinicians include neglecting to discuss newborn screening with parents, neglecting to document test results, failing to order a second test when needed, and assuming that a negative test result means there is no disease.

NOT DISCUSSING NEWBORN SCREENING WITH EXPECTANT PARENTS

Since newborn screening is conducted in the hospital, it is out of sight and often out of the minds of primary care clinicians. When expectant parents are not advised about newborn screening tests and their importance, they can be unprepared to make an informed decision if consent is required postpartum.

NOT DOCUMENTING RESULTS

It is important that the medical record of every newborn contain the results of the newborn screening tests. Keeping a record ensures that the tests were performed at the right time and that the results were documented. This documentation helps assure testing of those at high risk. Test results are frequently sent to hospitals rather than providers, and primary care clinicians need to institute a system to obtain them.

NOT ORDERING A SECOND TEST

The increasing proportion of newborns being discharged from the hospital before 24 to 48 hours presents a challenge to the newborn screening system. Primary clinicians often do not order second screening tests at 2 weeks when discharge takes place before 24 hours. This has led some states to implement mandatory second screening tests.

ASSUMING THAT A NEGATIVE TEST RESULT MEANS NO DISEASE

As mentioned previously in this chapter, a negative test result does not ensure lack of disease, and any newborn with suggestive signs and symptoms should undergo a complete workup to rule out possible metabolic disease or hemoglobinopathies. Clinicians can incorrectly assume that a negative newborn screening result rules out the metabolic disorder tested for.

Emerging Trends in Newborn Screening

Ongoing studies will better define and lead to improvement in test sensitivities and specificities and, in the case of unproven screening tests, will clarify whether early detection actually leads to improved outcomes. New screening technologies, such as tandem mass spectrometry, will expand the number of disorders that are candidates for newborn screening. Some of these disorders are listed in Table 7-10.

Technical and clinical resources are necessary to expand newborn screening programs, including laboratories, equipment, and personnel. Standardization and communication are crucial. It is critical that the rapidity of follow-up, diagnosis, and treatment of the screen-positive newborn remain appropriate, effective, and seamless. Tracking and treatment of more disorders will require well-defined access to the necessary clinical and laboratory expertise for definitive diagnosis and ongoing care.

The value of screening for rare metabolic disorders remains unclear, particularly when the clinical signs of many of these disorders manifest in the first few days of life, usually before the results of routine newborn screening would be available. There will need to be much research to prove the benefit of screening for

Table 7-10

Conditions That Are Candidates for Newborn Screening

3-Hydroxy-3-methyl glutaryl-CoA lyase deficiency

Adenosine deaminase deficiency

Argininemia

Arginosuccinate acidemia

Citrullinemia

Duchenne muscular dystrophy

Fatty acid enzyme deficiencies

Glucose-6-phosphate deficiency

Glutaric aciduria type 1

HIV

Isovaleric acidemia

Medium chain acyl-CoA dehydrogenase deficiency

Neuroblastoma

Proprionic acidemia

additional disorders as well as cost-benefit analyses to aid difficult decisions about how best to spend prevention resources. With the rapid accumulation of knowledge of the human genome, it is likely that gene therapies will be developed for metabolic disorders, leading to prenatal diagnoses and early definitive therapy.

Bibliography

American Academy of Pediatrics: Neonatal screening for congenital hypothyroidism: Recommended guidelines. *Pediatrics* 91:1203–1209, 1993.

American Academy of Pediatrics, Committee on Genetics: Health supervision for children with sickle cell diseases and their families. *Pediatrics* 98:467–472, 1996.

Charache S, Terrin ML, Moore RD, et al: Effect of hydroxyurea on the frequency of painful crisis in sickle cell anemia. *N Engl J Med* 332:1317–1322, 1995.

Chuang DT, Shih VE: Disorders of branched-chain amino acid ketoacid metabolism, in Scriver CR, Beaudet AL, Sly WS, Valle D (eds): *The Metabolic and Molecular Basis of Inherited Disease*, 7th ed. New York, NY, McGraw-Hill, 1995, pp 1239–1279.

Committee on Assessing Genetic Risks, Division of Health Sciences Policy, Institute of Medicine. Andrews LB, Fullarton JE, Holtzman NA, Motulsky AG (eds): *Assessing Genetic Risks: Implications for Health and Social Policy.* Washington, DC, National Academy Press, 1994.

Committee on Genetics, American Academy of Pediatrics: Issues on newborn screening. *Pediatrics* 89: 345–349, 1992.

Committee on Genetics, American Academy of Pediatrics: Newborn screening fact sheets. *Pediatrics* 98:473–501, 1996.

Council of Regional Networks for Genetic Services (CORN): Early hospital discharge: Impact on newborn screening, in Pass KA, Levy HL (eds):. Atlanta, Georgia, Emory University School of Medicine, 1995.

Elias S, Annas GJ: Genetic consent for genetic screening. *N Engl J Med* 330:1611–1613, 1994.

Elsas LJ, Langley S, Steele E, et al: Galactosemia: A strategy to identify new biochemical phenotypes and molecular genotypes. *Am J Hum Genet* 56:630–639, 1995.

Farrell PM, Kosorok MR, Laxova A, et al: Nutritional benefits of neonatal screening for cystic fibrosis. *N Engl J Med* 337:963–969, 1997.

Frank JE, Faix JE, Hermos RJ, et al: Thyroid function in very low birth weight infants: Effects of neonatal hypothyroidism screening. *J Pediatr* 128: 548–554, 1996.

Gregg RG, Wilfond BS, Farrell PM, et al: Application of DNA analysis in a population-screening program for neonatal diagnosis of cystic fibrosis: Comparison of screening protocols. *Am J Hum Genet* 52:616–626, 1993.

Guerina NG, Hsu HW, Meissner HC, et al: Neonatal serologic screening and early treatment for congenital toxoplasma gondii infection. *N Engl J Med* 330:1858–1863, 1994.

Hart PS, Hymes J, Wolf B, et al: Biochemical and immunologic characterization of serum biotinidase in profound biotinidase deficiency. *Pediatr Res* 31: 261–265, 1992.

Hilliges C, Awiszus D, Wendel U: Intellectual performance of children with maple syrup urine disease. *Eur J Pediatr* 152:144–147, 1993.

Kooistra L, Laane C, Vulsma T, et al: Motor and cognitive development in children with congenital hypothyroidism: A long-term evaluation of the effects of neonatal treatment. *J Pediatr* 124: 903–909, 1994.

Lieberman ER, Gomperts ED, Shaw KN, et al: Homocystinuria: Clinical and pathologic review, with emphasis on thrombotic features, including pulmonary artery thrombosis. *Perspect Pediatr Pathol* 17:125–147, 1993.

Mitchell GA, Lambert M, Tanguay RM: Hypertyrosinemia, in Scriver CR, Beaudet AL, Sly WS, Valle D (eds): *The Metabolic and Molecular Basis of Inherited Disease*, 7th ed. New York, NY, McGraw-Hill, 1995, pp 1077–1107.

New England Congenital Hypothyroidism Collaborative. Correlation of cognitive test scores and adequacy of treatment in adolescents with congenital hypothyroidism *J Pediatr* 124:383–387 1994.

Newborn Screening Committee, Council of Regional Networks for Genetics Services (CORN). *National Newborn Screening Report 1994.* Atlanta, Georgia, Council of Regional Networks for Genetics Services, 1999.

Reuss ML, Paneth N, Pinto-Martin JA, et al: The relation of transient hypothyroxinemia in preterm infants to neurologic development at two years of age. *N Engl J Med* 334:821–827, 1996.

Rouse B, Azen C, Koch R, et al: Maternal phenylketonuria collaborative study (MPKUCS) offspring: Facial anomalies, malformations and early neurologic sequelae. *Am J Med Genet* 69:89–95 1997.

Scriver CR, Kaufman S, Eisensmith RC, et al: The hyperphenylalaninemias, in Scriver CR, Beaudet AL, Sly WS, Valle D (eds). *The Metabolic and Molecular Basis of Inherited Disease*, 7th ed. New York, NY, McGraw-Hill, 1995, pp 1015–1077.

Segal S, Berry GT: Disorders of galactose metabolism, in Scriver CR, Beaudet AL, Sly WS, Valle D (eds). *The Metabolic Basis of Inherited Disease*, 7th ed. New York, NY, McGraw-Hill, 1995, pp 967–1000.

Sickle Cell Disease Guideline Panel: *Sickle Cell Disease: Screening, Diagnosis, Management and Counseling in Newborns and Infants*: Clinical Guideline Practice 6, AHCPR publication no 93-0562. Rockville, MD, US Department of Health and Human Services, Public Health Service, Agency for Health Care Policy and Research Publication, 1993.

Van Ommen GJ, Scheuerbrandt G: Neonatal screening for muscular dystrophy: Consensus recommendation of the 14th workshop sponsored by the European Neuromuscular Center. *Neuromuscul Disord* 3:231–239, 1993.

Woods WG, Tuchman M, Bernstein ML, et al.: Screening for neuroblastoma in North America: 2-year results from the Quebec Project. *Am J Pediatr Hematol Oncol* 14:312–319, 1992.

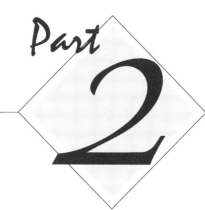

Part 2

Adolescents and Young Adults

Erica B. Monasterio
Jonathan M. Ellen

Chapter 8

Sexually Transmitted Diseases

Introduction

Adolescence and young adulthood are generally a time of good physical health. Morbidity and mortality among this age group can be linked primarily to individuals' involvement in behaviors that put their health at risk. The acquisition of sexually transmitted diseases (STDs), including human immunodeficiency virus (HIV) infection, and the morbidity and mortality associated with them are a case in point.

STDs are infections, conditions, and syndromes that are primarily though not exclusively acquired through sexual contact. These diseases are caused by viruses, bacteria, protozoa, and ectoparasites and result in not only localized genital-urinary tract infections but also systemic, and sometimes fatal, diseases and syndromes. Included among the bacterial STDs are chlamydia, gonorrhea, syphilis, bacterial vaginosis (a mixed sexually associated infection), chancroid, donovanosis, and shigellosis. Viral STDs include HIV infection, human papillomavirus (HPV) infection, herpes simplex, and hepatitis B and C (although use of blood products and use of injected drugs, not sexual contact, are the predominant modes of transmission of hepatitis C). Protozoal STDs include trichomoniasis, amebiasis, and giardiasis. The ectoparasitic diseases include scabies and pubic lice.

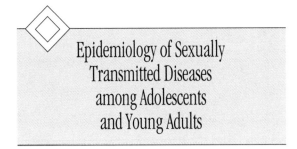

Epidemiology of Sexually
Transmitted Diseases
among Adolescents
and Young Adults

According to national prevalence data, adolescents and young adults are at higher risk for

acquiring a sexually transmitted disease than are children and older adults. These data are based on local surveillance activities and are aggregated and made publicly available by the Centers for Disease Control and Prevention (CDC) in Atlanta. These data may underestimate the true risk among adolescents. Prevalence rates are calculated as the number of reported cases per 100,000 adolescents in the United States. Because many adolescents are not sexually active, the prevalence of STDs among sexually active adolescents is higher.

National data are not available for all STDs. Diagnoses of chlamydia, gonorrhea, syphilis, and acquired immunodeficiency syndrome (AIDS), and in some states HIV are monitored and reported by the CDC. Prevalence rates of some other diseases are based on projections from smaller data sets. Herein we use the best data available to provide information about the prevalence of the various STDs.

Chlamydia

In 1995, there were 477,638 cases of chlamydia in the U. S., translating to a prevalence of 182.2 cases per 100,000 population. This case rate primarily reflects chlamydia identified through screening of women without symptoms who sought family planning services. The highest rates were reported in western and midwestern states. That a state had a markedly low rate, as did Mississippi and Arkansas, may reflect low rates of screening in states with very limited public health care dollars. There is definitely a "gender gap" in the prevalence of chlamydia. The overall rate among women (290.3/100,000) is nearly six times the rate for men (52.1/100,000). Again, this may reflect detection bias, because of the low national rates of screening of men who do not have symptoms. The prevalence of chlamydia is somewhat higher among minority youth with 15% of African Americans, 11% of Latinos, and 9% of whites with infections detected during screening of Job Corps applicants. There are no data available to describe the relation between socioeconomic status and chlamydia infection rate.

Most marked are variations in prevalence data by age. The age breakdown for the 1995 CDC surveillance data reveals 4% (2452) of the cases occurred among youths younger than 14 years, 46% (31,511) among youths 15 to 19 years of age, and 33% (22,540) among persons 20 to 24 years of age. This adds to 83% of reported instances of chlamydia occurring among persons 24 years of age or younger. Important is that the prevalence rates have decreased among all age groups over the last 10 years, including rates among women younger than 24 years.

International data on prevalence are limited because chlamydia screening programs are rare and the infection often is managed empirically without laboratory confirmation. The data that are available generally reflect rates comparable to those in the U. S., cases among adolescents and young adults constituting the bulk of infections.

Gonorrhea

Although the rates of gonorrhea have declined significantly since the peak in 1975, the rate of decline among adolescents and young adults has not come close to that for adults older than 25 years. In 1996, the highest age-specific gonorrhea rates were among girls and women 15 to 19 years of age. Young men in the same age group had the second highest age-specific rates. There has been a steady decrease in prevalence in the 1990s among male adolescents. The incidence decreased from 20.4/100,000 in 1993 to 9.9/100,00 in 1996 among boys 10 to 14 years of age (55% decline), 611.4 in 1993 to 394.3 in 1996 among boys and men 15 to 19 years of age (36% decline), and from 729.9 in 1993 to 522.4 in 1996 among men 20 to 24 years of age (28% decline). Rates among adolescent and young adult women also decreased, but not as impressively as among male adolescents and young

men. Among girls 10 to 14 years of age, the prevalence decreased from 78/100,00 in 1993 to 67.9/100,000 in 1996 (26% decline), from 851.6 in 1993 to 756.8 in 1996 among girls and women 15 to 19 years of age (11% decline), and from 629.2 to 522.9 among women 20 to 24 years of age (17% decline).

Prevalence rates by race and ethnicity are available only for Hispanics, African-Americans, and non-Hispanic Caucasians. Rates for African American youth are more than 25 times higher than rates for Caucasian youth of the same age. The reasons for this disparity are unknown. It is possible that racial and ethnic differences in access to care, probability of contact with an infected sex partner, and use of public health clinics (where STD reporting is more likely to occur) may contribute to this imbalance. There are no national data from direct studies of these factors, nor are there data on other racial and ethnic groups.

International data on the prevalence of gonorrhea are more widely available than data on chlamydia. In the developing world, rates also are markedly higher among adolescents than among adults. In industrialized nations, however, gonorrhea rates are significantly lower than in the U. S. Germany and Sweden report rates so low that the disease would probably die out without the importation of new cases from abroad.

Syphilis

Despite progress toward the elimination of syphilis in most of the developed world, the prevalence in the United States continues to be high. The highest rates for both primary and secondary syphilis occur among persons 20 to 24 years of age. After a steady national decline in cases of syphilis since the 1940s, there was a sudden and unexpected increase in the late 1980s, primarily in the southern states and among inner city residents nationwide. This surge in rates has been attributed to the so-called crack epidemic and its accompanying sexual behavior of trading sex for drugs of the late 1980s and early 1990s. Since peaking in 1990, the rate of syphilis has begun to decline slowly. The rates among persons 15 to 19 years of age dropped from 17.0/100,00 in 1993 to 6.4/100,00 in 1996. In the higher-prevalence group of persons 20 to 24 years of age, rates have dropped from 29.1 in 1993 to 10.8 in 1996.

Men have historically shown higher rates of syphilis than have women. A peak in disparity in 1970 is generally attributed to a high rate of transmission among homosexual men. With the epidemic of the 1980s (primarily representing heterosexual transmission), however, the case rate among women accelerated to the point that in 1993 six southern states reported higher syphilis rates for women than for men. Among 15 to 19 year old girls and women in 1991 the rate (35/100,000) was almost double that for their male age-mates. In the same reporting period, rates for girls 10 to 14 years of age were 5.5 times higher than those for adolescent boys of the same age.

Racial and ethnic differences in syphilis rates have persisted for the more than 50 years during which prevalence data have been collected. Even with controls for socioeconomic factors, which influence prevalence, the racial differences remain important. In 1991, the primary and secondary syphilis rates for African American boys and men 15 to 19 year of age was 11 times higher than the rate for Hispanic boys and men and 85 times higher than the rate for Caucasian boys and men of the same ages. Among African-American girls and women 15 to 19 years of age the syphilis rate increased 150% from 1986 to 1991, compared with a less than 50% increase in other racial and ethnic groups.

Since 1990, syphilis rates have decreased among all racial and ethnic groups except American Indians-Alaskan Natives. Rates of congenital syphilis, which reflects rates of syphilis among women of childbearing age who either enter late into prenatal care or do not receive any prenatal care, was 127.8/100,000 live births among African Americans, 36.4/100,000 among Latinos, and 3.2/100,000 among Caucasians. Again this disparity may be partially, but not entirely, explained by higher use of public sector clinics and hospitals, where reporting is more likely to occur by racial and ethnic minorities.

Syphilis has been almost eliminated in the rest of the industrialized world. The U.S. prevalence more closely resembles those of developing nations. Age-specific rates in the developing world are similar to those in the Untied States.

Pelvic Inflammatory Disease (PID)

Pelvic inflammatory disease is a disease of the upper reproductive tract primarily caused by gonorrhea or chlamydia, although these infections often are accompanied by co-infection with other aerobic and anaerobic bacteria. PID is not reported nationwide, is a diagnosis based on subjective clinical judgment, and often is managed on an outpatient basis. This makes prevalence data difficult to collect, and leaves us to extrapolate from hospital discharge and emergency department diagnostic data. Even with these limitations, two-thirds of reported cases of PID occur among women younger than 24 years, and most of these women are younger than 19 years. Like the infections that cause PID, prevalence data reflect a higher number of cases among noncaucasian women.

Human Immunodeficiency Virus (HIV)

National prevalence data on HIV infection among adolescents are based on extrapolation from AIDS case data, because HIV infection itself is not reportable in all jurisdictions. The CDC does report HIV infection rates for states with confidential HIV infection reporting (currently 30 of the 50 states but not New York and California, known epicenters of the HIV epidemic). Special populations at high risk for infection because of their behaviors, such as homeless or runaway youth, incarcerated youth, youth seeking services at STD clinics, and child-bearing adolescent women, have been studied to yield selective seroprevalence data, which reflect incidences higher than in the general population.

In states reporting HIV infection data, 18.2% (16,767 cases) of all new HIV infections occur among persons 13 to 25 years of age. The number of new cases among young men is almost double that among young women. AIDS case reports for 1997 showed a male to female ratio of 0.9:1 among persons 13 to 19 years of age, 1.6:1 among persons 20 to 24 years of age, and 3.8:1 among persons 25 years of age and older. Calculations based on projections of age at infection related to age at diagnosis indicate that between 1987 and 1991 25% of HIV infections were acquired by the age of 21 years.

There is an overrepresentation of minority populations in the AIDS data for adolescents. Among persons with AIDS who are 13 to 19 years of age, cumulative data through 1997 show that 36% are Caucasians, 41% African American, 21% Latino, 1% Asian-Pacific Islander, and less than 1% American Indian or Alaskan Native. New cases reported in 1997 showed an increased proportion among African Americans and Latinos and a decreased proportion among whites.

Human Papillomavirus (HPV)

Laboratory diagnosis of HPV infection by means of DNA typing is available in a few research centers, but cost and complexity of the laboratory process make it unrealistic in general practice. Diagnosis of HPV infection therefore depends on clinical identification of external genital warts and characteristic cytologic findings on Papanicolaou (Pap) smears for the identification of cervical HPV infection. In five studies in which attempts were made to calculate rates of recognizable anogenital warts

among sexually active female adolescents, rates ranged from 1% to 18%. Studies based on findings of the HPV genome in the lower genital tract of sexually active female adolescents have yielded rates of 13% to 33%. HPV is thought to be the most common viral STD among adolescents, but general adolescent population-based prevalence data are not available.

Herpes Simplex Virus (HSV)

Herpes simplex virus infection, like HPV infection, is not a reportable disease, making prevalence data difficult to obtain. Many persons with the infection do not have recognizable symptoms. In addition, the previous lack of serologic tests that could help differentiate HSV-1 from HSV-2 limited findings of past seroprevalence studies. Recent population-based serologic data with more specific tests are available from the National Health and Nutrition Examination Surveys. In this survey, investigators analyzed blood specimens from nationally representative samples of the U.S. population and included HSV-2 serologic results. In the report of HSV-2 seroprevalence rates among persons 12 to 19 years of age, female adolescents were more often infected than male adolescents and African Americans more often than Caucasians. There was a significant increase in infection between the reporting years of 1979 and 1991 among all groups. The proportion of Caucasian adolescent males infected increased from 0.5% to 4.6%, of Caucasian females from 1.3% to 4.3%, of African American adolescent males from 3.4% to 5.7%, and of African American females from 7.5% to 11.7%. This survey also showed that cumulative risk for HSV-2 increased with age.

Risk Factors

Certain specific behaviors put an individual at risk for acquisition of an STD. The most obvious risk behavior is sexual contact without the use of a protective barrier device (male condom, female condom, latex barrier for oral sexual contact). Unprotected sexual contact occurs in all age groups, however; this behavior alone cannot account for the prevalence patterns among young people. Biologic, social, and behavioral factors have been found to be associated with a higher risk for acquisition of an STD, and many of these risk factors are more prevalent among adolescents and young adults.

The biologic factors that influence disease transmission and acquisition are both host and agent related. Host factors include increased susceptibility to cervical infections among young women because of characteristics of the immature cervix. In adolescence and young adulthood, cervical ectopy is common. This is a normal variation in which the columnar epithelium, which lines the endocervical os in mature adult women, extends onto the face of the ectocervix. These cells are particularly susceptible to invasion by certain sexually transmitted organisms, and cervical ectopy has been found to be a risk factor for chlamydia and HIV infection. For men, although not specifically young men and adolescents, lack of circumcision has been associated with increased rates of STD. It has been hypothesized that the cells that line the foreskin are more prone to trauma and infection and that the foreskin "hides" genital lesions, increasing the likelihood that the lesions remain undetected. Asymptomatic infections, common with chlamydia and many viral STDs, including HIV infection, hepatitis B, genital herpes, and HPV infection, are agent factors that contribute to risk for transmission of STD. Because of lack of symptoms the infected person does not recognize the infection, seek care, or avoid transmission to others.

Earlier age at sexual debut has been associated with increased risk for STDs. With an earlier sexual debut, the person has a longer interval during which he or she can be exposed to different sexual partners. Added to this are the normative adolescent behaviors of sexual curiosity and experimentation, which often lead

to greater exposure to multiple sexual partners among sexually active adolescents. Taken together, these behaviors enhance the possibility of sexual contact with an infected partner.

Although reported condom use has increased among adolescents in the last 20 years, use is not consistent and tends to decrease with age and length of relationship. This is troublesome for disease prevention, because many STDs may be chronic and asymptomatic. Over time and with waning condom use the risk for infection may increase.

Natural History

The general category of STDs includes many diseases, each with its own natural history, recommended treatment, and sequelae. Each causative factor of an STD is presented separately. In general, however, the behaviors that put one at risk for acquisition of any one particular STD are the same as for any other. Where one STD is found there is an increased likelihood that others also may be diagnosed.

All treatment recommendations are drawn from the 1998 *Guidelines for Treatment of Sexually Transmitted Diseases,* published by the Centers for Disease Control and Prevention.

Chlamydia

Chlamydia, the most common bacterial STD, often is asymptomatic and may silently infect and scar the upper reproductive tract. Untreated this infection has the greatest repercussions for women. It causes urethritis, cervicitis, or PID, which may cause tubal factor infertility, ectopic pregnancy, and chronic pelvic pain. Men also show a high incidence of asymptomatic infections in addition to urethritis and acute epididymitis. Infants born to infected mothers may contract ophthalmia neonatorum and chlamydial pneumonia.

Because most chlamydia infections are asymptomatic, the infected population serves as a reservoir for new cases, never seeking care and unwittingly spreading the disease. The best predictor for chlamydia is age, the highest case rates occurring among adolescents and young adults.

In the treatment of chlamydia (Table 8-1) doxycycline and azithromycin are equally efficacious. Doxycycline is less expensive, but in the treatment of populations, such as adolescents, among whom treatment compliance may not be complete, it may be more cost effective to use azithromycin for single dose, observed therapy. Erythromycin is less efficacious than the recommended regimens, and the high incidence of gastrointestinal side effects may limit treatment compliance. Erythromycin is, however, safe in pregnancy. Doxycycline and ofloxacin are contraindicated in pregnancy, and the safety and efficacy of azithromycin in pregnancy have not

Table 8-1

Recommended Management of Chlamydia

RECOMMENDED REGIMENS
Azithromycin 1 g orally in a single dose *or* Doxycycline 100 mg orally twice a day for 7 days

ALTERNATIVE REGIMENS
Erythromycin base 500 mg orally four times a day for 7 days *or* Erythromycin ethylsuccinate 800 mg orally four times a day for 7 days *or* Ofloxacin 300 mg orally twice a day for 7 days

SOURCE: From Centers for Disease Control and Prevention, 1998.

yet been determined. Ofloxacin, a quinalone, is expensive, requires the same dosage as doxycycline, and is not approved for use among youth younger than 15 years.

A strong case has been made that regular screening of a population of women at risk for chlamydia will lower the incidence of PID in the population. In a randomized controlled study of chlamydia screening of members of a health maintenance organization, investigators concluded that ascertaining who was at risk, testing for chlamydia, and treating the women at increased risk for the disease were associated with a reduced incidence of PID.

Gonorrhea

Gonorrhea generally produces symptoms that provoke the infected person to seek care, although not always soon enough to prevent transmission to others. Among boys and men symptoms include purulent urethral discharge and dysuria 2 to 7 days after exposure. Among women and girls urethritis or cervicitis occurs, although often the symptoms are very mild. Among women, symptoms may not become evident until the infection has ascended to the upper genital tract and caused PID. There are also many asymptomatic infections, especially among women. With or without symptoms, gonorrhea can cause inflammation and scarring in the upper reproductive tract that lead to PID, tubal factor infertility, and ectopic pregnancy.

Infants born to mothers with gonorrhea may contract ophthalmia neonatorum, which can cause blindness and sepsis, including septic arthritis, and meningitis. Gonorrhea also can cause anal and pharyngeal infections, the latter of which can be more difficult to eradicate than anogenital infection. Some strains of *Neisseria gonorrhoeae,* found infrequently in the U. S. in the past 10 years, cause minimal genital symptoms but lead to disseminated gonococcal infection, a gonococcal bacteremia. Other complications of disseminated gonococcal infection include gonococcal meningitis and endocarditis. Clients with these complicated types of gonorrhea should be treated in the hospital with specialty consultation. Clients with uncomplicated gonorrhea can be treated on an outpatient basis.

Recommended therapies for gonorrhea are listed in Table 8-2. There is a high incidence of co-infection with chlamydia among persons with gonorrhea. For this reason, presumptive treatment of chlamydia when gonorrhea is diagnosed is recommended for populations where chlamydia testing is unavailable or for those who may not return for test results and treatment. Pregnant women should not be treated with doxycycline or quinalones but can be treated with any of the other regimens.

Syphilis

Syphilis is a complex systemic disease that untreated leads to chronic, progressive, and potentially fatal manifestations. The primary phase of the disease presents as a painless chancre at the site of inoculation on the genitalia, rectum, tongue, or lips. Secondary syphilis starts 6 to 12 weeks after exposure and presents as mucocutaneous lesions. The symptoms can include fever, malaise, lymphadenopathy, hepatitis, glomerulonephritis, uveitis, condylomata lata, and a generalized body rash. Between these phases, and for many years after the secondary manifestations, the disease becomes latent; causing no observable symptoms until tertiary phase end-organ damage occurs among as many as 33% of those infected. *Latent syphilis* is defined as the asymptomatic periods during which the person remains seroreactive. *Early latent syphilis* is defined as the period between primary and secondary manifestations, or up to 1 year after primary or secondary symptoms. *Late latent syphilis* refers to seropositivity documented more than 1 year after primary or secondary symptoms appear or as disease of

Table 8-2

Recommended Management of Gonorrhea

RECOMMENDED REGIMENS
Cefixime 400 mg orally in a single dose
or
Ceftriaxone 125 mg intramuscularly in a single dose
or
Ciprofloxin 500 mg orally in a single dose
or
Ofloxacin 400 mg orally in a single dose
plus
Azithromycin 1 g orally in a single dose
or
Doxycycline 100 mg orally twice a day for 7 days

SOURCE: From Centers for Disease Control and Prevention, 1998.

unknown duration. Tertiary syphilis manifests 10 to 40 years after the primary stage and can include aortic aneurysms, iritis, general paresis, tabes dorsalis, stroke, psychological symptoms, and gummatous lesions.

Infants of mothers with syphilis may acquire congenital syphilis. The manifestations include nonimmune hydrops fetalis, jaundice, hepatosplenomegaly, osteitis, mucocutaneous lesions, rash, and pseudoparalysis of an extremity. The risk for fetal infection is 70% to 90% if the mother has primary or secondary syphilis and 30% if she has latent syphilis. Fetal death occurs in approximately 25% of cases.

Diagnosis and management of neurosyphilis and syphilis among persons co-infected with HIV is beyond the scope of this book. Primary, secondary, and early and late latent syphilis can be managed on an outpatient basis as described in Table 8-3.

Human Immunodeficiency Virus

HIV disease is a systemic immunosuppressive process that renders the body essentially de-

Table 8-3

Recommended Management of Syphilis

PRIMARY, SECONDARY, AND EARLY LATENT SYPHILIS OF LESS THAN 1 YEAR DURATION RECOMMENDED REGIMENS
Benzathine penicillin G 2.4 million units intramuscularly in a single dose
ALTERNATIVE REGIMENS[a]
Doxycycline 100 mg orally twice a day for 2 weeks *or* Tetracycline 500 mg orally four times a day for 2 weeks
LATE LATENT SYPHILIS OR LATENT SYPHILIS OF UNKNOWN DURATION RECOMMENDED REGIMENS
Benzathine penicillin G 7.2 million units total administered as three doses of 2.4 million units intramuscularly each at 1-week intervals
ALTERNATIVE REGIMENS[a]
Doxycycline 100 mg orally twice a day for 4 weeks *or* Tetracycline 500 mg orally four times a day for 4 weeks

[a] For the treatment of persons who are allergic to penicillin and are not pregnant.

SOURCE: From Centers for Disease Control and Prevention, 1998.

fenseless in the face of other infections. There is specific cellular and systemic damage attributable to HIV itself, but most manifestations of HIV are related to the opportunistic infections contracted when the immune system is no longer competent. After a mild and transient acute retroviral syndrome characterized by flu-like symptoms, HIV has a prolonged asymptomatic period during which the immune system attempts to control the infection and remains relatively functional. In general, a period as long as 10 years can pass relatively symptom free before the immune system is so suppressed that a response to highly prevalent but usually non-pathogenic bacteria, viruses, fungi, and protozoa is not mounted, and these opportunistic infections cause severe and debilitating disease, eventually leading to death in most instances.

Management of HIV disease includes immune system monitoring, antiretroviral therapy to fight the virus itself, and medication to reduce risk for common opportunistic infections. Management of HIV disease is an evolving science and beyond the scope of this chapter. The reader is referred to the most current CDC recommendations for the management of HIV disease.

Human Papillomavirus

More than 20 types of HPV infect the genital tract, and persons with HPV infection may have a single or multiple types causing the infection. The manifestations of HPV range from asymptomatic, subclinical infections to visible genital warts to squamous cell carcinoma of the external genitalia, anus, and cervix. Pregnant women with HPV can transmit the virus to their infants, and the infection can result in laryngeal papillomatosis. The mechanism of transmission is not known.

Therapies for HPV infection are listed in Table 8-4. The goal of therapy for visible warts is eradication of symptomatic lesions. There is no evidence to indicate that therapy for visible warts results in eradication of the virus, affects the progression of disease, or reduces risk for cervical cancer. Untreated warts may resolve on their own, stay the same, or increase in size and number. There is no clear evidence that treatment affects infectivity. In general, persons with visible, symptomatic lesions want treatment. In pregnancy HPV-related lesions proliferate, and treatment is encouraged.

Table 8-4

Recommended Management of Human Papillomavirus (External Genital Warts)

RECOMMENDED REGIMENS
Patient Applied
Podofilox 0.5% solution or gel applied to visible lesions twice a day for 3 days followed by 4 days of no therapy. Cycle can be repeated as necessary for a total of four cycles,   *or*   Imiquimod 5% cream applied to visible lesions three times a week for up to 16 weeks. The treated area must be washed 6 to 10 hours after treatment.
Provider Applied
Cryotherapy with liquid nitrogen or cryoprobe. Treatment can be repeated every 1 to 2 weeks until resolved.   *or*   Podophyllin resin 10% to 20% in tincture of benzoin applied to each lesion. The treated area must be washed 1 to 4 hours after application. Treatment can be repeated weekly until lesions resolve.   *or*   Trichloroacetic acid or Bichloroacetic acid 80% to 90% applied to each lesion weekly until resolved   *or*   Surgical removal of lesions
ALTERNATIVE REGIMENS
Intralesional interferon   *or*   Laser surgery

SOURCE: From Centers for Disease Control and Prevention, 1998.

EXTERNAL GENITAL WARTS

None of the regimens described in Table 8-4 is superior to any other in terms of outcome, and choice of treatment depends on provider expertise, available modalities, client characteristics, and the extent and location of the lesions. In treating adolescents with genital warts, issues of compliance must be considered before utilizing client-applied modalities or treatments that require washing the genitals after treatment. Use of podophyllin as therapy for vaginal warts is controversial. This agent is contraindicated as therapy for anal warts because of concerns about systemic absorption.

Because genital warts often proliferate and can become friable in pregnancy, therapy for vulvar exophytic warts during pregnancy is recommended. Imiquimod, podophyllin, and podofilox are contraindicated in pregnancy. All other modalities are options, and the choice of treatment should be based on location of the lesions, how extensive they are, and the preference of provider and client. There is evidence that HPV types 6 and 11 can be transmitted to the infants of mothers with these types of HPV and cause laryngeal papillomatosis. The presence of genital warts is not an indication for cesarean delivery because the route of transmission is not yet well understood. The preventive value of cesarean delivery has not been determined.

CERVICAL HUMAN PAPILLOMAVIRUS

Diagnosis of cervical HPV may result from the direct observation of exophytic lesions on the cervix, or may be indicated on Pap smear findings and confirmed through cervical biopsy. Women with cervical lesions or abnormal Pap smear findings should undergo colposcopic examination, biopsy for grading of the extent of the visible or subclinical infection, and treatment appropriate to the findings. Treatment of the cervix should generally be avoided in pregnancy, unless maternal survival related to cervical cancer is a concern. Women with external genital warts can be followed with annual Pap smears; colposcopy is not indicated in the absence of cervical abnormalities.

Herpes Simplex Virus

Herpes simplex presents as small painful vesicles. It is a recurrent disease for which there is treatment to control symptoms and reduce recurrences, but there is no cure. Most persons with herpes simplex have asymptomatic or mild infections but still shed virus and can infect others, even in the absence of symptoms. In some cases, the initial episode of herpes simplex causes a systemic response that can be severe enough to necessitate hospitalization. Pregnant women with active symptoms of herpes simplex or its prodrome at the onset of labor should undergo cesarean section to avoid systemic herpes simplex in the newborn. A history of herpes simplex alone is not an indication for abdominal delivery.

Antiviral drugs can reduce the signs and symptoms of first episodes of herpes simplex (Table 8-5) and are indicated for use as suppressive therapy among persons with frequent out-

Table 8-5

Recommended Management of Genital Herpes

INITIAL EPISODE OF GENITAL HERPES RECOMMENDED REGIMENS
Acyclovir 400 mg orally three times a day for 7 to 10 days *or* Acyclovir 200 mg orally five times a day for 7 to 10 days *or* Famciclovir 250 mg orally three times a day for 7 to 10 days *or* Valacyclovir 1 g orally twice a day for 7 to 10 days.

EPISODIC RECURRENT INFECTION RECOMMENDED REGIMENS
Acyclovir 400 mg orally three times a day for 5 days *or* Acyclovir 200 mg orally five times a day for 5 days *or* Acyclovir 800 mg twice a day for 5 days *or* Famciclovir 125 mg orally twice a day for 5 days, *or* Valacyclovir 500 mg orally twice a day for 5 days.

DAILY SUPPRESSIVE THERAPY RECOMMENDED REGIMENS
Acyclovir 400 mg orally twice a day *or* Famciclovir 250 mg orally twice a day *or* Valacyclovir 500 mg orally once a day *or* Valacyclovir 1000 mg orally once a day

SOURCE: From Centers for Disease Control and Prevention, 1998.

breaks (six or more episodes per year). The intermittent use of antiviral drugs to reduce the intensity and duration of symptoms may be effective. These drugs do not eradicate the virus, nor do they affect the frequency or severity of outbreaks when the drug is discontinued.

Choice of regimen should take into account ease of administration. The more frequent the dosing and the longer the duration of therapy, the less likely it is that there will be compliance with the treatment regimen. The safety of acyclovir and related drugs in pregnancy has not been established, although to date there does not appear to be increased risk for serious birth defects when these drugs are taken during pregnancy.

Primary Prevention

Primary prevention of STDs is based in two distinct but complementary approaches. On a community-wide level, STD transmission can be reduced through community-based interventions that enhance knowledge about STDs and build skills to avoid or reduce risky behaviors. On an individual level, risk reduction counseling with an emphasis on behavioral changes can affect disease acquisition, transmission, and seeking care for treatment.

Unlike many of the health problems discussed in this book, STDs are communicable diseases. This is an important distinction. The interventions that can affect the prevalence of communicable diseases in a population are distinct from those that can affect the prevalence of noncommunicable diseases. Interventions that would be classified as secondary prevention on an individual level constitute primary prevention interventions from a population-based perspective. An example of this is teaching persons about early recognition of symptoms and seeking care if symptoms develop. At the individual

level, early management of an STD reduces risk for the negative outcomes of disease progression (secondary prevention). From a population-based perspective, these actions interrupt the chain of transmission and prevent additional infections among currently uninfected persons (primary prevention).

Models of transmission of communicable disease define factors that may reduce the incidence of infections in a community. According to these models, the rate of spread of an STD in a population is based on three factors; rate of exposure of susceptible persons to an infected person; efficiency of transmission, or probability that the disease will be acquired by a newly exposed person; and length of time that an infected person remains infected and can spread the infection to others. By developing interventions that influence each of these factors we can theoretically reduce the spread of an STD in a population.

Another important concept in the primary prevention of STDs from a community perspective is the concept of "core" groups. The essential ingredient in STD transmission is the presence of the infection. An individual can engage in all the behaviors that put him or her at risk for infection (e.g., unprotected sexual contact with multiple partners). If these behaviors take place within a social network that is disease-free, disease transmission and acquisition will not occur. The greater the number of partners, the greater is the likelihood of contact with an infected person. If infection is not present, however, it cannot be transmitted. It takes only one contact between a susceptible individual and an infected partner to achieve disease transmission and acquisition. Social networks that include infected persons and have high rates of partner change ("core" transmitter groups) disproportionately influence the rate of spread of disease and therefore are a logical focus of disease prevention interventions.

Public health measures in the primary prevention of communicable diseases have traditionally been heavily dependent on the use of vaccines. To date the only STD that can be prevented with vaccine is hepatitis B. A vaccine for herpes simplex is in trials, and vaccines for other STDs are in various stages of development. STD vaccines are currently far from a real option. Control of STDs has been dependent on biomedical interventions focused on ascertaining who is infected, treating infected persons, and locating and treating their partner or partners. Behavioral interventions also have been linked with biomedical interventions in an attempt to develop a more effective STD control program.

Risk Assessment and Risk Reduction Interventions

Sexually active adolescents and young adults are at risk for the acquisition of STDs. Primary care providers can be instrumental in helping clients identify their individual risk and determine actions that can reduce their risk for the acquisition of STDs. The first essential step in the process of risk reduction is assessment of risk. Because they are fundamentally healthy, adolescents and young adults do not often seek preventive care and are primarily seen for episodic illnesses, acute injuries, and health clearances at transitional times (secondary school or college entry, employment and sports participation exams, institutional clearances at incarceration, or entry into treatment programs). Sexually active young women may seek care for contraceptive methods or for a pregnancy diagnosis. Regardless of the motivation for seeking care, it is the responsibility of health care providers to discuss issues of sexuality and risk in order to provide adequate health guidance and counseling. This is a challenge for both providers and clients, because open discussion of sexuality is not a culturally acceptable activity, even, or especially, in the health care setting.

Compounding the problem of cultural reticence is the issue of confidentiality in the provision of sensitive services to underage clients. Adolescents often are hesitant to disclose behaviors which they believe their parents or other adults, such as the health care provider, may not approve. In the absence of guarantees of confidentiality, many young people will not discuss their risks, practices, or concerns. Although laws differ from state to state, most states have laws that allow adolescents to consent to the provision of confidential health services as they relate to testing and therapy for STDs. It is essential that providers be familiar with the laws in their states that pertain to adolescent consent, confidential services, and disclosure of confidential information to parents or guardians. Concerns about confidentiality and fear of disclosure of confidential information have been consistently identified by youth as the greatest barriers to seeking health care.

There are several behaviors that should be targeted as part of risk assessment and prevention counseling. Limiting the number of partners with whom one has sexual contact can effectively reduce risk for exposure to an infected individual. Consistent condom use can reduce the efficiency of transmission of an STD from an infected person to an uninfected person. Early recognition of symptoms, prompt seeking of care, and avoidance of unprotected sexual contact until the diagnosis is confirmed and treatment begun are activities an infected person can use to limit the amount of time he or she remains infected and can spread the disease to others (primary prevention from a population-based perspective). Each of these steps seems simple enough, yet we know that few persons use all of these risk reduction techniques in a consistent manner.

CLIENT-CENTERED COUNSELING

Evaluative research has shown that client-centered counseling that involves personalized risk reduction plans is more effective in increasing condom use and reducing acquisition of STDs (including HIV infection) than are didactic messages about risk reduction (Kamb et al, 1998). To design a personalized risk reduction plan with a client, the provider must enter into a conversation in which the client identifies his or her personal risk. This interactive process requires that the provider establish rapport and develop trust early in the interaction. Discussing confidentiality and giving a context to normalize the extremely personal questions that will be asked and issues that will be discussed can be very helpful in these first steps.

The provider must maintain a nonjudgmental stance, even when confronted with disclosure of sexual practices with which he or she may not feel comfortable. This requires vigilance on the part of the provider, who must monitor his or her verbal and nonverbal responses to information a client shares. For example, many providers operate under the assumption that their adolescent and young adult clients are heterosexual. Making this assumption communicates to the client that the provider can accept them only if they are heterosexual and is not willing or able to deal with them effectively if they are not. This kind of judgmental response can be avoided simply by asking all sexually active clients if they have sex with men, women, or both, regardless of how the client appears. Maintaining a nonjudgmental stance does not mean ignoring or not responding to clear indicators of risk with messages of concern and a focus on negotiating behavior change. It simply means keeping in check one's personal responses to a client's practices and beliefs, however different they may be from one's own.

Negotiation of a risk reduction plan must begin with assessment of the client's readiness for change. Sexual behavior and its modification are volitional activities. For change to occur clients must be interested in, motivated toward, and have the tools necessary for changing their behavior. Behavior change is difficult, and barriers to discarding old behaviors and adopting new ones must be examined with the client. Is the client's perception of his or her risk accurate? Is that of the partner or partners? Does the client have the skills needed to negotiate condom use? Does the client have the power and authority in the relationship to effectively negotiate safer sexual practices? Is this important to the client? Does it put the relationship at risk, and does the client believe the behavior change is worth the risk? These are just a few of the barriers that may interfere with a client's following through on a risk reduction plan. For these reasons and many more it is unrealistic to expect clients to radically modify their behavior on the basis of one interaction with a health care provider. It is not unrealistic, however, to support clients in taking small, achievable steps toward reducing risk, to obtain a commitment from them to try those small steps, and to follow up when possible to reinforce successes and plan the next steps.

Client-centered negotiation of risk reduction can be viewed in contrast to the traditional clinician-centered information and advice giving common in clinician-client interactions. Information is necessary but not sufficient to effect behavior change, yet many clinicians confine themselves to imparting oral or written information and advising the client about what they "should do" to avoid STD-related problems, as in "you really should use condoms every time you have sex". Many more clinicians never even obtain a sexual history or enter into the territory of risk reduction education, avoiding the issue altogether. They hope that parents or teachers will impart the necessary knowledge and that young people will independently conclude that they are at risk and take the necessary precautions. Studies have repeatedly shown, however, that Americans, particularly young Americans, underestimate their risk for STDs and often do not engage in any self-protective actions to avoid infection.

COMMUNITY INTERVENTIONS

Distinct from but complementary to individual-based primary prevention are community-based interventions. These interventions may target specific high-risk groups, such as adolescents, or may attempt to change community norms, often through advertising or "social marketing" campaigns. The logical place for community-based interventions that target adolescents is the schools. Although school-based interventions do reach most youth, they miss out-of-school youth (homeless, incarcerated, or otherwise marginalized young people), who may be at highest risk for STDs and may represent a core transmitter group. Evaluations of programs that target this high-risk population are scarce, and no studies provide long-term follow-up data which show sustained behavior change.

SCHOOL-BASED EDUCATION

In a review of 23 school-based STD and HIV education programs Kirby et al (1994) found that programs successful in changing behaviors shared the following characteristics:

- They provided basic, accurate information about the risks of unprotected intercourse and methods of avoiding unprotected intercourse through experiential activities designed to personalize this information.
- They included activities that address social or media influences on sexual behaviors.
- They reinforced clear and appropriate values to strengthen individual values and group norms against unprotected sex.
- They provided modeling and practice in communication and negotiation skills.

One of the debates currently affecting school-based risk-reduction education programs is the mandate in many states to teach "abstinence-based" sexuality education (the primary message being to delay sexual intercourse until marriage) rather then emphasizing harm reduction (the primary message being condom use to avoid unprotected sexual contact). Despite the evidence that promotion of condom use does not result in higher rates of initiation of sexual activity among adolescents, many school boards in communities across the country have opted for an abstinence-based model. When applied early (targeting pre-adolescents and early adolescents) this approach can be effective, because this seems to be the period for development of attitudes about sexuality and sexual intercourse. Unfortunately, most of these programs target high-school-aged youth. This can be troublesome because many of the young people being reached through these programs are already sexually active, and this model offers no tools for them to reduce their risk.

CONDOM AVAILABILITY

Condom availability programs in schools are controversial and comparatively rare. There are few data available on the effect of these programs on condom use or rates of unprotected intercourse. There are data to refute the fear that condom availability leads to initiation of sexual intercourse. One study of a high school condom availability program showed that the benefit of protecting sexually active students in avoiding STDs was three times greater than the risk for encouraging youth who are not sexually active to initiate sexual activity (Kirby et al., 1994). School-based condom availability programs, although supported by both the American Medical Association and the American Academy of Pediatrics Committee on Adolescence, remain contentious. Debates center on funding of such programs and the issues of parental and religious rights.

MASS MEDIA

Mass media campaigns have been shown to be effective in promoting awareness, increasing knowledge, and changing attitudes towards health issues such as smoking. A logical extension would be that well-designed mass media campaigns can have a positive effect on knowledge and attitudes about STDs and their prevention. A summary of empirical studies of 34 HIV prevention mass media campaigns in 13 countries indicated that generally knowledge increase and attitudes and behavior were positively influenced by many of these campaigns, although some showed no measurable effect. Cultural and political barriers to extensive national campaigns targeting adolescents and young adults are substantial in the U. S., but small-scale, population-specific media campaigns appear to be successful.

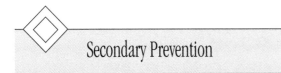

Secondary Prevention

The primary tool for the secondary prevention of STDs is screening an asymptomatic population for previously undiagnosed STDs. The efficacy of screening from a cost-effectiveness standpoint varies depending on the STD in question and the population being screened. The U. S. has extensive experience in screening programs targeting specific populations for gonorrhea, syphilis, and more recently chlamydia. HIV screening is a politically sensitive issue, and proposals for screening newborns, pregnant women, and other populations have been fraught with controversy. With changes in the effect of early diagnosis and therapy on HIV-related morbidity and mortality, the arguments for and against HIV screening have changed. Few would advocate screening for other viral STDs in the absence of treatment alternatives.

The U.S. Preventive Services Task Force in 1996 published recommendations for screening activities for primary care clinicians. These recommendations are based on the age and risk

behaviors of the client and take into account evidence of the effectiveness of prevention rather than cost effectiveness of screening interventions. A number of medical professional societies and other governmental agencies have published recommendations, which generally concur with those of the U.S. Preventive Services Task Force. The following information is based on the task force recommendations.

Chlamydia

Because of the high prevalence of chlamydia in the adolescent population and the fact that most cases among women are asymptomatic, it is recommended that all heterosexually active women in the general population younger than 20 years undergo screening for chlamydia infection. Additional recommendations include screening all sexually active women younger than 25 years who are pregnant or have multiple risk factors, including a history of STD, new or multiple sex partners, no use or inconsistent use of barrier contraceptives, and cervical ectopy. There are no screening recommendations for male adolescents and young men other than to consider local epidemiologic data and screen accordingly.

New technology in the laboratory diagnosis of chlamydia has made screening recommendations easier and more cost effective to carry out. Tissue culture once was considered the standard to which other diagnostic tests were compared. This was an expensive procedure with variable sensitivity (70% to 90%) and high specificity (100%) and required very careful handling of specimens on the part of the clinician, transporter, and laboratory personnel. Results were generally available in 3 to 5 days. Because of easier handling, lower cost, and shorter processing time, tests that do not require a culture, such as enzyme immunoassay, direct fluorescent antibody, and DNA probe have been more widely used in clinical practice. These tests have a reported sensitivity of 61% to 75% and a specificity of 99% to 100%. The newest diagnostic tests rely on nucleic acid amplification technology and include ligase chain reaction (LCR), polymerase chain reaction, and a transcription-mediated amplification. These nucleic acid amplification tests can be run on first-part-void urine (15 to 20 mL) of both men and women, avoiding the need for invasive procedures and facilitating screening of populations outside of clinical settings. A large multisite study of one LCR test showed a sensitivity of 94.4% to 98% and a specificity of 99.8% to 100%. Sensitivity depended on whether the collection site was cervical or urethral and whether the urine was from a male or a female client. The cost of LCR is comparable with that of other nonculture tests, but LCR has the advantage of higher sensitivity.

Chlamydia is an intracellular organism that colonizes the epithelial cells. For this reason, cervical and urethral specimens must be obtained with friction to assure gathering DNA fragments of the organism (or the organism itself if a culture is being performed) from inside the epithelial cells. Exudate alone is not adequate for sampling. Urine specimens should be obtained before a physical examination. Collection of a specimen from the first part of the urine flow rather than a clean-catch specimen is essential because collection of cellular debris is the goal.

All positive results to chlamydia screening tests should trigger treatment by means of one of the regimens discussed earlier. Notification and treatment of sexual contacts are discussed in the section on tertiary prevention. If a woman with chlamydia arrives for treatment more than one to two weeks after the diagnosis was made or has new symptoms such as lower abdominal pain or systemic symptoms, she should undergo a pelvic bimanual examination to rule out PID. If PID is suspected, further evaluation, a treatment regimen appropriate to PID, and hospitalization should be considered. As discussed earlier, diagnosis of and therapy for asymptomatic chlamydia have been shown to reduce risk for subsequent PID and can be postulated to reduce risk for tubal factor infertility and ectopic pregnancy. Screening during pregnancy can help prevent perinatal transmission and neonatal sequelae.

Gonorrhea

Although gonorrhea is not as prevalent a disease as chlamydia, age-specific gonorrhea rates are highest among girls and women 15 to 19 years of age and second highest among boys and men in the same age group. U.S. Preventive Services Task Force recommendations for gonorrhea screening include screening of girls and women younger than 25 years who meet any of the following criteria: are pregnant, have had two or more sex partners in the past year, have a sex partner who has had multiple sexual contacts, have exchanged sex for drugs or money; or have had gonorrhea in the past. Screening questions to determine whether a client meets the criteria may have a variable yield, because many young women are unaware of their partners' sexual practices. Gonorrhea infections among men tend to be symptomatic, and there are no screening recommendations for men and boys.

Screening tests for gonorrhea are quite inexpensive and readily available. Most microbiology laboratories have the capability to process specimens and identify positive gonorrhea culture results. Culture on selective media and maintained in an environment rich in carbon dioxide has been considered the standard for diagnostic testing for gonorrhea. DNA probe technology also exists and has been favorably compared with culture in terms of cost, sensitivity, and specificity, particularly among men and boys at high risk. Nucleotide amplification tests can be used for gonorrhea screening and can be run on first-void urine of both men and women.

As with chlamydia, this new technique facilitates screening of high-risk populations outside clinics and is highly sensitive and specific.

Gonorrhea is an intracellular organism, but unlike chlamydia it is found in the leukocytes. Specimens for gonorrhea cultures should contain exudate, and the swab should be left in the cervical os or urethra for at least 10 seconds to absorb exudate. As with chlamydia, to increase the yield of bacterial DNA fragments, first-part urine specimens rather than clean catch specimens should be used for LCR testing.

Selective screening of populations at high risk according to the foregoing criteria has been recommended to avoid progression of disease to PID and to reduce risk for tubal factor infertility and ectopic pregnancy. Selective screening also is effective in avoiding perinatal transmission and neonatal sequelae. Local epidemiologic factors, particularly the prevalence of gonococcal infections at the screening site, affect the cost effectiveness of screening. Data from the 1980s showed that screening would reduce overall costs in a population with a prevalence of 1.5%. Current diagnostic and treatment costs and the costs of sequelae in the 1990s and into the future are not reflected in this cost analysis, nor are any new data available.

As for chlamydia, all persons with positive results of screening tests for gonorrhea should be treated with one of the recommended regimens. If results of a chlamydia screening test are not available, a client with a positive gonorrhea culture result should be treated concurrently for chlamydia, because there is a high rate of co-infection. The cautions related to ruling out PID for women with chlamydia also pertain in the case of a positive gonorrhea test result. Notification and treatment of sexual contacts are discussed in the section on tertiary prevention.

Syphilis

Screening for syphilis is accomplished by means of serologic testing of a VDRL or rapid plasma reagin (RPR) test. From the time of exposure, a chancre, the symptom of primary syphilis can take from 9 to 90 days to develop. The average incubation period is 2 to 6 weeks, and during the incubation period VDRL or RPR test results may be negative. The VDRL and RPR tests are antibody tests subject to cross reactivity triggered by other diseases or syndromes. For this reason, all positive VDRL or RPR serologic results must be followed by a confirmatory test such as the MHA-TP, a microhemagglutination test specific for Treponema pallidum, the species of bacteria responsible for syphilis. The U.S. Preventive Services Task Force recommendations are for selective screening of persons 11 to 24 years of age. Criteria include screening of all pregnant women at their first prenatal visit, of persons (male and female) who exchange sex for money or drugs, of the sex partners of such persons, of persons with other STDs (including HIV infection), and of the sexual contacts of persons with active syphilis. A repeat VDRL or RPR test is recommended in the third trimester of pregnancy for women in any of the screening groups. The recommendation is to consider local epidemiologic factors when making screening decisions.

Syphilis is an example of an STD for which mandated premarital screening programs are probably not cost effective. Laws related to premarital and prenatal syphilis screening were enacted in the 1930s and 1940s to prevent the transmission of syphilis to sexual (marital) partners and infants. On the basis of data showing that only about 1% of cases of syphilis were detected with premarital screening, many states repealed laws requiring a blood test for syphilis as a condition of obtaining a marriage license. In 1996, however, 15 states still required premarital syphilis testing despite the low yield and lack of cost effectiveness. Prenatal testing for syphilis, however, has been shown to be cost effective. A study in Norway demonstrated significant cost savings attributed to a nationwide prenatal screening program.

The first step taken after a positive VDRL or RPR result, usually initiated by the testing laboratory, is to run a confirmatory test for syphilis. If the second test confirms past or present infection, the next step is a careful interview with the client to determine whether there is a history of a lesion, rash, or treatment in the past. Although many primary care providers are prepared to conduct this interview (and may be best suited to obtain this information because of their rapport with the client), a provider who does not feel prepared to manage syphilis staging should consult with local public health authorities and refer the client as appropriate. Staging is essential, because treatment is based on duration of infection. Treatment recommendations discussed earlier should be followed, and treatment of a pregnant client or a client with HIV infection usually triggers referral, as does any suspicion of neurosyphilis. Follow-up care includes serial VDRL or RPR testing and may be conducted by the primary care provider or public health specialist.

Selective screening for syphilis, a disease with prolonged asymptomatic infectious periods, can both reduce risk for transmission to uninfected persons (population-based primary prevention) and avoid progression of this serious, debilitating, and fatal disease. Prenatal screening in the first trimester can reduce risk for congenital syphilis and prevent perinatal transmission to the infant of an infected mother.

Human Immunodeficiency Virus

The screening criteria for HIV infection are similar to those for other STDs, yet HIV, much like syphilis in the past, is a highly stigmatized and politicized disease. Many primary care providers while following the screening recommendations for gonorrhea, chlamydia, and syphilis have had difficulty incorporating selective screening activities for HIV into their periodic health examination protocols. Early in the HIV epidemic,

before the disease and its transmission were well understood, there was an emphasis on risk groups (homosexual men, Haitians, and users of intravenous drugs) rather than risk behaviors. The influence of this early emphasis persists, and many providers continue (sometimes subconsciously) in using a risk group assessment to guide HIV screening recommendations.

Selective screening recommendations are to obtain a serologic test for HIV for persons 11 to 24 years of age if the client is a man or boy who has had sex with male partners or is a person (male or female) who has used or is currently using injected drugs, has traded sex for money or drugs, received a blood transfusion between 1978 and 1985, or is seeking treatment of an STD. All persons who have current or former partners who are using or have used injected drugs, are bisexual, exchange sex for money or drugs, or have HIV infection should be screened.

The CDC and the Preventive Services Task Force screening recommendations for pregnant women differ. The CDC recommends offering HIV testing to all pregnant women, and the Preventive Services Task Force recommends offering HIV testing on the basis of the prevalence of HIV disease in the area. Offering universal screening at the first prenatal visit is recommended in areas with a high prevalence of HIV among pregnant women. In low-prevalence areas, pregnant women who are past or present users of injected drugs, exchange sex for money or drugs, received a blood transfusion between 1978 and 1985, are seeking treatment of an STD, or have a partner who currently uses or in the past used injected drugs, is bisexual, or has HIV infection, should be offered HIV testing at the first prenatal visit. As always, local epidemiologic factors must be considered in the screening recommendations for all adolescents and young adults.

These recommendations are complex and depend on clients' knowing the behaviors and risks of their partners. This is a difficult issue in the care of adolescents and young adults, because sexual relationships often are transient and clients may disclose little about past or present practices and risk behaviors. This problem, which is compounded by a provider's persistence in viewing clients as at-risk or not on the basis of an unstated and often unconfirmed idea about the client's risk, results in underscreening of this population. HIV care is an evolving science and art. As treatment options change and increase, and the value of early diagnosis and treatment has become clearer, screening recommendations have changed. An example of this dynamic process is the screening recommendations for pregnant women. The proved efficacy of perinatal treatment of mother and child with antiretroviral drugs has reduced vertical transmission of HIV to neonates. As a result, providers of perinatal services have become far more aggressive in their screening recommendations. Over time, as providers and clients become less pessimistic about the meaning of an HIV diagnosis and view HIV disease as a chronic, manageable condition rather than a death sentence, attitudes toward screening all at-risk clients will most likely change.

The screening test for HIV is an HIV antibody test. As in the antibody test for syphilis, a positive HIV antibody test result must be confirmed with a second, more specific test to reduce the risk for cross reactivity and false-positive results. Further complicating the situation with HIV antibody testing is the window period, a 6 to 24 week period between infection and sufficient antibody production to yield a positive antibody test. Highly sensitive and specific diagnostic tests, such as the PCR, can be performed in special circumstances but because of expense are not used for screening purposes. Confirmation of a positive result of an HIV screening test should be followed by counseling, monitoring of immune status, and treatment as appropriate.

Recommendations for treatment of persons with HIV disease change rapidly as new drugs are developed and are beyond the scope of this

book. The latest treatment recommendations are available through the CDC. Many primary care providers provide follow-up care for clients with HIV infection through consultation and referral as necessary. The primary care provider must have a special interest in HIV care and be prepared to stay current in a constantly changing field. Referral to an HIV specialist may be appropriate for some clients or clinicians.

Human Papillomavirus

Screening activities related to cervical HPV infection are the secondary prevention recommendations for cervical cancer. Because of the high rates of spontaneous resolution of genital tract HPV infections, DNA assays for the presence of HPV are not recommended for use in nonexperimental settings. Screening for cervical cancer with a Pap test is discussed in Chapter 12.

Other Viral Sexually Transmitted Diseases

There are no general screening recommendations for herpes simplex, external HPV, or hepatitis B or C. The preventive goal for hepatitis B in the U. S. is universal immunization. In all likelihood, if a curative treatment is found for herpes simplex, screening recommendations will be developed to reduce morbidity and the rate of transmission of the disease.

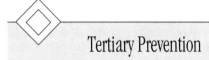

Tertiary Prevention

Early diagnosis, treatment, and prevention of transmission are the goals in tertiary prevention of STDs. These activities are undertaken when a client with symptomatic disease seeks STD-related care. Many young people delay seeking care for a variety of reasons. Because of a lack of knowledge of specific diseases and disease progression, a person with symptomatic disease may wait for spontaneous resolution of the symptoms, meanwhile continuing with unsafe sexual practices and adding links to the chain of transmission. Many STDs are asymptomatic or only mildly symptomatic until they have progressed considerably, again interrupting the process of care seeking. Some symptoms of STD, such as a syphilitic chancre or the lesions of herpes simplex, resolve spontaneously, which the individual may interpret as resolution of the problem unaware that despite the disappearance of the lesion the disease remains and progresses. There are many social reasons for delaying or avoiding care. Lack of knowledge of resources, fear of judgment on the part of the usual care provider, concern about confidentiality, cost, and the diagnostic process all mitigate against young persons' seeking immediate care for STD-related problems. Finally, the nature of the problem itself affects care seeking. STDs carry a stigma; young persons may feel too embarrassed to go to the customary care provider for STD-related services, and they may be unaware of other sources of care.

History, Physical Examination, Diagnostic Testing

Because of the stigma attached to an STD diagnosis, many youth use public sector STD clinics or family planning service providers rather than their primary care provider when faced with STD-related symptoms. Even when young persons do seek care from their customary care providers, if the provider does not ask the pertinent questions or responds in a judgmental way, the youth may not disclose their real reason for the visit and may not receive appropriate care.

Typical presentations of an STD are discharge from the vagina, urethra, or anus, dysuria, pain with intercourse, or genital lesions. Men and boys may report testicular pain, and women and girls may have menstrual irregularities and lower abdominal pain. When a client has these or similar symptoms, a thorough sexual history must be obtained. Areas to explore and sample questions are included in Table 8-6.

As with any other medical problem, the history of the present illness must be obtained. This includes questions related to the onset and duration of the problem, the nature of the problem, factors that aggravate or alleviate the condition, associated symptoms (fever and chills, lower abdominal pain, postcoital bleeding, dyspareunia, changes in normal bleeding pattern, testicular pain, genital or anal lesions, rash, rectal bleeding), and self-treatment.

Information gathered through history taking provides guidance for the physical examination, but certain things should be evaluated regardless of history. If a client describes an oral or anorectal disorder or a history of oral or anal sex, visual inspection and possible specimen collection of those orifices are necessary. A client who denies such activity does not need that intervention. In general, the physical examination for an STD-related problem should include the items listed in Table 8-7.

The diagnostic tests for STDs are the same as those used for STD screening. When a client has an STD-related problem, the clinician should test for gonorrhea and chlamydia. The clinician should prepare vaginal wet mounts for trichomoniasis, bacterial vaginosis, and moniliasis. The clinician also should consider testing for syphilis and HIV infection.

In many settings, syndromic diagnosis has traditionally been relied on in the diagnosis and management of urethritis, cervicitis, vaginal discharge, PID, and genital ulcers. The advantage of this approach is that it facilitates rapid treatment. The disadvantage is that syndromic diagnosis and treatment are nonspecific and often result in substantial overtreatment and lack of epidemiologic data. Nonetheless, to use this

Table 8-6

Sample Questions for a Sexual History

1. Sexual activity: Have you ever had sex?
2. Sex of sexual partners: Do you have sex with men, women, or both?
3. Age at sexual debut: How old were you the first time you ever had sex?
4. Number of sexual contacts in past 3 months and lifetime: How many different people have you had sex with in the last 3 months? How many different people have you had sex with in your whole life?
5. Sexual practices: What different kinds of ways do you have sex? Do you have vaginal (penis in the vagina), anal (penis in the butt), or oral (penis in the mouth or mouth on the woman's genitals) sex?
6. Contraception and risk reduction: Do you or your partner or partners do anything to reduce the changes of pregnancy or of getting sexually transmitted disease?
7. Condom use: Do you or your partner or partners use condoms? Out of 10 times you have sex, how many times do you or your partner use a condom? In what situations do you use condoms? In what situations don't you use condoms? Did you use a condom the last time you had sex?
8. History of STDs: Have you ever been told you had a sexually transmitted disease like gonorrhea, chlamydia, herpes, syphilis, genital warts, or HIV?
9. Details related to diagnosis: What disease? When? What treatment? Did you follow through with treatment? Was your partner treated?
10. Contact status: Has anyone you have had sex with told you that you might have a sexually transmitted disease?

approach effectively, the clinician must treat the client for the range of typical pathogens, choosing a regimen that will cover all probable causative organisms for the presenting syndrome. An example of this approach is the syndromic diagnosis of urethritis for a male client with dysuria and purulent urethral discharge. The clinician might (or might not) obtain a Gram stain consistent with gonococcus. He or she would then treat the client with a regimen to cover for gonorrhea and chlamydia, which also covers *Mycoplasma* and *Ureaplasma* organisms. Depending on resources and regional practice patterns, tests for chlamydia and gonorrhea might be processed, but treatment is initiated while results are pending.

If the current CDC treatment recommendations are followed, there is no indication for a laboratory test of cure. These treatment regimens, followed correctly, are curative of STDs.

The exception is syphilis, which requires serial VDRL or RPR titers to assure resolution of the disease. This does not preclude the need for follow-up care, however, particularly for adolescents and young adults. Rates of re-infection from an untreated partner or new partner in the same social (and STD) network are high, and compliance with complex regimens is difficult. A follow-up visit or telephone call is advisable to check on compliance, resolution of symptoms, and partner referral and treatment.

Behavioral Messages

Since the 1980s, the CDC has recommended a simple, clear, and programmatic approach to the disease-intervention behavioral messages that should be communicated to the client found to have a treatable STD. These behavioral messages are as follows:

Table 8-7

Physical Examination for STD-related Symptoms

WOMEN
Temperature
Skin check for rashes
Abdominal examination with attention to perihepatic and lower abdominal tenderness, rebound tenderness, inguinal lymphadenopathy
External genital examination with attention to erythema, excoriation, discharge, lesions
Pelvic examination with specimen collection and attention to vaginal and cervical erythema, vaginal and cervical discharge, odor, lesions
Bimanual examination with attention to uterine or adnexal tenderness, adnexal masses

MEN
Skin check for rashes
Genital examination with specimen collection and attention to inguinal lymphadenopathy, spontaneous urethral discharge, discharge with milking of the urethra, erythema of the meatus, epidydimal tenderness, genital lesions

1. Reduce risk
2. Respond to disease suspicion
3. Take medications (if applicable)
4. Return for follow-up tests (if applicable)

These simple messages must be communicated in an age appropriate manner and be individualized to the client engaged in the counseling session. Some of these interventions are informational; for example, the client must know the signs and symptoms of a disease to respond promptly to disease suspicion. The issue of risk reduction must be addressed with a client-centered approach with clients taking the lead in determining the steps they can take to

reduce their own risk. If the clinician remembers to address these four issues, risk for re-infection, future infection, and transmission to others can be reduced.

Sex Partner Management

Partner notification and treatment traditionally have been an integral part of public health disease control programs. The purpose of partner notification and treatment is that identification and treatment of the sexual contacts of an infected person (the index case) can prevent re-infection of the person treated for the index case and help find and treat the person with the source case (the sex partner or partners). This strategy prevents further transmission of disease from the source case to future sexual contacts. The client's role in this process can range from supplying accurate information about partner names and telephone numbers to bringing the partner into the office for treatment. There are three common methods of partner notification and treatment: provider referral, conditional referral, and patient referral. Provider referral entails an extensive interview between the person with the index case and the health care provider or member of the clinic team. The names of and information about how to locate sexual contacts are obtained. The provider takes the initiative of informing the sexual contacts of their STD contact status and need for treatment. This model has been used extensively in the public health sector. Patient referral puts the responsibility for partner notification on the person with the index case, who is advised by the provider to inform his or her sexual contacts that they have been exposed to an STD and need treatment. This is a classic private-sector approach. Conditional referral is a combined approach in which partner information is gathered by the clinician, but the patient is given a predetermined period of time to inform the partners. If the patient does not notify all partners within the predetermined time period, the provider takes on the task of partner notification.

There is little research evaluating the efficacy of partner notification in terms of effect on the incidence or prevalence of STDs in the general population, although it has been found to be an effective strategy in the control of focal outbreaks of specific STDs. A review of published studies (Oxman et al, 1994) on partner notification found the following:

1. There is strong evidence of the effectiveness of simple forms of patient assistance, such as a telephone call, directed at improving patient referral.
2. There is moderately strong evidence that provider referral results in more partners being notified than does patient referral for HIV infection.
3. There is weak evidence that provider or conditional referral is more effective than patient referral for syphilis.
4. There is conflicting evidence of the comparative efficacy of provider or conditional referral versus patient referral for gonorrhea and chlamydia.
5. There is weak evidence that trained interviewers are more effective than routine health care providers at identifying partners, and there is no evidence that employment of trained interviewers yields any important practical benefits.

The first essential step in any method of partner management is educating the client about the diagnosis and the nature of STDs. This means discussing with the client that the disease they have contracted is sexually transmitted, not caught from toilet seats or public showers. Emphasis on protecting the client's health by assuring partner notification and treatment, rather than a focus on the health of a sexual contact for whom the client may feel little more than anger at the time of diagnosis, may be a more fruitful approach in work with adolescents and young adults. The clinician should remember that this is a stigmatized and emotion-laden diagnosis that challenges basic trust in a relationship. The clinician must be prepared for emotional responses from disbelief to hurt and disappointment to anger and lashing out. It is the clinician's responsibility to address both the physical and emotional aspects of an STD diagnosis when providing STD-related care.

Reporting of Sexually Transmitted Diseases

Communicable disease reporting requirements vary from state to state. In general, gonorrhea, syphilis, and AIDS diagnoses are notifiable diseases, that is, reporting is required. Forty-eight states, Alaska and New York being the exceptions, also require chlamydia reporting, and 30 states require reporting of positive HIV test results. Compliance with reporting requirements is high in the public sector and highly variable in the private sector. This tends to skew data, because underreporting in the private sector leads to overrepresentation in the STD database of poor and ethnic minorities who receive public sector services.

The advantages to national monitoring of infectious diseases are numerous. Through monitoring, trends in STDs can be identified, leading to the identification of problems that need intervention. In response, money can be allocated to develop and implement programs to address these problems, and the effect of these programs can be evaluated.

All of the benefits of STD data collection on a local, state, and national level are clear to prevention-oriented health care providers. It is quite a different issue to the persons whose names and STD diagnoses are going to be reported to the public health department. How to discuss reporting requirements with a client is an important question for diagnosing clinicians. The ideal time to broach the topic of communicable disease reporting is at the beginning of the visit in the discussion of confidentiality. Drawing the parallel of the reporting requirements for nonstigmatized diseases such as measles and chickenpox may make the proposition somewhat more palatable to the client.

It is essential that the client understand that reporting by name with birth date, address, and other identifying information occurs at the local level. This information is handled confidentially by disease intervention specialists in the public health department and is necessary to assure that the same case is not reported multiple times (for example, by the laboratory and by the primary care clinician). Any further reporting, for example, data submitted by the local public health department to state or federal agencies, is done without personal identifiers. It is helpful to explain to the client that this information is important in tracking epidemics and watching for trends in STDs. Clinicians must know whether public health departments in their communities contact clients with an STD directly, so that they can prepare the client for that contact. Most health departments do little active case finding and limit their activities to clients within their own clinic system.

Local health department data systems can be helpful to primary care providers. Records of diagnoses and treatment can be accessed to aid in clinical decision making. An example of when this service might be appropriate is the case of a client who has a low-titer reactive RPR result, is a poor historian, but knows he or she received some treatment in the past. Confirmation of previous diagnosis and treatment can save that client the multiple injections and the monitoring that accompany a diagnosis of late latent syphilis. Public health STD clinics are staffed by experts in the clinical and laboratory diagnosis and management of STDs and are a good source for consultation when the primary care clinician encounters a clinical conundrum. These clinics also have diagnostic resources,

such as a dark-field microscope for the diagnosis of primary syphilis, which are not generally available in the primary care setting. For these reasons, cultivation of a good relationship with the local STD control program benefits both primary care providers and their clients.

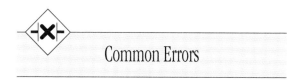

Common Errors

Inadequate Risk Assessment

A guiding principle in the work of health care is do no harm. In the area of STD diagnosis and management, we do great harm to our clients by inadequately assessing their risk for STDs. In a recent survey of sexually active youth it was found that although 91% had undergone a complete physical examination within the 2 years before collection of the survey data, only 42% had undergone screening for STDs (Ellen et al. 1998). The missed opportunities are clear. When assured of confidential, nonjudgmental services, adolescents and young adults disclose their risks, undergo STD screening, and engage in risk-reduction interventions. Through an adequate risk assessment process, clinicians can ascertain whether a client needs these services. If we do not ask, we will never know, and our clients may suffer by receiving insufficient or inappropriate services.

Assumptions about Sexuality

A second error concerns clinicians' common assumptions of heterosexuality, monogamy, and vaginal intercourse. If rather than assuming they ask clients about all risk behaviors, clinicians can avoid assumptions and give clients the opportunity to tell what they do and with whom. Interventions can then be geared to the specific risks of each individual client.

Not Using Client-centered Counseling

A third error is that clinicians use purely information-based interventions (e.g., the generic risk-reduction speech) even though research has demonstrated that this approach does not generate behavioral changes. Clinicians must challenge themselves to remain client centered, to listen to what the client tells them, and to plan *with* rather than *for* the client. The role of a clinician is to listen, to validate, to correct misperceptions, and to guide the decision-making process.

Failure to Stay Current

A fourth error involves a failure of clinicians to keep abreast of the latest information on diagnosis and management of STDs. New diagnostic techniques, new treatments, and new prevention approaches from vaccines to educational interventions are constantly being designed and tested. It is imperative that primary care clinicians remain aware of these advances. The CDC publishes regular updates on STD trends, treatment guidelines, and interventions. These resources can be obtained free of charge. All materials also are available on the Internet through the CDC home page at www.cdc.gov. Updates on the management of STDs are a popular topic at the annual meetings of professional societies. Practicing clinicians can keep on top of rapidly changing information by availing themselves of these educational opportunities. Local health departments often sponsor STD-related in-service education programs that are open to community providers. By remaining aware of changes in STD care, practicing clinicians can assure that they remain up to date and treat their clients properly.

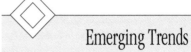

Emerging Trends

Vaccines

In the area of primary prevention of viral STDs, although there is continued interest and effort devoted to behavioral interventions to reduce risk for acquisition of disease, the increasing focus is on the development of vaccines. Using the traditional models of universal vaccination efforts in the U. S., there is great optimism that the incidence of hepatitis B as both a sexually transmitted and perinatally acquired infection will be substantially reduced. Currently, development of a vaccine for herpes simplex is underway. Human papillomavirus presents many challenges, because multiple types of HPV cause genital disease. The greatest challenge, however, is in development of vaccine against HIV, a rapidly mutating, evolving virus with extremely serious sequelae.

Behavioral Interventions

While vaccines are in development, behavioral interventions are still our most effective tool. New models of group and individual counseling, prevention education, and skills building for adolescents hold great promise. Client-centered counseling has been found to be most effective with adolescents and with persons who have a previous diagnoses of an STD. The task for clinicians is to look critically at their own counseling approach and work to integrate the tenets of client-centered counseling into their interventions.

Screening

In the area of secondary prevention, surely the most promising trend is the move toward highly sensitive and specific noninvasive screening tests. With the development of urine-based testing for gonorrhea and chlamydia, and oral specimens for HIV screening, access to STD screening for adolescent populations who do not use clinics is greatly enhanced. The barriers to care caused by time-consuming, anxiety producing, and sometimes painful procedures for specimen collection are eliminated.

Treatment

Treatment modalities used in tertiary prevention of bacterial STDs are changing. New drugs that can be administered in one dose as observed therapy are replacing complex and lengthy dosage regimens. This is a promising trend in the care of adolescents with STDs because it eliminates some concerns about compliance. Unfortunately, effective therapy for the viral diseases still eludes us, and the treatment regimens for viral STDs remain complex and demanding and do not offer a definitive cure.

Bibliography

Adolescent Health Program: *Sexually Transmitted Diseases amongst Adolescents in the Developing World,* WHO/ADH publication no. 93.1. Geneva, World Health Organization, 1993.

Aral SO, Holmes KK: Epidemiology of sexual behavior and sexually transmitted diseases, in Holmes KK, Mardh PA, Sparling PF, et al, (eds.): *Sexually Transmitted Diseases,* 2nd ed. New York, McGraw-Hill, 1990, pp 19–36.

Berman SM, Hein K: Adolescents and STDs. in, Holmes KK, Mardh PA, Sparling PF, et al, (eds.): *Sexually Transmitted Diseases,* 3rd ed. New York, McGraw-Hill, 1999, pp 129–142.

Cates W Jr: The epidemiology and control of sexually transmitted diseases in adolescents. *Adolesc Med* 3:409–428, 1990.

Centers for Disease Control and Prevention: 1998 Guidelines for treatment of sexually transmitted diseases. *MMWR* 48:RR-1, 1998.

Centers for Disease Control and Prevention: *HIV/AIDS Surveillance Report,* 9(no. 2). Atlanta, US Department of Health and Human Services, 1997.

Ciemins EL, Borenstein LA, Dyer IE, et al: Comparisons of cost and accuracy of DNA probe test and culture for the detection of *Neisseria gonorrhoeae* in patients attending public sexually transmitted disease clinics in Los Angeles County. *Sex Transm Dis* 24:422–428, 1997.

Critchlow CW, Wolner-Hanssen P, Eschenbach DA, et al: Determinants of cervical ectopia and cervicitis. *Am J Obstet Gynecol* 173:534–543, 1995.

Division of STD Prevention: *Sexually Transmitted Disease Surveillance, 1996.* US Department of Health and Human Services, Public Health Service. Atlanta, Centers for Disease Control and Prevention, 1997.

Division of STD/HIV Prevention: *STD Employee Development Guide.* US Department of Health and Human Services, Public Health Service. Atlanta, Centers for Disease Control and Prevention, 1992.

Ellen JM, McCright J, Garrett KA: Prevalence of asymptomatic STD screening among African American adolescents (abstr.). Presented at the International Congress of Sexually Transmitted Diseases, 12, 118, 1998.

Felman Y: Repeal of mandated premarital tests for syphilis: a survey of state health officers. *Am J Public Health* 71:155–159, 1981.

Gutman LT: Human papillomavirus infections of the genital tract in adolescents. *Adolesc Med* 6:115–126, 1995.

Hahn RA, Magder LS, Aral SO, et al: Race and the prevalence of syphilis seroreactivity in the United States population: A national sero-epidemiologic study. *Am J Public Health* 79:467–470, 1989.

Institute of Medicine: Prevention of STDs, in: Eng TR, Butler WT (eds.): *The hidden epidemic: confronting sexually transmitted diseases.* Washington, DC, National Academy Press, 1997, pp. 118–174.

Kamb ML, Fishbein M, Douglas JM, et al: Efficacy of risk-reduction counseling to prevent human immunodeficiency virus and sexually transmitted diseases. *JAMA* 280:1161–1167, 1998.

Kirby D, Short L, Collins R, et al: School-based programs to reduce sexual risk behaviors: A review of effectiveness. *Public Health Rep* 109:339–360, 1994.

Ku L, Sonnenstein FL, Fleck JH: The dynamics of young men's condom use during and across relationships. *Fam Plann Perspect* 26:246–251, 1994.

Mertz KL, Levine WC, Mosure DJ, et al: Screening women for gonorrhea: Demographic screening criteria for general clinical use. *Am J Public Health* 87:1535–1538, 1997.

Moss GB, Clemetson D, D'Costa L, et al: Association of cervical ectopy with heterosexual transmission of human immunodeficiency virus: Results of a study of couples in Nairobi, Kenya. *J Infect Dis* 164:588–591, 1991.

Oxman AD, Scott EA, Sellors JW, et al: Partner notification for sexually transmitted diseases: An overview of the evidence. *Can J Public Health* 85 (Suppl):S41–47, 1994.

Piot P, Islam M: Sexually transmitted diseases in the 1990s: Global epidemiology and challenges for control. *Sex Transm Dis* 21 (Suppl):S7, 1994.

Rosenberg PS, Biggar RJ Goedert JJ: Declining age at HIV infection in the United States (letter). *N Engl J Med* 33:89, 1994.

Schachter J, Moncada J, Whidden R, et al: Non-invasive tests for diagnosis of chlamydia infection: Application of ligase chain reaction to first-catch urine specimens of women. *J Infect Dis* 172:1411–1414, 1995.

Schafer MA, Sweer RL. Pelvic inflammatory disease in adolescent females. *Adolesc Med* 3:545–565, 1990.

Scholes D, Stergachis A, Heidrich FE, et al: Prevention of pelvic inflammatory disease by screening for cervical chlamydia infection. *N Engl J Med* 334:1362–1366, 1996.

US Preventive Services Task Force: *Guide to Clinical Preventive Services,* 2nd ed. Washington, DC, US Department of Health and Human Services, 1996.

Webster LA, Berman SM, Greenspan JR: Surveillance for gonorrhea and primary and secondary syphilis among adolescents, United States 1981-1991. *MMWR* 42:1–11, 1993.

Wolk LI, Rosenbaum R. The benefits of school-based condom availability-cross-sectional analysis of a comprehensive high school-based program. *J Adolesc Health* 17:184–188, 1995.

Elizabeth H. Morrison
Doug Campos-Outcalt

Chapter
9

Prenatal Care

Prevention of Toxoplasmosis
Prevention of Cytomegalovirus
Nutrition
Exercise
Injury Prevention
Breastfeeding
Prenatal Care Classes
Involvement of the Father and Other
　Family Members
Involvement of Doulas
Preparing Other Children for the
　New Arrival
Immunizations
　Non-live Vaccines
　Immunizations to Avoid: Live Viruses
Recommendations to Clinicians
　Approach to Patient Care
Common Errors

Lack of Periconception Counseling
Failure to Administer Anti-RhD
　Immunoglobulin
Prescribing Iron for All Women
Inaccurate Calculation of Dates
Performing Unnecessary Tests
Failure to Perform Third-trimester Syphilis
　Tests
Failure to Detect Breech Presentation
Emerging Trends
Screening for Down Syndrome and Other
　Anomalies
Gene Therapy
HIV Treatment
Immunizations
Gestational Diabetes
Folic Acid Supplementation

Introduction

Every year, nearly 4,000,000 infants are born in the United States. Each of the pregnancies and births offers clinicians opportunities to prevent disease and promote healthier families. Prenatal care is one of the most common reasons for patients to visit clinicians. There are more than 23 million prenatal care visits per year.

Out of 3,880,000 births in 1997, 110,874 were multiple births—104,137 sets of twins, 6,148 of triplets, 510 of quadruplets, and 79 of quintuplets or more. The multiple birth rate has doubled since 1991 (81.4 to 173.6 per 100,000) and has quadrupled since 1980. The continuous increase in multiple births over the past 20 years is illustrated in Table 9-1. The increase in multiple births is primarily due to use of fertility drugs and resulting multiple gestations.

Fertility rates by race and ethnicity are described as number of births per 1000 women 15 to 44 years of age in Table 9-2. Mexican-American women have the highest birth rates, 116.6 per 1000 in 1997.

The teen birth rate declined in 1997 to 52.3 births per 1000 girls and young women 15 to 19 years of age. As illustrated in Figure 9-1 and Table 9-3, birth rates among teens have been declining since 1991.

Birth rates by age of mother are described in Table 9-4. The highest rates occur among women 20 to 29 years of age. Although the birth rate among women older than 40 years of age is low compared with that of other age groups, it has been growing, as illustrated in Figure 9-1.

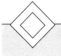

Natural History of Pregnancy

Although most pregnant women in the United States use prenatal services, some women face barriers to adequate prenatal care, including

Table 9-1

Number of Multiple Births: United States, 1989–1997

Year	Twins	Triplets	Quadruplets	Quintuplets and Other Higher Order Multiples
1997	104,137	6148	510	79
1996	100,750	5298	560	81
1995	96,736	4551	365	57
1994	97,064	4233	315	46
1993	96,445	3834	277	57
1992	95,372	3547	310	26
1991	94,779	3121	203	22
1990	93,865	2830	185	13
1989	90,118	2529	229	40

Source: From Ventura SJ, et al, 1999.

poverty, lack of health insurance, linguistic and cultural barriers, and poor geographic access to caregivers. The proportion of women obtaining prenatal care in the first trimester was 82.5% in 1997. This indicator has been improving for all women in recent years although African-Americans and Hispanics continue to receive care in the first trimester less often (72% and 74%) than do Caucasians (88%).

About 99% of births occur in a hospital; 92.3% are attended by a physician and 7% by a certified nurse midwife. The overall rate of cesarean delivery in 1997 was 20.8%.

Outcome of Pregnancy

Maternal death is a rare event in the United States, occurring in 5 out of 100,000 live births. The prevalence varies by race and level of prenatal care, as shown in Table 9-5.

The low-birth weight rate in 1997 was 7.5% and has increased slightly in recent years largely due to the increase in multiple births. There are marked differences in low-birth weight rates by race—6.5% for Caucasians, 13.1% for African-Americans, 6.4% for Hispanics. The preterm birth rate (proportion of infants born before 37 weeks of gestation) also rose in 1997, from 11.0% to 11.4%. Preterm birth rates by ethnicity are 10.2% for Caucasians and 17.6% for African-Americans.

Table 9-2

U.S. Birth and Fertility Rates, 1997

Race	Birth Rates[a]	Fertility Rates[b]
All races	14.5	65.0
Caucasian	13.9	63.9
African-American	17.7	70.7
Native American	16.6	69.1
Asian/Pacific Islander	16.9	66.3
Total Hispanic	24.2	102.8
Mexican-American	26.8	116.6

[a] Per 1000 population.
[b] Per 1000 women 15 to 44 years of age.
Source: Ventura SJ, et al, 1999.

Table 9-3

Birth Rates for Teenagers by Age, Race, and Hispanic Origin of Mother: United States, 1991, 1996, and 1997

		NONHISPANIC		
YEAR AND AGE GROUP	TOTAL	CAUCASIAN	AFRICAN-AMERICAN	HISPANIC
10–14 YR				
1997	1.1	0.4	3.4	2.3
1996	1.2	0.4	3.8	2.6
1991	1.4	0.5	4.9	2.4
15–17 YR				
1997	32.1	19.4	62.6	66.3
1996	33.8	20.6	66.6	69.0
1991	38.7	23.6	86.7	70.6
18–19 YR				
1997	83.6	61.9	134.0	144.3
1996	86.0	63.7	136.6	151.1
1991	94.4	70.5	163.1	158.5

NOTE: Rates per 1000 women in specified group.
SOURCE: Ventura SJ, et al, 1999.

Table 9-4

Birth Rate by Age of Mother

AGE (YR)	BIRTH RATE/1000 WOMEN
15–17	32.1
18–19	83.6
20–24	110.0
25–29	113.8
30–34	85.3
35–39	36.1
40–44	7.1

SOURCE: Ventura SJ, et al, 1999.

More than 1600 babies were born with Down syndrome in 1995. Another 1000 were born with neural tube defects and 4500 with heart defects.

It is difficult to conduct good studies to prove the benefits of prenatal care, because it would be unethical to randomize women to control groups that would receive no care. The author of one critical review using rigorous methodology could not prove that prenatal care improves outcomes (Fiscella, 1995). Yet many observational studies suggest that prenatal care benefits pregnant women and their infants. Fetal mortality is much higher among women who do not receive prenatal care than among women who receive at least some prenatal care. This trend holds true among women of all ages, ethnic groups, and educational levels (Figure 9-2, Table 9-5). In retrospective studies, mothers who lacked prenatal care delivered infants with significantly lower birth weights, longer neonatal hospital stays, and lower Apgar scores than

Figure 9-1

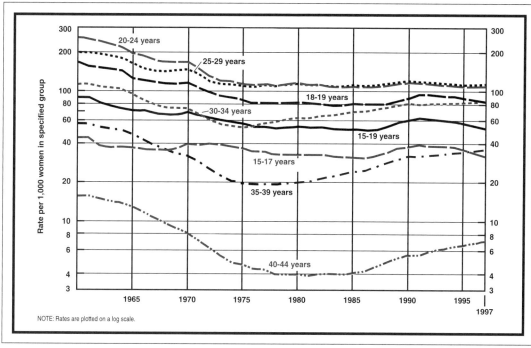

Birth rates by age of mother: United States, 1960–1997. *(Reproduced from Ventura SJ, et al, Natl Vital Stat Rep 47:1–96, 1999.)*

did women who had prenatal care. It seems clear that prenatal care is an important resource to which all pregnant women should have adequate access.

Risk Factors for Poor Pregnancy Outcomes

Many risk factors can worsen pregnancy outcomes. Risks for adverse pregnancy outcomes include young age of mother, older age of mother, low socioeconomic status, being unmarried, smoking, illicit drug use, and lack of prenatal care. Women 30 years and older are at increased risk for fetal demise, having low-birth weight babies, and preterm birth. After 30 years of age, the magnitude of these risks increases.

Women 40 years and older are at four times greater risk for death caused by pregnancy-related conditions than women younger than 30 years.

Ethnicity, race, and socioeconomic status interact with each other in complex ways. In some ethnic groups, foreign-born women have better pregnancy outcomes than their counterparts born in the United States. Women from ethnic minority groups in the United States generally have poorer outcomes, even with controls for socioeconomic status. African-American women, for example, on average have higher rates of preterm birth and maternal death. Yet Mexican-American women overall have better perinatal outcomes than the general population.

Table 9-5

Crude Pregnancy-related Mortality Rate[a], by Race[b] and Adequacy of Prenatal Care[c]–United States,[d] 1987–1990

ADEQUACY OF PRENATAL CARE	RACE			ALL DEATHS
	CAUCASIAN	AFRICAN-AMERICAN	OTHER[e]	
No care	19.0	26.5	49.5[f]	23.0
Inadequate	3.3	10.3	6.6	5.0
Adequate	2.4	7.0	3.7	3.0
Adequate plus	5.5	14.8	10.7	7.3
All levels of care	**3.6**	**11.2**	**7.1**	**5.1**

[a] Pregnancy-related deaths among women who delivered a live-born infant per 100,000 live births.
[b] Hispanic women were classified according to reported racial group.
[c] Levels of prenatal care were based on a modification of the adequacy of prenatal care use index developed by Kotelchuck, and they were defined as follows: adequate plus, care began at ≤4 months of pregnancy, and ≥110% of recommended prenatal care visits were made (in accordance with standards established by the American College of Obstetricians and Gynecologists); adequate, care began at ≤4 months of pregnancy, and <80% of recommended visits were made, or care began at ≥5 months of pregnancy (recommended number of visits not applicable); no care, no prenatal care obtained.
[d] Excludes California for 1987–1988.
[e] Includes Asian/Pacific Islander, Native American/Alaskan native, and those reported as "other."
[f] This rate was based on fewer than five deaths and should be interpreted with caution.
SOURCE: Koonin LM, et al. 1997

Figure 9-2

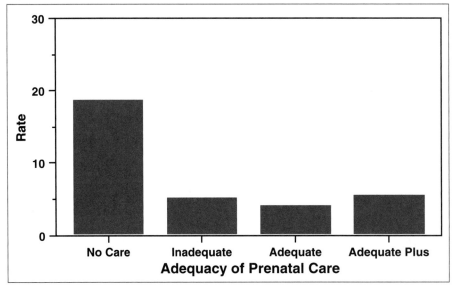

Adjusted pregnancy-related mortality rate, by adequacy of prenatal care: United States, 1987–1990.
(Reproduced from Centers for Disease Control and Prevention, MMWR Morb Mortal Wkly Rep 45:1–24, 1996.)

Periconception Care

Because patients often do not seek maternity care until after the first trimester, when the critical period of organogenesis is already completed, many health professionals advocate *periconception care.* This is health care provided before and around the time of conception that is specifically designed to improve pregnancy outcomes. Although limited evidence exists to support most periconception interventions, many clinicians choose to provide this care while awaiting better evidence. If periconception care is to be provided, it must be offered at all routine visits by patients of reproductive age, because patients rarely make specific appointments for periconception care. Items that should be addressed include folic acid supplementation, use of other vitamins and minerals, avoidance of teratogens, immunizations, and prevention of infectious diseases (Table 9-6).

Table 9-6

Recommended Periconception Interventions

Daily folic acid supplementation for all women of reproductive age
Genetic screening and counseling as appropriate
Multivitamin supplementation
Rubella screening and immunization as appropriate
Varicella screening and immunization as appropriate
Tetanus-diphtheria (dT) immunization if needed
Avoidance of teratogens
Prevention of infectious disease (toxoplasmosis, cytomegalovirus infection)

Folic Acid Supplementation

Folic acid supplementation is one periconception intervention supported by excellent evidence. The infants of women who take 0.8 mg of folate daily around the time of conception are at significantly reduced risk for neural tube defects. Unfortunately, since the U.S. Public Health Service recommended in 1995 that all U.S. women of childbearing age take folate supplements, there has been little change in most women's folate intake, indicating that more effective ways are needed to carry out this intervention. To facilitate population-wide folate supplementation, the U.S. Food and Drug Administration recently mandated folate supplementation of certain grain and cereal products.

Other Vitamin and Mineral Supplements

Periconceptional use of multivitamins and minerals has not been found helpful in randomized, controlled trials. Case-control studies, however, indicate that periconceptional multivitamin supplementation, with or without folic acid, may help prevent certain birth defects. Many clinicians recommend the use of a folate-containing multivitamin supplement for women before and after conception.

Avoidance of Teratogens

For both women and men, increasing evidence suggests that many chemical exposures are potentially teratogenic. These include occupational exposures such as those to organic solvents, anesthetic gases, and antineoplastic agents. Young families should be informed that tobacco products might cause birth defects. The American College of Obstetricians and Gynecologists (ACOG) recommends that pregnant women avoid taking more than 5000 IU of vitamin A daily because in high doses this vitamin can act as a teratogen. Alcohol is a known teratogen and should be avoided around conception and during pregnancy. Other substances of abuse such as cocaine and heroine should also be avoided. It is good advice to avoid all medications unless the potential for teratogenicity is checked and ruled out.

Infectious Diseases

As recommended by the U.S. Preventive Services Task Force, the American Academy of Pediatrics, and the Centers for Disease Control and Prevention (CDC), all women of reproductive age should be screened for rubella immunity and be immunized if not immune. Immunization before pregnancy prevents the numerous severe birth defects that occur with congenital rubella syndrome. Multiple missed screening opportunities have been found for many women who give birth to children with congenital rubella syndrome. Because of a theoretical risk from the live virus vaccine, women who are not pregnant who receive rubella immunization should not attempt pregnancy for 3 months, although there are no reports of adverse outcomes among women who have received rubella vaccine while pregnant.

Clinicians also should consider screening women for varicella in the periconception period or simply immunizing women who have no history of varicella infection. Nine percent of pregnant women with varicella infection contract varicella pneumonia. Fetal varicella resembles congenital rubella syndrome and occurs with about 5% of first-trimester varicella infections. Neither rubella nor varicella immunizations should be given during pregnancy but may be given before conception or postpartum. The periconception period also is an excellent time to ensure that tetanus and diphtheria vaccination is current.

Toxoplasma gondii infection can cause fetal growth retardation and numerous physical anomalies. It is controversial whether women should undergo screening for this infection before conception or even during pregnancy, because the diagnostic evaluation carries considerable morbidity and there is no evidence that treatment prevents congenital disease. Cytomegalovirus acts as a similar teratogen. It is a common infection among infants and children and is passed through infectious secretions. Women who work in hospitals should use universal precautions and those who work in daycare centers should adopt high standards of hygiene and hand washing. Counseling to prevent exposure to these infectious agents is the preferred option. This topic is discussed later in Anticipatory Guidance.

Diabetes

The evidence is clear that for mothers with diabetes, strict diabetes control around the time of conception results in fewer congenital defects and better outcomes of pregnancy for both mother and baby. This issue should be discussed with all diabetic women with childbearing potential.

Prenatal Care

Once a pregnancy occurs and a woman seeks prenatal care, the clinician needs to address a number of issues. These include risk assessment and risk reduction, screening tests, immunizations, the initial physical examination, follow-up visits, and anticipatory guidance. The goal is to maximize the potential for a good outcome for both mother and baby.

Risk Assessment and Risk Reduction

An important part of prenatal care is to assess risk factors so that risks may be reduced. Risk assessment can be complex because a variety of risk factors may affect pregnancy.

ALCOHOL

As many as one-third of U.S. women report drinking alcohol during pregnancy, fewer than 10% of them more than once a month. In the United States, the incidence of fetal alcohol syndrome (FAS) is 1.95 per 1000 live births; 4.7 per 1000 births among daily drinkers. Each year in the United States more than 2000 infants are born with FAS. FAS causes a number of physical and behavioral problems among affected children, including developmental and learning difficulties that may persist throughout the school years. The physical problems include growth retardation, characteristic facial features, hearing and visual impairment, and other birth defects. Although only high levels of alcohol intake during pregnancy appear to cause FAS, lower levels can cause persistent neurobehavioral deficits. Children of mothers who drink alcohol during pregnancy are smaller in weight, height, head circumference, and palpebral fissure width.

A positive answer to any of the CAGE questions (see Table 11-3) correlates strongly with alcohol abuse and other substance abuse by both pregnant and nonpregnant patients. Alcohol treatment programs are mandated to accept pregnant women. Counseling programs for pregnant drinkers seem to be at least somewhat effective, but studies are limited because it would be unethical to randomize pregnant substance abusers to a no-treatment arm of a study.

SUBSTANCE ABUSE

Abuse of illegal drugs during pregnancy is common, occurring among more than 5% of pregnant women in some communities. The most commonly used drugs are marijuana, cocaine, and opiates. Pregnant drug users are at risk for numerous complications, including

sexually transmitted diseases, preeclampsia, chorioamnionitis, and postpartum hemorrhage. Infants of cocaine users carry increased risk for low-birth weight, prematurity, abruptio placentae, and perinatal death. Intrauterine growth retardation is more than twice as common among pregnant users of "crack" cocaine than it is for the general population of pregnant women.

Few data exist on the efficacy of risk assessment for substance abuse. Women with poor records of attending prenatal care are at higher risk for using cocaine and should be screened carefully, as should pregnant smokers. The CAGE questionnaire also is valid for substance abuse during pregnancy. Clinicians can consider urine toxicologic screening, with the patient's informed consent. Some substance abuse treatment programs are tailored to pregnant patients. It is difficult to assess the effectiveness of drug treatment programs for pregnant women. In observational studies, various types of treatment programs seem to be at least somewhat effective. These programs usually include intensive counseling and supervision. Pregnant drug abusers in some counseling programs who obtain prenatal care have babies with higher birth weights than do drug abusers who avoid prenatal care.

Drug abuse treatment of pregnant women is cost effective. A case-control study compared outcomes among 100 pregnant women undergoing drug treatment with outcomes among 46 matched controls who were not in treatment. The mean net savings for the treated group was $4644 per mother-infant pair, because the savings in neonatal intensive care costs exceeded the modest costs of drug treatment (Svikis, et al, 1997). Unfortunately, many clinicians are not aware of local resources for pregnant substance abusers and often do not refer these women for treatment. Even when patients are referred appropriately, many drug treatment programs lack adequate funding and must defer potential clients.

TOBACCO

According to the National Center for Health Statistics, as many as 18% of pregnant women report smoking tobacco. Tobacco smokers are at increased risk for abruptio placentae, placenta previa, preeclampsia, and preterm birth. In case-control studies, pregnant smokers also show more than double the baseline risk for delivering infants with congenital anomalies. Maternal smoking during pregnancy appears to confer independent risk for sudden infant death syndrome after the birth and for developmental delay. Complicated births have been estimated to cost at least $4000 more for smokers than for nonsmokers, creating a nationwide cost of $1.4 billion a year attributable to smoking during pregnancy.

To assess risk, clinicians generally rely on maternal self-reports about smoking, although these are not as accurate as measuring urinary cotinine concentration. Various smoking cessation programs are available for pregnant patients. Numerous randomized controlled trials have examined whether intervention programs generally succeed in helping pregnant women stop smoking. It appears that approximately one-half of pregnant smokers stop smoking when they participate in structured intervention programs. Relapse prevention programs focused on brief counseling have had modest but statistically significant success, emphasizing that clinicians should reinforce cessation among women who have previously stopped smoking during pregnancy. Chapter 10 discusses smoking cessation in depth.

CAFFEINE

In some studies, pregnant women who exceeded a certain level of caffeine consumption (one to 1.5 cups of coffee or tea a day or about three caffeine-containing soft drinks per day) doubled their risk for spontaneous abortion and increased their risk for delivering low-birth weight infants. Caffeine intake in the month before conception, if greater than about three cups daily, also may increase risk for spontaneous abortion. Although other studies showed less or no apparent risk, many clinicians caution pregnant patients to limit their caffeine intake.

OCCUPATIONAL EXPOSURES

Occupational toxins, including dry-cleaning chemicals and organic solvents, may cause spontaneous abortion. Prospective studies show that walking or standing for more than 5 hours a day greatly increases risk for preterm birth. Other potentially harmful exposures include prolonged noise exposure, exposure to electric and magnetic fields, and biologic agents found in day care and health care settings. Prospective parents, both men and women, should be screened for occupational exposure early in pregnancy, although there are no data to prove or disprove whether counseling about occupational risks improves pregnancy outcomes.

OBSTETRIC HISTORY

Patients with a history of preterm birth remain at very high risk for preterm birth in subsequent pregnancies. There are no good methods to prevent preterm birth among women at high risk. Targeted prevention programs have failed to date, although it may be helpful to identify precipitating infections early, before they lead to preterm birth. (See discussion of Asymptomatic Bacteriuria and Bacterial Vaginosis.)

Unlike type I and type II diabetes mellitus, gestational diabetes by definition occurs only during pregnancy, but it recurs in subsequent pregnancies in up to 35% of patients. Women with recurrent gestational diabetes tend to have higher-fat diets than women who do not have a recurrence, so it may help to counsel these women about diet early in pregnancy. (See discussion of Gestational Diabetes.)

For patients who want to attempt vaginal birth after cesarean section (VBAC), as long as the previous operation involved only a nonextended, low transverse uterine incision, the risk for uterine rupture in a subsequent pregnancy is low. The American Academy of Family Physicians (AAFP) recommends that clinicians allow a pregnant woman to choose a trial of labor or elective repeat cesarean section because the two options are equally safe and have similar maternal and infant outcomes. Even women with one low-segment, nonextended, vertical uterine incision may consider VBAC. No special prenatal interventions are necessary for VBAC other than comprehensive counseling and informed consent about the risks and benefits of a trial of labor versus elective repeat cesarean birth. VBAC births should take place in hospitals where emergency cesarean section can be readily performed.

MEDICAL COMPLICATIONS

Part of risk assessment involves asking about chronic and past medical conditions that can affect the course and outcome of pregnancy. Table 9-7 contains a list of disease categories that should be covered in the initial history.

Screening Tests

RECOMMENDED SCREENING TESTS FOR AN EARLY PRENATAL VISIT

Many clinicians choose to perform a set of screening tests at an early prenatal visit, often before or during the visit when the prenatal history and physical examination are performed (Table 9-8).

ASYMPTOMATIC BACTERIURIA   Asymptomatic bacteriuria (ASB) occurs among 2% to 7% of pregnancies. ASB during pregnancy often leads to urinary tract infection, which has been correlated with prematurity, low-birth weight, hypertensive complications, and chorioamnionitis. To screen for ASB, a midstream, clean-catch voided urine specimen or a specimen collected with a

Table 9-7

Medical Conditions That Can Complicate Pregnancy

Diabetes, including gestational diabetes
Hypertension
Asthma and other respiratory diseases
Cardiovascular disease, including thromboembolic disease
Hematologic disorders
Gastroenterologic disease
Seizure disorders and other neurologic disease
Infectious diseases, including HIV infection
Renal failure and other renal and urologic disorders
Nondiabetic endocrine disease, including thyroid disorders
Connective tissue disorders such as rheumatoid arthritis and lupus erythematosus
Dermatologic conditions
Malignant tumors
Psychiatric disorders

catheter can be used to obtain a sample for urine dipstick testing, culture, and sensitivity testing.

The urine culture is the standard against which other tests are measured. Urine Gram stain is the next most accurate test and is reportedly 91.7% sensitive and 89.2% specific in the detection of ASB with a positive predictive value of 45%. Urine dipstick tests may not be sufficiently accurate for optimal screening. Nitrite and leukocyte esterase tests are 43% to 50% sensitive and 77% to 96.9% specific with a positive predictive value of only 18 to 62%. Many clinicians obtain a urine culture at an early prenatal visit and then repeat if signs or symptoms of a urinary tract infection develop. A positive urine culture contains at least 100,000 colonies of a single pathogen per milliliter of urine. Treatment is based on the bacterial pathogen and sensitivity results.

Table 9-8

Recommended Screening Tests and Interventions to Offer to Pregnant Patients

AT AN EARLY PRENATAL VISIT
Asymptomatic bacteriuria
Bacterial vaginosis
Blood typing, Rh, and antibodies
Iron deficiency anemia
Chlamydia
Gonorrhea
Herpes
Hepatitis B
HIV
Cervical dysplasia (Papanicolaou test)
Rubella immunity
Syphilis
Urine toxicology, as appropriate

AT 15–20 WEEKS' GESTATIONAL AGE
Triple marker screening

AT 24–28 WEEKS' GESTATIONAL AGE
Gestational diabetes
Sexually transmitted disease if high risk
Rh antibody if RhD-negative

AT 35–37 WEEKS' GESTATIONAL AGE
Group B streptococci

BACTERIAL VAGINOSIS Bacterial vaginosis is an overgrowth of anaerobic bacteria in the vaginal flora. It often causes a malodorous vaginal discharge and can trigger a cascade of inflammatory mediators. This infection appears to confer 40% increased risk for preterm birth, at least among women at high risk. The following criteria are used to diagnose bacterial vaginosis: (1) vaginal pH greater than 4.5, (2) clue cells on saline mount, (3) a positive whiff test result with 10% potassium hydroxide, and (4) a thin, uniform vaginal discharge. Diagnosing bacterial vaginosis requires three of these four criteria.

In a landmark randomized, controlled trial of bacterial vaginosis treatment during pregnancy, Hauth, et al (1995) diagnosed bacterial vaginosis using the aforementioned strict criteria. Pregnant women with and without bacterial vaginosis were randomized to receive oral metronidazole and erythromycin or placebo. Among women with bacterial vaginosis, treatment decreased the rate of preterm births by 18%. Women without bacterial vaginosis did not benefit from the antibiotics.

When the result of a bacterial vaginosis screen is positive, typical treatment is metronidazole with or without oral erythromycin. Topical metronidazole and clindamycin may relieve symptoms but have not been shown to decrease risk for preterm labor. Some clinicians defer oral therapy until after the first trimester of pregnancy. A follow-up wet mount and vaginal pH may be checked for test of cure after antibiotic therapy.

BLOOD TYPE, RH STATUS, AND ANTIBODIES Rhesus, or Rh, status includes five major antigenic loci-C, D, E, c, and e. Persons with D antigens are said to be Rh-positive, and the others are Rh-negative. When Rh-negative mothers carry Rh-positive fetuses, they risk development of anti-RhD antibodies that can attack fetal red blood cells in subsequent pregnancies, causing hemolytic disease of the newborn. To prevent this problem, pregnant women undergo routine screening for blood type and antigen-antibody status by means of standard screening techniques or polymerase chain reaction. Blood typing and serum antigen-antibody screening are highly sensitive and specific. The U.S. Preventive Services Task Force (USPSTF), American Academy of Pediatrics, and ACOG support this routine prenatal screen and administration of anti-RhD immunoglobulin at 28 weeks' gestational age to unsensitized RhD-negative women after a repeat screen confirms the absence of the antibody. It should be given again within 72 hours after delivery to mothers whose baby is RhD-positive. This prophylaxis regimen decreases the rate of isoimmunization among RhD-negative women from 30% to less than 0.2%.

The 28-week anti-RhD injection should be given regardless of the father's blood type because paternity is not always known or reported accurately. Anti-RhD immunoglobulin should also be administered after elective abortion, spontaneous abortion, and amniocentesis to RhD-negative, antibody negative women.

If the antibody screen shows Rh antibodies in an RhD-negative woman, she has Rh isoimmunization. Primary care clinicians should obtain obstetric or perinatologic assistance with such patients. Antibodies other than anti-Rh may or may not be clinically significant, and advice regarding their importance can be obtained from the laboratory or perinatologist.

IRON DEFICIENCY ANEMIA Moderate to severe anemia (hemoglobin <9.0 to 10.0 g/dL) is associated with increased risk for low-birth weight, preterm delivery, and perinatal death. Whether this association is caused by anemia or other associated variables is not clear. There is some evidence of benefit to treating anemic pregnant women with supplemental iron. Although this evidence is not the strongest, the USPSTF still recommends checking a hemoglobin level or hematocrit at the first prenatal visit and providing iron supplementation to women with a hemoglobin level less than 10 g/dL once iron deficiency has been confirmed by means of serum ferritin measurement.

CHLAMYDIA AND GONORRHEA Chlamydial cervicitis is a common infection, especially among teens. Chapter 8 discusses the prevalence, screening, diagnosis, and management of chlamydia and gonorrhea. Both infections have a greater effect on the neonate than they do on the mother, although there is reasonable evidence that screening and therapy for chlamydia during pregnancy improve the outcome for both mother and baby.

Gonorrhea causes eye infections among 30% to 50% of exposed newborns. Gonococcal oph-

thalmia usually appears as conjunctivitis but also can cause corneal scarring, eye perforation, and blindness. Chlamydial infection can cause endometritis both before and after delivery as well as neonatal conjunctivitis and pneumonia.

There is some debate whether all pregnant women or only those at high risk should undergo screening for gonorrhea and chlamydia. Risk factors include age younger than 30 years, two or more sex partners in the previous year, sexual contact with partners who have sexually transmitted diseases, and age at first intercourse of 16 years or younger.

It is not clear whether treating pregnant women for gonorrhea and chlamydia improves pregnancy outcomes, but a study to look at this question definitively is unlikely to be performed.

HERPES Genital herpes at the time of delivery can cause newborn disseminated herpes, which has a high fatality rate. There is a much higher risk from primary infection than recurrent infection. All women should be asked about past genital herpes. Herpes cultures of suspicious lesions should be taken to confirm the diagnosis. Routine cultures are not recommended in the care of patients who are not infected or do not have symptoms. The presence of a herpes lesion at the time of delivery is an indication for cesarean section.

HEPATITIS B Approximately 20,000 infants are born each year in the United States to women with active hepatitis B. Infections contracted during childhood and infancy constitute 42% of cases of chronic hepatitis B. When they reach adulthood, many of these persons die of hepatocellular carcinoma or hepatic cirrhosis. The presence of hepatitis B surface antigen in the blood indicates active infection with hepatitis B virus, either acute or chronic, including the carrier state.

Universal hepatitis B screening for all pregnant women is recommended by the AAFP, ACOG, the American Academy of Pediatrics, and the Advisory Committee on Immunization

Practices. ACOG recommends that women at high risk for contracting hepatitis B virus infection during pregnancy be immunized. All 50 states now sponsor programs to prevent perinatal transmission of hepatitis B.

Chapter 1 contains a description of how to prevent hepatitis B among infants born to women who have positive test results for hepatitis B surface antigen.

HIV   A description of the prevalence and epidemiologic features of HIV infection among young adults is located in Chapter 8, as is a discussion of screening tests.

The purpose of prenatal screening is to reduce risk for perinatal transmission of HIV from mother to child. The chance of mother-to-infant transmission is 13 to 35%. There is good evidence that administration of zidovudine to the mother starting between 14 and 34 weeks' gestation and continued through delivery along with zidovudine treatment of the newborn reduces the rate of transmission to about 8%. It is likely that this rate of transmission can be reduced even further with combination antiretroviral therapy. Because HIV can be passed in breast milk, mothers in the United States who have positive results of tests for HIV should be advised not to breast feed their babies.

As with other sexually transmitted diseases, there is some controversy about whether to offer HIV screening to all pregnant women or only to those at high risk. Because of the important of the disease to both mother and child and good evidence for the effectiveness of screening and treatment, the CDC recommends that all pregnant women be encouraged to undergo HIV testing. The USPSTF recommends screening only for those at high risk—those with other sexually transmitted diseases, past or present users of injected drugs, those who exchange sex for money or drugs, those with past or present sex partners with HIV infection or sex partners at risk for HIV infection, and those with a history of a blood transfusion between 1978 and 1985.

PAPANICOLAOU TESTING   Although screening for cervical cancer during pregnancy is not proven to lead to better birth outcomes, it is a proven beneficial screening test for women. Perinatal care offers an excellent opportunity to conduct screening. If cervical cancer is detected during pregnancy, consideration can be given to performing hysterectomy at the delivery or terminating the pregnancy. Chapter 12 covers the epidemiologic features and prevalence of cervical cancer, screening methods, and follow-up care after positive test results are obtained.

RUBELLA   The purpose of rubella screening is to prevent congenital rubella syndrome. Rubella, congenital rubella syndrome, and rubella screening tests are discussed in Chapter 1.

Pregnant women who are not immune to rubella should be immunized postpartum to provide protection against rubella in subsequent pregnancies. If a rash with a febrile illness develops during pregnancy, rubella can be confirmed with a fourfold rise in serum rubella IgG titer or the presence of rubella IgM antibodies. If infection during pregnancy is confirmed, the mother can choose whether to terminate the pregnancy on the basis of the timing of the infection and her personal beliefs and preferences.

Rubella screening is a routine part of prenatal care. Yet once immunity is established, it is not clear that screening during subsequent pregnancies is necessary. The USPSTF recommends screening for rubella susceptibility through a documented history of vaccination or by serologic testing for all women of childbearing age at their first clinical encounter. The ACOG recommends prenatal screening for all women not known to be immune.

SYPHILIS   Congenital syphilis occurs among 70 to 90% of newborns if the mother has untreated primary or secondary syphilis during pregnancy. The complications of congenital syphilis include hydrops fetalis, jaundice, hepatosplenomegaly, osteitis, mucocutaneous lesions, and rash. Fetal death occurs in 25% of cases.

Chapter 8 contains a description of the screening tests for syphilis. To screen for asymptomatic syphilis, nontreponemal serum tests are used. These include the VDRL or rapid plasma reagin (RPR) tests. A positive screening test result should be followed by a test for treponemal antibodies, either the fluorescent treponemal antibody absorption test (FTA-ABS) or microhemagglutination test for *Treponema pallidum* (MHA-TP). A positive treponemal antibody test confirms syphilis.

If the screening test result is positive but the antibody test result is negative, one of two situations exists: (1) the result is falsely positive because of another type of infection, drugs, or autoimmune disease, or (2) it is an early infection and the antibody test result has not yet changed to positive. The antibody test and VDRL or RPR titer should be repeated in 1 to 2 months.

Once syphilis is confirmed, a decision to treat or not to treat should be based on the history of syphilis and syphilis treatment along with the result of the VDRL or RPR titer. A woman with a history of syphilis adequately treated, with adequate follow-up care, and no rise in titer since adequately responding to treatment probably does not have new, active syphilis. If there is any doubt about the adequacy of past response to treatment or whether there is a new infection, treatment is indicated. If syphilis treatment is given during pregnancy, repeat VDRL or RPR titers should be performed monthly to document the fourfold decrease in titer that indicates adequate response to therapy. A description of syphilis treatment is found in Chapter 8.

TUBERCULOSIS Tuberculosis (TB) occurs in one of two forms—asymptomatic infection or active disease. Persons with asymptomatic infection have positive TB skin test results, which indicate the presence of *Mycobacterium tuberculosis* in the body but no signs of active disease. Persons with symptomatic pulmonary TB generally have weight loss, productive cough, hemoptysis, and evidence of pulmonary disease on a chest radiograph. TB also can occur in a number of extrapulmonary sites.

There are approximately 15,000 to 20,000 new cases of active TB in the United States each year. Persons at higher risk include immigrants from developing countries, residents and staff of correctional and long-term care institutions, health care workers, persons with HIV infection or AIDS, users of illicit intravenous drugs, and persons who are socioeconomically disadvantaged. Pregnant women who are in a high-risk group should undergo screening early in pregnancy for two reasons—to detect infection and to detect active disease among persons who may not have classic symptoms.

Tuberculin skin testing, also known as the purified protein derivative (PPD) or Mantoux test, involves injecting a purified form of the *M. tuberculosis* antigen intradermally and observing the injection site in 48 to 72 hours for a local inflammatory reaction that indicates TB infection. PPD test results usually become positive about 6 weeks after infection, so testing may miss early infections. False-positive test results occur when there is infection with other mycobacteria.

The PPD dose is 0.1 mL and is injected intradermally in the volar forearm. According to CDC criteria, an induration reaction of at least 5 mm is considered positive for persons at high risk—those with HIV infection, close contacts of persons with active TB, users of intravenous drugs who have unknown HIV status, and patients whose chest radiographic findings show evidence of old, healed TB. A 10 mm reaction is positive among immigrants from TB-endemic areas (Asia, Africa, Central and South America), persons living in poverty, users of intravenous drugs who have negative HIV test results, residents and workers in nursing homes, and persons with chronic medical conditions. For all other persons, a 15 mm reaction is considered positive. (See Table 20.3 for a description of tuberculosis skin test criteria.)

Positive tuberculin skin test results are followed with a chest radiograph, usually deferred until after 20 weeks' gestation and performed with an abdominal shield. Pregnant patients with active TB are treated as nonpregnant patients are. If the chest radiograph is normal, pregnant patients usually are offered prophylaxis with isoniazid (INH) postpartum because an increased rate of INH-associated hepatitis has been reported among pregnant women and because earlier prophylaxis is not known to be more effective. Those who should receive INH during pregnancy because of higher risk for reactivation include those with HIV infection, close contacts of persons with active cases of TB, and persons whose skin test result has recently converted. Pregnant women with positive skin test results and no active disease should be advised to seek care should symptoms of TB develop.

RECOMMENDED SCREENING TESTS AT 15 TO 20 WEEKS' GESTATIONAL AGE

MATERNAL SCREENING FOR NEURAL TUBE AND CHROMOSOMAL DEFECTS Neural tube defects include anencephaly, encephalocele, and spina bifida. They occur in 1 in 1000 births in the United States. Down syndrome, the most common human malformation, occurs in 1 in 800 live births. The triple marker screen is a maternal serum screen for three analytes—α fetoprotein (AFP), human chorionic gonadotropin (hCG), and conjugated estriol. The screen is used to detect neural tube defects, Down syndrome, and less common trisomy syndromes. A few laboratories still conduct AFP testing alone.

The sensitivity of the AFP screen in detecting a neural tube defect is 56% to 91%. The positive predictive value of a positive test result, however, is low, 5% or less. The cutoff values used to define an abnormal test result depend on gestational age and the presence of other congenital defects, growth retardation, or multiple gestations, all of which can cause false-positive results. If the AFP level is low or the triple screen indicates increased risk for Down syndrome, follow-up testing includes a repeat triple screen and high-resolution sonography to confirm fetal age and to search for visible defects. If no identifiable cause of the abnormal results is detected, amniocentesis should be offered to measure amniotic fluid AFP and for chromosomal analysis.

The combination of low levels of AFP and estriol and elevated hCG level is 79% sensitive and 82% specific in detecting fetal Down syndrome. This combination, however, results in a positive predictive value of 1 per 200 to 270, the same risk for Down syndrome among pregnant women older than 35 years.

The potential harm from screening includes psychological effects on parents who have positive test results, complications of amniocentesis, and risk for elective abortion of a normal fetus because of a false-positive test result. Amniocentesis can result in fetal loss, but the rate is low (as low as 0.04 % in some studies, but as high as 0.8% in others).

Maternal serum screening offers families the option of detecting neural tube defects and trisomy syndromes early in pregnancy. Although some patients may not want to have this information before delivery, others use information from a positive test result to terminate pregnancy or to plan for care of the infant's medical problems. Although a controlled trial of screening has not been conducted, both the USPSTF and ACOG recommend that all pregnant women be offered analyte screening if adequate counseling and follow-up services are available. The screening must be performed between 15 and 20 weeks' gestational age and is most accurate between 16 and 18 weeks. Whether or not they choose testing, families should be counseled about the test and sign informed consent documents. They should understand that if the screen result is positive, ultrasonography and amniocentesis are the common follow-up tests.

RECOMMENDED SCREENING TESTS AND INTERVENTIONS AT 24 TO 28 WEEKS' GESTATIONAL AGE

GESTATIONAL DIABETES   Gestational diabetes mellitus is the most common medical complication of pregnancy, affecting 3 to 6% of pregnancies. If the woman is not treated, gestational diabetes may result in substantial morbidity for the neonate, including macrosomia and birth injuries.

In the standard screening test for gestational diabetes, the pregnant patient takes a 50 g oral glucose load, usually as a glucose cola drink. One hour later, a phlebotomist draws a blood sample for serum glucose measurement. Maximum sensitivity (88%) and specificity (85%) are achieved when the cutoff for a positive plasma glucose screen is set at 140 mg/dL, which yields a positive predictive value of 29.1%. However, 12% of cases of diabetes are missed. With 135 mg/dL as the cutoff, the positive predictive value is 24.3%, and very few cases are missed. A cutoff of 130 mg/dL leads to little gain in sensitivity and an increase in the number of false positive results, leading many providers to select a cutoff of 135 mg/dL. Screening generally is performed between 24 and 28 weeks' gestational age. Diabetes among patients at high risk usually can be diagnosed with a screen between 12 and 24 weeks' gestation, but 16% of patients who develop diabetes have a normal screen at this gestational age but will have a positive screen result at 28 weeks. Screening before 12 weeks is too insensitive to be of value.

Patients with an abnormal 1-hour screen result should undergo a 3-hour oral glucose tolerance test (GTT) unless the 1-hour, 50 g glucose screen result exceeds 216 mg/dL. Almost all such patients have class A2 gestational diabetes and need insulin, so these patients do not need confirmatory tests.

The National Diabetes Data Group (NDDG) standards for an abnormal GTT are two values at or above the following cutoffs: 105 mg/dL fasting, 190 mg/dL at 1 hour, 165 mg/dL at 2 hours, and 145 mg/dL at 3 hours. If the fasting value is abnormal, the patient has class A2 gestational diabetes and will likely need insulin. If the fasting value is normal, she has class A1 gestational diabetes and can likely be treated with diet. Data conflict on whether a single abnormal value on the GTT confers increased risk for macrosomia. Depending on standards of practice in the community, many primary care providers obtain obstetrical or perinatology consultation for class A2 gestational diabetes.

Recognition and management of gestational diabetes reduces the risk for macrosomia. Screening is not risk free, however. Women with false-positive screen results may experience emotional stress. Some experts have argued that not all pregnant women need screening. The incidence of gestational diabetes is low, for example, among adolescents. Some clinicians screen only women with risk factors such as advanced maternal age, family history of diabetes, and obesity (Table 9-9). In a population at low risk, only 1% of patients in prenatal care who lack risk factors for gestational diabetes have gestational diabetes. ACOG and the National Diabetes Data Group recommend universal screening for gestational diabetes; the USPSTF does not.

Table 9-9

Risk Factors for Gestational Diabetes Mellitus

Advanced maternal age (>35 years)
Family history of diabetes, including gestational diabetes
Obesity
Nonwhite ethnicity
Previous gestational diabetes

SEXUALLY TRANSMITTED DISEASES   As part of the care of women who are at high risk for sexually transmitted diseases in the third trimester, clinicians should consider a repeat screen for gonorrhea, chlamydia, and syphilis. Because gonorrhea and chlamydia have more implications for the newborn it is reasonable to test for these diseases later in the trimester to minimize the risk for infection after the last screening test. Rescreening for syphilis has more implications for the fetus and the pregnancy. Earlier screening (28 to 30 weeks' gestation) is recommended for women at high risk and for all women in geographic areas where syphilis rates are high.

RH ANTIBODY IN RHD-NEGATIVE WOMEN   A repeat Rh antibody screen is recommended for RhD-negative women before anti-RhD immunoglobulin is administered. After anti-RhD immunoglobulin is given, the antibody test has positive results, making differentiation between isoimmunization and passive immunization difficult if a preliminary level has not been measured.

RECOMMENDED SCREENING TESTS AT 35 TO 37 WEEKS' GESTATIONAL AGE

GROUP B STREPTOCOCCI   Group B streptococcus (GBS), or *Streptococcus agalactiae*, is a leading cause of serious bacterial infection among newborns. It causes sepsis, pneumonia, meningitis, and shock and has a case-fatality rate of 5% to 20%. Colonization with GBS can be identified with a vaginal-perineal culture. GBS prevention is controversial because the evidence has been conflicting. Administering antibiotics to all women before the onset of labor has not proved effective, nor has postpartum administration of antibiotics to all newborns. However, intrapartum administration of intravenous antibiotics (penicillin or ampicillin) to women colonized with GBS can decrease risk for invasive disease among newborns.

Ascertaining whether a patient is a carrier of GBS is accomplished by means of vaginal cul-

tures late in pregnancy, near term. A positive GBS culture early in pregnancy correlates poorly with risk for sepsis at delivery. The risk for neonatal sepsis, however, is approximately 1 in 200 if GBS cultures are positive at 36 weeks' gestation. GBS is best isolated by means of a culture performed with selective media. Anorectal colonization is most common, so the swab should be taken from the outer one-third of the vagina and then the perineal and anal areas. Once positive, always positive is the rule. A positive GBS culture any time during pregnancy or GBS disease in a prior infant should lead the clinician to consider the mother to have positive GBS status at delivery.

The CDC recommends either of two approaches to GBS prevention. The first, illustrated in Figure 9-3, entails a combination of risk factor-triggered prophylaxis and universal screening at 35 to 37 weeks' gestation for those without risk. The second approach does not involve screening cultures and is illustrated in Figure 9-4. The recommendations for intrapartum prophylaxis are listed in Table 9-10.

OPTIONAL SCREENING TESTS

AMNIOCENTESIS FOR WOMEN OF ADVANCED MATERNAL AGE   Down syndrome, caused by a trisomy of chromosome 21, causes mental and growth retardation, heart defects, and characteristic physical abnormalities. Women 35 years of age and older are at higher risk than are younger women for delivering an infant with Down syndrome. Women of "advanced maternal age" (35 years and older) and those with a prior Down syndrome pregnancy traditionally have been offered screening amniocentesis at 15 to 16 weeks' gestational age according to guidelines of the USPSTF and ACOG, but this policy has become increasingly controversial. Under ultrasound guidance, the clinician taps a pocket of amniotic fluid to obtain a fluid sample for chromosomal analysis.

Even though amniocentesis at 15 to 16 weeks is highly sensitive and specific, it can result in

Figure 9-3

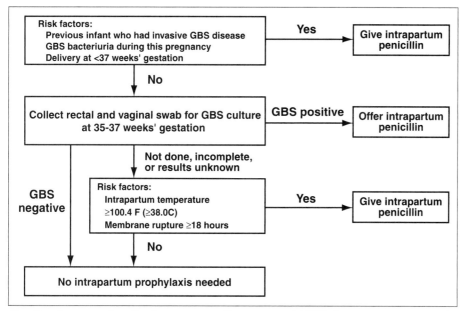

Algorithm for prevention of early-onset group B streptococcal (GBS) disease among neonates by means of prenatal screening at 35 to 37 weeks' gestation. *(Reproduced from Centers for Disease Control and Prevention, MMWR Morb Mortal Wkly Rep 45:1–24, 1996.)*

Figure 9-4

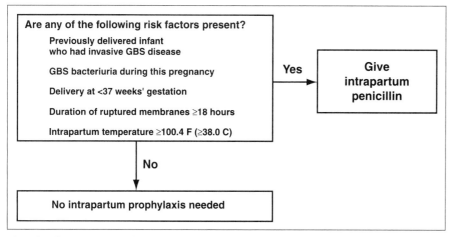

Algorithm for prevention of early-onset of group B streptococcal (GBS) disease among neonates by use of risk factors. *(Reproduced from Centers for Disease Control and Prevention, MMWR Morb Mortal Wkly Rep 45:1–24, 1996.)*

Table 9-10

Recommended Regimens for Intrapartum Antimicrobial
Prophylaxis for Perinatal Group B Streptococcal Disease

Recommended	Penicillin G 5mU IV load, then 2.5 mUs IV every 4 h until delivery
Alternative	Ampicillin 2 g IV load, then 1 g IV every 4 h until delivery
IF PENICILLIN-ALLERGIC	
Recommended	Clindamycin 900 mg IV every 8 h until delivery
Alternative	Erythromycin 500 mg IV every 6 h until delivery

NOTE: If patient is receiving treatment for amnionitis with an antimicrobial agent active against group B streptococci (e.g., ampicillin, penicillin, clindamycin, or erythromycin), additional prophylactic antibiotics are not needed.
SOURCE: Centers for Disease Control, 1996.

fetal loss in 0.04% to 0.8% of pregnancies. This can equate to one normal fetus lost for every one to two fetuses with Down syndrome found in women 35 years of age. If amniocentesis is performed only on women whose triple marker screens indicate a greater than 1 in 200 risk for Down syndrome, 89% of cases of Down syndrome will be identified with a 25% false-positive rate, eliminating 75% of amniocenteses and the attendant complications. These data make triple marker screening of older women with amniocentesis for those beyond a threshold of risk an attractive alternative to universal amniocentesis.

TOXICOLOGY TESTING   Clinicians who choose to screen their pregnant patients for drug abuse may use urine toxicologic studies, which measure levels of commonly used and abused drugs. Metabolites of most drugs of abuse are present in the urine a few hours after use and

persist for one or more days. In general, clinicians should document informed consent before requesting a toxicologic screen for an adult. Consent is not mandatory before testing of infants and children. Referral for substance abuse treatment is appropriate if test results indicate abuse. Many communities offer follow-up programs for infants of substance-abusing mothers.

ULTRASONOGRAPHY FOR ROUTINE SCREENING   Routine ultrasound screening for fetal anomalies or establishing fetal age is controversial. The sensitivity of ultrasound screening in the detection of fetal anomalies varies between 16.6 and 85%. Its specificity is greater than 99% in most studies. There is no evidence that routine ultrasound screening changes perinatal outcomes or increases the live birth rate. The USPSTF does not recommend routine screening ultrasonography of women at low risk. ACOG advocates the use of ultrasonography only for specific clinical indications. If ultrasonography is performed for pregnancy dating, it is more accurate before 12 weeks' gestational age. A fetal anatomic survey can be completed at 18 to 20 weeks.

Initial Physical Examination

HEIGHT, WEIGHT, BLOOD PRESSURE, PREGNANCY DATING

Most clinicians measure the patient's height, weight, and blood pressure during the initial prenatal visit. After the prenatal history is taken, a complete physical examination with pelvic examination is performed early in pregnancy. Clinical pelvimetry may be done at this time. Little research has examined the benefit of these common practices.

The first prenatal examination also focuses on accurate estimation of pregnancy dating. Accurate dating is critical because complications such as postdates gestation and preterm labor can appear without warning later in pregnancy and can be diagnosed accurately only if the correct gestational age is known. ACOG offers the following criteria for accurate pregnancy dating that also are appropriate for determining a date for elective cesarean section: fetal heart tones auscultated for 20 weeks by means of nonelectronic fetoscope or for 30 weeks by means of Doppler evaluation, positive urine or serum hCG test results for 36 weeks, ultrasound measurement of embryonic crown-rump length at 6 to 11 weeks' gestational age, or ultrasonographic findings at 12 to 20 weeks' gestational age that support a clinically determined estimated date of delivery. Except for the first-trimester ultrasound scan, the results of these tests must match dating according to last menstrual period to yield accurate dates. Bimanual examination is notoriously unreliable for pregnancy dating.

A patient who has had a prior cesarean section should undergo first-trimester ultrasonography for accurate pregnancy dating. If the patient chooses or needs cesarean section later in the pregnancy, the operation often is performed during the 39th week of gestation, and an early ultrasound scan is the best way to establish accurate dates before this gestational age.

Ultrasonography is not necessary to date most normal pregnancies if the mother obtains early prenatal care. If Doppler evaluation is used for pregnancy dating, the clinician should attempt to auscultate fetal heart tones by the 12th week of gestation to meet the ACOG criteria (30 weeks of fetal heart tones by the 42nd week). If heart tones are not heard before the 13th week, a dating ultrasound scan should be obtained.

Follow-Up Visits

WEIGHT

Although clinicians typically follow pregnant patients' weight gain at follow-up prenatal visits, there is little evidence that routine weighing of

mothers improves pregnancy outcomes. The Institute of Medicine (IOM) in 1990 offered the following recommendations for weight gain during pregnancy: women with a body mass index (BMI; weight in kilograms divided by the square of height in meters) less than 19.8 are advised to gain 28 to 40 pounds during the pregnancy; those with a BMI of 19.8 to 26 to gain 25 to 35 pounds; those with a BMI of 26.1 to 29 to gain 15 to 25 pounds; and those with a BMI greater than 29 to gain up to 15 pounds. The IOM guidelines have been criticized for their lack of evidence basis. In recent studies, more than one-half of healthy pregnant women with good outcomes did not meet the IOM guidelines for weight gain during pregnancy. Once pregnant women become overweight, additional weight gain leads only to maternal obesity without appreciably increasing infant birth weight.

African-American women are at risk for delivering low-birth weight infants even if they gain weight in the upper half of the range recommended by the IOM. African-American women who follow the IOM guidelines retain significantly more weight post-partum than do Caucasian women, which may cause health problems later in life. Until evidence-based guidelines are available, clinicians may continue to use the IOM guidelines and temper them with clinical judgment.

Evidence does suggest that markedly inadequate maternal weight gain can lead to low-birth weight among infants and may increase risk for preterm birth. Pregnant adolescents are at especially high risk for inadequate weight gain and delivering low-birth weight infants. Protein- and calorie-restricted diets are unsafe and do not decrease risk for preeclampsia. They do result in lower birth weights.

BLOOD PRESSURE

Many maternity care providers follow the USPSTF guidelines that suggest periodically monitoring patients' blood pressure throughout pregnancy. Although there is nothing wrong with this practice, it alone cannot be relied on to predict preeclampsia. There is a statistically significant, albeit small, difference in blood pressure between women with normal blood pressure and those who will become preeclamptic, but there is considerable overlap. Unfortunately, there is no reliable way to predict or prevent preeclampsia. Patients with elevated blood pressure should be examined for other warning signs of preeclampsia such as edema and proteinuria. Elevated blood pressure often is defined as 140 mm Hg systolic or 90 mm Hg diastolic pressure.

FUNDAL HEIGHT

Another common practice in prenatal visits is to follow the growth of the fundal height. There is no solid evidence that routine measurement of fundal height leads to improved pregnancy outcomes, but several observational studies have suggested that this screen helps identify at least half of cases of fetal growth retardation. This method is most accurate when one examiner records multiple measurements over time.

URINE PROTEIN AND GLUCOSE

Urinary protein and glucose levels often are checked at each prenatal visit, presumably to help identify preeclampsia, gestational hypertension, and gestational diabetes as early as possible. Urine dipstick screening is not accurate for these purposes. A normal urine dipstick result can miss marked proteinuria. In one study (Hooper, 1996), only 17.7% of pregnant women who later had preeclampsia had proteinuria that preceded the hypertension. Of the participants who later had gestational diabetes, only 36% had glycosuria first. Pregnant women who exhibit proteinuria or glycosuria during prenatal visits should undergo screening for complications of hypertension or diabetes. An occasional patient with gestational diabetes, for example, has normal results of glucose screening tests

early in pregnancy only to manifest diabetes later with glycosuria. Because urine dipstick screening is relatively inexpensive, many clinicians continue to offer it at each prenatal visit.

FETAL PRESENTATION

When patients approach term, it is important to perform Leopold's maneuvers to verify a cephalic presentation. Depending on the standards of the individual clinician and medical community, breech presentations may be handled by means of external cephalic version (usually at approximately 37 weeks' gestation), elective cesarean section, or vaginal breech delivery. These decisions ideally should be made before delivery.

CLINICAL ESTIMATION OF FETAL WEIGHT

Another purpose of Leopold's maneuvers is to estimate fetal weight at term. In one study, 72% of clinically estimated fetal weights estimated during labor by a senior obstetrics resident were within 10% of actual birth weight, whereas only 69% of concurrent ultrasound examinations achieved this goal. No recommendations for clinical intervention have been based on these findings because cesarean section for macrosomia has not been proved to be beneficial except when the mother has gestational diabetes and the estimated weight of the baby is 4500 g.

Anticipatory Guidance

The ongoing care provided throughout the pregnancy offers clinicians the opportunity to discuss and counsel patients about a number of different health promotion and disease prevention interventions. It also is an opportunity for clinicians to develop a solid bond with their patients and families and to make plans for labor, delivery, and future care of the baby.

Although very few studies have been conducted to determine the effectiveness of this anticipatory guidance or of any one specific intervention other than in tobacco and alcohol use, these topics are offered as possible discussion items (Table 9-11).

STAGES OF PREGNANCY AND COMMON SYMPTOMS

Most maternity care providers spend time during prenatal visits discussing common symptoms that patients may experience during the different stages of pregnancy. Charts and diagrams that depict the fetus and mother at different developmental stages can be useful.

Table 9-11

Recommended Topics for Anticipatory Guidance of Pregnant Patients

Stages of pregnancy and common symptoms
Symptoms of premature labor
Avoiding unnecessary substances
Prevention of toxoplasmosis
Prevention of cytomegalovirus
Nutrition
Exercise
Injury prevention
Breastfeeding
Prenatal care classes
Involvement of the father and other family
   members
Involvement of doulas
Preparing other children for the new arrival
Other topics
   Sexual activity during and after pregnancy
   Maternal serum screening and other testing
   Fetal movement precautions
   Preparation for labor and delivery
   Control of labor pain
   Infant care and safety

SYMPTOMS OF PREMATURE LABOR

It is wise to counsel pregnant patients about symptoms of preterm labor and rupture of membranes. Overt preterm labor is preceded by subjective symptoms that can be used diagnostically, but in prospective studies these symptoms are noticeable only on the same day that the preterm labor is diagnosed. These symptoms include uterine contractions, menstrual-type cramps, backache, and increased vaginal discharge. Patients with ruptured membranes occasionally have a slow fluid leak rather than a gush of fluid. All pregnant patients need to be educated to recognize and promptly report any symptoms that suggest preterm labor or rupture of membranes.

AVOIDING UNNECESSARY SUBSTANCES

Early in pregnancy, women should be counseled to avoid over-the-counter medications, tobacco, alcohol, and illicit drugs. If they use these substances, they should stop; if they do not use them, they should not start. Even brief counseling programs appear effective in stopping existing alcohol use during pregnancy. The same holds true for smoking cessation during pregnancy. What is not known is whether pregnant women who do not already smoke or drink are less likely to start when their clinicians tell them not to.

PREVENTION OF TOXOPLASMOSIS

Toxoplasmosis is a protozoan infection that causes generalized, nonspecific symptoms such as fever, anorexia, lymphadenopathy, and fatigue. Infection during pregnancy can cause fetal demise or congenital toxoplasmosis characterized by chorioretinitis, brain damage, intracerebral calcifications, hydrocephaly, microcephaly, jaundice, rash, and hepatosplenomegaly. Animal hosts for *Toxoplasma* organisms include cats, sheep, goats, rodents, pigs, cattle, and birds, among others. Infected cats excrete infectious cysts in their feces. Infection can be contracted by means of eating raw or undercooked meat, drinking unpasteurized milk, and ingesting cysts acquired in sandboxes, playgrounds, and yards.

The ACOG does not recommend routine screening for toxoplasmosis during pregnancy because both prevention and treatment strategies are uncertain. Pregnant women can be counseled, however, about avoiding exposure. The following practices increase risk for toxoplasmosis: eating or preparing raw, undercooked, or minced beef, pork, or mutton, changing cat litter, and failing to wash kitchen knives after preparing raw meat. Research indicates that pregnant women can be effectively counseled to avoid these practices and decrease toxoplasmosis seroconversion.

PREVENTION OF CYTOMEGALOVIRUS

Congenital cytomegalovirus (CMV) infection occurs in 1% of all live births in the United States, causing major illness among 5 to 10% of the infants and minor illness among the others. Major illness consists of mental retardation, microcephaly, hearing loss, and motor disabilities. Minor illness includes symptoms of generalized infection. As many as 90% of congenital infections are asymptomatic, but of these 10% eventually cause some form of neurosensory deficit. Most illness is caused by primary infection during pregnancy. The annual cost of treating CMV complications in the United States is $2 billion. CMV is excreted in the urine and saliva for months to as long as 6 years by neonates and is contracted by means of mucosal contact with infectious excretions. Preschool personnel are at high risk for infection.

Counseling to avoid possible exposure through good hand washing, wearing gloves when changing diapers of infants who have or are likely to have CMV infection, and avoiding exposure to urine and saliva is advised. The effectiveness of this advice is unknown, but the advice has the added advantage of helping prevent exposure to other infections, such as parvovirus. Women at risk may choose to undergo screening and modify their risks if the serologic results are negative.

NUTRITION

Pregnant women often are sensibly counseled to eat a healthful diet and avoid weight-loss dieting during pregnancy. Yet little evidence guides us in dietary counseling. There are few clear data to suggest that any dietary interventions improve outcomes of pregnancy. With the notable exception of folate (see section on Periconception Care), most special dietary interventions in pregnancy are of unclear benefit. A Cochrane Collaboration systematic review (Kramer, 1998) found that high-protein supplementation during pregnancy does not improve weight gain and is associated with an insignificant increase in the rate of neonatal death. Neither is there evidence to support routine prophylaxis with zinc, iron, magnesium, or pyridoxine.

Although it is common for clinicians to prescribe prenatal vitamins and iron during pregnancy, there is limited evidence to support these practices. The USPSTF does not recommend iron supplementation during pregnancy unless anemia is present. Other nutritional interventions have been tested, including prophylactic administration of vitamin D to prevent neonatal hypocalcemia, but none can be recommended for routine use at this time.

EXERCISE

More than one-third of U.S. women reportedly choose to exercise during pregnancy. Except for occupational exposures that involve prolonged standing, moderate exercise seems to be reasonably safe during pregnancy, but research has been limited. Regular aerobic exercise during pregnancy improves maternal fitness, although the benefits or risks to mother or baby are unclear. Women who exercise regularly do not seem to have an increased rate of preterm birth, as previous observational data suggested. Few data shed light on particular exercise guidelines, but ACOG recommends that pregnant women keep their heart rate less than 140 beats per minute and avoid high-impact sports.

INJURY PREVENTION

Pregnant women should receive at least some counseling about specific safety issues, such as falls that can easily occur with weight and balance changes in late pregnancy, motor vehicle crashes, and risks for violence. Car safety restraints are an especially important issue during pregnancy; motor vehicle crashes account for as many as one-third of all injury-related maternal deaths. More than three-fourths of pregnant women killed in one study were not wearing seat belts at the time of the crash (Schiff, et al, 1997). Surviving a motor vehicle crash doubles a woman's risk for giving birth within 48 hours of the crash and giving birth to a low-birth weight baby. Many pregnant women stop using seat belts because they fear fetal injury or death. However, there is no evidence that safety restraints increase risk for fetal or uteroplacental injury when properly used. It is important to explain to pregnant women that they should place the lap part of the seat belt low across the lap, not across the abdomen, to avoid transmitting force through the uterus. Counseling pregnant women to wear seat belts appears to be effective, increasing the rate of seat belt use from 65% to 80% and increasing proper placement of safety belts.

Families should be counseled about obtaining an infant car seat before the birth. Specific teaching may be needed for less experienced parents. New families taught to use "loaner" car seats before hospital discharge can demonstrate correct use of the seats much more effectively than families who are not taught these skills.

BREASTFEEDING

Breastfeeding is the preferred form of infant feeding because it prevents neonatal infections and allergic conditions while providing excellent, economical nutrition. Although increasing breastfeeding rates across the country is one of the goals of the U.S. Public Health Service Healthy People 2000 initiative, breastfeeding rates lag far behind these goals. Only 59.4% of eligible U.S. women were breastfeeding in 1995, and only 21.6% were doing so when their infants were 6 months old. Lower-income women in particular tend to resist breastfeeding. Because breastfeeding education appears effective in increasing breastfeeding rates, it is important for clinicians to include this intervention in prenatal care. Fathers as well as mothers must be educated. Whether a father approves of breastfeeding can be an important factor in whether a mother chooses to breastfeed.

PRENATAL CARE CLASSES

Many pregnant women and their families participate in prenatal care classes. Few studies have examined the efficacy of these interventions. Limited evidence suggests that families who participate in parenting classes before delivery have better intrapartum and postpartum outcomes, such as reduced anxiety and better marital adjustment, than do control families.

INVOLVEMENT OF THE FATHER AND OTHER FAMILY MEMBERS

Fathers frequently attend the births of their children. They often feel relegated to a supporting role when they prefer being more actively involved in the births. Women often state that their partners are important sources of support during labor and delivery. Although limited evidence exists in this area, it seems logical to invite the father or other partner to take an active role in prenatal care, prenatal classes, and deliveries whenever appropriate.

INVOLVEMENT OF DOULAS

During prenatal care, expectant families may benefit from discussions of the presence of doulas (lay women trained to provide comfort and support during labor and delivery) and other sources of labor support. In a representative randomized study in the United States, having a doula involved in the births greatly decreased the rate of cesarean section and use of epidural analgesia and oxytocin (Kennell, et al, 1991). Such outcomes have led more U.S. birth attendants to work with doulas during labor and delivery.

PREPARING OTHER CHILDREN FOR THE NEW ARRIVAL

Many families now include siblings during prenatal classes and labor and delivery. There is some research to support this approach as a mechanism to decrease sibling rivalry but not enough to make a universal recommendation on this practice.

Immunizations

NON-LIVE VACCINES

Non-live vaccines may be safely administered during pregnancy if necessary, including immunizations for influenza, hepatitis B, pneumococcus, tetanus toxoid-diphtheria, and rabies. Because pregnant women are at higher risk for hospitalization with influenza than is the general population, the CDC Advisory Committee on Immunization Practices recommends that all women who will be beyond 14 weeks' gestation during influenza season should be immunized.

IMMUNIZATIONS TO AVOID: LIVE VIRUSES

Live-virus immunizations are contraindicated during pregnancy because of theoretical risks.

These vaccines include measles, mumps, rubella, oral polio vaccine, varicella, and yellow fever. There is no evidence, however, that women who accidentally receive these immunizations during pregnancy suffer ill effects or that the infants are affected.

Recommendations to Clinicians

Approach to Patient Care

It is a constant challenge to follow the many scientifically based recommendations for pregnancy care and to avoid engaging in needless, potentially harmful interventions. A helpful approach is to remember that most pregnancies are normal and end with the uneventful births of healthy infants. Although perfect outcomes cannot be guaranteed, an evidence-based approach to pregnancy care helps clinicians and families view pregnancy as a generally normal process. In this way, caregivers can review each family's particular needs and wishes to help the patient and family decide on a course of pregnancy care that is agreeable to all parties.

Clinicians need to stay abreast of new evidence as it develops. Several organizations review evidence and make recommendations to assist busy clinicians. These include the CDC, AAFP, ACOG, and USPSTF.

Implementing recommendations consistently can be a challenge in a busy practice. Systems in which specific tasks are assigned to all members of the health care team and in which flow sheets and periodic quality assurance checks are used can help ensure that each woman receives all preventive services.

Common Errors

Lack of Periconception Counseling

Perhaps the most common mistake made is for clinicians and patients not to discuss plans for conception. Women usually seek care when already pregnant, sometimes well into pregnancy, and an important prevention opportunity is lost.

Failure to Administer Anti-RhD Immunoglobulin

RhD-negative women who are anti-RhD seronegative should receive anti-RhD immunoglobulin whenever there is a potential for the mother to be exposed to fetal blood. Anti-RhD therapy can be overlooked after amniocentesis, miscarriage, or abortion. The dose at 28 to 32 weeks sometimes is administered before a repeat antibody level is confirmed to be negative. Probably the most common mistake is to assume the mother will not need anti-RhD therapy because the presumed father also is Rh-negative. The key word here is *presumed* because who the father is may not always be clear. The only circumstance in which a mother should not receive anti-RhD treatment is when the newborn baby is Rh-negative.

Prescribing Iron for All Women

It is a common practice to prescribe prenatal iron universally. There is no proven benefit to iron supplementation during pregnancy unless the mother has clinically significant iron deficiency anemia. Iron ingestion can cause gastrointestinal upset during pregnancy and is a potential source of toxic ingestion for infants and children in the mother's home.

Inaccurate Calculation of Dates

Failure to calculate a reliable estimate of date of delivery can have serious consequences if a preterm or postterm fetus is delivered unknowingly. Errors occur because of overreliance on uterine size for dating and not considering the inaccuracy of late ultrasound scans.

Performing Unnecessary Tests

Blood tests frequently ordered as screening tests during pregnancy that have no proven value include toxoplasmosis and CMV titers, complete blood cell counts, and some chemistry studies. These tests should be reserved for diagnostic purposes to confirm or rule out suspected disease.

Failure to Perform Third-trimester Syphilis Tests

Women at high risk for syphilis include those who have multiple sex partners, exchange sex for money or drugs, use illicit drugs, are homeless, have recently contracted another sexually transmitted disease or live in an area with high syphilis prevalence. These women should undergo a syphilis test at the first prenatal visit and again at the beginning of the third trimester. A syphilis test also should be requested whenever there is an unexplained fetal death.

Failure to Detect Breech Presentation

Breech presentation should be detected and prepared for before labor or impending delivery. This diagnosis can be missed when clinicians do not perform Leopold's maneuvers or inaccurately assess fetal position.

Emerging Trends

A number of new approaches to pregnancy care are on the horizon. These include improved screening tests for Down syndrome and other anomalies, gene therapy to correct chromosomal disorders, new therapies for HIV, immunizations against infectious diseases, alternative ways to increase folic acid use, and advances in knowledge about gestational diabetes.

A family-centered and evidence-based approach helps ensure that these new technologies and approaches will help clinicians continue to promote healthier mothers, infants, and families.

Screening for Down Syndrome and Other Anomalies

Chorionic villus sampling is being used with increasing frequency and offers the prospect of karotyping at 10 to 12 weeks' gestation. Improvements in ultrasound technologies may make this an option for screening for congenital anomalies. As new serum markers are tested and diagnostic cutoffs refined for women in different age and risk groups, there will likely be improvement in the accuracy of prediction. Multistep screening protocols will involve risk assessment, serum screening with ultrasonography, amniocentesis, and chorionic villus sampling.

Gene Therapy

The explosion in knowledge about the human genome holds promise for intrauterine gene therapy to correct genetic causes of diseases. Cystic fibrosis and sickle cell anemia are two examples.

HIV Treatment

The rapid development of new antiretroviral agents will have several effects on pregnancy care. The increased survival periods these agents offer persons with HIV infection and current epidemiologic trends will lead to an increase in the number of women of childbearing age who have HIV infection. Although the use of zidovudine and other antiretroviral agents appears to result in markedly reduced risk to newborns, a large proportion still are infected. Trials of new agents and combination therapy should lead to even more improvement.

Immunizations

Immunizations against CMV and GBS are being developed. These hold promise for dramatically decreasing the incidence of congenital infections, just as rubella immunization has accomplished with congenital rubella syndrome.

Gestational Diabetes

New thresholds for diagnosing gestational diabetes are being discussed. The debate over universal or selective screening will probably continue until a clear benefit of universal screening is demonstrated.

Folic Acid Supplementation

Because many women do not plan or anticipate pregnancy, it will be difficult to obtain the maximum potential from folic acid supplementation. To reduce the risk for neural tube defects, the U.S. Food and Drug Administration mandated that enriched grain products be fortified with 140 µg folic acid per 100 g of product starting in 1998. This policy will be evaluated for effectiveness and will be refined.

Bibliography

Abma JC, Chandra A, Mosher WD, et al: *Vital and Health Statistics: Fertility, Family Planning, and Women's Health: New Data From the 1995 National Survey of Family Growth.* Hyattsville, MD, Division of Vital Statistics, National Center for Health Statistics, 1997.

Adams EK, Solanki G, Miller LS: Medical-care expenditures attributable to cigarette smoking during pregnancy—United States, 1995. *MMWR Morb Mortal Wkly Rep* 46:1048, 1997.

Adler SP, Finney JW, Manganello AM, et al: Prevention of child-to-mother transmission of cytomegalovirus by changing behaviors: A randomized controlled trial. *Pediatr Infect Dis J* 15: 240–246, 1996.

Bachman JW, Heise RH, Naessens JM, et al: A study of various tests to detect asymptomatic urinary tract infections in an obstetric population. *JAMA* 270:1971–1974, 1993.

Bader TJ, Macones GA, Asch DA: Prenatal screening for toxoplasmosis. *Obstet Gynecol* 90:457–464, 1997.

Bobrowski RA, Bottoms SF, Micallef JA, et al: Is the 50-gram glucose screening test ever diagnostic? *J Matern Fetal Med* 5:317–320, 1996.

Centers for Disease Control and Prevention: Prevention of perinatal group B streptococcal disease: A public health perspective. *MMWR Morb Mortal Wkly Rep* 45:1-24, 1996.

Chandler S, Field PA: Becoming a father: First-time fathers' experience of labor and delivery. *J Nurse Midwifery* 42:17–24, 1997.

Chitty LS: Ultrasound screening for fetal abnormalities. *Prenat Diagn* 15:1241–1257, 1995.

Coustan DR: Screening and testing for gestational diabetes mellitus. *Obstet Gynecol Clin North Am* 23: 125–136, 1996.

Czeizel AE: Controlled studies of multivitamin supplementation on pregnancy outcomes. *Ann NY Acad Sci* 678:266–275, 1993.

Daniel Y, Gull I, Peyser R, et al: Congenital cytomegalovirus infection. *Eur J Obstet Gynecol Reprod Biol* 63:7–16, 1995.

Division of Vital Statistics, National Center for Health Statistics, Centers for Disease Control and Prevention: Preliminary data on births and deaths—United States, 1995. *MMWR Morb Mortal Wkly Rep* 45:914–919, 1996.

Dolan-Mullen P, Ramirez G, Groff JY. A meta-analysis of randomized trials of prenatal smoking cessation interventions. *Am J Obstet Gynecol* 171:1328–1334, 1994.

Fiscella K. Does prenatal care improve birth outcomes? A critical review. *Obstet Gynecol* 32: 468–479, 1995.

Haddow JE, Palomaki GE, Knight GJ, et al: Reducing the need for amniocentesis in women 35 years of age or older with serum markers for screening. *N Engl J Med* 330:1114–1118, 1994.

Hauth JC, Goldenberg RL, Andrews WW, et al: Reduced incidence of preterm delivery with metronidazole and erythromycin in women with bacterial vaginosis. *N Engl J Med* 333:1732–1736, 1995.

Helton MR, Arndt J, Kebede M, et al: Do low-risk prenatal patients really need a screening glucose challenge test? *J Fam Pract* 44:556–561, 1997.

Henshaw SK: Teenage abortion and pregnancy statistics by state, 1992. *Fam Plann Perspect* 29:115–122, 1997.

Hooper DE. Detecting GD and preeclampsia. *J Reprod Med* 41:885–888, 1996.

Kennell J, Klaus M, McGrath S, et al: Continuous emotional support during labor in a U.S. hospital: A randomized controlled trial. *JAMA* 265:2197–2201, 1991.

Koonin LM, MacKay AP, Berg CJ, et al: Pregnancy related mortality surveillance—United States, 1987–1990. *MMWR Morb Mortal Wkly Rep* 46:17–36, 1997.

Koonin LM, Smith JC, Ramick M, et al: Abortion surveillance—United States, 1995. *MMWR Morb Mortal Wkly Rep* 47:31, 1998.

Kramer MS: High protein supplementation in pregnancy, in: Neilson JP, Crouther CA, Hodnett ED, Hofmeyr GJ (eds.): *Pregnancy and Childbirth Module of the Cochrane Database of Systematic Reviews*, [updated December 12, 1997]. Available in the Cochrane Library database on disk and CD-ROM. The Cochrane Collaboration. Updated quarterly. Issue 1. Oxford, UK Update Software, 1998.

Kramer MS. Regular aerobic exercise during pregnancy, in: Neilson JP, Crouther CA,, Hodnett ED, Hofmeyr GJ (eds.): *Pregnancy and Childbirth*

Module of the Cochrane Database of Systematic Reviews, [updated December 12, 1997]. Available in the Cochrane Library database on disk and CD-ROM. The Cochrane Collaboration. Updated quarterly. Issue 1. Oxford, UK, Update Software, 1998.

Lee SH, Ewert DP, Frederick PD, et al: Resurgence of congenital rubella syndrome in the 1990s: Report on missed opportunities and failed prevention policies among women of childbearing age. *JAMA* 267:2616–2620, 1992.

Mahomed K, Gulmezoglu AM: Vitamin D supplementation in pregnancy, in: Neilson JP, Crouther CA, Hodnett ED, Hofmeyr GJ (eds.): *Pregnancy and Childbirth Module of the Cochrane Database of Systematic Reviews*, [updated December 12, 1997]. Available in the Cochrane Library database on disk and CD-ROM. The Cochrane Collaboration. Updated quarterly. Issue 1. Oxford, UK, Update Software, 1998.

Meyer WJ, Carbone J, Gauthier DW, et al: Early gestational glucose screening and gestational diabetes. *J Reprod Med* 41:675–679, 1996.

Moses RG, Shand JL, Tapsell LC: The recurrence of gestational diabetes: Could dietary differences in fat intake be an explanation? *Diabetes Care* 20:1647–1650, 1997.

Neilson JP: Routine symphysis-fundal height measurement during pregnancy, in: Neilson JP, Crouther CA, Hodnett ED, Hofmeyr GJ (eds.): *Pregnancy and Childbirth Module of the Cochrane Database of Systematic Reviews*, [updated December 12, 1997]. Available in the Cochrane Library database on disk and CD-ROM. The Cochrane Collaboration. Updated quarterly. Issue 1. Oxford, UK, Update Software, 1998.

Pearlman MD, Phillips ME: Safety belt use during pregnancy. *Obstet Gynecol* 88:1026–1029, 1996.

Pearlman MD, Viano D: Automobile crash simulation with the first pregnant crash test dummy. *Am J Obstet Gynecol* 175:977–981, 1996.

Ray JG: Lues-lues: Maternal and fetal considerations of syphilis. *Obstet Gynecol Surv* 50:845–850, 1995.

Reifsnider E, Eckhart D: Prenatal breastfeeding education: Its effect on breastfeeding among WIC participants. *J Hum Lact* 13:121–125, 1997.

Schieve LA, Cogswell ME, Scanlon KS: An empiric evaluation of the Institute of Medicine's pregnancy weight gain guidelines by race. *Obstet Gynecol* 91:878–884, 1998.

Schiff M, Albers L, McFeeley P: Motor vehicle crashes and maternal mortality in New Mexico: the significance of seat belt use. *West J Med* 167:19–22, 1997.

Scholl TO, Hediger ML, Bendich A, et al: Use of multivitamin/mineral prenatal supplements: Influence on the outcome of pregnancy. *Am J Epidemiol* 146:134–141, 1997.

Schorling JB: The prevention of prenatal alcohol use: A critical analysis of intervention studies. *J Stud Alcohol* 54:261–267, 1993.

Sherman DJ, Arieli S, Tovbin J, et al: A comparison of clinical and ultrasonic estimation of fetal weight. *Obstet Gynecol* 91:212–217, 1998.

Svikis DS, Golden AS, Huggins GR, et al: Cost-effectiveness of treatment for drug-abusing pregnant women. *Drug Alcohol Depend* 45:105–113, 1997.

Thorp JM: Management of drug dependency, overdose, and withdrawal in the obstetric patient. *Obstet Gynecol Clin North Am* 22:131–142, 1995.

Ventura SJ, Peters KD, Martin JA, et al: Births and deaths: United States, 1996. *Mon Vital Stat Rep* 46:1–40, 1997.

Ventura SJ, Martin JA, Curtin SC, et al. Births: Final data for 1997. *Natl Vital Stat Rep* 47:1–96, 1999.

Waller DK, Lustig LS, Smith AH, et al: Alphafetoprotein: A biomarker for pregnancy outcome. *Epidemiology* 4:471–476, 1993.

Wenstrom KD, Owen J, Chu DC, et al: Alpha-fetoprotein, free beta-human chorionic gonadotropin, and dimeric inhibin A produce the best results in a three-analyte, multiple-marker screening test for fetal Down syndrome. *Am J Obstet Gynecol* 177:987–991, 1997.

Wolf ME, Alexander BH, Rivara FP, et al: A retrospective cohort study of seatbelt use and pregnancy outcome after a motor vehicle crash. *J Trauma* 34:116–119, 1993.

Yalcin HK, Zorlu CG: Threshold value of glucose screening tests in pregnancy: Could it be standardized for every population? *Am J Perinatol* 13:317–320, 1996.

Adults

A. Substance Abuse

B. Cancer

C. Chronic Disease

D. Infectious Disease

Smoking Prevention and Cessation

Today, nearly 3,000 young persons across our country will begin smoking regularly. Of these 3,000 young persons, 1,000 will lose that gamble to the diseases caused by smoking. The net effect of this is that among children living in America today, 5 million will die an early preventable death because of a decision made as a child.

Donna E. Shalala, PhD
Secretary, U.S. Department of Health and Human Services
Testimony before the Senate Labor and Human Resources Committee
September 25, 1997

Introduction

By virtue of their direct access to a large population of smokers, credibility with patients, and ability to provide effective intervention, primary care clinicians have a unique and powerful opportunity to contribute to the control of tobacco abuse.

The purpose of this chapter is to describe the prevalence and effect on health of smoking, describe community-based approaches used to prevent smoking and promote smoking cessation, and introduce the most important aspects of brief smoking cessation counseling interventions. This chapter emphasizes knowledge, but success depends on one's ability to incorporate these recommendations into everyday routines.

Tobacco abuse is a common chronic illness, not unlike hypertension and diabetes. The key is not to expect immediate success with smokers, just as one will not expect immediate adoption of dietary and physical activity recommendations with diabetic and hypertensive patients. Smoking is also an addiction and shares the challenge of terminating any other drug addiction.

This chapter concentrates on the prevention of tobacco smoking. Tobacco can also be used by chewing and smoking cigars. These forms of tobacco use also have significant consequences on morbidity and mortality; many of the prevention interventions described for smoking can be applied to them.

Prevalence of Smoking

Tobacco use continues to be the most important preventable cause of morbidity and mortality in the United States. It is responsible for more than 400,000 deaths each year and more than $50 billion in direct medical costs. In 1994, 48 million adult Americans were current smokers—25 million men and 23 million women. The overall 1994 prevalence of tobacco use among persons 18 years and older in the United States was 26%–28% among men and 23% among women. Among men, those who were between 35 and 54 years of age had the highest prevalence at 32%. Among women, those between 25 and 44 years of age had the highest prevalence at 27%. Prevalence was lowest among persons 65 years of age and older (14% for men and 11% for women).

Risk Factors for Smoking Initiation

Surveys of current adult smokers reveal that almost 80% began smoking regularly at 16 years of age or earlier. Initiation of cigarette smoking is associated with multiple factors. Environmental factors include availability of cigarettes, the perception that tobacco use is the norm, peer and sibling attitudes, and lack of parental support during adolescence. The influence of parental smoking is not clear because only about half of prospective studies have shown a clear predictive relation between parental smoking and teenage smoking. Behavioral factors include low academic achievement, rebelliousness, alienation from school, and lack of skills to resist offers of cigarettes. Personal factors include low self-esteem and a belief that smoking confers future advantages in social life. Other factors associated with initiation of smoking include price of cigarettes, cigarette advertising and promotions, and degree of exposure to effective counteradvertising and school-based prevention programs.

Racial and Ethnic Differences in Smoking Prevalence

Among adults, American Indians and Alaskan Natives have the highest prevalence (36%), followed by African Americans (27%) and Hispanics (18%) (Table 10-1). Asian Americans and Pacific Islanders have the lowest rate (14%). In all racial and ethnic minority groups, men have a higher prevalence of smoking than do women. Among adolescents, Caucasians smoke at higher rates than African Americans and Hispanics. Minority smokers as a group smoke fewer cigarettes per day than do Caucasian smokers.

These figures point to the need to develop programs that appeal to these racial and ethnic minority groups to decrease the burden of disease related to tobacco use.

Socioeconomic Characteristics of Smokers and Nonsmokers

There is an inverse relation between income level and smoking prevalence; the lower the income, the higher is the prevalence of smoking (Table 10-2). Across categories of occupation, marital status, and military status, the highest prevalences of cigarette smoking are found in the following subgroups: blue collar workers, persons separated or divorced, and active-duty military personnel. Large numbers of Americans stopped smoking during the decades that followed the early surgeon-general warning about the dangers of smoking. Wealthier and more educated persons were more likely to stop smoking. By 1991 only 3% of physicians and 18% of nurses were smokers.

Poverty appears to have an independent effect on smoking prevalence. Persons with incomes under the poverty threshold are about 30% more likely to be cigarette smokers and 19% to 36% less likely to stop smoking. This effect is seen even after control for education, sex, age, race-ethnicity, employment status, marital status, and geographic region. It is likely that persons who are poor are not exposed to changing social norms regarding smoking behavior and may need more focused efforts to reduce smoking.

U.S. Geographic Differences

Tobacco-growing states in the southeastern United States have the highest rates of smoking. Kentucky, with a rate of 28% has more than twice the prevalence of smoking as Utah, at 13%. Among the 50 states, Utah is the only state to have achieved the Healthy People 2000 objective to reduce the prevalence of smoking to no more than 15%.

U.S. Rates for the Past 20 to 30 Years

Since 1965, the prevalence of cigarette smoking is one of the measures collected yearly in the United States as part of the National Health Interview Survey. This survey also allows determination of the prevalence of cessation (also

Table 10-1

Age-adjusted Prevalence of Current Cigarette Smoking[a] among Adults, Overall, and by Race-ethnicity and Sex, National Health Interview Surveys, United States, 1994 and 1995 Aggregate Data

CHARACTERISTIC	AFRICAN AMERICAN		AMERICAN INDIANS, ASLASKA NATIVE		ASIAN AMERICANS, PACIFIC ISLANDER		HISPANIC		WHITE	
	%	±CI[b]	%	±CI	%	±CI	%	±CI	%	±CI
Total	26.5	1.7	36.0	6.0	14.2	2.7	18.0	1.5	26.4	0.7
Men	31.4	2.6	39.3	9.5	23.8	5.1	21.7	2.3	28.1	1.0
Women	22.2	1.8	32.9	8.0	5.4	2.1	14.6	1.8	25.0	0.9

[a] Current cigarette smokers are persons who reported smoking at least 100 cigarettes in their lives and who reported at the time of survey that they currently smoked every day or on some days. Data were age-adjusted to the 1990 U.S. census population.
[b] 95% confidence interval.
SOURCE: National Care Center for Health Statistics, public use data tapes, 1994–1995.

Table 10-2

Prevalence (%) of Smoking by Income Level for Adults 18 Years of Age and Older by Race and Sex

FAMILY INCOME	ALL RACES		WHITE, NON-HISPANIC		BLACK, NON-HISPANIC		HISPANIC	
	MALE	FEMALE	MALE	FEMALE	MALE	FEMALE	MALE	FEMALE
Poor	38	31	42	39	41	29	26	17
Near poor	34	28	38	32	40	25	20	15
Middle income	28	25	25	22	22	16	16	14
High income	18	17						

known as the *quit ratio*) defined as the number of former smokers among ever smokers. During the last 20 to 30 years, U.S. residents have stopped smoking in great numbers. The proportion of ever smokers who are exsmokers changed from 24% in 1965 to 49% in 1994. The prevalence of smoking changed from 42% in 1965 to 26% in 1994.

Not only have Americans stopped smoking in increasing numbers, but also fewer have started or ever tried smoking. The proportion of U.S. adults who have never smoked increased from 44% in 1965 to 50% in 1991. These improvements, however, were due to changes in smoking prevalence among men. The proportion of women who never smoked remained stable (58% in 1965 to 57.6% in 1991). If these trends continue, in the near future the prevalence of smoking among women might be greater than that among men.

Intensity of smoking also has declined among smokers. The proportion of smokers who were heavy smokers (25 or more cigarettes per day) was 25% in 1974, 29% in 1980, and 22% in 1991. The number of cigarettes smoked daily by smokers declined from 20 in 1974 to 18 in 1991. Similar declines were observed for most members of racial and ethnic minority groups. From 1978 to 1995, the prevalence of cigarette smoking declined among African Americans, Asian Americans and Pacific Islanders, and Hispanics. However, among American-Indians and Alaskan Natives, current smoking prevalence did not change for men from 1983 to 1995 or for women from 1978 to 1995.

There were significant improvements in smoking rates among adolescents between 1976 and 1989. Between these years the rate of smoking among high school seniors declined 34%. However, the rate was 2% higher in 1993 than in 1984. Cigarette smoking increased in the 1990s among male adolescents except African Americans, after several years of substantial decline among all racial and ethnic groups (Table 10-3). There also has been an increase in smoking among college students. Their preva-

lence of smoking rose from 22.3% to 28.5% from 1993 to 1997. Increases occurred in all age and race groups and both sexes.

Global Prevalence of Smoking

The World Health Organization estimates that about one-third of the world's population 15 years or older are smokers; about 1.1 billion persons. About 800 million smokers live in developing countries, and most, 700 million, are men. China alone has as many smokers as all developed countries combined, about 300 million. The global prevalence of smoking is 47% for men and 12% for women. There is a striking contrast in the pattern of smoking by women living in less developed countries compared with that for women in more developed countries. The prevalence of smoking among women in less developed countries is 7% compared with 24% in more developed countries. The global prevalence of smoking among men varies from less than 30% in the African region to 60% in the Western Pacific region, mostly reflecting the 61% prevalence of smoking in China. There is also considerable variation even among more developed countries. In countries with well-established market economies, the prevalence of smoking among men averages 37% compared with 60% in the former socialist countries of central and eastern Europe.

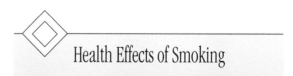

Health Effects of Smoking

Smoking-related Diseases and Rates

Since the early 1950s and 1960s a massive body of epidemiologic evidence has accumulated to demonstrate the negative consequences of smoking. Each year in the United States there are about 120,000 deaths of lung cancer, 31,000

Table 10-3

Trends in Percentage of High School Seniors Who Were Previous-month Smokers by Race, Ethnicity, and Sex, United States, 1976–1979, 1980–1984, 1985–1989, 1990–1994

SEX AND RACE OR ETHNICITY	1976–1979	1980–1984	1985–1989	1990–1994
MALE				
African American	33.1	19.4	15.6	11.6
American Indian and Alaskan Native	50.3	39.6	36.8	41.1
Asian American and Pacific Islander	20.7	21.5	16.8	20.6
Hispanic	30.3	23.8	23.3	28.5
White	35.0	27.5	29.8	33.4
FEMALE				
African American	33.6	22.8	13.3	8.6
American Indian and Alaskan Native	55.3	50.0	43.6	39.4
Asian American and Pacific Islander	24.4	16.0	14.3	13.8
Hispanic	31.4	25.1	20.6	19.2
White	39.1	34.2	34.0	33.1

SOURCE: U.S. Department of Health and Human Services. 1998

of other cancers, 99,000 of ischemic heart disease, 65,000 of chronic lung disease, 23,000 of strokes, and 80,000 of other disorders directly attributed to cigarette smoking. It is estimated that more than 10 million Americans have died prematurely of causes attributed to smoking since the first surgeon-general report of the health effects of smoking was published in 1964.

The more than 4000 chemicals in cigarette smoke include more than 40 known carcinogens. In addition to lung cancer, smoking is directly related to cancer of the oral cavity, pharynx, larynx, pancreas, kidney, bladder, and cervix. Smoking promotes arteriosclerosis and is a major risk factor for myocardial infarction, coronary artery disease, stroke, and peripheral vascular disease. Close to one-fifth of deaths due to cardiovascular disease are related to smoking. Cigarette smoke has direct toxic effects on the respiratory tissue of all smokers that results in paralysis of ciliary epithelia and increased difficulty clearing respiratory irritants and carcinogens. Cigarette smoke accelerates the decline in lung function among patients with chronic obstructive pulmonary disease. Use of smokeless tobacco and cigars also increases risk for cancer of the lung, larynx, esophagus, and oral cavity. Tobacco use also is associated with gum disease and tooth decay.

Some effects of cigarette smoking may not cause death but produce considerable pain and suffering. Persons who continue to smoke after receiving a diagnosis of peptic ulcer disease have more difficulty healing despite administration of appropriate medications. Smoking is an important risk factor for the development of osteoporosis. Less well known effects of smoking include decreases in testosterone levels, decrease in percentage of sperm with normal morphologic features, and increased risk for impotence among men. There also is consistent evidence that cigarette smoking causes facial wrinkling that could make smokers appear unattractive and prematurely old and may contribute to the development of cataracts. Smoking during pregnancy causes increased rates of low birth weight, preterm delivery, perinatal death, miscarriage, and fetal growth retardation.

Risks from Secondhand Smoke

Smoking affects the health of nonsmokers. Environmental tobacco smoke (ETS), the most important contaminant of indoor air, is composed of both *sidestream smoke*, directly contributed by the smoldering cigarette, and exhaled *mainstream smoke*. The Environmental Protection Agency declared ETS as a group A (known human) carcinogen, in the same group as asbestos, vinyl chloride, and radon. Exposure to ETS is widespread. Traces of cotinine, a metabolite of nicotine, are detected in the blood of 88% of nonsmokers in the United States. It is estimated that ETS causes about 3000 deaths per year from lung cancer and increases risk for coronary artery disease among nonsmokers. Exposure to ETS increases the risk for middle ear effusion, bronchitis, and pneumonia among children. It causes 8000 to 26,000 new cases of asthma a year and contributes to increased symptoms of asthma among 200,000 to 1,000,000 children a year.

Smoking-related Mortality

On average, cigarette smokers die nearly 7 years earlier than nonsmokers. Smoking triples the risk for dying from heart disease among middle-aged men and women. Men and women who smoke are 10 times more likely to die of bronchitis and emphysema. Eighty-five percent of deaths of lung cancer are caused by smoking. After a delay of about 20 years, mortality rates for diseases associated with smoking have shown increases that reflect historical changes in smoking prevalence (Figs. 10-1, 10-2). For example, between 1960 and 1990, the mortality from lung cancer among women increased by 400%. By the mid 1980s more women died of lung cancer than from breast cancer every year. Women who smoke increase their risk of dying

Figure 10-1

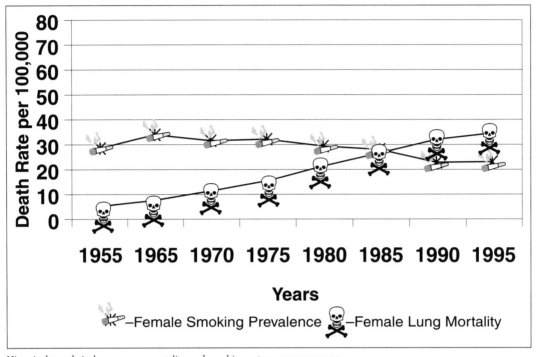

Historical trends in lung cancer mortality and smoking rates among women.

of lung cancer nearly 12 times, men more than 22 times.

Every year premature deaths of smoking steal more than 5 million years from the potential life span of those who have died. It is estimated that about half of yearly deaths in the United States are preventable and of these tobacco use accounts for 40%. Overall, one in five deaths in the United States are associated with smoking. Smoking-related disease kills 16% of heavy smokers by the age of 65 years, 28% by 74 years, and 36% by 84 years.

The Global Toll of Smoking

The estimated body count related to tobacco use in the world in 1995 was more than 3 million; two-thirds of these deaths occurred among residents of more developed countries. Projections for the year 2030 are that by then 10 million citizens of the word will be dying of tobacco use every year unless massive numbers stop smoking. Seventy percent of this death toll is likely to include residents of less developed countries.

 Primary Prevention of Smoking and Exposure to Secondhand Smoke

Nicotine is one of the most addicting substances known, and smoking is an addictive behavior. Most smokers want to stop and have tried to

Figure 10-2

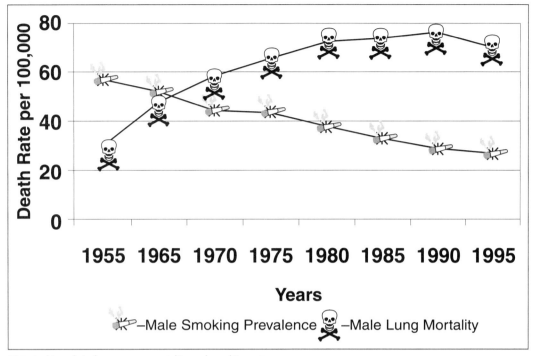

Historical trends in lung cancer mortality and smoking rates among men.

stop smoking. In light of this reality, primary prevention of smoking is critical. Eighty percent of smokers start smoking as adolescents. If a person reaches adulthood as a nonsmoker, it is unlikely he or she will start smoking. Therefore smoking prevention efforts should be aimed at children and adolescents. With the increasing incidence of the adverse health effects of secondhand smoke, prevention of exposure of nonsmokers to secondhand smoke has also received more attention.

Primary prevention programs can be classified into health education options and health policy options (Table 10-4). Health education options include clinician advice not to smoke, school-based education programs, community-based education programs, and advertising.

Health Education

Although there is little evidence that clinician advice not to smoke is effective in preventing smoking among children and adolescents, the U.S. Preventive Services Task Force still recommends that this issue be discussed with children, adolescents, and young adults.

School-based education programs can reduce by 30% to 50% the prevalence of smoking among students under experimental conditions. These programs are difficult to sustain in nonexperimental settings because of the curriculum time and staff effort needed. The Centers for Disease Control and Prevention lists seven strategies for school-based prevention of tobacco use and recommends that schools

Table 10-4

Primary Prevention Interventions for Smoking Initiation and Exposure to Secondhand Smoke

	SMOKING PREVENTION	REDUCING EXPOSURE TO SECONDHAND SMOKE
HEALTH EDUCATION		
	Clinician advice	
	School-based education programs	
	Community-based education	
	Media advertisements	
	Health warnings on tobacco products	
HEALTH POLICY		
	Prohibition of tobacco sales to minors	Prohibit smoking in public places
	Licensure of tobacco retailers	
	Vending machine restrictions	
	Location	
	Locks	
	Required supervision	
	Advertising restrictions	
	Prohibition of free samples	
	Health warnings on tobacco products	
	Increasing the price of cigarettes through taxes	

adopt all seven. The strategies are as follows: (1) development and enforcement of a school policy on tobacco use; (2) instruction on the physiologic and social consequences of tobacco use and refusal skills, (3) education in prevention of tobacco use in kindergarten through 12th grade with intensive instruction in middle school and reinforcement in high school, (4) specific training for teachers on tobacco prevention curricula, (5) involvement of parents and families in support of school programs, (6) support of the cessation efforts of students and staff who smoke, (7) regular assessment of the prevention program.

Community-wide efforts have also proved effective, especially if they are comprehensive and include increases in taxes on tobacco and enforcement of minor-access laws along with advertising and school-based programs.

Health Policy

Youth-oriented mass media campaigns have been implemented to counter tobacco industry advertising. The degree of success of these efforts in preventing smoking initiation is not clear.

Health policy options are listed in Table 10-4. Policies that aim to decrease the access of minors to cigarettes do succeed in making it more difficult for adolescents to purchase tobacco products and to decrease the prevalence of teenage smoking, although this effect is small. Smokers, however, especially teens, are extremely sensitive to the price of cigarettes. For every 1% increase in real price, per capita consumption of cigarettes falls 0.5%. Whether this is the result of smoking cessation, lower intensity of smoking or a decline in initiation of smoking is not clear.

Laws prohibiting smoking in public places have proliferated over the past decade. By 1989 44 states and 50% of cities with a population of 25,000 or more had adopted some kind of smoking restriction. In 1995, 41 states had laws restricting smoking in state government work sites, 21 states restricted smoking in private work sites, and 31 states regulated smoking in restaurants. The strength and enforcement of the laws varied considerably, however.

These laws not only decrease nonsmokers' exposure to secondhand smoke but also encourage smoking cessation and a lower intensity of smoking among smokers. There is evidence that when such laws are extended to private enterprises such as restaurants there is no detrimental effect on business.

Support for tobacco control efforts is consistently undermined by the $45 billion tobacco industry. Every year this industry spends more than $4 billion in the United States in advertising and promotions, making them the biggest health educators in this country. They also spend large amounts of money lobbying state and federal politicians to support initiatives opposing tobacco control. One strategy used is to pass state legislation preempting or prohibiting more restrictive local ordinances.

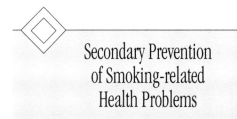

Secondary Prevention of Smoking-related Health Problems

Evidence That Smoking Cessation Reduces Risk for Smoking-related Illness

The benefits of smoking cessation are not limited to smokers who have smoked for a short time. Even smokers who stop smoking after 70 years of age experience substantial benefits from cessation. Smokers who stop smoking experience short-term and long-term benefits from cessation. Short-term benefits include a reduction in carbon monoxide levels in about 12 hours, return of olfactory function and related ability to taste food, recovery of lost ciliary function, a decrease in smoker's cough, and improved dental health. Pregnant women who stop smoking during the first trimester eliminate risk for fetal death and low birth weight.

Long-term benefits of smoking cessation include a reduction in the morbidity and mortality of most tobacco-related diseases. One year after cessation the risk for myocardial infarction and heart disease is cut in half. After 15 years the risk for cardiovascular disease approaches that of someone who never smoked. Risk for stroke returns to the level among persons who have never smoked within 5 to 15 years after smoking cessation. After 10 years of abstinence the risk for lung cancer is 30% to 50% of the risk among those who continue to smoke. After 15 years the risk for lung cancer approaches the risk of someone who never smoked. Smoking cessation also reduces risk for cancers of the larynx, mouth, esophagus, pancreas, and urinary bladder. The rate of decrease in pulmonary function improves dramatically for patients with chronic obstructive pulmonary disease who stop smoking, regardless of the severity of their disease. Risk for influenza, pneumonia, and bronchitis also is reduced. Smoking cessation also reduces the risk for dying of abdominal aortic aneurysm and for development of gastric or duodenal ulcers.

Smokers who already have smoking-related disease also can benefit from smoking cessation. This is especially true of those with coronary artery disease, chronic lung disease, and peptic ulcer disease.

Community-based Approaches to Smoking Cessation

All of the interventions listed in Table 10-4 for the prevention of smoking initiation also apply to smoking cessation. All appear to work to some degree. In California, where there has been 10 years of experience with a program that combines increased taxes on cigarettes with antismoking mass media advertising, school-based tobacco prevention programs, community intervention by local health departments, and projects aimed at high-risk groups, there has been a decline in tobacco consumption and the prevalence of smoking. It is not clear whether the benefits have been caused by less smoking initiation, more smoking cessation, or both.

There is also evidence that initial gains obtained by such programs tend to plateau with time.

How to Elicit an Accurate Smoking History

When seeing patients in a primary care setting it is important to obtain an accurate representation of current and past smoking behavior and readiness to change. Table 10-5 details questions that can be useful in obtaining a smoking history. Because exsmokers are always at risk for

Table 10-5
Sample Questions Useful in Obtaining a Smoking History

QUESTIONS	USE OF INFORMATION
Smoking status as a vital sign Have you ever used tobacco?	If never smoker, used to congratulate positive health choice. If former user, used to congratulate success and encourage continued abstinence. If current user, is introduction to the following questions.
How much do you smoke now?	Provides baseline and monitoring window into intensity of smoking.

Was there a time when you smoked more?
    If yes, when?
    Why did you cut down?
	Helps assess efforts to cut down as part of the continuum of cessation.
	Provides information on proximity of recent attempts.
	Is motivation for reduction and possible anchor for message relevance.

Have you ever been off cigarettes since you started smoking regularly?
    If yes, when?
    How long were you off?
    What made you go back to smoking?
	Helps assess past cessation attempts.
	Opportunity to provide guidance related to relapse prevention in the context of previous attempts.

Are you planning to quit smoking?
    If yes, when?
	Allows staging in terms of readiness to change.
	    Guides type of brief intervention to use: motivational or cessation.
	If next month, preparation stage.
	If next six months, contemplation stage.
	If more than 6 months or never, precontemplation stage.

relapse, and 80% of smokers start by the age of 16 years, primary care clinicians should ask about tobacco use at every visit. A practical and effective way to do this is to include tobacco use (current, former, or never) with other vital signs measured routinely.

In view of the competing demands of practice experienced by most primary care clinicians, it makes sense that this function be delegated to other members of the clinical team such as nurses or medical office assistants. These other team members can initiate counseling interventions that are reinforced and expanded by the primary care clinician. There is good evidence that screening systems that systematically identify and document smoking status result in higher rates of smoking intervention by clinicians.

Readiness-to-change models describe smoking cessation as a process rather than a discrete event. These models divide current smoking into three stages: precontemplation, contemplation, and preparation. Population studies describe a relatively constant proportion of smokers in each of the stages. Precontemplation (40% of smokers) includes those who are not planning to stop smoking in the next 6 months or have no intention to ever stop. Contemplation (40% of smokers) includes those who are planning to stop smoking in the next 6 months but not in the next 30 days. Preparation (20% of smokers) includes those who plan to stop smoking in the next 30 days. Smokers in each stage differ in terms of expected positive outcomes from quitting and belief in their ability to stop smoking successfully. However, they do not differ in number of cigarettes smoked daily, nicotine dependency score, or number of years smoked. Stages of change are, however, highly predictive of quitting behavior.

The basic approach in obtaining a smoking history does not change with age. It is important to assess smoking status at the first visit by a newborn. The smoking status of caregivers influences the health of young children and is a critical area for intervention to lessen the harm of ETS. If smoking cessation is not possible for caregivers, we must teach them to smoke outside. Smoking in the basement, bathroom, or another room is not sufficiently protective in homes that are insulated and have poor ventilation patterns.

Given the natural history of smoking initiation it makes sense to start asking about tobacco use when patients are 11 years of age. Those 65 years of age or older who have never smoked are not likely to start smoking. Once their never-smoking status is established, there is no need to continue asking about tobacco use at every visit.

Laboratory and Other Diagnostic Tests

Carbon monoxide monitors can discriminate between current smokers and nonsmokers by measuring carbon monoxide concentration in expired air. These tests are useful in validating self-reports of cessation in research studies. Although carbon monoxide monitoring allows detection of continued smoking and modification of smoking cessation interventions, their effectiveness in improving results is not proved. Other routinely available diagnostic and laboratory tests are not useful for screening in the evaluation of smoking patients. The U.S. Preventive Services Task Force advises against screening for lung cancer with chest radiography or sputum cytologic examination among persons who do not have symptoms because use of these modalities does not lead to improved outcomes. Smokers should be advised to observe the same frequency of screening for breast, cervical, and colon cancer as any other patient.

Smoking Cessation Clinical Practice Guidelines

In 1996 a panel convened by the Agency for Health Care Policy and Research (AHCPR) published a set of clinical practice guidelines for smoking cessation. This panel reviewed more than 3000 articles published between 1975 and 1994. More than 300 articles met inclusion criteria and were used in 50 meta-analyses to support clinical recommendations. The strength of the evidence for each recommendation had one of three ratings. (A) recommendations were supported by multiple well-designed, randomized clinical trials directly related to the recommendation and yielding a consistent pattern of findings. (B) recommendations were supported by evidence from a randomized clinical trial, but the scientific support was not optimal. (C) recommendations were reserved for important clinical situations in which the panel achieved consensus in the absence of relevant randomized clinical trials. The panel declined to make recommendations when there was no relevant evidence or the evidence considered was too weak or inconsistent. The guideline recommends specific strategies to deliver smoking cessation interventions including the 4 A's (*ask, advise, assist,* and *arrange*), follow-up if the patient is ready to stop smoking, and the 4 Rs (*relevance, risks, rewards,* and *repetition*) if the patient is not ready to stop smoking.

Clinician Actions to Enhance Smoking Cessation

The first step is to *ask* about tobacco use at every visit. The second step is to *advise* smoking cessation for every smoker. It is important that this advice be clear, strong, and personalized. Table 10-6 gives examples of phrases that can be useful. The AHCPR panel found (A) evidence for this recommendation. A meta-analysis of seven randomized clinical trials estimated that the cessation rate increased significantly going from 8% with no advice to 10% when clinicians offered advice to stop smoking. Given the large number of smokers who visit a clinician every year, the potential public health effect of this increase is substantial.

Table 10-6

Advise: Strongly Urge All Smokers to Quit

ACTION	STRATEGIES FOR IMPLEMENTATION
In a clear, strong, and personalized manner, urge every smoker to stop.	Advice should be: Clear. "I think it is important for you to quit smoking now and I will help you." "Cutting down while you are ill is not enough."
	Strong. "As your clinician, I need you to know that quitting smoking is the most important thing you can do to protect your current and future health." "If you need a doctor to tell you that you need to quit, I'm it."
	Personalized. "I know that you're concerned about your cough and the fact that your son gets so many colds. If you stop smoking, your cough should improve, and your son might get fewer colds." "You asked me for help with your acne, if you stop smoking you will also get fewer wrinkles in your face."

Because four of five smokers are not ready to stop smoking at any particular moment, it is important to establish whether a smoker is ready to stop smoking before proceeding. Providing precontemplators and contemplators with cessation assistance is not effective. If a smoker is not ready to stop, the clinician should offer a brief motivational intervention such as the 4 R's recommended by the AHCPR panel. This intervention requires that the clinician connect the advice message to a relevant topic and allow the patient to list risks of continued smoking and

rewards of cessation. This intervention should be repeated at every visit. Table 10-7 outlines and gives examples of this type of intervention.

If the patient is ready to stop smoking, the next step is to *assist*. Table 10-8 provides

Table 10-7

Components of Clinical Interventions Designed to Enhance Motivation to Stop Smoking: The 4Rs

Relevance	Motivational information given to a patient has the greatest influence if it is relevant to a patient's disease status, family or social situation (e.g., having children in the home), health concerns, age, sex, and other important patient characteristics (e.g., prior cessation experience).
Risks	The clinician should ask the patient to identify the potential negative consequences of smoking. The clinician may suggest and highlight those that seem most relevant to the patient. The clinician should emphasize that smoking low-tar, low-nicotine cigarettes or use of other forms of tobacco (e.g., smokeless tobacco, cigars, pipes) will not eliminate these risks. Example of risks are as follows: *Acute risks*: Shortness of breath, exacerbation of asthma, impotence, infertility, increased serum carbon monoxide level. *Long-term risks*: Heart attack and stroke, lung and other cancer (larynx, oral cavity, pharynx, esophagus, pancreas, bladder, cervix, leukemia), chronic obstructive pulmonary diseases (chronic bronchitis and emphysema). *Environmental risks*: Increased risk for lung cancer in spouse and children; high rates of smoking by children of smokers; increased risk for SIDS, asthma, middle ear disease, and respiratory infections among children of smokers.
Rewards	The clinician should ask the patient to identify the potential benefits of quitting smoking. The clinician may suggest and highlight those that seem most relevant to the patient. Examples of rewards are as follows: Improved health Improved taste of food Improved sense of smell Saving money Feeling better about yourself Better-smelling, home, car, breath Freedom from worrying about quitting Setting a good example for children Having healthy babies and children Freedom from worrying about exposing others to smoke Feeling better physically Freedom from addiction Better in sports performance
Repetition	The motivational intervention should be repeated every time an unmotivated patient visits the clinic.

Table 10-8

Assist: Aid the Patient in Cessation

ACTION	STRATEGIES FOR IMPLEMENTATION
Help the patient with a cessation plan.	Set a quit date. Ideally, the quit date should be within 2 weeks, taking patient preference into account. Advise patients preparing to stop smoking to • Inform family, friends, and co-workers of the intention to quit and request understanding and support. • Remove cigarettes from their environment. Before quitting, avoid smoking in places where they spend a lot of time (e.g., home, car). • Review previous cessation attempts. What helped? What led to relapse? • Anticipate challenges to the planned cessation attempt, particularly during the critical first few weeks. These include nicotine withdrawal symptoms.
Encourage nicotine replacement therapy or other pharmacotherapies except in special circumstances.	Encourage the use of a nicotine patch or nicotine gum or sustained release buprorion therapy for smoking cessation. Give specific information regarding use and side effects and clarify expectations.
Give key advice on successful quitting.	Abstinence. Total abstinence is essential. "Not even a single puff after the quit date." Alcohol. Drinking alcohol is highly associated with relapse. Those who stop smoking should review their alcohol use and consider limiting or abstaining from alcohol during the cessation process. Other smokers in the household. The presence of other smokers in the household, particularly a spouse, is associated with lower success rates. Patients should consider stopping smoking with their significant others or developing specific plans to stay abstinent in a household where others still smoke.
Provide supplementary materials.	Sources. Federal agencies, including AHCPR; nonprofit agencies (American Cancer Society, American Lung Association, American Heart Association), or local and state health departments. Type. Culturally, racially, educationally and age appropriate for the patient. Location. Readily available in every clinic office.

strategies for helping patients with a cessation plan, encouraging use of nicotine replacement or other effective pharmacologic aids, giving key advice on successful cessation, and providing supplementary materials. The content of the advice is best if focused on training in problem-solving skills and on social support, as outlined in Tables 10-9 and 10-10.

Most smokers gain weight after smoking cessation. The average weight gain is about 10 pounds, but as many as 10% of persons who stop smoking may gain more than 30 pounds. Weight gain is likely to be related to a decrease in basal metabolic rate once nicotine is removed. Smokers who are stopping should be advised against dieting during the cessation

Table 10-9

Common Elements of Problem Solving and Skills Training for Smoking Cessation

PROBLEM-SOLVING TREATMENT COMPONENT	EXAMPLES
RECOGNITION OF DANGER SITUATIONS	
Identification of events, internal states, or activities that are thought to increase the risk for smoking or relapse.	Being around other smokers Being under time pressure Getting into an argument Experiencing urges or negative moods Drinking alcohol
COPING SKILLS	
Identification and practice of coping or problem-solving skills. Typically, these skills are intended to come with danger situations.	Learning to anticipate and avoid danger situations Learning cognitive strategies that will reduce negative moods Accomplishing lifestyle changes that reduce stress, improve quality of life, or produce pleasure Learning cognitive and behavioral activities that distract attention from smoking urges
BASIC INFORMATION	
Provision of basic information about smoking and successful cessation.	The nature and time course of withdrawal The addictive nature of smoking The fact that any smoking (even a single puff) increases the likelihood of full relapse

attempt. Patients should be advised to not attempt weight loss until they are secure about their cessation behavior.

The next step is to *arrange* follow-up. Follow-up visits after the cessation date are important interventions to improve success. The first follow-up contact, either in person or by telephone, should be scheduled within the first week after the cessation date, when the risk for relapse is highest. The second follow-up contact should be scheduled within the first month after the cessation date, if possible. Additional contacts should be scheduled as necessary. On average, most exsmokers have had three or more serious attempts at cessation. The follow-up visits provide opportunities to prevent relapse and to support maintenance of cessation. Table 10-11 provides details of potential action during follow-up visits.

Referral to Intensive Smoking Cessation Programs

Because the average visit to a primary care clinician lasts only 12 minutes, intensive counseling on smoking cessation is not possible during routine visits. Although the brief clinician interventions described earlier are effective in increasing smoking cessation rates, more intensive smoking cessation programs can increase this rate from 10% to 25%.

Table 10-10

Common Elements of Supportive Smoking Cessation Treatments

SUPPORTIVE TREATMENT COMPONENT	EXAMPLES
Encourage the patient in the cessation attempt.	State that effective cessation treatments are now available. State that half of all people who have ever smoked have now quit. Communicate belief in the patient's ability to quit.
Communicate caring and concern.	Ask how the patient feels about quitting. Directly express concern and willingness to help. Be open to the patient's expression of fears of quitting, difficulties experienced, and ambivalent feelings.
Encourage the patient to talk about the quitting process.	Ask about Reasons the patient wants to quit Difficulties encountered while quitting Success the patient has achieved Concerns or worries about quitting
Provide basic information about smoking and successful cessation.	Ask about The nature and time course of withdrawal The addictive nature of smoking The fact that any smoking (even a single puff) increases the likelihood of full relapse

The AHCPR panel evaluated the content of intensive counseling interventions. Categories examined included cigarette fading, relaxation and breathing exercises, contingency contracting, exercise and fitness interventions, weight and nutrition, motivation, social support outside treatment, establishing a cessation day, problem solving and skills training, social support within treatment, and aversive smoking. Only problem solving and skills training, social support within treatment, and aversive smoking were found effective. The use of problem solving and social support is described in Tables 10-9 and 10-10. Aversive smoking sessions involve the patient's smoking intensely, often to the point of discomfort or malaise. Some aversive smoking techniques, such as rapid smoking, may present a health risk and should be conducted only under direct medical supervision and screening. Hypnosis and acupuncture are popular approaches for smoking cessation, but evidence from randomized clinical trials is too sparse to allow a judgment regarding efficacy.

There is a direct relation between the duration and intensity of intensive programs and cessation rates. Patients who participate in group counseling are 2 times more likely to stop smoking, those who participate in four to seven sessions are 2.5 times more likely to stop smoking, and those who are in treatment for more than 8 weeks are 3 times more likely to stop than smokers not participating in these sessions.

Both individual and group counseling are effective formats, and nicotine replacement increases cessation rates. Intensive programs are effective for both men and women, for all racial and ethnic groups, and for all ages. AHCPR recommendations regarding intensive smoking cessation programs are listed in Table 10-12.

Intensive programs are offered by many nonprofit organizations, including the American Cancer Society and the American Lung Associa-

Table 10-11

Arrange: Schedule Follow-Up Contact

ACTION	STRATEGIES FOR IMPLEMENTATION
Schedule follow-up contact, either in person or via telephone.	Timing. Follow-up contact should occur soon after the cessation date, preferably during the first week. A second follow-up contact is recommended within the first month. Schedule additional follow-up contacts as indicated.
	Actions during the follow-up visit. Congratulate success. If smoking occurred, review circumstances and elicit recommitment to total abstinence. Remind patient that a lapse can be used as a learning experience. Identify problems already encountered and anticipate challenges in the immediate future. Assess use of and problems with nicotine replacement therapy. Consider referral to a more intense or specialized program.

Table 10-12

Recommendations Regarding Intensive Smoking Cessation Programs

Assessment: Assessments should determine whether smokers are motivated to stop smoking through an intensive smoking cessation program. Other assessments can provide information useful in counseling (e.g., stress level, presence of comorbidity).

Program clinicians: Multiple types of clinicians should be used. One strategy would be to have a medical or other health care clinician deliver messages about health risks and benefits and nonmedical clinicians deliver psychosocial or behavioral interventions.

Program intensity: Because of evidence of a strong dose-response relation, the program should be at least 20 to 30 minutes long[a], should include at least 4 to 7 sessions, and should last at least 2 weeks, preferably more than 8 weeks.

Program format: Either individual or group counseling may be used. Use of adjuvant self-help material is optional. Follow-up assessment procedures should be used.

Counseling content: Counseling should involve problem-solving or skill-training content or both and social support delivered during treatment sessions. In addition, the content should target motivation to stop smoking and relapse prevention.

Pharmacotherapy: Except in special circumstances, every smoker should be offered nicotine replacement therapy. The clinician should encourage the use of NRT or bupropion for smoking cessation.

Population: Intensive intervention programs may be used with all smokers willing to enter such programs.

[a] A session length of 20 to 30 minutes is recommended because most trials of effective smoking cessation counseling entailed sessions of at least this length.

tion. The time commitment involved with intensive programs is a barrier. In a clinical practice many patients are unwilling or unable to participate. Brief smoking cessation interventions are especially important for these patients.

Nicotine Replacement and Other Pharmacologic Aids

The AHCPR panel gave an (A) level of evidence for the effectiveness of nicotine replacement therapy (NRT) for smoking cessation with either nicotine gum or patches. NRT appears to reduce cravings and to blunt the withdrawal symptoms, which include nausea, irritability, restlessness, nervousness, difficulty concentrating, insomnia, hunger, and weight gain. NRT is recommended for all smokers except in the presence of serious medical contraindications, such as recent myocardial infarction, serious arrhythmia, and severe angina. Patients with these conditions should use NRT only after carefully considering the risks and benefits. Clinical trials of NRT in the treatment of patients with underlying, stable coronary artery disease suggest that nicotine does not increase cardiovascular risk. There is no support for the notion that wearing a nicotine patch causes myocardial infarction.

Pregnant smokers should be encouraged to attempt cessation without pharmacologic treatment. NRT should be used in pregnancy only after a determination that smoking cessation with its potential benefits outweighs the risk of nicotine replacement and potential concomitant smoking. Similar considerations are necessary for lactating mothers.

NICOTINE PATCHES

The nicotine patch is applied daily on awakening in an area that is relatively hairless between the waist and neck. There are no restrictions on activity, but smokers are encouraged not to smoke while using the patch,

mainly to avoid relapse. It is important to start with the highest dose. Although it is recommended that patients be treated for 8 weeks, duration of therapy can be individualized. Recommended doses and duration of treatment of different nicotine patches are described in Table 10-13.

GUM

Proper chewing technique is essential for success with nicotine gum. Chewing nicotine gum as one would in a manner similar to conventional chewing gum produces nicotine toxicity (nausea, hiccups, dyspepsia). Gum should be chewed slowly until a peppery taste emerges then "parked" between cheek and gum to facilitate nicotine absorption through the oral mucosa. Gum should be slowly and intermittently "chewed and parked" for about 30 minutes. Acidic beverages such as coffee, juices, and soft drinks interfere with the buccal absorption of nicotine and should be avoided for 15 minutes before and during gum use.

Nicotine gum comes in two doses: 2 mg and 4 mg. The 4 mg dose is most appropriate for highly dependent smokers—those who smoke more than 20 to 25 cigarettes per day or who smoke within 30 minutes of awakening. Patients who are particularly concerned about weight

Table 10-13

Dosage and Duration of Action of Nicotine Patches

BRAND	DURATION, (WK)	DOSAGE, (MG/HR)
Nicoderm,	4	21/24
Habitrol	Then 2	14/24
	Then 2	7/24
Prostep	4	22/24
	Then 4	11/24
Nicotrol	4	15/16
	Then 2	10/16
	Then 2	5/16

gain can benefit from using nicotine gum to prevent weight gain.

INHALERS AND SPRAYS

Other delivery systems for NRT include a nicotine inhaler and a nasal spray. The AHCPR panel did not have enough information to make recommendations regarding these modalities. Nicotine inhalers deliver 4 mg nicotine from cartridges with a porous plug containing 10 mg nicotine. Patients may self-titrate to the level of nicotine they need and use at least 6 cartridges per day for the first 3 to 6 weeks of treatment. Frequent continuous puffing is recommended for best effects. Nicotine nasal spray delivers a spray containing 0.5 mg nicotine. One dose is 1 mg nicotine (2 sprays, one in each nostril). Patients should start with 1 to 2 doses per hour, which may be increased to a maximum of 40 doses per day (5 doses per hour).

SUCCESS RATES

NRT achieves the best results when combined with cessation counseling, either brief or intensive. The nicotine transdermal patch doubles the 6 to 12 month abstinence rates over those produced with placebo interventions. This conclusion is supported by five meta-analyses including 6 to 16 randomized clinical trials. Nicotine gum increases smoking cessation rates 40% to 60% compared with control interventions through 12 months of follow-up. This conclusion is supported by three meta-analyses. Other forms of NRT appear to achieve similar cessation rates.

OTHER PHARMACOLOGIC APPROACHES

Bupropion, in a slow-release (SR) formulation, is the first nonnicotine drug approved by the U.S. Food and Drug Administration for smoking cessation. The mechanism of action is not clear, but it may be related to increases in serotonin, dopamine, and norepinephrine. Dopamine and noradrenergic pathways are believed to be involved in nicotine addiction and withdrawal. For some smokers, bupropion appears to blunt the pleasure pathway related to nicotine intake. One smoker described its effects as feeling like "sucking hot air" when using the drug.

Bupropion SR is started 150 mg every day for 3 days and then increased to a maximum dose of 300 mg a day in divided doses. Smokers should start bupropion 1 week before their cessation day because it takes 5 days to achieve steady-state plasma levels. To prevent insomnia, a common side effect, doses can be separated by only 8 hours, giving a second dose 3 to 4 hours before bedtime. Contraindications include seizure disorder, current or history of bulimia or anorexia nervosa, concomitant use of monoamine oxidase inhibitors, concomitant use of other forms of bupropion, current other substance abuse, and any other medical condition that lowers the seizure threshold.

A large randomized clinical trial found rates of abstinence at 1 year of 23% with use of bupropion compared with cessation rates of 12% with placebo. This trial excluded smokers with depression. It also demonstrated a reduction in weight gain among those who remained abstinent. One study showed that bupropion SR, either alone or in combination with nicotine patches, resulted in higher 1-year abstinence rates (35%) at 6 months than did use of patches alone (16%). Abstinence rates with bupropion alone were 30%.

HOW TO CHOOSE

How does the clinician decide which patients are good candidates for nicotine replacement or other pharmacologic approaches? In view of the evidence of equal effectiveness of NRT and bupropion, the patient's preference is the most important consideration. Some patients prefer to take a pill and are likely to prefer bupropion.

Others prefer to use over-the-counter medications and chose NRT. If a patient shows evidence of depression, bupropion has the added advantage of being an antidepressant. A smoker who has unsuccessfully tried multiple approaches to cessation may benefit from combined therapy.

Advice to Clinicians

Smoking prevention and cessation should be a priority for primary care clinicians. Office staff and procedures should facilitate documenting the smoking status of each patient, encouraging nonsmokers to remain abstinent, and assisting smokers in cessation. Clinicians should *ask* each patient about their smoking status, *advise* smoking cessation for every smoker, *assist* in developing a cessation plan, and *arrange* for follow up contact.

Every smoker should be treated with a cessation or motivational intervention and offered NRT, except in special circumstances. Follow-up contact should be scheduled after initiation of a cessation plan.

Common Errors

Not Asking about Smoking

Primary care clinicians often do not document the smoking status of their patients. Not developing a partnership with other members of the clinical team is a common error whereby many smokers do not receive the smoking cessation advice they deserve. There are so many competing opportunities for intervention in the office that it is easy to forget to address smoking. Del-

egating this function to another member of the team and including smoking status as part of assessing vital signs are efficient ways to ascertain who smokes.

Not Offering Smoking Cessation Advice

Only half of smokers report that their primary care clinician has advised them to stop smoking. Even less have received specific advice on how to stop smoking. Only about 25% of smokers receive smoking cessation advice at every visit. Clinicians often believe that there is not sufficient time to advise every smoker during every visit. On average, it takes about 1½ minutes per patient for smoking cessation counseling during primary care visits. If a clinician sees 30 patients a day and about 25% of them are smokers, counseling each patient about smoking would add 11 minutes to the entire day.

Forgetting to Follow Up

Most relapses occur within the first month of cessation. Once a smoker has made the serious effort to try to stop smoking, he or she needs all the help available. A quick telephone call or short visit is an excellent opportunity to address early failure and support success. Some pharmaceutical companies offer telephone support systems for smokers. Linking patients with these services also helps in improving success.

Giving Up Too Early

Smoking is a complex behavioral and addictive pattern that is difficult to break. Smokers need to be ready and willing to stop before any progress is made. Even then, multiple attempts are often necessary to successfully achieve cessation. No smoking cessation specialist or program can ever force an unmotivated smoker to stop smoking. The trick is to be patiently persistent and to not spend too much time encouraging smoking cessation if the patient is not ready.

Not Using Pharmacologic Aids

Clinicians often forget to advise their patients to use NRT or to prescribe bupropion. If a patient is motivated and wants to use NRT or bupropion, it is important not to discourage this therapy unless there are serious medical contraindications.

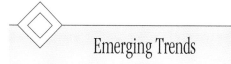

Emerging Trends

An emerging concept in smoking cessation is that of harm reduction with alternative nicotine delivery devices. In the context of smoking and nicotine dependence, this concept recognizes that some smokers are not able to stop smoking altogether and are therefore at increased risk for death from tobacco-related diseases. One proposed solution is to give smokers alternative, safer ways to satisfy their nicotine addiction. Some advocate the use of long-term NRT; others the use of alternative nicotine delivery systems. One example of an alternative nicotine delivery system is the Eclipse cigarette in the United States. This cigarette heats but does not burn tobacco or deliver tobacco in the vapor phase. Because there is no burning of tobacco, there is less sidestream smoke and less tar. The balance of risks and benefits for these alternatives is not yet clearly established.

It is likely that other medications that block the symptoms of nicotine withdrawal and increase the rate of success of smoking cessation will be discovered and marketed.

There has been a remarkable shift in public attitudes toward smoking over the past decade. There is now much less tolerance of smoking in public places and the resulting secondhand smoke. However, the renewed popularity of cigars and higher rates of smoking among college students may be the first signs of a pendulum swing in public attitudes and acceptance of smoking.

Legal battles will continue at all levels of government—local, state, and federal—to concentrate on decreasing the effectiveness of the tobacco industry in attracting new, mostly youthful, smokers. Whether state and federal tobacco financial settlements and marketing restrictions result in the eventual decline of tobacco use in the United States or guarantee a continued, albeit lower, level of tobacco use by means of precluding stronger government regulation by agencies such as the Food and Drug Administration will be seen with time.

The legal and financial culpability of tobacco companies will be determined by individual liability suits by victims of smoking-related diseases and their families. Public health efforts will focus on how to decrease smoking initiation rates among adolescents. These legal and public health efforts are likely to yield larger gains in the struggle against smoking-related mortality and morbidity than are efforts by clinicians to promote smoking cessation, but attacking the problem of smoking-related disease at all levels is necessary.

Bibliography

Benowitz NL, Gourlay SG: Cardiovascular toxicity of nicotine: Implications for nicotine replacement therapy. *J Am Coll Cardiol* 29:1422–1431, 1997.

Centers for Disease Control and Prevention: State-specific prevalence of cigarette smoking—United States, 1995. *MMWR Morb Mortal Wkly Rep* 45:962–966, 1996.

Centers for Disease Control and Prevention: Cigarette smoking among adults—United States, 1994. *MMWR Morb Mortal Wkly Rep* 45:588–590, 1996.

Centers for Disease Control and Prevention: Guidelines for school health programs to prevent tobacco use and addiction. *MMWR Morb Mortal Wkly Rep* 43:RR-2, 1994.

Centers for Disease Control and Prevention: Smoking-attributable mortality and hears of potential life lost—United States, 1990. *MMWR Morb Mortal Wkly Rep* 42:645–648, 1993.

Department of Health and Human Services: *The Health Benefits of Smoking Cessation: A Report of the Surgeon General*, DHHS publication no CDCA 90-8418. Rockville, MD, Department of Health and Human Services, 1990.

Department of Health and Human Services: *Reducing the Consequences of Smoking: 25 Years of Progress—A Report of the Surgeon General*, DHHS publication no CDC 89-8411. Rockville, MD, Department of Health and Human Services, 1989.

Farrelly MC, Bray JW: Response to increases in cigarette prices by race/ethnicity, income and age groups—United States, 1996–1993. *MMWR Morb Mortal Wkly Rep* 47:605–609, 1998.

Fiore MC, Bailey WC, Cohen SJ, et al: *Smoking Cessation*, Clinical Practice Guideline no 18, AHCPR publication no 96-0692. Rockville, MD, US Department of Health and Human Services, Public Health Service, Agency for Health Care Policy and Research, 1996.

Flint AG, Novotny TE: Poverty status and cigarette smoking prevalence and cessation in the United States, 1983–1993: The independent risk of being poor. *Tob Control* 6:14–18, 1997.

Giovino GA, Henningfield JE, Tomar SL, et al: Epidemiology of tobacco use and dependence. *Epidemiol Rev* 17:48–65, 1995.

Herdman R, Hewitt M, Laschober M: *Smoking-related deaths and financial costs: Office of Technology Assessment estimates for 1990*. Washington, DC, Congress of the United States. Office of Technology Assessment, 1993.

Hurt RD, Sachs DPL, Glover ED, et al: A comparison of sustained-released buproprion and placebo for smoking cessation. *N Engl J Med* 337:1195–1202, 1997.

Jaén CR: Protecting nonsmokers from environmental tobacco smoke. *J Fam Pract* 43:530–532, 1996.

Jaén CR, Crabtree BF, Zyzanski SJ, et al: Making time for tobacco cessation counseling. *J Fam Pract* 46:425–428, 1998.

Jaén CR, Stange KC, Nutting PA: Competing demands of primary care: a model for the delivery of clinical preventive services. *J Fam Pract* 38:166–171, 1994.

Jaén CR, Stange KC, Tumiel LM, Nutting PA: Missed opportunities for prevention: Smoking cessation advice and the competing demands of practice. *J Fam Pract* 45:348–354, 1997.

Lichtenstein E, Hollis J: Patient referral to a smoking cessation program: who follows through? *J Fam Pract* 34:739–744, 1992.

McGinnis JM, Foege WH: Actual causes of death in the United States. *JAMA* 270:2207–2212, 1993.

National Cancer Institute: *Strategies to Control Tobacco Use in the United States: A Blueprint for Public Health Action in the 1990's*, NIH publication no 92-3316. (Smoking and tobacco control monograph no 1). Bethesda, MD, US Department of Health and Human Services, National Institutes of Health, 1991.

Pierce JP, Gilpin EA, Emery SL, et al: Has the California tobacco control program reduced smoking? *JAMA* 280:893–899,1998.

Pirkle JL, Flegal KM, Bernett JT, et al: Exposure of the US population to environmental tobacco smoke: The Third National Health and Nutrition Examination Survey, 1988 to 1991. *JAMA* 275:1233–1240, 1996.

Reid DJ, McNeill AD, Glenn TJ: Reducing the prevalence of smoking in youth in western countries: an international review. *Tob Control* 4:266–277, 1995.

Thorndike AT, Rigotti NA, Stafford RS, Singer DE: National patterns in the treatment of smokers by physicians. *JAMA* 279: 604–608, 1998.

US Department of Health and Human Services: *Preventing Tobacco Use among Young People: A Report of the Surgeon General*. Atlanta, US Department of Health and Human Services, Public Health Service, Centers for Disease Control and Prevention, Office on Smoking and Health, 1994.

US Department of Health and Human Services: *Tobacco Use among US Racial/Ethnic Minority Groups, African Americans, American Indians and Pacific Islanders, Hispanics: A report of the Surgeon General*. Atlanta, US Department of Health and Human Services, Centers for Disease Control and Prevention, Office on Smoking and Health, 1998.

US Environmental Protection Agency: *Respiratory Health Effects of Passive Smoking: Lung Cancers and Other Disorders*. NIH publication no 93-3605. (Smoking and tobacco control monograph no. 4). Washington DC, Indoor Air Division, Office of Air and Radiation, US Environmental Protection Agency, 1993.

US Preventive Services Task Force: *Guide to Clinical Preventive Services*, 2nd ed. Baltimore, Williams & Wilkins, 1996.

Velicer WF, Fava JL, Prochaska JO, et al: Distribution of smokers by stage in three representative samples. *Prev* Med 24: 401–411, 1995.

Wechsler H, Rigotti NA, Gledhill-Hoyt J, Lee H. Increased levels of cigarette use among college students. *JAMA* 280:1673–1678, 1998.

Williamson DF, Madans J, Anda RF, et al: Smoking cessation and severity of weight gain in a national cohort. *N Engl J Med* 324:739–745, 1991.

World Health Organization: *Tobacco or Health: A Global Status Report.* Geneva, World Health Organization, 1997.

Daniel C. Vinson

Alcohol and Drug Abuse

Introduction

Alcohol and drug abuse are common problems, are commonly overlooked, and even when recognized are commonly untreated. However, we have effective and efficient screening tools to find the problems; brief interventions with problem drinkers can make a difference; and even patients with severe alcohol or drug dependence can experience remarkable recovery.

Definitions

The word *alcoholism* implies a dichotomous disease state with severely alcohol-dependent patients on one side and perfectly safe social drinkers on the other side of some ostensible dividing line. Reality is quite different. The spectrum of problems includes at-risk drinkers, whose consumption puts them at risk for adverse consequences not yet encountered, and harmful drinkers, who have experienced some consequences (alcohol abuse) and alcohol dependence, both psychological and physical (Tables 11-1, 11-2). In this chapter, we describe all these drinkers as *problem drinkers*.

Table 11-1

Definition of At-risk Drinking from the National Institute on Alcohol Abuse and Alcoholism (NIAAA)

For men: More than 14 drinks per week or more than 4 drinks per occasion
For women[a]: More than 7 drinks per week or more than 3 drinks per occasion
One standard drink is 12 oz (360 mL) of beer, 5 oz (150 mL) of wine, or 1.5 oz (45 mL) of liquor.

[a] The threshold for women is less because they absorb and metabolize alcohol differently from men. It takes less alcohol to cause the same blood level, even after adjustment for body weight.

The term *drug abuse* covers more ground than we usually realize. Illicit use of psychoactive drugs, whether prescription medications or street drugs, is illegal and therefore always carries the potential for substantial adverse consequences. Even here there is a spectrum, from infrequent use with relatively few risks to self-destruction. Standard definitions imply a certainty often lacking in clinical settings, where diagnoses of these problems often are fuzzy. Recognizing, however, where a patient is on the spectrum of these disorders can assist practitioners in helping patients sort out the realities of their own lives and work out a reasonable therapeutic plan.

Prevalence

ALCOHOL USE

In 1992, the National Longitudinal Alcohol Epidemiologic Survey found a past-year prevalence of alcohol abuse and dependence (according to DSM-IV criteria) among adults of 7.4%, higher for men (11.0%) than for women (4.1%). Younger adults were more likely to meet criteria for an alcohol-use disorder, but no age group was exempt. At-risk drinking is even more common. The Behavioral Risk Factor Surveillance System in 1994–1995 found that 13.9% of all adults reported drinking five or more drinks on at least one occasion in the past month. In a clinical trial in Wisconsin, 16.5% of adult patients in 17 family practices had positive screen results for drinking problems. A problem was considered drinking beyond the National Institute on Alcohol Abuse and Alcoholism (NIAAA) safe-drinking limits and answering at least two of the CAGE questions affirmatively (Table 11-3). A national survey in 1997 confirmed earlier findings that at-risk drinking is very common among college students; 42.6% of those surveyed in 1997 said they had had at least five (for men) or four (for women) drinks on one occasion in the past 2 weeks. One of

Table 11-2

DSM-IV Diagnostic Criteria for Substance Abuse and Dependency

SUBSTANCE ABUSE
A. A maladaptive pattern of substance use leading to clinically significant impairment or distress, as manifested by one or more of the following within a 12-month period: 1. Recurrent substance use resulting in a failure to fulfill role obligations at work, school, or home 2. Recurrent substance use in situations in which it is physically hazardous 3. Recurrent substance-related legal problems 4. Continued substance use despite having persistent or recurrent social or interpersonal problems caused or exacerbated by the effects of the substance B. The symptoms have never met the criteria for substance dependence for this class of substance.

SUBSTANCE DEPENDENCE
A. A maladaptive pattern of substance use that leads to clinically significant impairment or distress as manifested by three or more of the following occurring at any time in the same 12-month period: 1. Need for markedly increased amounts of the substance to achieve intoxication or desired effect, or markedly diminished effect with continued use of the same amount of the substance 2. The characteristic withdrawal syndrome for the substance, or the same (or a closely related) substance is taken to relieve or avoid withdrawal symptoms 3. The substance often is taken in larger amounts or over a longer period than the person intended 4. Persistent desire or one or more unsuccessful efforts to cut down or control substance use 5. A great deal of time spent in activities necessary to obtain the substance, to use it, or to recover from its effects 6. Important social, occupational, or recreational activities given up or reduced because of substance use 7. Continued substance use despite knowledge of having a persistent or recurrent physical or psychological problem that is likely to be caused or exacerbated by the substance B. No duration criterion separately specified. However, three or more dependence criteria must be met within the same year and must occur repeatedly as specified by duration qualifiers associated with criteria (e.g., "often," "persistent," "continued"). C. Physiologic dependence 1. With physiologic dependence. Evidence of tolerance or withdrawal (either of items A1 or A2 above is present). 2. Without physiologic dependence. No evidence of tolerance or withdrawal (neither of items A1 or A2 above is present).

five had consumed that much on three or more occasions in the past 2 weeks, and more than half the students (52.3%) said that when they drink, they drink to get drunk.

In the United States, apparent per capita consumption of alcohol declined from 2.76 gallons of absolute ethanol in 1980 to 2.21 gallons in 1994, but the level in 1994 was still higher than

Table 11-3
CAGE Questions

> 1. Have you ever felt you should *cut* down on your drinking?
> 2. Have people *annoyed* you by criticizing your drinking?
> 3. Have you ever felt bad or *guilty* about your drinking?
> 4. Have you ever had a drink first thing in the morning to steady your nerves or to get rid of a hangover (*eye-opener*)?

for any year from 1935 to 1964 except 1946. That level of consumption is the equivalent of 49 gallons of beer per year per person 14 years or older; roughly 10 beers per week on average. Not everyone drinks, of course; 10% of the population drinks about 50% of the alcohol.

ILLICIT DRUG USE

Illicit drug use is prevalent. Two national surveys in the early 1990s showed a past-year prevalence of illicit drug use of 11% to 15%. The past-year prevalence of illicit drug dependence was about 2%. In the 1993 National Household Survey on Drug Abuse, 14.2% of men and 9.6% of women reported past-year use of illicit drugs; 5.6% of the population 12 years and older reported past-month illicit drug use. In 1995, 24% of 18-year-olds acknowledged past-month use of an illicit drug; 10% used a drug other than marijuana. Those figures declined with age so that among persons 31 and 32 years of age, only 13% had used an illicit drug in the past month and 4% a drug other than marijuana. Figure 11-1 shows trends in past-year use of drugs by high school seniors from 1975 through 1998.

Use of marijuana accounts for much of reported use of illicit drugs. Other drugs used frequently include cocaine, heroin, phencyclidine, methaqualone, a variety of hallucinogens, amphetamines, and inhalants such as amyl nitrite, gasoline, glue and paint. Some estimates place the number of heroin users at half a million. Close to 5% of high school seniors use marijuana daily and an estimated 1.4 million Americans use cocaine.

Although it is a vexing problem, the prevalence of prescription-drug abuse is unknown. Many medications have a potential for abuse, the most common being narcotics, benzodiazepines, and barbiturates. Little is known about the characteristics of patients likely to misuse prescription drugs, but men and women appear equally involved. One estimate is that 2 million adults 65 years and older may be addicted to sleeping medicines or tranquilizers. Systematic studies, even descriptive ones, are few, and we know little about how to screen for, recognize, or treat these patients.

Morbidity and Mortality

ALCOHOL

Alcohol abuse accounts for approximately 100,000 deaths each year in the United States. The threshold of alcohol consumption at which risk begins to rise is low. In prospective cohort studies, drinking more than two or three drinks a day significantly increased overall mortality. Those who drink six or more drinks per day have mortality rates 50% higher than those for matched controls.

Alcohol use is related to several other diseases. Drinking increases risk for breast cancer and is causally related to several other types of cancer, including cancer of the mouth, larynx, esophagus, and liver. Hepatic cirrhosis and pancreatitis are much more likely among heavy drinkers, and alcohol increases risk for hemorrhagic stroke. Alcohol has also been implicated in gastritis, cardiomyopathy, neuropathy, low birth weight, and fetal alcohol syndrome. Drink-

Figure 11-1

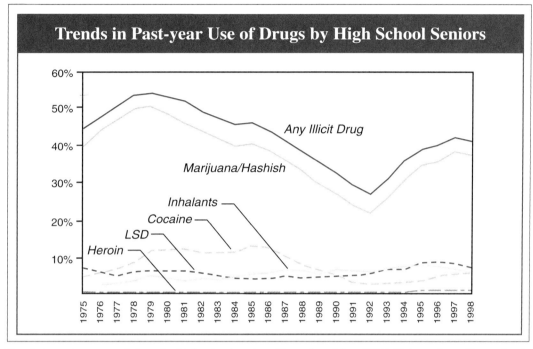

Trends in Past-year Use of Drugs by High School Seniors

Trends in past-year use of drugs by high school seniors. (Reproduced from NIDA Notes, volume 14, number 1. Bethesda, MD, National Institute on Drug Abuse, 1999.)

ing increases risk for injury, even with blood levels less than 0.08 to 0.1 g/dL, the legal limit for driving in most states. Alcohol is a factor in one-third to one-half of all injury-related deaths. It is a major contributor to suicides, homicides, violent crimes, and deaths from motor vehicle crashes and often is involved in spouse and child abuse. However, low amounts of alcohol consumption appear to reduce risk for coronary heart disease, approximately 12%. The amount needed to obtain that benefit is on the order of two to six drinks per week, fewer than one a day.

Alcohol-related harm (defined as social, legal, financial, and other personal problems) is common, and there is no threshold of consumption below which the risk is zero. Among drinkers who seldom or never drink more than five drinks on one occasion, 5% to 13% report two or more alcohol-related adverse events in the past 12 months in their social relationships, marriage, work, finances, or health, even among those whose average consumption is less than one drink a day. Among those who report binge drinking at least once a month, 20% to 33% report two or more alcohol-related harmful events. Binge drinkers are 72% more likely to experience that level of harm, compared with nonbinge drinkers, when adjustment is made for total consumption and demographic factors. With control for frequency of binge drinking and demographic factors, an increase in average consumption of one drink per day increases risk for alcohol-related harm by 16%.

ILLICIT DRUGS

Illicit drug use sometimes involves using non-sterile injection equipment, sometimes shared with others. This can lead to HIV infection, hepatitis B, endocarditis, and skin abscesses. Cocaine can directly cause cardiac arrhythmia and precipitate infarction and is associated with cerebral hemorrhage as well as minor problems such as nasal septal perforation. Chronic marijuana use can lead to pulmonary disease and decreased motivation. The incidence of these complications is not well understood. Illicit drug trafficking may be responsible for much of the recent increase in the incarceration rates of young men and contributes to the spread of HIV infection, hepatitis, and syphilis through trading sex for drugs or for money to purchase drugs.

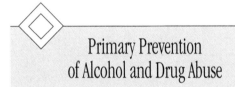

Primary Prevention of Alcohol and Drug Abuse

Advice to Avoid or Delay

Alcohol abuse and dependence are partially genetically determined; the heritability estimate from twin studies is 50% to 60%. However, the predictive value of a family history of alcohol abuse is low, and there are no tests to predict who will become an alcoholic. Advising children, adolescents, and young adults with a family history of alcoholism to delay the initiation of drinking—or to avoid it altogether—seems prudent, but such a strategy has not been tested.

Family Interventions

Family interventions by public health nurses appear to be effective in preventing alcohol use in both the short and the long term. In a randomized, controlled trial, women and their babies who met certain social and economic criteria received either home visits from nurses or usual prenatal and well-child care. Women in the intervention group received an average of 9 visits during pregnancy and 23 from the child's birth to 2 years of age. In a follow-up study when they were 15 years of age, the children in the intervention group reported less than half as many arrests, less smoking, and less than half the prevalence of alcohol use than did those in the control group. Relatively modest investments with the mother during pregnancy and early childhood had substantial benefits in the children's lives even more than 10 years later (Olds, et al, 1998).

Although it has not been proved with a randomized trial, improved parenting behaviors often follow management of alcohol and drug abuse. That improvement might reasonably be assumed to improve the children's outcomes. Some alcohol and drug-abuse treatment programs for women accommodate their young children, providing therapy not only for the substance abuser but also for her family. There are potential benefits for the children, and there are demonstrated benefits for the women themselves. Women in a long-term residential treatment program for cocaine abuse stayed three times as long (300 versus 100 days) if their children were with them compared with others whose children were placed with the best available caretaker. Substance-use disorders may best be thought of as family illnesses. Providing care for all the affected members of the family probably improves outcomes.

Government Policies

The effects of governmental policies on alcohol and drug problems are often debated, partly because they have never been tested in any randomized clinical trial. Some research has taken advantage of natural experiments to compare, for example, states that have low thresholds for defining drunk driving with states that do not.

Such analyses have consistently shown benefits. The number of traffic-crash deaths is reduced by means of increasing taxes on alcoholic beverages, raising the minimum drinking age, and enforcement of zero-tolerance laws that set the maximum blood alcohol concentration for drivers younger than 21 years at 0.02% or less. The effects appear to be enduring. In New York, the proportion of adults 18 through 20 years of age who purchased alcohol in the previous month declined from approximately 70% before the minimum age was raised to 21 years, to 30% or less afterward. Past-month alcohol use dropped from approximately 70% to less than 50%. These effects were still evident 10 years later.

Community and School-based Programs

Primary prevention programs based in the community or school have a small but important effect. Community-based educational programs that involve schools, the media, businesses, citizen groups, and health-care providers reduce alcohol consumption and drunkenness among adolescents. Programs that seek to engender fear may arouse curiosity, especially among risk takers, and lead to heavier drinking. Although most school-based programs show little benefit, one program that provided a total of 30 class sessions in 7th through 9th grades showed a considerably lower risk for drug abuse among the intervention groups compared with risk among controls. The primary focus of the program was teaching skills for resisting social influences to use drugs.

Secondary Prevention

Screening for Problem Drinking

On the basis of a review of current evidence, the U.S. Preventive Services Task Force recommends screening to detect problem drinking among adults and adolescents by means of a careful history interview, standardized screening questionnaire, or both. Screening for problem drinking is quick and effective at ascertaining whether someone is a problem drinker. Many screening instruments are appropriate for primary care practice, and use of these instruments leads to increased detection of problem drinking.

CAGE

The most commonly used screening test is the four CAGE questions (see Table 11-3). They are less sensitive, however, in the detection of problem drinking among younger persons and women than among older persons and men. They also do not deal with consumption and therefore may miss at-risk drinkers.

TWEAK

The TWEAK screen (Table 11-4) is a set of five questions similar to those used in the CAGE screen. They may, however, be more sensitive and specific and can help detect at-risk drinking. The first question, focusing on tolerance, has two versions, one given in Table 11-4. The other version is, "How many drinks does it take before you begin to feel the first effects of the alcohol?" Three or more drinks is considered a positive response and given 2 points in scoring.

AUDIT

The Alcohol Use Disorders Identification Test (AUDIT; Table 11-5) is a 10-item instrument designed for primary care practitioners to detect both at-risk drinking and alcohol-use disorders. Although it takes a little more time to administer and score than the CAGE questions, the AUDIT is equally effective for men and women and different countries and ethnic groups. Scoring only AUDIT items 1, 2, 4, 5, and 10 and using a score of 5 or greater as a cutoff results in a sensitivity

Table 11-4

TWEAK Questions

1. How many drinks does it take before the alcohol makes you fall asleep or pass out? (*Tolerance.* Any answer of 5 or more drinks is counted as 2 points.)
2. Have your friends or relatives *worried* or complained about your drinking in the past year? (An affirmative answer is counted as 2 points.)
3. Do you sometimes take a drink in the morning when you first get up? (*Eye-opener.* Counted as 1 point.)
4. Are there times when you drink and afterward you can't remember what you said or did? (*Amnesia.* Counted as 1 point.)
5. Do you sometimes feel the need to *cut* down on your drinking? (*K.* Counted as 1 point.)

NOTE: A score of 3 or more is considered positive.

of 79% with a specificity of 95%. Although this smaller subset of AUDIT items may have clinical utility, they were selected from *a posteriori* analyses, a process that may capitalize on chance associations.

SINGLE QUESTION

It also is possible to screen patients for problem drinking with a single question: "On any single occasion in the last 3 months, have you had more than five drinks containing alcohol?" (four drinks for women). Although in original testing the specificity of this question for problem drinking (past-year alcohol-use disorder or at-risk drinking) was 93%, the sensitivity was only 62%. On the other hand, it detected all the patients who had engaged in at-risk drinking in the past month and those who had a diagnosis of past-year alcohol-use disorder. The question is short and simple enough for routine use, and

repetition may help find affected individuals who initially deny recent binge drinking. It fits well with similar screening questions about other risk behaviors ("Do you use tobacco?" for example) and could be included as part of intake assessment with every patient for whom the answer to this question is not already known. A simpler version of the question also works: "When was the last time you had more than five drinks?"

INTERPRETATION OF SCREENING TEST RESULTS

All these screening instruments work better at identifying problem drinking than do usual rates of clinician recognition. It is important to understand, however, what positive and negative results do and do not mean. Table 11-6 shows the sensitivity and specificity of each test. In a population with a prevalence of alcohol dependence of 10%, using the AUDIT (with a score of 5) would provide a positive predictive value of 48% and a negative predictive value of 98%. Thus a negative test result comes close to ruling out alcohol dependence but a positive result indicates an alcohol problem only half of the time. This could falsely label half of those with positive results. In a population with a prevalence of 5% the positive predictive value would be only 30%. It is therefore important to remember that the results of these screening tests are not diagnostic of a problem but are one indication that a problem may exist. Specific questions have to be asked. Higher screening test scores are more likely to indicate a real problem than are marginal or borderline scores.

Screening for Drug Abuse

In contrast to the large number of useful screening instruments available for detecting at-risk drinking and alcohol-use disorders, few have been developed or studied for detecting drug abuse. Brown, et al, (1995) expanded the CAGE questions to include screening for drug abuse

Table 11-5

The Alcohol Use Disorders Identification Test (AUDIT)

1. How often do you have a drink containing alcohol?
   - __0__ Never
   - __1__ Once a month or less
   - __2__ 2 to 4 times a month
   - __3__ 2 to 3 times a week
   - __4__ 4 or more times a week
2. How many drinks containing alcohol do you have on a typical day when you are drinking?
   - __0__ 0
   - __0__ 1 or 2
   - __1__ 3 or 4
   - __2__ 5 or 6
   - __3__ 7 to 9
   - __4__ 10 or more
3. How often do you have six or more drinks on one occasion?
   - __0__ Never
   - __1__ Less than monthly
   - __2__ Monthly
   - __3__ Weekly
   - __4__ Daily or almost daily
4. How often during the last year have you found that you were unable to stop drinking once you had started?
   - __0__ Never
   - __1__ Less than monthly
   - __2__ Monthly
   - __3__ Weekly
   - __4__ Daily or almost daily
5. How often during the last year have you failed to do what was normally expected from you because of drinking?
   - __0__ Never
   - __1__ Less than monthly
   - __2__ Monthly
   - __3__ Weekly
   - __4__ Daily or almost daily
6. How often during the last year have you needed a first drink in the morning to get yourself going after a heavy drinking session?
   - __0__ Never
   - __1__ Less than monthly
   - __2__ Monthly
   - __3__ Weekly
   - __4__ Daily or almost daily

(Continued)

Table 11-5

The Alcohol Use Disorders Identification Test (AUDIT) *(Continued)*

---

7. How often during the last year have you had a feeling of guilt or remorse after drinking?

  _0_ Never

  _1_ Less than monthly

  _2_ Monthly

  _3_ Weekly

  _4_ Daily or almost daily

8. How often during the last year have you been unable to remember what happened the night before because you had been drinking?

  _0_ Never

  _1_ Less than monthly

  _2_ Monthly

  _3_ Weekly

  _4_ Daily or almost daily

9. Have you or someone else been injured as a result of your drinking?

  _0_ No

  _2_ Yes, but not in the last year

  _4_ Yes, during the last year

10. Has a relative, friend, doctor, or other health worker been concerned about your drinking or suggested you cut down?

  _0_ No

  _2_ Yes, but not in the last year

  _4_ Yes, during the last year

NOTE: Items are scored as indicated and summed. A total score of 8 or more usually is considered positive. Some studies have used a higher or lower threshold.

by adding the phrase "or drug use" to each of the four questions. The adapted CAGE was substantially more sensitive than the standard CAGE questions in identifying drug abuse (86% for persons with drug abuse only) with no loss of sensitivity in detecting alcohol-use disorders.

In another study, Brown, et al, tested nine questions and selected the two that functioned best in identifying drug or alcohol problems: "In the last year, have you ever drank [*sic*] or used drugs more than you meant to?" and "Have you felt you wanted or needed to cut down on your drinking or drug use in the last year?" A positive answer to either of these two questions had a sensitivity of 81% and specificity of 81% in detecting a past-year substance-use disorder (alcohol, drugs, or both), as judged with a structured psychiatric interview. Although the utility of these questions has not yet been validated in a separate sample, they show considerable promise.

Although the position of the U.S. Preventive Services Task Force is that there is insufficient evidence to recommend or not recommend routine screening for drug abuse, including questions about drug use, when taking a history, can be recommended on the basis of the prevalence of drug abuse and its consequences.

Table 11-6

Screening Tests for Problem Drinkers

Test	Sensitivity (%)	Specificity (%)
CAGE (Buchsbaum, et al, 1991)		
1 positive answer	89	81
2 positive answers (Cherpitel, 1995)	75	88
TWEAK (Chan, et al, 1993)	93–94	80–89
AUDIT		
Score ≥5 (Piccinelli, et al, 1997)	84	90
Score ≥6 (Barry, et al, 1993)	72	71
Score ≥ 8 (Cherpitel, 1995; Barry, et al, 1993)	61–85	88–90
Single questions (Taj, et al, 1998)	62	93

Physical Examination and Laboratory Tests

Physical examination and laboratory testing are of little value in screening tests for alcohol- or drug-use disorders. The following equation combines results of several ordinary blood tests and clinical measurements: $MCV + (0.31 \times BMI) + (0.08 \times \text{systolic BP}) + (0.239 \times \text{HDL in mg/dL}) + (0.02486 \times \text{fasting triglyceride level in mg/dL})$, where MCV is mean corpuscular volume, BMI is body mass index, BP is blood pressure, and HDL is high-density lipoprotein level. Use of this equation had a sensitivity of 75% and a specificity of 64% in the derivation cohort in Caerphilly, Wales, and 66% and 71% in the validation cohort in Speedwell, England, with a score of 126.22 or greater. However, the definition of heavy drinking was the equivalent of more than 35 standard U.S. drinks per week, considerably above the NIAAA threshold for at-risk drinking; and these sensitivities and specificities are lower than those of verbal screening tests. Carbohydrate-deficient transferrin level also can be used to detect heavy drinking, but it is usually not abnormal unless consumption exceeds about five drinks per day. Self-reported history is usually sufficiently sensitive, even at lower levels of consumption, to be more useful than these tests. In addition, gathering information about consumption patterns can lead into a discussion of alcohol-related problems and from there into a brief intervention. Blood test results, however, remain unknown to the patient until the follow-up visit and are less likely to facilitate an open discussion about alcohol use.

Brief Interventions with Problem Drinkers Found with Screening

Brief interventions with problem drinkers in primary care practice have been studied in more than a dozen randomized, controlled trials. Most have shown a substantial benefit. Approximately 40% of the patients in the intervention group reduced their drinking compared with approximately 20% of controls.

Successful brief interventions take 5 to 15 minutes. They can be conducted either by the physician at an office visit scheduled to discuss health-related behaviors or by another health team member. Successful interventions are characterized by feedback about how the patient's drinking pattern compares with that of persons whose drinking is not problem drinking. Information is provided about ways that drinking may be related to the patient's problems. Specific advice is given about cutting down or stopping drinking and alternative approaches to the problem. A clear statement should be made that doing something about the problem is the patient's responsibility and is possible. There is evidence that checking γ-glutamyltranspeptidase level every 3 months and giving feedback to the patient is associated with reductions in drinking and its consequences. The NIAAA has published a useful physician's guide to brief interventions, available on line at http://silk.nih.gov/silk/niaaa1/publication/physicn.htm.

Not all controlled clinical trials of brief interventions have shown them to be successful. Brief interventions in primary care settings have been shown to work only with at-risk drinkers and those who abuse alcohol, not with alcohol-dependent patients. Some unsuccessful programs included screening and intervention in the same visit. This opportunistic approach resembles what would happen in an actual office setting but perhaps is not as effective as scheduling the intervention for a later visit.

Although the best approach to problem drinkers has not been identified, the weight of evidence is clearly in favor of screening all patients and intervening with those who are found to have an alcohol problem. Those who are alcohol-dependent should be referred to a treatment program.

Brief Interventions with Patients Who Abuse Drugs

No studies have been performed on brief interventions with patients who use illicit drugs. It is reasonable, however, to apply an intervention approach similar to those used with problem drinkers. Drug-dependent patients are likely to be similar to alcohol-dependent patients and respond less well to brief interventions. The goal probably should be to get these patients to a consultant or a treatment program. Research is needed into effective ways of facilitating acceptance of the referral.

Readiness to Change

Patients with drug and alcohol problems sometimes are not interested in changing their drinking or drug use. They might not even be interested in discussing it. A helpful way of thinking about this is provided by the concept of stages of change. Some patients do not see the problem at all and are not open to talking about it. They are called *precontemplators*. Others, *contemplators*, are thinking about it. Some are planning to do something about the problems or are already taking action. Some have entered recovery and are in a maintenance stage. The clinician's job is to recognize where patients are along this continuum and help them move toward the next stage. Trying to move a precontemplator into action may not be possible and may instead lead to increased resistance, which we sometimes label as denial. Helping a precontemplator move into contemplation—"I would like for you to think about it"—may be a more realistic and achievable goal. Scales are available for measuring readiness to change, but often a conversation about change will make it clear enough to guide the clinician's approach.

Tertiary Prevention

Alcohol and Drug Withdrawal

Alcohol withdrawal is common in medical settings. It is potentially dangerous, especially for patients with severe medical or surgical conditions. Knowing that a patient has been drinking heavily is key, and that requires thoughtful, empathic inquiry. Pulse and blood pressure do not correlate well with outcomes. A score on a scale that focuses on somatic symptoms and signs (nausea, tremor, sweating) and psychological disturbances (anxiety, agitation, hallucinations, disorientation) is a better predictor of the course of withdrawal and can be used to improve outcomes.

Benzodiazepines reduce the severity of withdrawal symptoms and the risk for delirium and seizures. Long-acting benzodiazepines can accumulate in patients with liver disease and in the elderly and cause excessive sedation; use of a short-acting preparation may be preferable. When an intramuscular route of administration is needed, as for severely agitated patients, lorazepam is the drug of choice. For most other patients, however, longer-acting benzodiazepines may provide a smoother course of withdrawal. Benzodiazepines with a rapid onset of action (such as diazepam, lorazepam, and alprazolam) may have greater potential for abuse. Moreover, costs of these drugs vary more than 20-fold. Outpatient pharmacotherapy for alcohol withdrawal can be successful. A short-acting benzodiazepine such as oxazepam is dispensed one day at a time. Table 11-7 suggests several medication regimens.

Clonidine and β-blockers relieve many of the symptoms of mild alcohol withdrawal, but their effect on seizures and delirium is unknown. Magnesium supplementation has no effect on the course of alcohol withdrawal and is unnecessary, even if the blood level is low. Because some severely alcohol-dependent patients have thiamine deficiencies, giving one dose of thiamine is reasonable and may help prevent the neuropsychiatric complications of alcoholism. There is, however, no evidence that this treatment affects the course of withdrawal.

The main aim of management of withdrawal from illicit drugs is to replace the main effects of the drug in question. Withdrawal from sedative hypnotics can be managed with substitution of a long-acting benzodiazepine. Narcotic withdrawal in an acute-care hospital setting can be managed with any narcotic, but oral methadone may provide a smoother course. Clonidine also is useful in managing narcotic withdrawal.

Harm Reduction

Patients with alcohol or drug abuse or dependence can be helped with interventions to

Table 11-7

Examples of Benzodiazepine Dosing for the Management of Alcohol Withdrawal

DRUG	TYPICAL DOSE	COMMENTS
Chlordiazepoxide	25 to 50 mg orally every 4 hr as needed, for high withdrawal scores	Inexpensive and effective; standard. May accumulate, especially in elderly or patients with liver impairment.
Diazepam	10 to 20 mg orally every 1 to 2 hr until sedated, then no further doses	Loading with this long-lasting drug simplfies care. Appropriate for patients for whom withdrawal is the primary problem.
Lorazepam	1 to 2 mg orally, IV, or IM every 4 hr	The only benzodiazepine absorbed when given IM; therefore, useful in treament of very agitated patients. Short acting; won't accumulate.
Oxazepam	15 to 30 mg orally 4 times a day, then taper	When dispensed one day at a time, effective in the management of withdrawal among outpatients.

minimize the harm they might cause themselves or others even though they continue drinking or using illicit drugs. Decreasing the frequency or intensity of use may be of some benefit, and altering the circumstances may reduce harm. Although they usually are only partially successful, at best an intermediate goal representing a step toward abstinence, and have not been tested very often in randomized clinical trials, these harm-reduction strategies are worth trying with patients who are unwilling or unable to stop using drugs or drinking. This is the philosophy behind designated-driver programs and community efforts to encourage bar patrons to call a cab instead of driving home while under the influence of alcohol.

PUBLIC POLICY

Governmental policies can focus on harm reduction or "use reduction" to reduce the number of people who drink or use illicit drugs and reduce the frequency or intensity of use. Examples of use reduction policies are minimum age laws for drinking, licensing of liquor outlets, taxes on alcohol products, and forbidding sales after certain hours or on certain days. Harm reduction policies include laws against driving while intoxicated, lowering the blood alcohol level definition of impairment, and needle and syringe exchange programs. The goals of risk reduction and harm reduction sometimes are presented as antithetical to one another, and sometimes they may be. For example, in quasi-experimental studies, syringe-exchange programs have been shown to reduce the incidence of bloodborne infections in some populations. However, some policy makers still worry, in spite of a lack of evidence, that offering an unlimited supply of sterile needles may increase the frequency of use of injected drugs, which would be followed by an increase in other adverse outcomes. The issues are complex and solutions difficult. Even measuring outcomes is difficult, and the difficulty complicates research efforts. As Caulkins and Reuter (1997) pointed

out in a recent article, perhaps the best way to achieve harm reduction is through use reduction, and achieving reductions in both harm and use may be possible. For example, increasing the age limit for drinking to 21 years appears to decrease the number of motor vehicle crash deaths among young adults.

METHADONE MAINTENANCE

For patients addicted to narcotics, methadone maintenance therapy reduces the rate of illicit opiate use, HIV-risk behaviors, and criminal activity. For the most part, the effects are moderate; but for drug-related criminal activity, the reduction with methadone maintenance is substantial, 85% of those undergoing treatment show improvement. In Scotland, some general practitioners manage methadone maintenance in their offices, but in the United States methadone maintenance for narcotic addicts is allowed only in clinics that are federally licensed to provide it. An NIH consensus panel concluded that methadone maintenance treatment is effective and should be made more readily available to persons addicted to opiates.

PREVENTION OF COMPLICATIONS

A focus of harm reduction efforts is preventing secondary consequences of heavy drinking or illicit drug use. For example, persons with severe alcohol or drug dependence are at increased risk for acquiring infections, such as hepatitis B and C, HIV infection, and tuberculosis. Preventing, diagnosing, and managing these diseases can provide benefit not only to the affected patient but also to the community. Hepatitis B vaccination should be offered to all users of injected drugs who do not already have infections. Influenza, pneumococcus, and tetanus booster vaccinations are appropriate for this group of patients. Consideration should be given to offering hepatitis A vaccine to heavy drinkers or users of illicit drugs. Any person with chronic hepatitis B or C should receive hepatitis A vaccine.

SCREENING FOR INFECTION

Routine screening for HIV should be offered to all users of illicit intravenous drugs and to anyone with multiple sex partners or who exchanges sex for money or drugs. Counseling about safe sex should be provided to all patients. Anyone who has HIV infection or hepatitis B should be advised not to share needles and syringes and counseled about safe sex in an effort to prevent transmission of these diseases. Those with chronic hepatitis B, hepatitis C, and HIV infection should be monitored and treated according to current guidelines to prevent liver failure and immunosuppression.

Purified protein derivative (PPD) skin testing for tuberculosis should be considered on a regular (every 1 to 2 years) basis. In PPD testing for tuberculosis among drug abusers, use of a lower threshold (5 mm of induration) to define a positive test result is recommended if HIV status is unknown. Those who are infected with *Mycobacterium tuberculosis* and do not have active disease, should receive isoniazid therapy. Those with active disease should be treated with a four-drug regimen as recommended by the local health department. Direct observation of patients' taking antituberculosis medications three times a week can improve compliance and thereby the success of treatment.

Emotional Problems

Depression is common in primary care, probably more so among patients with drug or alcohol dependence. Depression often is part of drug and alcohol withdrawal and may require only supportive care and continuing therapy for the addiction. A patient with depression, however, especially if the depression continues, may benefit from treatment with counseling and pharmacotherapy. Treatment of depression helps maintain abstinence, so the threshold for starting therapy should be low. Management of anxiety disorders is more difficult because of the addictive potential of many antianxiety medications. Although the onset of clinical benefit may take weeks, buspirone is not addicting and has been shown effective in improving anxiety and retention in treatment of alcohol-dependent patients, though not in reducing alcohol consumption.

Specialized Treatment

Treatment of patients for alcohol and drug abuse works. As in other chronic diseases, some patients respond better than others do. Some patients are not successful despite multiple attempts at treatment, and relapse is common even among those who respond. But some patients with addiction succeed. Unlike the situation with most other chronic diseases, the outcome can look like a total cure with cessation of drinking and drug use and resolution of the resulting problems. Although the patients often refer to themselves as being "in recovery" rather than "recovered," long-term success does occur among patients with addiction and can be facilitated by treatment.

There are a variety of types of specialized treatment programs. Although they differ in treatment approach (medical, psychological, sociocultural), treatment setting (inpatient, residential, outpatient), and techniques used (pharmacotherapy, psychological intervention, behavioral therapies, self-help groups), the programs all have similar goals: (1) reducing substance abuse or achieving abstinence, (2) maximizing all aspects of life function, and (3) preventing or reducing relapses.

ALCOHOL

In the management of alcoholism, several approaches are available. If well done, they all work about equally well for just about any kind of patient. Project MATCH (Matching Alcoholism Treatment to Client Heterogeneity) randomized more than 1700 patients into three therapies: (1)

motivational enhancement therapy, which seeks to mobilize the person's own desire and ability to change; (2) cognitive behavioral therapy, which trains patients in skills to cope with situations that carry risk for drinking; or (3) 12-step facilitation, designed to promote involvement in Alcoholics Anonymous. Outcomes were equivalent across all patient groups and for almost all patient characteristics examined, with a slight advantage for the 12-step facilitation group in some comparisons. In comparisons with untreated control groups, several approaches have been shown effective, including behavioral self-control training, behavioral marital and family therapy, and the community reinforcement approach (Miller, et al, 1998). Given this information, it is reasonable for a primary care provider to encourage an alcohol-dependent patient to enter treatment, any treatment, as long as the program appears to fit the patient's needs from both the clinician's and the patient's perspectives. Inpatient treatment in a residential setting may be provided if there are severe coexisting medical or psychiatric problems, risk for harm to self or others, or a severely dysfunctional social or family situation that is a barrier to recovery. Insurance coverage may be a deciding factor for some patients.

Drug Use

As in other areas of our understanding of these problems, we know much less about the effectiveness of therapy for drug dependence than we do for alcohol dependence. Contingency contracting, which provides positive reinforcement for appropriate behavior and negative reinforcement for inappropriate behavior, benefits some patients. Multiple addictions are common, and many patients are involved with both alcohol and illicit drugs. Until more definitive results are available to guide treatment, it is reasonable to extrapolate from Project MATCH and involve patients closely in choosing which treatment they will undergo.

Pharmacotherapy for Alcohol Dependence

Two drugs are available in the United States that are effective in the management of alcohol dependence.

Disulfiram

Disulfiram blocks an essential step in the metabolism of alcohol, leading to accumulation of toxic amounts of acetaldehyde. This causes an unpleasant and potentially serious reaction characterized by vomiting, headache, hypotension, sweating, and, if enough alcohol is consumed, syncope, arrhythmia, and cardiac arrest. Disulfiram prevents drinking not through pharmacologic action but through the psychological threat of adverse side effects. The usual dose is 250 mg daily.

In one study, disulfiram showed little advantage over placebo, but the outcome is better if the drug is given as part of a broader intervention that includes the family or community. For example, married male alcoholics whose wives observed their disulfiram dosing each day had outcomes almost as good as those for a comparison group who received multidimensional community-reinforcement therapy. The outcomes were much better than those for a third group who received conventional outpatient counseling (weekly for 5 weeks then monthly) and a prescription for disulfiram. Although this approach has not been tested in a primary care practice with the physician providing (probably briefer) counseling, it may be worth trying in the care of a patient who declines referral for specialized treatment and whose spouse is willing to participate. Disulfiram can affect the liver, but the risk for hepatic damage is greater with continued heavy drinking than with disulfiram.

Naltrexone

Naltrexone is a narcotic-receptor blocker usually given 50 mg daily. Why it works in the management of alcohol dependence is still largely a matter of speculation, but it does work. In two independent randomized, clinical trials, both lasting 12 weeks, use of naltrexone reduced the risk for relapse, defined as drinking more than five drinks on one occasion for men and four for women, from 54% to 23% in one study and from almost 90% to less than 50% in the other. In both trials, naltrexone was provided as part of standard alcoholism treatment. Studies of the use of naltrexone in primary care settings are in progress. Pending the results of those studies, it is reasonable to consider naltrexone along with supportive counseling and frequent follow-up contact for a patient who is unwilling to accept a referral for specialty care. This drug is becoming a regular part of alcohol-treatment programs, and primary physicians are likely to encounter patients who are taking it.

Advice to Clinicians

An Approach to the Problem Drinker

The following steps are based in part on recommendations from the NIAAA Physicians' Guide.

ASK

Ask every patient about his or her use of alcohol. Simply ask, "Do you drink?" If the answer is yes, ask, "When was the last time you drank more than four drinks on one occasion?" (four for women, five for men). The CAGE questions also are a good screening device if supplemented with questions about the quantity and frequency of drinking, such as the first three AUDIT questions.

ASSESS

Patients who have drunk heavily sometime in the past year are at least at-risk drinkers. Inquire

further about the maximum amount on one occasion, the frequency of heavy drinking, and the frequency of lighter drinking. Ask the CAGE or TWEAK questions. Assess possible alcohol-related consequences by asking about medical, social, employment, or legal problems. You can start your assessment with, "Have you ever had any problems because of your drinking?" followed immediately with "Any job or family problems? Arrests for driving while intoxicated? Medical problems?" Simply asking the question may help patients begin to understand the situation they are in.

Assess not only the *quantity and frequency* of drinking and the *severity* of alcohol-related adverse consequences but also the patient's *readiness to change*. Is this patient a precontemplator, or is he or she ready to take some action toward change?

ADVISE

Conduct a brief intervention as described earlier. If the patient is an at-risk drinker without serious consequences or dependence, a goal of cutting down may be appropriate. Negotiate a specific quantity and frequency. "What do you think about cutting down to, say, no more than three drinks a day, 3 days a week?" If the patient insists on a limit above what is safe, go with it, but leave the door open. "I think it would be better to set a lower, safer limit, but let's see how you do with that."

If the patient is alcohol-dependent, abstinence is a better goal. Referral to a specialist or treatment program for evaluation and treatment is indicated. Of course, the patient may not be ready for that; and a temporary goal of cutting down or even just thinking about the issues may be the best the patient will accept.

FOLLOW UP

In primary care, we are used to routine follow-up care of patients with chronic diseases. It is the same for patients with alcohol and drug problems, for whom regular follow-up contact can be valuable. A patient who is not willing to accept a referral for alcohol dependence during one visit may be willing to do so a few visits later. A patient who insists on a goal of controlled drinking but then does not meet it may accept a goal of abstinence.

Follow-up care also is important after a patient returns from specialty treatment for drug or alcohol problems. Supportive, nonjudgmental care can help maintain sobriety. Be prepared to deal with relapses. Expect them.

An Approach to the Patient Who Uses Illicit Drugs

Less is known about what is effective in a primary care practice in dealing with patients with drug problems. It is, however, reasonable to build on the foregoing approach with problem drinkers. Whether they have evident drug-related problems, such as infected injection sites, or their drug use is discovered almost incidentally, empathetic discussion of their drug use and the availability of treatment may help.

Recognition and management of prescription-drug abuse is more difficult. A desire to help can sometimes tend to overrule the clinician's suspicions. Rather than acquiescing to unreasonable requests for controlled drugs, or trying to "prove" drug abuse and angrily confronting the patient, it may be effective simply to say, "I do not think [the controlled drug the patient is seeking] will be helpful for you in the long run. Let's try some other approaches." Or say, "No. I feel pushed to write a prescription that is not indicated, and I am concerned about you and your use of medications." Antidepressants help some patients. Referrals to a psychiatrist or psychologist and to a specialist in the area of the patient's symptoms may not be acceptable to the patient but are worth discussing.

Complicating this matter further is the debate about long-term use of narcotics to treat patients who are not terminally ill. As Portenoy, et al, (1997) pointed out, "Although most pain specialists now endorse the use of long-term opioid therapy for selected patients with chronic non-malignant pain, this issue also remains controversial." Consultation and caution are appropriate.

Common Errors

Lack of Detection

Detecting and managing alcohol and drug dependence and abuse are areas in which many clinicians are not well trained or with which they are not comfortable. Perhaps the most common error is not asking about alcohol and drug use. It is easy to overlook these hidden problems in a busy clinical practice. Less than half of patients with alcohol problems are recognized as such by their physicians. In a national survey of general internists in the United States, 45% of the physicians did not routinely ask patients how much they drank daily. Gathering data from the patients' perspective, the 1991 National Health Interview Survey found that only 39% of patients who had seen a physician in the previous 2 years had been asked about alcohol use. In one randomized clinical trial, routine screening for problem drinking increased the frequency of physician counseling from 33% to 50%. It is relatively unimportant which screening approach is used as long as one of them is used to screen all patients routinely.

Errors in Counseling

Other frequent errors include not taking the time needed to effectively counsel about drug and alcohol use and not using effective counseling techniques. If they do not understand the chronic nature of alcohol and drug dependence, clinicians can become discouraged and cynical with patients who have relapses.

Errors in Prescribing

Clinicians can overprescribe narcotics and sedatives as a convenient, albeit ineffective, way to manage the symptoms of drug dependence. This is not appropriate therapy except in the context of formal substance abuse programs such as methadone maintenance. Although overprescribing of narcotics and sedatives is common, underprescribing of disulfiram and naltrexone also is common. Many primary care clinicians are neither familiar with nor comfortable using these pharmacotherapies.

Neglecting Tertiary Prevention

It is common for clinicians to neglect tertiary prevention in the care of patients addicted to drugs and alcohol by not thinking about hepatitis vaccines, HIV testing, and tuberculosis screening.

Emerging Trends

Genetics

Alcohol dependence is inheritable. Studies of twins raised in different adoptive families indicate two types of alcoholism. Type I usually begins after 25 years of age and is characterized by psychological dependence symptoms. Type II is more common among men, begins in the teens or twenties, and is associated with antisocial activity. Although some candidate genes or markers for these two types have been found in

some studies, multiple genes are probably involved in these diseases. As genes associated with alcohol or drug dependence are found, questions of predictive value must be addressed before widespread application of any screening technology. Primary care providers will need to be alert to avoid misuse of genetic information either by individuals (to avoid, for example, legal responsibility for their actions) or by third parties such as insurers or potential employers. This explosion of genetic understanding of the causes of drug and alcohol problems may lead to more focused and effective interventions, both behavioral and pharmacologic.

Pharmacotherapy

The success of naltrexone is likely to lead to intense efforts to develop other drugs that can reduce the craving for alcohol or illicit drugs or that can safely meet the neuropsychiatric biochemical need that leads to drug use. Acamprosate is one example. It has been approved for use in Europe and appears to decrease drinking frequency, but its effects on abstinence are not clear. The mechanism of action is unknown. These new therapies are likely to be available to primary care clinicians in the future, which may lead to closer working relationships between addiction treatment specialists and primary care clinicians.

Public Policy

At the community level there will continue to be debate over use reduction and harm reduction. Programs with a combined approach, such as linking education about and therapy for drug dependency with needle and syringe exchange programs, will have to have their effectiveness proved to overcome political resistance.

Social attitudes toward substance abuse and dependency are likely to shift. Before the mid 1980s, smoking in public places was commonly accepted. Nonsmoking sections in commercial airplanes covered half the plane. A dramatic shift in public opinion accompanied by restrictive policies has occurred. Predicting the timing and direction of such trends is risky. In recent years we have seen the beginning of an attitude change about drinking and driving, with the public becoming less tolerant of it. We also have seen the passage of medical marijuana initiatives, indicating perhaps a more tolerant attitude toward this drug, at least for some medical purposes.

Conclusion

Problem drinking and illicit drug use are common among primary care patients. Though often hidden, and seldom the presenting problem, substance-use disorders can be recognized with routine screening and empathetic discussion. Many randomized, controlled trials in primary care settings have demonstrated the value of brief interventions with less severely affected problem drinkers, making screening and intervention skills essential for any primary care provider. We know less about how to help patients who are alcohol dependent or use illicit drugs, but specialized treatment, including Alcoholics Anonymous, helps. Even among severely addicted patients, recovery is possible.

Bibliography

American Psychiatric Association: Substance-related disorders, in *Diagnostic and Statistical Manual of Mental Disorders*, 4th ed. Washington, DC, American Psychiatric Association, 1994:175–183.

Barry KL, Fleming MF: The Alcohol Use Disorders Identification Test (AUDIT) and the SMAST-13: Predictive validity in a rural primary care sample. *Alcohol Alcohol* 28:33–42, 1993.

Bien TH, Miller WR, Tonigan JS: Brief interventions for alcohol problems: A review. *Addiction* 88:315–335, 1993.

Botvin GJ, Baker E, Dusenbury L, et al: Long-term follow-up results of a randomized drug abuse prevention trial in a white middle-class population. *JAMA* 273:1106–1112, 1995.

Bradley KA, Curry SJ, Koepsell TD, Larson EB: Primary and secondary prevention of alcohol problems: US internist attitudes and practices. *J Gen Intern Med* 10:67–72, 1995.

Brown RL, Rounds LA: Conjoint screening questionnaires for alcohol and other drug abuse: criterion validity in a primary care practice. *Wis Medical Journal* 94:135–140, 1995.

Buchsbaum DG, Buchanan RG, Centor RM, et al: Screening for alcohol abuse using CAGE scores and likelihood ratios. *Ann Intern Med* 115:774–777, 1991.

Caulkins JP, Reuter P: Setting goals for drug policy: harm reduction or use reduction? *Addiction* 92:1143–1150, 1997.

Chan AW, Pristach EA, Welte JW, Russell M: Use of the TWEAK Test in screening for alcoholism/heavy drinking in three populations. *Alcohol Clin Exp Res* 17:1188–1192, 1993.

Cherpitel CJ: Analysis of cut points for screening instruments for alcohol problems in the emergency room. *J Stud Alcohol* 56:695–700, 1995.

Clements R: A critical evaluation of several alcohol screening instruments using the CIDI-SAM as a criterion measure. *Alcohol Clin Exp Res* 22:985–993, 1998.

Deitz D, Rohde F, Bertolucci D, Dufour M: Prevalence of screening for alcohol use by physicians during routine physical examinations. *Alcohol Health Res World* 18:162–168, 1994.

Fleming MF, Barry KL, Manwell LB, et al: Brief physician advice for problem alcohol drinkers. *JAMA* 277:1039–1044, 1997.

Friedmann PD, Saitz R, Samet JH: Management of adults recovering from alcohol or other drug problems: Relapse prevention in primary care. *JAMA* 279:1227–1231, 1998.

Grant BF, Harford TC, Dawson DA, et al: Prevalence of DSM-IV alcohol abuse and dependence: United

States, 1992. *Alcohol Health Res World* 18:243–248, 1994.

Gruer L, Wilson P, Scott R, et al: General practitioner centred scheme for treatment of opiate dependent drug injectors in Glasgow. *BMJ* 314:1730–1735, 1997.

Kitchens JM: Does this patient have an alcohol problem? *JAMA* 272:1782–1787, 1994.

Malec TS, Malec EA, Dongier M: Efficacy of buspirone in alcohol dependence: A review. *Alcohol Clin Exp Res* 20:853–858, 1996.

Marsch LA: The efficacy of methadone maintenance interventions in reducing illicit opiate use, HIV risk behavior and criminality: A meta-analysis. *Addiction* 93:515–532, 1998.

Mayo-Smith MF: Pharmacological management of alcohol withdrawal: A meta-analysis and evidence-based practice guideline. *JAMA* 278:144–151, 1997.

Midanik LT, Tam TW, Greenfield TK, Caetano R: Risk functions for alcohol-related problems in a 1988 US national sample. *Addiction* 91:1427–1437, 1996.

Miller WR, Andrews NR, Wilbourne P, Bennett ME: A wealth of alternatives: Effective treatments for alcohol problems, in, Miller WR and Heather N (eds): *Treating Addictive Behaviors*, 2nd ed. New York, Plenum Press, 1998, pp 203–216.

National Consensus Development Panel on Effective Medical Treatment of Opiate Addiction: Effective medical treatment of opiate addiction. *JAMA* 280:1936–1943, 1998.

National Institute on Alcohol Abuse and Alcoholism: *The Physician's Guide to Helping Patients with Alcohol Problems.* Bethesda, MD, National Institutes of Health, 1995.

O'Connor PG, Schottenfeld RS: Patients with alcohol problems. *N Engl J Med* 338:592–602, 1998.

Olds D, Henderson CR, Jr., Cole R, et al: Long-term effects of nurse home visitation on children's criminal and antisocial behavior: 15-year follow-up of a randomized controlled trial. *JAMA* 280:1238–1244, 1998.

Piccinelli M, Tessari E, Bortolomasi M, et al: Efficacy of the alcohol use disorders test as a screening tool for hazardous alcohol intake and related disorders in primary care: A validity study. *BMJ* 314: 420–424, 1997.

Portenoy RK, Dole V, Joseph H, et al: Pain management and chemical dependency: evolving perspectives. *JAMA* 278:592–593, 1997.

Prochaska JO, DiClemente CC, Norcross JC: In search of how people change: Applications to addictive behaviors. *Am Psychol* 47:1102–1114, 1992.

Project MATCH Research Group: Matching alcoholism treatments to client heterogeneity: Project MATCH three-year drinking outcomes. *Alcohol Clin Exp Res* 22:1300–1311, 1998.

Richmond R, Heather N, Wodak A, et al: Controlled evaluation of a general practice-based brief intervention for excessive drinking. *Addiction* 90:119–132, 1995.

Saitz R, Mayo-Smith MF, Roberts MS, et al: Individualized treatment for alcohol withdrawal: a randomized double-blind controlled trial. *JAMA* 272:519–523, 1994.

Saunders JB, Aasland OG, Babor TF, et al: Development of the Alcohol Use Disorders Identification Test (AUDIT): WHO Collaborative Project on Early Detection of Persons with Harmful Alcohol Consumption—II. *Addiction* 88:791–804, 1993.

Sellers EM, Naranjo CA, Harrison M, et al. Diazepam loading: simplified treatment of alcohol withdrawal. *Clin Pharmacol Ther* 34:822–826, 1983.

Steinbauer JR, Cantor SB, Holzer CE III, Volk RJ: Ethnic and sex bias in primary care screening tests for alcohol use disorders. *Ann Intern Med* 129:353–362, 1998.

Taj N, Devera-Sales A, Vinson DC: Screening for problem drinking: Does a single question work? *J Fam Pract* 46:328–335, 1998.

Thakker KD: An overview of health risks and benefits of alcohol consumption. *Alcohol Clin Exp Res* 22: 285S–298S, 1998.

Thun MJ, Peto R, Lopez AD, et al: Alcohol consumption and mortality among middle-aged and elderly US adults. *N Engl J Med* 337:1705–1714, 1997.

Tractenberg AI, Fleming MF, Jarris R, et al (eds): *Diagnosis and Treatment of Drug Abuse in Family Practice.* New York, Health Science Communications, 1994.

Volpicelli JR, Alterman AI, Hayashida M, O'Brien CP: Naltrexone in the treatment of alcohol dependence. *Arch Gen Psychiatry* 49:876–880, 1992.

Warner LA, Kessler RC, Hughes M, et al: Prevalence and correlates of drug use and dependence in the United States: Results from the National Comorbidity Survey. *Arch Gen Psychiatry* 52: 219–229, 1995.

Wechsler H, Dowdall GW, Maenner G, et al: Changes in binge drinking and related problems among American college students between 1993 and 1997: Results of the Harvard School of Public Health College Alcohol Study. *J Am Coll Health* 47: 57–68, 1998.

White D, Pitts M: Educating young people about drugs: a systematic review. *Addiction* 93:1475–1487, 1998.

WHO Brief Intervention Study Group: A cross-national trial of brief interventions with heavy drinkers. *Am J Public Health* 86:948–955, 1996.

Wilk AI, Jensen NM, Havighurst TC. Meta-analysis of randomized control trials addressing brief interventions in heavy alcohol drinkers. *J Gen Intern Med* 12:274–283, 1997.

Yu J, Shacket RW: Long-term change in underage drinking and impaired driving after the establishment of drinking age laws in New York State. *Alcohol Clin Exp Res* 22:1443–1449, 1998.

Paul Gordon

Chapter
12

Cervical Cancer

Introduction

Epidemiology of Cervical Cancer

Cervical cancer is the second most common cancer among women worldwide. In 1996, 471,000 new cases were diagnosed and there were 213,000 deaths. In developing countries, where 80% of the cases occur, cervical cancer is the most common cancer among women and the most common cancer-related cause of death.

Worldwide rates vary markedly with a tenfold difference between the high- and low-incidence areas. The high-incidence areas include Latin America, Southern Africa, and Melanesia. The low-incidence areas include Western Europe, North America, Japan, Western Asia, and China (Table 12-1). Rates per hundred thousand women vary from a low of 4.2 among Jewish women in Israel to a high of 54 in Peru. Incidence and mortality have decreased over the past 40 years in western Europe, the United

States, Canada, Australia, New Zealand, Japan, Hong Kong, and Singapore. This is believed to be related in part to screening, reductions in parity, and better access to treatment. A reversal of this trend, however, over the past 20 years among women younger than 50 years has been found in England, Wales, Scotland, Ireland, New Zealand, and Australia. This worsening rate is thought to be related to changes in sexual behavior and increases in the prevalence of sexually transmitted diseases.

In the United States, cervical cancer is the seventh most common cancer among women. The incidence in 1992 was 8.1/100,000 women, and the mortality rate was 2.6/100,000. Since 1950, the incidence and mortality have decreased by about 75%, but in 1995 there were still 15,800 cases of invasive cervical cancer, 65,000 cases of carcinoma in situ (CIS), and 4800 deaths of cervical cancer.

There are marked differences in U.S. incidence and mortality rates for cervical cancer by race. In 1992 the rate of cervical cancer was 7.6 per 100,000 Caucasian women and 12.0 per 100,000 African American women. The mortality rate for cervical cancer was 2.2 per 100,000 Caucasian women and 5.7 per 100,000 African American women. Disease among African American women is diagnosed at more advanced stages than that among Caucasian women. Five-year survival rates also differ. Among African American women the survival rate is 56.4%, whereas among Caucasian women it is 69.9% with little change over time. There are also racial differences in stage at diagnosis. Between 1983 and 1990, of all invasive cancers, 39% were still localized in African American women, whereas 53% were localized in Caucasian women. Incidence by race is presented in Table 12-2. Hispanic, Korean American, and Alaskan Native women and those from Vietnam have elevated rates compared with others.

There are also state by state differences in the rate of cervical cancer. The areas with the highest rates per 100,000 include Washington, D.C. (4.9), Kentucky (4.1), Alabama (4.0), South Car-

Table 12-1

Incidence of Cervical Cancer in Selected World Regions

REGION	RATE/100,000
Central America	44.4
Malaysia	43.4
Southern Africa	40.4
Tropical South America	31.8
Temperate South America	27.7
Middle Africa	26.6
Southeast Asia	18.6
Eastern Europe	13.7
Western Europe	10.9
Japan	9.7
North America	9.1
Western Asia	5.5
China	4.9

SOURCE: Parkin, et al., 1999.

Table 12-2

Cervical Cancer Rates in the United States

GROUP	RATE/100,000
White	8.7
Black	13.2
Hispanic	16.2
American Indian	9.8
Alaskan Native	15.8
Korean American	15.2
Vietnamese American	43.0
Japanese American	5.8
Hawaiian	9.6

SOURCE: Miller, et al., 1996.

Table 12-3

Risk Factors for Cervical Cancer

RISK FACTOR	RELATIVE RISK
Menarche to first coitus <1 yr	26.4
Age at first coitus <16 yr	16.1
More than 3 partners before age 20	10.2
Never having a Pap smear	8.0
Cigarette smoking >20 yr	4.0
History of genital warts	2.5
Lower socioeconomic status	Uncertain
Use of oral contraceptives	Uncertain

olina (3.9), and Delaware (3.7). These areas have large proportions of African American women, rural poor, or both. The areas with the lowest incidence include North Dakota (2.1), Nebraska (2.1), Hawaii (2.0), Idaho (1.8), and Minnesota (1.6).

The distribution of cervical cancer by stage diagnosed in the United States between 1986 and 1991 was 51% localized, 33% regional, 8% metastatic, and 7% unstaged. The histologic distribution of diagnosed cervical cancer includes squamous cell carcinoma (77.1%), adenocarcinoma (10.9%), other carcinoma not otherwise specified (8.4%), adenosquamous or adenocarcinoma with squamous metaplasia (2.5%), and other rare histologic types (1.1%). The incidence of squamous cell cancer is decreasing while that of adenocarcinoma is increasing, particularly in most developed countries and particularly among young women.

Risk Factors

Epidemiologic risk factors for cervical cancer have been well known and documented for years. These risk factors with their relative risks are included in Table 12-3.

HUMAN PAPILLOMAVIRUS

Over the last 15 years, the role of human papillomavirus (HPV) has become better understood. It is known that the link between HPV and cervical cancer is stronger than the link between tobacco use and lung cancer. HPV has been detected in 96% of high-grade cervical intraepithelial neoplasms (CIN). Only 3% to 30% of women with normal cytologic findings have HPV infection, and the presence of HPV-negative cancers is uncommon.

The presumed mechanism of HPV infection involves inactivation of p53 (tumor suppressor gene) and pRB proteins by products of E6 and E7 regions of HPV 16. Of the various HPV subtypes, numbers 16, 18, 45, and 56 have been found to be high-risk types; 31, 33, and 35 are intermediate risk; and 6, 11, 42, 43, and 44 are considered low risk in that they are almost never found in association with malignant tumors. In the presence of cofactors such as smoking, use of oral contraceptives, parity, and other sexually transmitted diseases, the persistence of high-risk HPV types has been found to lead to CIN and invasive cancer.

HPV infection resolves within 2 years in most women because most are able to eliminate the infection through immunologic mechanisms.

The persistence of high-risk HPV types leads to progression of cervical lesions, which is not observed in the absence of HPV DNA or in the presence of low-risk subtypes. The reason for persistent infection, which is a necessary condition for the progression to a high-grade lesion, remains unclear.

OTHER FACTORS

Identification of HPV as a cause specific to most cases of cervical cancer has helped to explain the contribution of some of the other risk factors. Early onset of sexual activity and large numbers of sexual partners place women at high risk for exposure to HPV.

It is thought that prostitutes may be an important reservoir of HPV infections, and sexual contact by husbands with prostitutes may be a more important source of HPV infection than a woman's lifetime number of sex partners.

Uncertainty continues about the role of use of oral contraceptive agents in cervical cancer. It appears that use of oral contraceptives moderately increases risk for cervical neoplasms. Recent studies with accurate DNA technique to identify HPV lesions have helped elucidate possible mechanisms, such as promotion of HPV by contraceptives. It also is possible that women who use contraceptives have more sexual exposure to HPV.

Lack of cervical cancer screening is a risk for cervical cancer. Fifty percent of all cervical cancers diagnosed occur in women who have never undergone screening, and 60% occur in women who have not had a Papanicolaou (Pap) smear in the past 5 years. The higher rate of cervical cancer among women of low socioeconomic status may be related to poor access to medical care and screening. Minority and elderly populations have a higher proportion of cancers diagnosed at an advanced stage. This may relate to lower rates of Pap smear screening because cervical cancer screening rates vary by age and by insurance status. Women who remain unscreened or underscreened include the elderly,

those of low socioeconomic status, and ethnic minorities (especially older African American, Hispanic, and Native American women). Barriers to screening include a lack of knowledge on the part of the patient or the provider, economic barriers, barriers inherent in the group's culture or belief system, and logistical barriers.

A statistically significant association between cigarette smoking and cervical cancer was shown in a meta-analysis of case-control studies that examined this issue (Sood, 1991). Smoking increases a woman's risk for cervical cancer 42% to 46%.

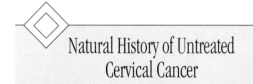

Natural History of Untreated Cervical Cancer

Current cervical cancer control strategies are based on the belief that cervical cancer develops in a series of successive, progressive stages starting with squamous atypia, progressing through CIN1, CIN2, and CIN3 and ending at CIS and invasive cancer. Baron and Richart (1968) published results of the first large-scale study of the natural history of cervical cancer. They showed that more than 50% of women with a low-grade lesion had CIN3 within 5 years, almost none showing regression. This was the basis of the CIN1 through CIN3 continuum and the belief that these various morphologic changes on Pap smears and at biopsy represented successive and increasingly abnormal stages in the pathogenesis of cervical cancer.

Other natural history studies did not support the concept of uniform progression but showed that low-grade squamous intraepithelial lesions (LGSIL) were generally benign and often reverted to normal. We now know that CIN1 progresses to CIN2 or CIN3 in 10% to 15% of women if left untreated; 60% regress to normal, and 30% persist at CIN1. In one study, 1.6% of screened adolescents had abnormal cytologic findings. In 10 years, 65% of these had reverted to normal; 20% revealed no change, and 15% had progressed to CIN3. None of these progressed to invasive cancer before the age of 21 years. Among women slightly older but younger than 34 years, 84% of cases regressed spontaneously (Guidozzi, 1996). The original study by Baron and Richart required women to have had multiple Pap smears with CIN1 lesions as a condition of participation. This may have biased their outcomes because many first smears with CIN1 regress. Nonetheless, the CIN1 to CIN3 continuum took hold and served as the rationale for aggressive management of early lesions.

There also is a question about the frequency with which CIS progresses to invasive cancer. Because it has long been accepted that CIS progresses to invasive cancer, it has been seen as unethical to study the natural history of CIS. What we know comes from patients who inadvertently were not treated. CIS regresses in 10% to 30% of women if left untreated, and only 12% to 70% of women have cancer within a normal life span (Kiviat, 1996). The Swedish Cancer Registry has been tracking cervical cancer cases for many years. They report the average sojourn time (CIS to invasive cancer) is 13 years. The preclinical time (the length of time elapsed before invasive cancer is detected) is 3 to 4 years. The total sojourn time is 17 years. The Swedish Registry has an unusually high fraction of cases of preinvasive cancer, and this potential overrepresentation of CIS cases is believed to lead to overestimation of the likelihood of regression. However, the sojourn time would remain the same.

Mitchell et al (1994) found that 36% of cases of CIS progress on to invasive cancer. They also found that in patients with CIN1 to CIN3, 14% of lesions progressed to CIS and 1.4% progressed to invasive cancer. Other investigators found that less than 2% of CIN (excluding CIS) progressed to invasive cervical cancer; however among patients with CIN3-CIS, this rate was 16%

to 36% (Ostor, 1993). The time for progression from CIN to CIS to invasive cancer was 10 to 22 years, with progression taking longer in younger women.

We now know that most low-grade lesions do not progress to cervical cancer and that even higher-grade lesions such as CIN1-3 and CIS do not inevitably progress to cervical cancer. This knowledge has caused a revision in the way low-grade lesions are managed. This is discussed later with follow-up after abnormal Pap smears.

Primary Prevention

Several interventions involving behavior change would possibly decrease an individual woman's risk for cervical cancer and, if adopted widely, possibly result in a lower incidence of cervical cancer. These interventions include delaying the onset of sexual intercourse, limiting the number of sex partners, using barrier contraception, avoiding or stopping smoking, and avoiding long-term (more than 5 years) use of oral contraceptives. Interventions to delay the onset of sexual activity are discussed in Chapter 8. Smoking cessation and prevention are discussed in Chapter 10. Although these interventions are advisable for other reasons, such as decreasing risk for HIV infection and other sexually transmitted diseases and smoking-related disease, none have been specifically tested in prospective studies as a way to prevent cervical cancer.

Although there is a statistical association between use of oral contraceptives and cervical cancer, there remains much about this association that is not understood. The relation may be causal or it may be due to confounding by other variables related to sex partners. Because of this uncertainty and because of the multiple other benefits afforded by oral contraceptives, avoiding or limiting use of oral contraceptives cannot be recommended as a strategy for prevention of cervical cancer.

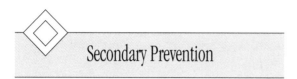

Secondary Prevention

Papanicolaou Tests

The Pap smear was introduced as a screening test for cervical cancer in the late 1940s. Papanicolaou, recognizing that Pap smear results cannot always be judged as positive or negative, described the earliest classification system in 1954. This was the class I through V system. Other classifications have since been developed (Tables 12-4, 12-5).

Although the Pap smear was never studied in a randomized, controlled trial with mortality as an end point, results of case control and observational studies support the effectiveness of Pap smear screening in preventing cervical cancer. The best observational studies on the effectiveness of Pap screening were performed in the Nordic countries. Investigators compared mortality before and after the introduction of screening in different countries. For example, in Norway, which had the lowest participation rate, the mortality of cervical cancer remained comparatively unchanged. In Iceland, which has an aggressive screening program and had a high rate of participation, there was a 73% reduction in mortality. These data are considered so strong that it would now be considered unethical to conduct a randomized trial of the effectiveness of Pap smear screening.

ACCURACY OF PAP TESTS

Determining the sensitivity and specificity of Pap smears is difficult because of difficulties identifying a standard of comparison. The U.S. Preventive Services Task Force reviewed this issue and reported that the most frequently used

figures are a sensitivity of 55% to 80% and a specificity of 90% or higher. Other investigators have reviewed Pap smear studies and report a sensitivity of 56% to 58% and a specificity of 66% to 69% (Fahey, et al, 1995; Wilkinson, 1990).

The lack of 100% sensitivity concerns many experts and leads to the disagreements about the recommended frequency of screening (see later). The accuracy of Pap smears is influenced by multiple factors, including the skill and thoroughness of the examiner, which influences the adequacy of the specimen; proper preparation and fixation of the smear; and the accuracy and skill of cytotechnologists and pathologists. Even when all involved are functioning at maximum levels of quality, there are still false-negative results.

OBTAINING A PAP SMEAR

Obtaining an adequate cervical smear for a Pap test is a skill acquired through practice. The uterine cervix must be completely visualized with a vaginal speculum without lubricant. Visual inspection of the cervix is an important step in the examination, and abnormalities found at inspection should be evaluated even if the Pap smear results are normal.

The exocervical sample is obtained with a spatula. The spatula must be rotated around the entire cervix with pressure applied and the tip of the spatula in the endocervix. To ensure that the squamocolumnar junction is sampled, an endocervical specimen is obtained with an endocervical brush. Samples without endocervical cells often are considered inadequate, although there is no evidence of any differences in clinical outcomes when endocervical cells are or are not collected.

The smear should be prepared by means of pressing both sides of the spatula against a glass slide and rolling the swab or brush on another portion of the slide. The smear should be fixed rapidly by means of immersing the slide into, or spraying it with, a fixative.

Table 12-4

Relation Between the Bethesda System and Previous Classifications

System	Within Normal Limits	Benign Cellular Changes	Epithelial Cell Abnormalities				
			ASCUS AGUS	LGSIL	HGSIL		Invasive carcinoma
Bethesda		Infection Reactive Repair	ASCUS AGUS	LGSIL HPV	HGSIL		Invasive carcinoma
Reagan				Mild dysplasia[a]	Moderate dysplasia[a]	Severe dysplasia[a] CIS[a]	
Richart				CIN1[b]	CIN2[b]	CIN3[b]	
Papanicolaou	I		II		III	IV	V

ABBREVIATIONS: The Bethesda System Terminology. ASCUS, atypical squamous cells of unknown significance; AGUS, atypical glandular cells of unknown significance; LGSIL, low-grade squamous intraepithelial lesion; HGSIL, high-grade squamous intraepithelial lesion; HPV, human papillomavirus.

SOURCE: [a] Terminology from Reagan et al. CIS, carcinoma in situ. [b] Terminology from Richart. CIN, cervical intraepithelial neoplasia.

Other Suggested Screening Tests

Three other suggested screening tests for detection of cervical cancer are cervicography (a photograph of the cervix), colposcopy (examination of the cervix under high magnification), and screening for the presence of HPV. Each has disadvantages compared with Pap smears, including lack of standardization, technical difficulty, cost, and no better or worse accuracy.

None is recommended for routine screening of women who do not have symptoms.

Controversies Regarding Pap Smear Screening

Although Pap smear screening has been available for many decades in the U. S., the ideal use of this screening test remains an area of contro-

Table 12-5

The 1991 Bethesda System

ADEQUACY OF THE SPECIMEN
Satisfactory for evaluation Satisfactory for evaluation but limited by [specify reason] Unsatisfactory for evaluation [specify reason]

GENERAL CATEGORIZATION (OPTIONAL)
Within normal limits Benign cellular changes; see descriptive diagnosis Epithelial cell abnormality; see descriptive diagnosis

DESCRIPTIVE DIAGNOSES

Benign Cellular Changes
  Infection
    Trichomonas vaginalis
    Fungal organisms morphologically consistent with *Candida* sp
    Predominance of coccobacilli consistent with shift in vaginal flora
    Bacteria morphologically consistent with *Actinomyces* sp
    Cellular changes associated with herpes simplex virus
    Other
  Reactive changes
  Reactive cellular changes associated with
    Inflammation (includes typical repair)
    Atrophy with inflammation ("atrophic vaginitis")
    Radiation
    Intrauterine contraceptive device (IUD)
    Other   *(Continued)*

Table 12-5

The 1991 Bethesda System *(Continued)*

Epithelial Cell Abnormalities
  Squamous cell
    Atypical squamous cells of undetermined significance (ASCUS): qualify[a]
    Low-grade squamous intraepithelial lesion (LSIL) encompassing human papillomavirus (HPV)[b] mild
      dysplasia/CIN1
    High-grade squamous intraepithelial lesion (HSIL) encompassing moderate and severe dysplasia.
      CIS/CIN2 and CIN3
    Squamous cell carcinoma
  Glandular cell
    Endometrial cells, cytologically benign, in a postmenopausal woman
    Atypical glandular cells of undetermined significance; qualify[a]
    Endocervical adenocarcinoma
    Endometrial adenocarcinoma
    Extrauterine adenocarcinoma
    Adenocarcinoma, not otherwise specified
  Other malignant neoplasms: specify

HORMONAL EVALUATION (APPLIES TO VAGINAL SMEARS ONLY)

Hormonal pattern compatible with age and history
Hormonal pattern incompatible with age and history: specify
Hormonal evaluation not possible because of [specify]

---

[a] Atypical squamous or glandular cells of undetermined significance should be further qualified as to whether a reactive or a premalignant or malignant process is favored.
[b] Cellular changes of HPV (previously termed *koilocytotic atypia* or *condylomatous atypia*) are included in the category of low-grade squamous intraepithelial lesion.

versy. The areas of uncertainty include the following: At what age should screening start? How frequently should screening be conducted? At what age should screening stop? Should all women be screened?

WHEN SHOULD SCREENING START?

Pap smear screening ideally should take place when the prevalence of abnormalities is high. The optimal age for starting and stopping screening also is connected with the number of screening tests performed. If only one Pap test is performed, it should be done close to the age of the most proximate precursor of invasive cancer-CIS. A screening program starting at the age of 25 years is more effective than one starting at the age of 35 years because high-grade abnormalities such as CIS can occur in women around 25 years of age. The benefit of moving testing from 25 years to 20 years is negligible because invasive cancer is rare at young ages. The additional costs of starting screening at a younger age are substantial because of the high prevalence of preclinical lesions and the cost of follow-up evaluation of these lesions. Most of these lesions regress.

Although the sexual activity of younger Americans has increased, the age-specific incidence curve has not shifted. There is still very little cervical cancer (1 to 3 cases per 100,000) among women younger than 25 years.

Although the value of screening women younger than 20 years is open to question, most authorities recommend starting screening when sexual activity begins or at 18 years of age if there is any question about whether the patient has had sexual relations.

FREQUENCY OF SCREENING

Evidence is convincing that much more benefit would be gained overall by increasing the proportion of women who undergo screening than by increasing the frequency of screening among women who already undergo periodic screening. A large retrospective study in seven European countries and Canada showed that annual screening decreased the risk for cervical cancer 93.5%, biennial screening 92.5%, screening every 3 years 90.8%, every 5 years 83.6%, and every 10 years 64.0% (Austoker, 1994; Morrison, 1997). A U.S. study showed biennial screening, compared with annual screening, had a relative risk of 1.01 for cervical cancer whereas screening every 3 years had a relative risk of 3.9 (Morrison, 1997). Although data in the epidemiologic literature support less frequent monitoring, there is a lack of consensus on this issue.

Some authorities believe that women who are at high risk (those with multiple sex partners, those with an early age at onset of sexual activity) should undergo more frequent screening than should women not at high risk. There is little evidence to support this belief. Although women at high risk do have a higher rate of abnormal Pap smears, these women are not at increased risk for more aggressive, faster growing cancers. The lead time and natural history of cervical neoplasia is the same for these women as for others. One countering argument, however, is that because a Pap test is not 100% sensitive, more frequent testing of women at high risk is indicated to ensure that precancerous lesions are not missed.

Women with HIV infection should undergo screening at least once a year. There is good evidence that this group of women is at risk for a rapidly progressing, aggressive form of cervical cancer.

WHEN SHOULD SCREENING STOP?

There is little evidence to help answer this question. Elderly women who have had regular Pap smears with normal results probably benefit little from continued testing. Unfortunately, many elderly women are not in this category; they have been screened sporadically and infrequently. An estimated 20% to 40% of women older than 65 years have never undergone testing. Because of the lead time for cervical cancer to develop, the benefit of screening markedly diminishes for women each year after 65 years of age.

SHOULD ALL WOMEN UNDERGO SCREENING?

Women who have never had sexual intercourse probably do not benefit from screening for cervical cancer. Evidence is mounting that women who have undergone complete hysterectomy do not benefit from Pap smears. Women whose cervix was not removed during hysterectomy probably should continue to undergo screening, as should women who have undergone hysterectomy because of cervical cancer.

Current Recommendations

Because of the uncertainties described earlier and the confusion generated by conflicting recommendations, the American Cancer Society, National Cancer Institute, American College of Obstetricians and Gynecologists, American Medical Association, American Nurses Association, American Academy of Family Physicians, and American Medical Womens Association came together in 1998 and agreed on a standardized set of recommendations. They recommended starting Pap smear screening at the onset of sexual activity or 18 years of age, whichever is earlier, and annual screening for 3 years, then less frequently. The U.S. Preventive Services Task Force concurs with the recommendations.

There is still disagreement about whether women at high risk should undergo screening more frequently, the age to stop, and whether screening is needed after hysterectomy. The current recommendations of four authoritative groups are listed in Table 12-6.

Follow-up after Abnormal Results

Near consensus exists regarding the evaluation and treatment of patients with high-grade dysplasia or carcinoma. They are referred for colposcopy-directed biopsy.

There is, however, controversy regarding the evaluation and treatment of patients with low-grade lesions. Few low-grade lesions progress to high-grade lesions. For those that do progress, the process tends to be slow. There is no consensus on how to follow-up management of these lesions, and it is likely that we are much more aggressive than is necessary. Nevertheless there is little evidence to support one approach over another.

Figure 12-1 illustrates an algorithm for follow-up management of low-grade lesions. It is a conservative approach based on findings from a working group of the National Cancer Institute (Kurman, et al, 1994). The recommended follow-up management of each type of abnormality is as follows.

ATYPICAL SQUAMOUS CELLS OF UNKNOWN SIGNIFICANCE (ASCUS)

Patients who receive a diagnosis of ASCUS that is not qualified, or when the pathologist favors a reactive process, can undergo Pap smears every 6 months as long as subsequent test results are negative and the samples are sat-isfactory for interpretation. At the end of 2 years normal screening frequency can be resumed. A second ASCUS, or an LGSIL (see below), report during the 2-year period should result in consideration of colposcopic evaluation.

A report of ASCUS with inflammation should lead to a follow-up test in 2 to 3 months after specific therapy for any infection found. Nonspecific therapy for undiagnosed infections is not recommended. ASCUS in postmenopausal women not taking hormone replacement can be managed with topical estrogen before re-evaluation. If the pathologist favors a neoplastic process with the diagnosis of ASCUS, or if the patient has had a previous ASCUS diagnosis, she should be treated according to the LGSIL recommendations.

LOW-GRADE SQUAMOUS INTRAEPITHELIAL LESION (LGSIL)

Two options are acceptable for women with LGSIL: (1) Follow-up tests every 6 months, as for patients with ASCUS, or (2) colposcopy with directed biopsy and endocervical curettage. If biopsy results show CIN1 the following three options are available: excision or ablation, repeat colposcopy, or repeat Pap smears every 6 months until they are repeatedly normal. CIN2 or more severe abnormalities at biopsy should be managed by means of excision, ablation, or cervical conization.

HIGH-GRADE SQUAMOUS INTRAEPITHELIAL LESION (HGSIL)

Colposcopy with directed biopsy and endocervical curettage is recommended for HGSIL. CIN1 and CIN2 and greater results on biopsy can be handled as shown in Figure 12-2. For pregnant patients, therapy for biopsy-confirmed HGSIL can wait until after delivery.

The optimal frequency of repeat Pap tests after excision or ablation is unknown. Many clinicians repeat a Pap test every 3 to 6 months until a series of normal results are obtained. The

Table 12-6

Selected Pap Smear Guidelines from Various Medical Organizations

GUIDELINE	U.S. PREVENTIVE SERVICES TASK FORCE	AMERICAN ACADEMY OF FAMILY PHYSICIANS	AMERICAN COLLEGE OF OBSTETRICIANS AND GYNECOLOGISTS	AMERICAN CANCER SOCIETY
When to start	At the onset of sexual activity or age 18 years	At the onset of sexual activity or age 18 years	At the onset of sexual activity or age 18 years	At the onset of sexual activity or age 18 years
When to stop	Insufficient evidence to recommend for or against an upper age limit	Age 65 years if documented evidence of previously normal smears	No age stated	No age stated
Frequency of screening	At least every 3 years	Less frequently after three or more annual smears have been normal, at the discretion of the physician	Less frequently after three or more annual smears have been normal, at the discretion of the physician	Less frequently after three or more annual smears have been normal, at the discretion of the physician
Women at high risk	No statement	No statement	Annually for women with high-risk factors	No statement
Women who have undergone hysterectomy	If cervix was removed, no Pap testing unless the hysterectomy was performed because of cervical cancer or its precursors	If cervix was removed, no Pap testing unless the hysterectomy was performed because of cervical cancer or its precursors	If cervix was removed, no Pap testing unless the hysterectomy was performed because of cervical cancer or its precursors or risk factors are present	If cervix was removed, no Pap testing unless the hysterectomy was performed because of cervical cancer or its precursors

Figure 12-1

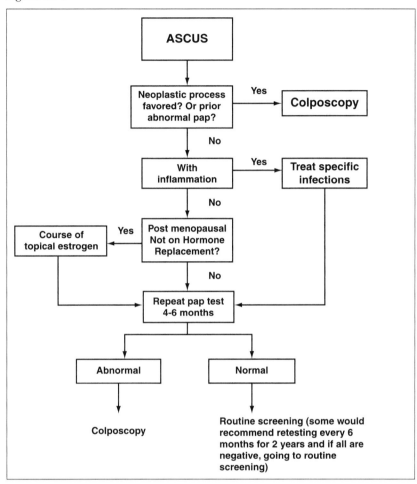

Algorithm for follow-up after ASCUS Pap test result.

optimal frequency of routine testing after completion of treatment and follow-up testing also is unknown. Many clinicians recommend annual testing after therapy for HGSIL (Fig. 12-3).

ATYPICAL GLANDULAR CELLS OF UNKNOWN SIGNIFICANCE (AGUS)

An AGUS result that is unqualified or classified as reactive can be evaluated in one of three ways: (1) repeat test of a specimen obtained with a cytobrush, (2) endocervical and endome-trial curettage, (3) hysteroscopy. Persistent AGUS or AGUS with suspicion of adenocarcinoma in situ should probably be evaluated by means of cone biopsy (Fig. 12-4).

UNSATISFACTORY FOR EVALUATION

The test should be repeated.

SATISFACTORY BUT LIMITED BY . . .

The tests may or may not be repeated depending on clinical judgment. The absence of

Figure 12-2

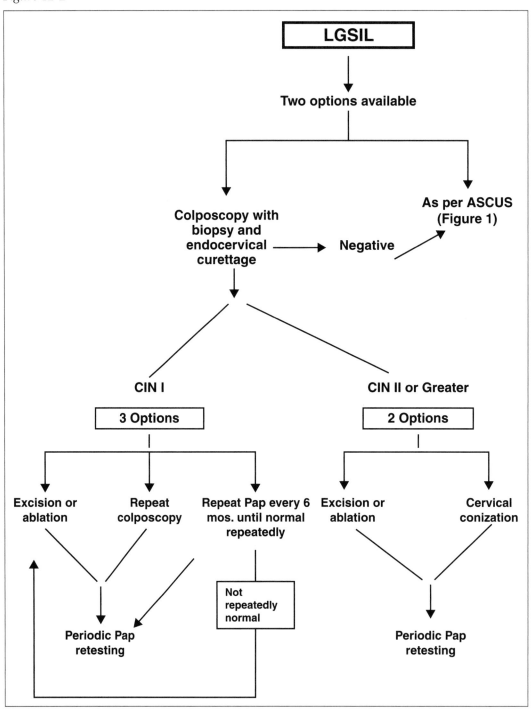

Algorithm for follow-up after LGSIL Pap test and CIN I, CIN II or greater colposcopic biopsy.

Figure 12-3

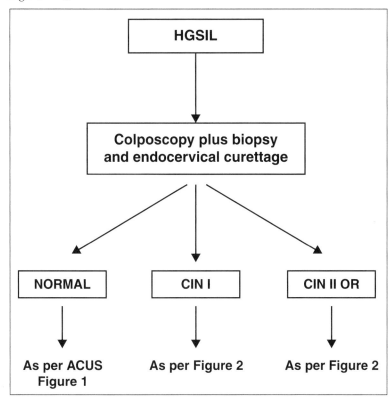

Algorithm for follow-up after HGSIL Pap test result.

endocervical cells alone should not necessitate a repeat test.

Barriers to Pap Smear Testing

For a system of cervical cancer screening to work at maximum efficiency all women at risk (including all women who have been or are sexually active and all women who have not undergone hysterectomy for an indication other than cancer) should undergo routine screening. All women with abnormal test results should undergo follow-up treatment or evaluation according to guidelines.

In spite of the efficacy of Pap testing in the detection and prevention of cervical cancer, many women do not undergo screening or undergo tests irregularly and infrequently. Although more than 90% of American women have undergone at least one Pap test, there are demographic subgroups that have lower rates. Norman et al (1991) reviewed the literature and found that characteristics associated with lower rates of Pap-test screening include age (fewer older women have been tested), rural residence, race (African American and Hispanic women are less likely to have undergone a test), and income (poorer women are less likely to have been tested). Age and race act jointly. Older,

Figure 12-4

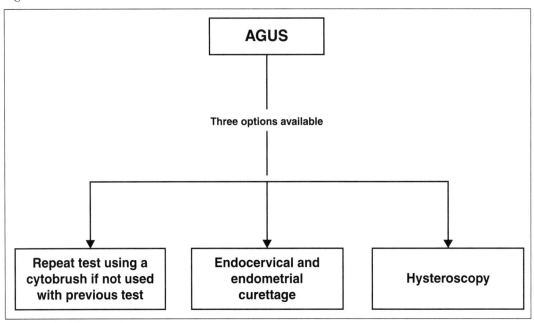

Algorithm for follow-up of AGUS

minority women are least likely to have undergone testing; 40% of African American and Hispanic older women have never been tested.

Frequency of Pap testing also is associated with certain characteristics. Women less likely to have undergone a Pap test in the past 3 or 4 years include those with low incomes and less education and those who are single. Race also is associated with less frequent testing but in a surprising way—minority women are more likely than Caucasian women to have undergone a recent test.

Women who view Pap testing positively as a mechanism for detecting cancer at a curable stage are more inclined to undergo screening; women who are more fatalistic are less likely. Other barriers to screening include misunderstanding the importance of Pap testing, fear of embarrassment and pain, and lack of encouragement by family or physician.

Women who have frequent contact with the health care system, those who have a regular source of care, and those who have visited a clinician for a problem that requires a pelvic examination are more likely to have undergone a Pap test.

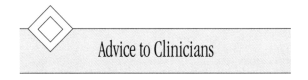

Advice to Clinicians

Primary care clinicians are the front line in the battle to decrease mortality from cervical cancer. A systematic approach will help to ensure that all patients undergo screening and that follow-up treatment and evaluation of abnormal test results is comprehensive, allowing a more conservative approach to low-grade lesions.

Deciding on Testing Frequency

Each clinician needs to review the scientific data and guidelines and decide on the frequency of screening to recommend to patients. Every clinician should discuss Pap testing with every woman, and the two together should determine the frequency of testing.

Adolescents should be asked about sexual activity so that Pap testing can begin at the appropriate age. Older women should be asked about previous frequency of Pap testing and whether any results were abnormal to decide when Pap testing can cease.

Encouraging Women to Undergo Pap Testing

Clinicians should remember that their advice is one of the most important influences on a woman's decision to be tested for cervical cancer and should encourage patients to undergo regular testing. If a woman is hesitant about or refuses testing, the clinician should ask about her fears and concerns and make sure that the patient fully understands the importance of testing and how the test is performed. Revisiting the issue at later visits may eventually lead the patient to undergo the test.

Integrating Cervical Cancer Prevention into a Comprehensive Health Maintenance Plan

Cervical cancer screening is only one component of a comprehensive plan to promote health and prevent disease among women. Other components include risk assessment, risk reduction counseling, other screening tests, and immunizations. Coordinating Pap testing with other screening tests and including the primary prevention of cervical cancer in risk assessment and risk reduction helps to achieve not only cervical cancer prevention but also overall prevention because Pap testing can serve as an incentive for women to address prevention issues.

Developing Office Systems to Enhance Prevention

Office or clinic systems that are properly designed can ensure that all patients have the opportunity for maximum and appropriate prevention interventions. Components of such a system include history or intake forms that ask about cervical cancer risks and past testing, protocols that ensure Pap testing within a set number of visits and then at an agreed upon frequency, reminder systems for both patient and clinician when tests are due, and a tracking system for abnormal tests to ensure recommended follow-up care is completed.

Establishing a Fail-safe System to Ensure Follow-up

Abnormal Pap test results should be tracked to ensure that patients receive recommended follow-up care. This is particularly important if a more conservative approach to low-grade lesions is adopted. Assigning this responsibility to one staff person can ensure that no abnormalities are overlooked.

Even with an excellent system of tracking and follow up, some women with abnormal results do not undergo recommended examinations. McKee (1997) suggested strategies to help improve patient adherence to recommendations. They include discussing abnormal results in person, emphasizing the precancerous and curable nature of most lesions, asking about fears and concerns, and emphasizing that most lesions can be managed on an outpatient basis with minimal morbidity.

Common Errors

Inadequate Specimen Collection

Proper specimen collection for a Pap test requires proper preparation and technique. Errors at any step can produce a less than optimum specimen for evaluation. The most common errors are not visualizing the entire cervix, not applying pressure while the spatula is rotated around the entire cervix, pressing only one side of the spatula against the slide (leaving part of the specimen on the other side of the spatula), and not properly sampling the endocervix with a brush.

Laboratory Error

Without proper laboratory methods, Pap test specimens can be interpreted as higher or lower grade than they are. In most populations, a diagnosis of ASCUS should occur in approximately 5% of tests, or about two to three times as frequently as squamous intraepithelial lesions. Overuse of the ASCUS diagnosis can cause unneeded patient anxiety and the expense and morbidity of follow-up treatment and evaluation.

Overly Aggressive Follow-up of Low-grade Lesions

Automatic referral for colposcopy, biopsy, and attempts to manage all low-grade lesions costs the U.S. health care system about $6 billion annually (Kurman, et al, 1994). Most of these low-grade lesions resolve without treatment, and several authors have offered guidelines that provide adequate protection for both patient and clinician while avoiding colposcopy for every low-grade lesion (Kurman, et al, 1994; McKee, 1997; Nuovo, et al, 1995).

Over- and Underscreening of Older Women

The issue of when to stop Pap testing is discussed earlier. It is appropriate to stop Pap testing at 65 to 70 years of age if the woman has undergone regular Pap tests and had normal results up to that age. Many women, however, continue to undergo Pap tests into their later years in spite of little benefit and, often, considerable discomfort and difficulty.

On the other hand, many older women have been inadequately tested throughout their life and it is not appropriate to delete Pap tests from their health maintenance until they have had a series of normal test results.

Screening of Women Who Have Undergone Hysterectomy

Many clinicians are reluctant to give up Pap tests for women who have undergone hysterectomy for a condition not related to cancer. The rationale is that these women need periodic pelvic examinations anyway, so why not obtain a Pap smear? First, there is no proven value of a periodic pelvic examination. Second, there is nothing wrong with performing a pelvic examination and testing for other diseases, such as sexually transmitted diseases, if indicated, without collecting a Pap specimen. Third, a Pap test is an added cost that is unnecessary and may lead to a false-positive result, which leads to an unnecessary and expensive evaluation.

Emerging Trends

Several promising trends in prevention of cervical cancer will improve the system of early detection and management of this highly preventable condition. They include methods to improve screening, improved laboratory methods, and HPV screening.

Methods to Improve Screening

The method receiving the most attention is cervicography. It has an advantage over colposcopy of being less expensive and noninvasive. However, it has a high false-positive rate (about 40%) and currently it is experimental. Cervicography may prove to be a useful second step after Pap testing that might help avoid unnecessary colposcopy. It may also be useful in remote rural areas where colposcopy is not readily available.

Much research is being conducted on the system and behavioral aspects of Pap testing to increase the proportion of women tested. A greater reduction in cervical cancer mortality would be achieved by screening of more women than by screening more frequently. This will lead to ways to improve the system of providing preventive services to all women and more knowledge about how to overcome personal barriers that prevent women from undergoing screening.

Improved Laboratory Methods

Several laboratory methods are being developed to improve the sensitivity of Pap tests. They include automated microscopy with computerized analysis and semiautomated slide preparation methods. These methods are promising and may help improve laboratory accuracy to the extent that less frequent testing (every 3 years) can receive the confidence and endorsement of most authoritative groups. It is possible that the higher costs of these technologies can be offset by less frequent screening (Brown and Garber, 1999).

HPV Testing

One of the most exciting and promising potentials for the future of cervical cancer screening is

HPV testing by means of polymerase chain reaction. A finding that HPV of a high-risk type is present in a cervical specimen might indicate that a low-grade lesion is more likely to progress to cancer, whereas detection of low-risk subtypes might indicate low or no risk for progression.

It is possible that HPV testing can become routine combined with Pap testing to offer a way to increase both sensitivity and specificity of testing. On the other hand, it might prove to be more useful as a secondary screening modality, to be used to clarify the potential of low-grade lesions. The final role of HPV testing remains to be determined.

HPV Vaccine

Another exciting new potential for the primary prevention of cervical cancer is an HPV vaccine. The ideal vaccine would be assembled from pseudovirions that lack viral DNA. If such a vaccine were used before the onset of sexual activity, the initial cervical infection might be prevented. If infection were to occur, efforts could be aimed at cell-mediated immunity with HPV type-specific peptides from E6 and E7 with the intention of causing regression of the disease. Although work on the vaccine continues, the lack of an effective HPV culturing system will have to be overcome to make vaccine production a reality.

Bibliography

Austoker J: Cancer prevention in primary care: Screening for cervical cancer [published correction appears in *BMJ* 309:452, 1994]. *BMJ* 309:241–248, 1994.

Baldauf JJ, Dreyfus M, Ritter J, et al: Cervicography: Does it improve cervical cancer screening? *Acta Cytol* 41:295–301, 1997.

Baron BA, Richart RM: A statistical model of the natural history of cervical carcinoma based on a prospective study of 557 cases. *J Natl Cancer Inst* 41:1343–1353, 1968.

Brown AD, Garber AM: Cost-effectiveness of 3 methods to enhance the sensitivity of Papanicolaou testing. *JAMA* 281:347–353, 1999.

Brown CL: Screening patterns for cervical cancer: how best to reach the unscreened population. *J Natl Cancer Inst Monogr* 7–11, 1996.

Conway K: Attitudes to Papanicolaou smears. *J Psychosom Obstet Gynaecol* 17:189–194, 1996.

Coutlee F, Mayrand MH, Provencher D, Franco E: The future of HPV testing in clinical laboratories and applied virology research. *Clin Diagn Virol* 8:123–141, 1997.

Cox JT: Clinical role of HPV testing. *Obstet Gynecol Clin North Am* 23:811–851, 1996.

de Sanjose S, Bosch FX, Munoz N, Shah K: Social differences in sexual behaviour and cervical cancer. *IARC Sci Publ* 309–317, 1997.

Dubois G: Cytologic screening for cervix cancer: Each year or each 3 years? *Eur J Obstet Gynecol Reprod Biol* 65:57–59, 1996.

Faggiano F, Partanen T, Kogevinas M, Boffetta P: Socioeconomic differences in cancer incidence and mortality. *IARC Sci Publ* 65–176, 1997.

Fahey MT, Irwig L, Macaskill P: Meta-analysis of Pap test accuracy. *Am J Epidemiol* 141:680–689, 1995.

Guidozzi F: Screening for cervical cancer. *Obstet Gynecol Surv* 51:247–252, 1996.

Herbert A: Is cervical screening working? A cytopathologist's view from the United Kingdom. *Hum Pathol* 28:120–126, 1997.

Herrero R: Epidemiology of cervical cancer. *J Natl Cancer Inst Monogr* 1–6, 1996.

Kiviat N: Natural history of cervical neoplasia: Overview and update. *Am J Obstet Gynecol* 175:1099–1104, 1996.

Kurman RJ, Henson DE, Herbst AL, et al: Interim guidelines for management of abnormal cervical cytology. The 1992 National Cancer Institute Workshop. *JAMA* 271:1866–1869, 1994.

La Vecchia C, Tavani A, Franceschi S, Parazzini F: Oral contraceptives and cancer: A review of the evidence. *Drug Saf* 14:260–272, 1996.

Mandelblatt JS, Phillips RN: Cervical cancer: How often—and why—to screen older women. *Geriatrics* 51:45–58, 1996.

McIntyre-Seltman K: The abnormal Papanicolaou smear. *Med Clin North Am* 79:1427–1442, 1995.

McKee D: Improving the follow up of patients with abnormal Papanicolaou smear results. *Arch Fam Med* 6:574–577, 1997.

Meyskens FL Jr, Manetta A: Prevention of cervical intraepithelial neoplasia and cervical cancer. *Am J Clin Nutr* 62:1417S-1419S, 1995.

Miller BA, Kolonel LN, Bernstein L, et al: *Racial/Ethnic Patterns of Cancer in the United States 1988–1992.* NIH Publication no 96-4104. Bethesda, MD, National Cancer Institute, 1996.

Mitchell MF, Hittelman WN, Hong WK, et al: The natural history of cervical intraepithelial neoplasia: An argument for immediate endpoint biomarkers. *Cancer Epidemiol Biomarkers Prev* 3:619–626, 1994.

Mitchell MF, Tortolero-Luna G, Wright T, et al: Cervical human papillomavirus infection and intraepithelial neoplasia: a review. *J Natl Cancer Inst Monogr* 17–25, 1996.

Morris M, Tortolero-Luna G, Malpica A, et al: Cervical intraepithelial neoplasia and cervical cancer. *Obstet Gynecol Clin North Am* 23:347–410,1996.

Morrison EH: Controversies in women's health maintenance. *Am Fam Physician* 55:1283–1290, 1997.

Morrow CP, Cozen W: Perspective on cervical cancer: Why prevent? *J Cell Biochem Suppl* 23:61–70, 1995.

National Institutes of Health consensus development conference statement on cervical cancer, April 1–3, 1996. *Gynecol Oncol* 66:351–361, 1997.

Norman SA, Talbott EO, Kuller LK, et al: Demographic, psychosocial and medical correlates of Pap testing: A literature review. *Am J Prev Med* 7:219–226, 1991.

Nuovo J, Melnikow J, Hutchison B, Paliescheskey M: Is cervicography a useful diagnostic test? A systematic overview of the literature. *J Am Board Fam Pract* 10:390–397, 1997,

Nuovo J, Melnikow J, Paliescheskey M: Management of patients with atypical and low-grade Pap smear abnormalities. *Am Fam Phys* 52:2243–2250,1995.

Ostor AG: Natural history of cervical intraepithelial neoplasia: A critical review. *Int J Gynecol Pathol* 12:186–192, 1993.

Parkin DM, Pisani P, Ferlay J: Global cancer statistics. *CA Cancer J Clin* 49:33–63, 1999.

Perlman SE, Kahn JA, Emans SJ: Should pelvic examinations and Papanicolaou cervical screening be part of preventive health care for sexually active adolescent girls? *J Adolesc Health* 23:62–67, 1998.

Ponten J, Adami HO, Bergstrom R, et al: Strategies for global control of cervical cancer. *Int J Cancer* 60:1–26, 1995.

Reagan JW, et al: The cellular morphology of carcinoma in situ and dysplasia or atypical hyperplasia of the uterine cervix. *Cancer* 6:224–235, 1953.

Richart RM: Cervical intraepithelial neoplasia. *Pathol Annu* 8:301–328, 1973.

Richart RM: Screening: The next century. *Cancer* 76: 1919–1927, 1995.

Segnan N: Socioeconomic status and cancer screening. *IARC Sci Publ* 369–376, 1997.

Shafer MA: Annual pelvic examination in the sexually active adolescent female: What are we doing and why are we doing it? *J Adolesc Health* 23:68–73, 1998.

Shingleton HM, Patrick RL, Johnston WW, Smith RA: The current status of the Papanicolaou smear. *CA Cancer J Clin* 45:305–320, 1995.

Singer A: Cervical cancer screening: State of the art. *Baillieres Clin Obstet Gynaecol* 9:39–64, 1995.

Sood AD: Cigarette smoking and cervical cancer: Meta-analysis and critical review of recent studies. *Am J Prev Med* 7:208–213, 1991.

Stanley MW: Quality and liability issues with the Papanicolaou smear: The role of professional organizations in reform initiatives. *Arch Pathol Lab Med* 121:321–326, 1997.

US Preventive Services Task Force: *Guide to Clinical Preventive Services*, 2nd ed. Baltimore, Williams & Wilkins, 1996.

Vellozzi CJ, Romans M, Rothenberg RB: Delivering breast and cervical cancer screening services to underserved women, I: Literature review and telephone survey. *Womens Health Issues* 6:65–73, 1996.

Villa LL: Human papillomaviruses and cervical cancer. *Adv Cancer Res* 71:321–341, 1997.

Walker B, Figgs LW, Zahm SH: Differences in cancer incidence, mortality, and survival between African Americans and whites. *Environ Health Perspect* 103(Suppl 8):275–281, 1995.

Wheeler CM. Preventive vaccines for cervical cancer. *Salud Publica Mex* 39:283–287, 1997.

Lorne Becker
Pamela Horst
Pamela Vnenchak

Chapter
13

Breast Cancer

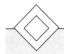

How Common
Is Breast Cancer?

Breast Cancer in the U.S.

Approximately 178,700 American women are diagnosed with breast cancer each year, and the disease causes 43,000 deaths annually. Only non-melanoma skin malignancies occur more frequently than breast cancer in American women, and since 1987 breast cancer is second only to lung cancer as a cause of cancer death in women. Twenty-nine percent of new cancers each year and 16% of cancer deaths in women are due to breast cancer. The incidence of breast cancer increases with increasing age, with the rate leveling off slightly after menopause (Table 13-1). Women in the U.S. have a 1 in 8 chance of developing breast cancer over their lifetime and a 3.6% chance of dying of the disease. Because of the presence of other competing causes of mortality, however, the lifetime risk for breast cancer begins to decrease for women in their 60s.

Breast cancer incidence has been gradually increasing over the last 25 years in the U.S. and worldwide. A portion of this increase has been ascribed to detection of small tumors related to publicity about early detection generated by famous people developing the disease, breast cancer awareness campaigns, and improved mammography equipment that has permitted better resolution causing an increase in diagnosis of breast tumors less than 2 cm in diameter.

International and Interethnic Comparisons

Not all countries have breast cancer rates as high as those found in the U.S. In Japan the overall incidence is only one-fifth that seen in the U.S. Developing countries also have lower age-specific rates than the U.S. Over the past few years, breast cancer incidence and mortality rates have stopped their increase and may be decreasing in some parts of the developed world, including the U.S., Sweden, and the U.K.

African American women have worse survival rates and less localized disease than Caucasian women do. Thus, although the incidence of breast cancer in African American women is lower, their mortality rate is higher than Caucasian women. Screening mammography rates are also lower for African American women. Men do develop breast cancer, but account for less than 1% of cases.

Table 13-1

Breast Cancer Risk by Age

CURRENT AGE (IN YR)	CHANCE OF DIAGNOSIS OF INVASIVE BREAST CANCER IN THE NEXT 10 YR	CHANCE OF DEATH FROM INVASIVE BREAST CANCER IN THE NEXT 10 YR	LIFETIME RISK FOR BREAST CANCER
30	1 in 250 (0.4%)		1 in 8 (12.8%)
40	1 in 70 (1.6%)	1 in 300 (0.3%)	1 in 8 (12.5%)
50	1 in 40 (2.4%)	1 in 150 (0.7%)	1 in 9 (11.3%)
60	1 in 30 (3.6%)	1 in 100 (1%)	1 in 10 (9.6%)
70	1 in 25 (4.1%)	1 in 70 (1.4%)	1 in 14 (7.1%)

SOURCE: Adapted from Feuer et al. 1993 and Landis et al. 1998

Risk Factors

A number of factors have been associated with an increased risk of breast cancer. These (Table 13-2) can be divided into two groups: those that are modifiable and those that are not. This classification is not always straightforward and has been based on a judgment as to what is practical. For instance, high socioeconomic status, age of first pregnancy, nulliparity, and residence are theoretically modifiable, but they are in the non-modifiable category because it is not considered practical to change these characteristics. The modifiable risk factors will be discussed more in the section on primary prevention.

An association between a risk factor and increased risk of breast cancer does not imply causation. Risk factors are simply those variables found to be associated with an increased risk. The association may or may not be causal.

Family History

Women with a family history of breast cancer are at higher risk of developing the disease themselves. Estimates of the proportion of breast cancer cases associated with this risk factor range from 6% to 19%. The risk is increased if the family includes multiple affected members, or relatives who developed their cancers before the age of 50.

Approximately 4%–5% of the breast cancers diagnosed each year are due to highly penetrant dominant genes (BRCA1 and BRCA2) that promote oncogenesis. These genes also increase the risk of ovarian and colon cancer.

Personal History

Conditions that increase a woman's lifetime exposure to estrogen during menstrual cycles are associated with increased breast cancer risk. Thus, early menarche (ages 11—14 years) is associated with a relative breast cancer risk of 1.3; at 15 years a relative risk of 1.1. A first pregnancy at age less than 20 years is protective because it decreases the presence of normal menses early in life. Because later pregnancy results in persistence of normal menstrual cycles a first pregnancy at age 25–29 carries a relative risk of 1.6 and a first pregnancy at age 30 or more has a relative risk of 1.9. Menopause at age 45 years or less is protective (relative risk [RR] of 0.7) while menopause at age 55 or more is a risk (RR 1.5).

A history of benign breast biopsy is also a risk factor. The risk is higher if the biopsy showed atypical hyperplasia (RR 4.0) than proliferative disease (RR 1.5).

Table 13-2

Risk Factors for Breast Cancer

MODIFIABLE	NONMODIFIABLE
Alcohol intake	Early menarche
Lack of exercise	Family history
High-fat diet	High socioeconomic status
Hormone therapy	History of atypical hyperplasia
Obesity	History of proliferative breast disease
Radiation exposure	History of breast cancer
	Late age of first pregnancy
	Nulliparity
	Older age
	Residence in North America or northern Europe

Natural History of Breast Cancer

Breast cancer has a heterogeneous clinical course and the survival of patients with breast cancer can be relatively long. In a series of 250 British patients diagnosed between 1805 and 1933, the median survival time from onset of symptoms was 2.7 years; eighteen percent of untreated patients survived 5 years and 4% survived 10 years. With current treatment, results are much better. Survival data collected by the National Cancer Institute demonstrate a biphasic curve. One subgroup of patients with histologically confirmed breast cancer has a median survival of more than 10 years, representing a force of mortality (the percentage of remaining patients who die each year) of 2.5% per year. This subgroup represents approximately 60% of the entire group. The other subgroup demonstrates, a more aggressive course, with a force of mortality rate of 25% per year and a median survival of 10 years. Survival rates are better for patients with smaller tumors. The 5-year survival rate for localized breast cancer is 97%. In patients with regional spread, the 5-year survival rate declines to 76% and when there is distant metastasis, the rate is 21%. The 10-year breast cancer survival rate is 67% and the 15-year rate is 56%.

Primary cancer of the breast is typically described by its location in the breast. One series of 696 cases found 48% of breast cancers were in the upper outer quadrant, 17% in the central region, 15% in the upper inner quadrant, 11% in the lower outer quadrant, 6% in the lower inner quadrant, and 3% of patients had diffuse disease.

Breast cancer spreads directly into the breast parenchyma, along the mammary ducts and by way of the lymphatic system. These multiple mechanisms of spread increase the probability that the cancer will be present beyond the palpable limits of the tumor.

The clinical size of the primary tumor is highly correlated with prognosis. Breast cancer grows in an exponential fashion, with a doubling time of approximately 100 days. A single malignant cell requires 8 years to become a 1-cm clinically detectable mass. The interval from mammographic detectability to clinical detectability is 1.3 to 2.4 years. Increasing size of primary tumor is correlated with an increased likelihood of distant metastasis.

Approximately half of patients with clinically palpable breast cancer have axillary lymph node involvement. The axillary lymph node region is the most common site of regional breast cancer involvement, followed by the internal mammary and supraclavicular areas. Bone, lung, and liver are the most common sites of distant metastasis. The time from initial diagnosis of breast cancer to detection of distant metastasis can be long. It may take 10 or more years for distant disease to become apparent. The time to detection of metastasis is related to the size of the primary tumor. By the time a breast cancer has reached a diameter of 4 cm approximately 50% of patients will have metastases.

Treatment is individualized and typically is directed at the breast, regional lymph nodes, and sites of distant metastasis. Treatment regimens include lumpectomy (local removal of the tumor), simple or radical mastectomy, axillary lymph node dissection, radiation, chemotherapy, or hormone therapy. These methods may be used alone or in combination. In early stage breast cancer, long-term survival rates after lumpectomy plus radiotherapy are similar to those of modified radical mastectomy. There are several options for breast reconstruction available at the time of, or in the months that follow, surgery.

Primary Prevention of Breast Cancer

Primary prevention refers to the eradication of risk factors to prevent cancer from developing. It can also include preventive therapy, genetic testing and prophylactic surgery. Table 13-3 lists the factors that are targets for primary prevention, the intervention that addresses the risk, and a summary of the current evidence for or against effectiveness from clinical trials.

Risk Factor Modification

For many potentially modifiable risk factors, the association with breast cancer is weak or questionable. Obesity, alcohol, and lack of exercise are exceptions. All three have been shown in observational studies to have statistically significant and clinically meaningful associations with breast cancer risk.

Unfortunately changing modifiable risk factors does not always lead to changes in disease rates. In fact, we have no good studies to date that show decreases in breast cancer rates or outcomes resulting from alterations to any of

Table 13-3

Targets for Primary Prevention

RISK FACTOR	INTERVENTION	EVIDENCE OF EFFECTIVENESS FROM CLINICAL TRIALS	STUDY IN PROGRESS
Obesity	Weight loss	None	—
Diet	Low-fat diet ↑ Soy (plant?)	Conflicting	Women's Health Trial results expected in 2007
Exercise	↑ Recreational exercise	None	—
Alcohol	↓ Use	None	—
Oral contraceptives	No use	Relative risk increases by 2.3% for each year of use	—
HRT	Avoid use	Yes, see text	Women's Health Trial
Ionizing radiation	Avoid exposure	None	—
Genetic history			3 European trials
First degree relative with breast cancer	Tamoxifen	Yes, see text	—
BRCA1&2	Prophylactic mastectomy	Yes, see text	—
	Prophylactic oophorectomy	None	

these risk factors. For women at high risk of developing breast cancer, other primary prevention strategies such as chemoprophylaxis with such drugs as tamoxifen, or prophylactic mastectomy or oophorectomy have been considered. Unfortunately, there is much uncertainty about the effectiveness of these strategies as well.

Diet

Obese women are more likely to develop breast cancer. The relative risk increases by 3.1% for every kg/m^2 above ideal body weight. This association holds true only among postmenopausal women. For premenopausal women, obesity is actually slightly protective.

While obesity is a breast cancer risk, no evidence is available for the effectiveness of weight loss in reducing breast cancer risk for women at any age. However, several specific components of the diet have been suggested as risk factors for development of breast cancer. Evidence for these has been conflicting and unconvincing.

Adoption of a low fat diet is probably not an effective method of breast cancer prevention. Dietary intake of fat, and in particular of saturated fats, was once thought to be an important risk. Dietary fat intake and estrogen levels are directly related in postmenopausal women, and in international comparisons, higher rates of breast cancer are found in countries in which high fat diets are consumed. This presumed association disappears in studies using increasing methodologic rigor. Case control studies in general show only a weak association, and a recent pooled analysis of existing cohort studies found no evidence for an association between total dietary fat intake and breast cancer risk. The association noted in international and case control studies may have been spurious and related to the inaccuracy of dietary self-report instruments. No randomized trials addressing this question have been completed, but one trial is currently in progress. The Women's Health

Initiative has randomly assigned a group of postmenopausal women to their regular diet or a low fat diet. Results should be available in 2007.

Because some Mediterranean countries have breast cancer incidence rates that are half those in other developed countries, studies have investigated the beneficial effects of other components of the "Mediterranean diet." Results have been conflicting. Some studies have suggested that high intakes of olive oil have a small beneficial effect on breast cancer, decreasing incidence rates by 13% to 33%. Diets high in fiber from fruits and vegetables have been found protective in some studies; reducing cancer incidence rates by 34% to 52%, but having no protective effect in others. Studies of the proposed protective effects of other dietary components such as vitamins A, C, E, and beta-carotene have also shown very mixed results. Plant estrogens, found in soy products such as tofu, have been suggested as one of the factors responsible for the low rate of breast cancer in Asian women, but no formal studies have been conducted.

Given this uncertainty, and the lack of association in the strongest studies, there is no reason to hold out hope to women that dietary modifications will substantially change their risk of breast cancer. A diet low in saturated fats may be advised, however, as a means of preventing coronary disease, which is a much larger cause of death for women than breast cancer.

Exercise

Physical activity in adolescence and young adult life has been associated with a reduced risk of breast cancer in premenopausal and perimenopausal women. The observation that physical activity delays the onset of menarche and decreases the number of menstrual cycles may provide a partial explanation for this association. A systematic review of observational studies found that 7 of 9 demonstrated an association between higher levels of occupational physical activity and reduced breast cancer risk, while 11 of 16 found a similar decrease in risk among women who reported higher recreational exercise levels. The association was present in both case-control and cohort studies, but no dose-response trend was evident in most studies. In these studies, regular recreational exercise decreased breast cancer risk by 12%–60%. While there are no randomized trials demonstrating that exercise programs can improve breast cancer incidence or mortality rates, it is reasonable to advise regular exercise because of its beneficial effects on other health conditions.

Alcohol

Two systematic reviews of case-control and cohort studies have shown a linear association between breast cancer risk and alcohol intake, with breast cancer risk rising by 11% when alcohol intake rises by one drink per day. (One drink is equivalent to a bottle of beer, a glass of wine, or 1½ oz of spirits.) The relationship appears to plateau at 4 drinks per day, although few women drinking this amount were included in the studies. The biological mechanism for this association is not well understood. Some studies have shown correlations between alcohol intake and estrogen levels, but others have not. It has also been suggested that alcohol may act as a co-carcinogen, improving the permeability of membranes to carcinogens, inhibiting the detoxification of carcinogens, and activating pro-carcinogens. No trials of the effect of modification of alcohol intake have been conducted.

Oral Contraceptives and Hormone Replacement Therapy

Because endogenous hormones are known to influence the risk and prognosis of breast cancer, a number of studies have investigated the association of oral contraceptives (OCs) or post-menopausal hormone replacement therapy (HRT) and breast cancer risk. These studies have reached conflicting conclusions, and many have been too small to show statistically significant results.

This confusing situation has recently been resolved with a large collaborative reanalysis of the original data from 51 different studies involving over 52,000 women with breast cancer, and 108,000 controls. Data from both case-control and cohort studies were included. Data from cohort studies were used by means of a "nested case-control" design, with four controls randomly selected for each woman with breast cancer. Use of either OCs or HRT was associated with a statistically significant increase in breast cancer risk while the hormonal preparation was being taken. In both cases, the risk decreased after stopping the medication. Furthermore, the cancers diagnosed in women taking these preparations were less advanced than those diagnosed in controls, and were less likely to have spread to lymph nodes or to have metastasized.

While taking oral contraceptives, women have a 24% increase in their relative risk of having a breast cancer diagnosed. This excess breast cancer risk decreases to 16% in the first years after discontinuing OCs, to 7% in the next 5 years, and disappears after 10 years. Since breast cancer is relatively rare in women of childbearing age, the actual number of cancers involved is quite small. If 10,000 women used OCs from age 20 through age 24, only 1.5 additional breast cancers would be diagnosed.

For current HRT users, the relative risk of breast cancer increases by 2.3% for each year of use. In terms of absolute risk, if 1000 50-year-old women used HRT for 10 years, 6 additional cases of breast cancer would be diagnosed. This excess risk disappears 5 years after discontinuing use of HRT.

This association of hormone use with breast cancer risk has a number of rather unusual features. Women taking hormones are at highest risk soon after their exposure to the drugs, with their risks returning to normal after they stop taking them. Their tumors are smaller, and less likely to have spread. This pattern suggests the possibility that hormone users may not be developing more breast cancers, but simply having their cancers diagnosed earlier. A "detection bias" of this sort is reasonably plausible, since users of OCs or HRT must visit physicians to receive prescriptions for these medications, and may have more cancer detection maneuvers performed at those visits.

Ionizing Radiation

Exposure of the breast to ionizing radiation is associated with an increase in cancer risk, which increases with decreasing age at the time of exposure. In the past, sources of exposure have included radiation treatments for acne or thymic enlargement. Currently, clinically significant levels of exposure rarely occur except in women treated with mantle radiation for Hodgkin's disease. The higher risks of radiation for younger women have raised some concerns about adverse effects of screening mammography. By one estimate, screening women biennially between the ages of 45 and 50 would lead to one additional death from radiation induced cancer for every 20 breast cancer deaths prevented. While some radiation exposure is unavoidable, avoidance of unnecessary or occupational radiation exposure should be advised.

Preventive Drug Therapy for High-Risk Women

Estrogen receptor antagonists such as tamoxifen have been shown to be effective in preventing recurrences in women after treatment for primary breast cancer. This effectiveness has led to hopes that treatment of high-risk women prior to the diagnosis of breast cancer might decrease their chance of developing or dying from breast cancer. Recent reports from randomized trials in

the U.S. and Europe have reached conflicting conclusions, leaving significant uncertainty about the effectiveness of this approach.

In the United States, the National Cancer Institute's Breast Cancer Prevention Trial (BCPT) enrolled women who were over the age of 60 or had the breast cancer risk of a 60-year-old woman due to risk factors such as the presence of first-degree relatives with breast cancer, age at menarche, parity, age at delivery of first child, number of breast biopsies, or history of lobular carcinoma in situ (CIS) or atypical hyperplasia. Women randomized to take tamoxifen had a 45% reduction in the incidence of invasive breast cancer when compared with those taking a placebo.

The decreased cancer incidence came at some cost, since women in the tamoxifen group experienced more endometrial cancers, deep vein thromboses (DVT), and pulmonary emboli. These results suggest that for every 1000 women who took tamoxifen for 4 years, 10 cases of invasive cancer, 3 cases of ductal carcinoma in situ (DCIS), and 10 fractures would be prevented. However among this group of 1000 women, there would be 3 additional cases of endometrial cancer, 1–2 additional cases of DVT and 2 additional pulmonary emboli.

Because of early beneficial effects, the BCPT was halted early and it is unclear whether these initial benefits will translate into longer-term improvements in survival. Concerns have been raised that tamoxifen may selectively avert neoplasms with a better prognosis, and that women taking tamoxifen prophylaxis may obtain less benefit from adjuvant therapy with tamoxifen if they later develop breast cancers. While the benefits of tamoxifen therapy may decrease with longer follow up, the risks will probably increase, as longer exposure to the drug produces more endometrial cancers, DVTs, and pulmonary emboli. The average length of follow up in the BCPT was only 4 years, leaving clinicians and patients in a quandary about whether tamoxifen will lead to more harm or more benefits if prescribed for women with a life expectancy of 10 to 20 years or more. Finally, since women using HRT were not enrolled in the BCPT, the trial gives no information about the benefits of tamoxifen in the important subset of women who are taking HRT.

Two European trials have reported preliminary results. Neither was able to confirm the benefits of tamoxifen found in the BCPT. Several possible explanations for this discrepancy have been discussed. The European trials were smaller and included more women under the age of 60 or taking HRT. More of the women included in these trials had a family history of breast cancer, and tamoxifen may be less effective for some familial cancers. These trials also followed women for longer periods than the BCPT, again raising the possibility that the early results of the BCPT may overestimate the long-term benefits of tamoxifen.

Given these uncertainties, it is inappropriate to urge women, whatever their level of risk, to start tamoxifen prophylaxis. Instead, women should be advised of the results of these 3 studies, and the trade-offs of potential benefits and risks. Some women may wish to start tamoxifen in spite of these uncertainties. Others may wish to wait for longer-term results from the 3 European trials that are currently under way.

Genetic Testing

Approximately 4–5% of the breast cancers diagnosed each year are due to highly penetrant dominant genes (BRCA1 and BRCA2). Should women with a family history of breast cancer be tested for the presence of these genes?

Many women with breast cancer (perhaps as many as 19%) have other family members with the disease. Women with a family history of breast cancer can be divided into moderate risk and high-risk groups. High-risk families have three or more close relatives with breast cancer in a pattern of inheritance consistent with autosomal dominant genetics. Cancers in these families appear at a relatively early age (before 45), and there may be cases of ovarian cancer in relatives as well. Moderate risk families have a less striking family history with fewer affected members, cancer onset at a later age, and an absence of ovarian cancer cases. Genetic testing in high-risk families will often reveal one of the breast cancer susceptibility genes, but these are much less likely to be found in moderate risk than in high-risk families.

Whether or not to offer genetic testing to women in high-risk families provides an uncomfortable dilemma. A woman carrying one of these genes is clearly at high risk of breast cancer. Approximately 20% of BRCA1 mutation carriers will develop breast cancer by age 40, 51% by age 50, and 71% by age 70. Unfortunately, no interventions have clearly been shown to reduce the risk born by these women other than prophylactic mastectomy. Regular surveillance with mammograms, Clinical Breast Examination (CBE), and Breast Self-Examination (BSE) may be recommended, although none of these interventions has been tested in this high-risk population. There is some evidence that BRCA-related tumors grow more quickly than sporadic cancers. Thus screening efforts may be less effective, suggesting that shorter intervals between tests should be considered. Indeed, some authorities recommend mammography every 6 months starting at age 25–35 for women known to be carriers. Bilateral prophylactic mastectomy or oophorectomy have been advocated by some. While these procedures probably lower cancer risks, they are not universally effective, since current surgical technique does not allow removal of all breast tissue. Chemoprophylaxis with such drugs as tamoxifen has been shown to reduce the risk of cancer by 45% among high-risk women, but we do not know as yet whether these drugs will provide a similar benefit in women at risk of BRCA-related disease.

While it is unclear whether testing brings any benefits, there are a number of known negative effects for women offered BRCA testing. In one study of high-risk families, almost half of the women tested chose not to return to receive their results. One quarter of those receiving their results refused to release test results to their physicians because of concerns about future discrimination by insurance companies. Women with positive results suffer the emotional stress of facing their increased risks, and the uncertainty arising from the incomplete penetrance of the genes. For some women, a positive result led to a very strong fear of finding a breast cancer. These women refused mammograms or breast examinations, and would not touch their breasts or allow their partners to do so. Even those receiving negative results had some adverse effects. Some women refused to believe a negative test and continued to be anxious about their increased risk, having already decided that they were carrying the gene. Others felt "survivor guilt" and worried about how they would discuss their favorable results with other family members who had been found to carry the gene. Still others expressed regret about decisions they had already made (e.g., sterilization or prophylactic surgery) based on their perceived susceptibility.

Because of the many unresolved issues, patients requesting such testing should be encouraged to seek it in the context of a clinical study which has received institutional review board approval. This will maximize the possibility that issues of confidentiality and informed consent will be appropriately addressed.

Prophylactic Mastectomy and Oophorectomy

Women found to be carriers of one of the BRCA genes are faced with a difficult decision about how to proceed. Three choices have been suggested—increased breast cancer surveillance, chemoprevention, or prophylactic mastectomy or oophorectomy. All 3 options have their problems. Many women are unconvinced that routine mammography and CBE will offer them

adequate protection. Some authorities feel that mammography should be performed more frequently (as often as every 6 months) in these patients, since there is evidence that BRCA-1 related tumors may have faster rates of growth. The concerns and uncertainties about prolonged chemoprophylaxis with such drugs as tamoxifen are outlined above. In addition to these concerns, there is some suggestion that tamoxifen may be less effective in some women with a strong family history of breast cancer.

Some women at high risk have chosen to have prophylactic mastectomy or oophorectomy to lessen their chances of developing breast cancer. This decision involves trade offs between the potential benefits of these procedures, and the psychological and physical traumas involved in pursuing them. The potential for increases in life expectancy from these procedures is greatest for women in their 30s, and decreases continuously for older women.

A good description of the patient's perspective is provided in a recent article by Eales, in which one of the authors describes her decision and experiences with prophylactic mastectomy. In addition to the postoperative pain and discomfort, which she described as lasting "for a long time" and producing "a sensation of 'cut glass' under the skin, plus extreme tightness across the pectoral muscles," she described a number of other adverse effects. These included the lack of sensation in her breasts following the procedure, the experience of being a "non-cancer" patient in a cancer ward, the emotional sense of loss of sexuality and femininity, and the long period required before she was able to accept "the new breasts not being as before." The author described the supportive relationship with her primary care clinician as an invaluable aide in her adaptation to the after effects of the procedure.

While this is only one patient's story, many other women may share her sentiments. In one study, women estimated that their quality of life following a diagnosis of breast cancer would be higher than their quality of life with no cancer but having had an oophorectomy and a mastectomy. Unfortunately, we have limited evidence about the effectiveness of these preventive procedures. Neither provides absolute protection against cancer, since new breast cancers are known to arise from breast tissue remaining after prophylactic mastectomy, and ovarian cancers can arise spontaneously in the peritoneal reflection after oophorectomy.

While there are no randomized trials of the effectiveness of prophylactic mastectomy, a recent study from the Mayo Clinic provides some evidence for its effectiveness. Women at moderate to high risk had an estimated 90% reduction in their breast cancer rates when compared with the rates predicted by a risk model or the rates experienced by their sisters who did not have prophylactic mastectomies. Oophorectomy may be less effective, with estimates suggesting that it may reduce ovarian cancer risk by about 50%.

Two recent decision analyses, using these data, project an average gain of 3 to 5 years in life expectancy for a 30-year-old BRCA carrier who elects prophylactic mastectomy. Increases in quality adjusted life expectancy (QALY) were expected only for women with a high cancer risk (85% breast cancer, 63% ovarian cancer). The gains in life expectancy were less for women choosing mastectomy at later ages, and disappeared by age 60. These results were very sensitive to changes in assumptions about risk and about quality of life. Thus, different women may come to very different conclusions about the appropriateness of prophylactic surgery, based on their levels of concern about developing cancer, and their feelings about their anticipated quality of life following the procedures.

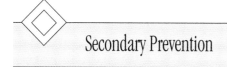

Secondary Prevention

Secondary prevention involves tests designed to diagnose breast cancer early, in the hope that early treatment will lead to better outcomes. The three screening maneuvers currently in favor for breast cancer prevention include mammography, breast examination by a clinician, and breast self-examination. Other potential screening tests (such as thermography) have been abandoned because of ineffectiveness. Still other potential candidates (e.g., MRI and ultrasound) are being evaluated, but as yet have not shown sufficient promise to warrant recommendations for their widespread use.

Mammography

Mammography involves the use of x-rays to detect small tumors. Until recently, there was little standardization in the way the procedure was performed or interpreted. In 1999 the Mammography Quality Standards Act (MQSA) regulations become effective, helping to standardize the quality monitors for the x-ray technique of mammography including personnel training, interpretation, equipment standards, radiation exposure (maximum 0.1 mrads), and tracking data. State health departments will certify facilities meeting these standards, and patients should be referred to such facilities wherever they are available.

According to MQSA, screening exams should include standard craniocaudal and oblique views of each breast performed on women with no breast problems. The interpreting physician must have at least three months of formal training in interpretation of mammograms and then earn 15 category I CME credits every 3 years in mammography. Double reading by 2 radiologists has been used in studies but is not the standard for certification by MQSA.

Referring clinicians need to be aware that high-density breasts in young women and women with implants make interpretation more difficult. Patients should be advised not to schedule the test just before and during their menses due to increase pain with the compression that is necessary for adequate exams. Two piece clothing makes the study more convenient for the woman.

Clinical Breast Examination

While mammography can detect small tumors that are not yet palpable, it can also miss tumors that can readily be detected on a careful breast examination by a physician, other clinicians, or a patient. In one study, breast examination by a skilled clinician was as effective as mammography plus breast examination in reducing breast cancer mortality in postmenopausal women. A complete breast examination involves both inspection and palpation of both breasts in a systematic fashion.

Inspection begins with the woman sitting with her arms relaxed by her side. The breasts are compared, looking for any discrepancies in shape, size, color or contour, dimpling, puckering, or nipple retraction. The inspection is then repeated with the woman's hands raised over her head. Finally, a third observation is made after asking the woman to rest her palms on her hips, press down firmly to flex her chest muscles, and roll her shoulders slightly forward.

Palpation should be done twice, once with the woman sitting, and a second time with her lying down. Palpation is always done using the palmar finger pads of the three middle fingers. With the woman sitting, palpation begins with a careful and systematic examination of the chest wall from the collarbone to the nipple. Three downward strokes should cover the entire chest wall. Next, the breast is cupped firmly between both hands, with the fingers of the upper hand gently walking across the breast in a semi-circle. Finally, the axilla is palpated, after asking the woman to place one hand on her hip and to roll her shoulder slightly forward. The entire procedure is then repeated for the opposite breast.

The woman is next asked to lie flat on her back with her left arm over her head. A pillow or folded towel may be placed under her left shoulder to spread breast tissue more evenly over the chest wall. Again using the pads of the middle three fingers, the examiner's hand is moved in small circular motions (about the size of a dime) from one area to another until the entire breast and axilla have been covered. The procedure is then repeated for the right breast.

Breast Self-Examination

The procedure for breast self examination is exactly the same as that described above for examination by a clinician. Women are taught to use a mirror for self-inspection, and to examine each breast using the finger pads of the middle three fingers of the opposite hand. They are encouraged to report any mass, skin dimpling, asymmetry, or change from a previousself-examination.

Accuracy and Predictive Values of Breast Cancer Screening Tests

MAMMOGRAPHY

In a recent meta-analysis, the sensitivity of screening mammography in published reports was found to range from 83% to 95%. Specificity ranged from 93.5% to 99.1%. Actual performance of community radiologists may fall short of these numbers. Beam et al. sent the same set of 79 randomly selected screening mammograms to 108 radiologists, and found wide variations in interpretation. Sensitivities ranged from 46.7% to 100% (median, 80.0%). Specificities ranged from 36.3% to 99.3% (median 92.7%). Specificity was much lower for films from patients with benign breast disease (median 60%, range 13.3–100%). Mammogram sensitivity is lower in premenopausal women, and mammograms performed on women in their 30s have lower sensitivities (54%–91%) than those of women in their 40s (72%–94%). For women over 50, mammogram sensitivity varies with breast density. Sensitivity is higher for women with primarily fatty breast tissue than in those with dense breasts. For women under 50 years of age, breast density is not related to sensitivity of mammography. Specificity of mammography appears not to vary with age of the woman being screened.

The sensitivity of screening mammography can be increased by approximately 5%–10% by having two radiologists independently review each film. The additional cancers detected by this method are smaller and of lower stage than those noted by both reviewers. If all films identified as possibly abnormal by either radiologist are considered positives, then specificity decreases, and many more women are subjected to follow up testing. However, if the two radiologists are asked to form a consensus opinion on each questionable film ("consensus double reading") specificity actually improves along with sensitivity. This approach was found to be less costly than single reading in one study, since the extra cost of the second radiologist was more than outweighed by the decreased follow-up costs resulting from the improved specificity. The consensus double-reading approach, when used in England, identified 9 additional cancers while saving 4,853 pounds for each 10,000 women screened.

Because the prevalence of breast cancer rises with age, the predictive value of a positive screening mammogram rises with age as well. Table 13-4 indicates the probability of breast cancer (in percent) after an initial mammogram abnormality, interpreted by the radiologist as needing additional evaluation, suspicious for malignancy, or clearly malignant.

While many of these predictive values are rather low (especially those in the "additional evaluation needed" column), they were obtained from a program in an academic medical center. Community predictive values may be even lower. In one study of 50 randomly selected community mammography facilities, between 3% and 57% of screening mammograms were reported as abnormal. Two-thirds of the facilities reported abnormalities in 5%–15%

Table 13-4

Risk of Breast Cancer Based on Age and Mammographic Interpretation

Age	Additional Evaluation Needed	Suspicious of Malignancy	Malignant
30–39	1%	9%	57%
40–49	2%	30%	87%
50–59	5%	39%	92%
60–69	7%	54%	90%
>69	7%	63%	97%

SOURCE: From Kerlikowske K et al., 1996.

of mammograms performed. The number of cancers detected per 1000 examinations was somewhat less than those reported for academic centers, but many more women were subjected to invasive follow-up procedures. The number of cancers detected per follow-up procedure was therefore rather low, particularly for women under the age of 50 (Table 13-5).

All of the above analyses concern only the effects of a single mammogram. Women receiving repeated mammography on an annual or biennial basis experience additional risks of a false positive with each new examination. A study of patients in a Boston health maintenance organization estimated the cumulative risk of a false-positive result as 49.1% (95% confidence interval, 40.3% to 64.1%) after 10 mammograms. By their estimate, 18.9% of women with no breast cancer would have 1 or more biopsies recommended as a result of 10 mammograms.

CLINICAL BREAST EXAMINATION

The best estimates of CBE sensitivity come from the two Canadian National Breast Screening studies. In both trials, carefully trained nurses performed CBE using the methods outlined above. While the combination of mam-

Table 13-5

Percentage of Patients with Cancer Detected Following Specific Follow-up Procedures

PROCEDURE	<50 YR OLD	>50 YR OLD
Additional mammographic views	1.9%	3.8%
Sonography	0.3%	4.4%
Clinical breast exam	0.0%	1.2%
Needle aspiration	3.6%	11.8%
Needle biopsy	8.7%	26.2%
Open surgical biopsy	9.5%	29.8%

SOURCE: From Brown et al., 1995.

mography and CBE detected more cancers than CBE alone, the sensitivity of CBE was higher in women under 50 (68%) than in older women (63%). The specificity of CBE appears to be similar to that of mammography, about 95%.

BREAST SELF-EXAMINATION

It is estimated that BSE sensitivity decreases as patient age increases, from 41% for women aged 35–39 to 21% for women aged 60–74. Specificity is thought to be lower than that of mammography or CBE.

Evidence That Screening Reduces Mortality

PITFALLS IN THE EVALUATION OF BREAST CANCER SCREENING STUDIES

Much of the enthusiasm about specific screening tests arises from observational studies that show that women participating in a screening program have smaller tumors detected at earlier stages, and live longer following detection of their tumors. While suggestive, observational studies cannot provide strong evidence of benefit because of 3 important biases—leadtime bias, length bias, and compliance bias. Only randomized clinical trials (RCT) can avoid these biases, and therefore estimates of the effective-

ness of breast cancer screening should rely on RCT evidence where available.

Unfortunately, because breast cancer deaths are relatively rare events, particularly in younger women, such trials must have large samples and long follow-up periods, and are generally difficult and expensive to perform. This has left us in a situation in which, for many proposed breast cancer screening interventions, we have evidence only from observational studies, or conflicting evidence from randomized trials. This uncertainty has resulted in many debates about breast cancer screening between those who insist that any intervention shown to be potentially effective must be forcefully recommended to all women, and others who advise caution whenever RCTs have not shown a clear advantage. The approach advocated in this chapter is that women should be provided with the necessary information to make their own decisions.

MAMMOGRAPHY

For women between the ages of 50 and 70, screening mammograms (used alone or in conjunction with CBE) lead to a 34% reduction in breast cancer mortality. This finding has been confirmed in 8 different RCTs, and is apparent within the first 7 years of follow-up. Studies using a 2-year interval between mammograms have shown benefits similar to those using annual screening.

The picture for women in their 40s is not so promising. Seven randomized trials of the effectiveness of mammography have included women under the age of 50. None of the trials showed any benefit after 7 years of follow-up. After 10–12 years of follow-up, the combined results of these trials show a 15% reduction in breast cancer deaths. This optimistic finding must be approached with caution for a number of reasons. Because breast cancer is an uncommon condition in women of this age group, a 15% reduction would translate into only 4 fewer cancer deaths for every 10,000 women screened regularly throughout their 40s. With one exception, the studies were not designed primarily to evaluate the effectiveness of mammography in women in this age range, and estimates of effectiveness therefore depend on analysis of results of a subset of the women participating in the trial. Since the reductions in cancer mortality did not become evident until the women involved were more than 50 years old, it is unclear whether the reductions were due to the screening provided to women during their forties, or could have been achieved by delaying regular mammograms until the women reached their 50s. Even if mammography is effective for women in their 40s, it is clearly much less effective in preventing cancer deaths than it is for women over the age of 50.

Two possible explanations have been advanced for the clear difference in effectiveness of mammography for women before versus after the age of 50. Fifty is the average age at which women experience menopause. Premenopausal women's breasts are more mammography dense, making mammograms more difficult to interpret. Breast cancers arising in premenopausal women grow more quickly than cancers developing in older women. Thus, the pre-symptomatic interval during which cancers are amenable to early detection is shorter. Some experts believe that offering screening mam-

mograms more frequently can alleviate this problem.

While the benefits of screening mammograms are uncertain for women in this age group, there are very clear negative effects. An abnormal mammogram in a younger woman is much more likely to be false positive. In one of the trials, the ratio of benign to malignant biopsy results (after the first screening mammogram) was 9.0 for women 40–45 compared with 3.6 for 50–54-year-old women, and 1.7 for women 55 and older. As noted above, the problem of false positives increases with repeated examinations. Women in their 40s have a 30% risk of having at least one false positive after 5 screening mammograms and a 56% risk after 10 mammograms. These risks decrease somewhat with age. For women over 50, the corresponding rates are 24% and 47%.

DUCTAL CARCINOMA The question of whether mammography leads to net negative effects or benefits in women under the age of 50 is further muddied by the issue of ductal carcinoma in-situ (DCIS). This term refers to lesions arising from cells within the milk duct, with no extension through the basement membrane surrounding the ducts. In the past decade, the frequency of diagnosis of DCIS has increased 5 fold—mainly due to screening mammography. Almost one-third of all breast neoplasms diagnosed by mammography in the U.S. are DCIS. This proportion is highest among younger women. In one screening program, 43% of mammograms detected cancers in 40–49-year-old women, and 92% of those detected in 30–39 year olds were DCIS. Unfortunately, the natural history of this condition is poorly understood, and most of our knowledge comes from studies of women whose DCIS presented in the days before widespread screening mammography, with symptoms such as nipple discharge, mass, or Paget's disease of the nipple.

We have no good data to predict which (or even how many) women with mammographically detected DCIS will have their lesions progress to invasive cancers. Clearly not all DCIS will lead to clinically significant disease, since the condition has been found at autopsy in up to 16% of completely asymptomatic women. (One study, which used postmortem breast x-rays to determine areas to sample found DCIS in 40% of asymptomatic women at autopsy.) On the other hand, some cases of DCIS clearly do progress. In one small case series study, 35% of women with DCIS treated by biopsy alone developed invasive cancer in the same breast within 10 years.

In addition to our ignorance about natural history, there is no clear evidence about how DCIS should be treated. Breast conserving surgery with or without radiation, and mastectomy are all options. At present, 40%–50% of American women treated for DCIS receive a mastectomy, although this proportion is falling slowly. Thus the risk of being subjected to disfiguring surgery to treat a disease that might never have led to symptoms must be included among the potential harms of mammography.

NIH SUMMARY   In January 1997, the National Institutes of Health convened a panel of experts at a consensus development conference to review the existing evidence on screening mammography. Their recommendation included the following statement: "The data currently available do not warrant a universal recommendation for mammography for all women in their forties. Each woman should decide for herself whether to undergo mammography. Given both the importance and the complexity of the issue involved in assessing the evidence, a woman should have access to the best possible relevant information regarding both benefits and risks, presented in an understandable and usable form."

This recommendation became the subject of intense political debate and resulted in a flurry of raised voices in favor of screening mammography for women in their forties—including a 98 to 0 vote in the U.S. Senate in favor of a nonbinding resolution supporting mammography for women in their 40s.

CLINICAL BREAST EXAMINATION

There are no RCTs available that compare CBE with no screening. Mammography detects more cancers than CBE, suggesting that, if only one modality can be used, it should be mammography. However, studies of breast cancer screening have consistently shown that mammography and clinician breast examination both detect cancers missed by the other procedure.

One randomized clinical trial showed no difference in mortality rates among postmenopausal women offered CBE alone vs. those offered CBE plus mammography. However, the authors of this trial, in a recent literature review, have concluded that screening with a combination of mammography and clinical examination results in higher cancer detection rates, and improved 10-year survival when compared with screening using clinical examination alone. The addition of CBE to mammography is particularly important for premenopausal women who choose to have regular breast screening, because of the poorer sensitivity of mammograms in this age group.

BREAST SELF-EXAMINATION

A number of observational studies have found that women who report performing BSE on a regular basis are more likely to have tumors under 2 cm in diameter and less likely to have nodal involvement. These findings, while suggesting that BSE may be beneficial, could be due to compliance or lead-time bias. A recent case-control study found that women who use one or more of three specific techniques in their BSE have a lower risk of death or distant metastatic disease. The three techniques were visual examination of their breasts, use of finger pads for palpation, and use of their three middle fingers. Women who examined their breasts more frequently did not have better outcomes however, women who perform it more proficiently did, suggesting that BSE may be effective.

Two randomized trials of the effectiveness of BSE, involving more than 380,000 women, are being conducted in Russia and in China. Both have reported disappointing preliminary results. In the Shanghai study, women in the intervention group demonstrated a high level of participation, showed a greater proficiency in detecting lumps in breast models, and detected more benign breast lesions than the control group (1457 versus 623, respectively). Cumulative breast cancer mortality rates through 5 years from entry into the study were nearly equivalent for the two groups, and the breast cancers detected in the instruction group were not diagnosed at an appreciably earlier stage or smaller in size than those in the control group. In the Russian study, women randomized to the self-examination group had 10% higher 5- and 9-year survival rates. These differences were not statistically significant, and were much less than the 30% improvement in mortality expected when the study was designed.

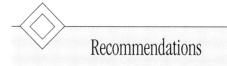

Recommendations

Age 50

Table 13-6 summarizes breast cancer screening recommendations from different organizations. The U.S. Preventive Task Force (USPTF), the American Cancer Society (ACS), the National Cancer Institute (NCI), American Academy of Family Physicians (AAFP) and the Canadian Task Force (CTF) all agree that after age 50 mammography and CBE should be performed every 1 to 2 years. The USPTF does note that mammography alone is acceptable.

Ages 40–49

For those between the ages of 40 and 49, organizations differ in their recommendations. The USPTF does not recommend routine mammography or CBE due to insufficient evidence for its benefit but does note that, in high-risk individuals, clinicians may chose to screen. The CTF also does not recommend screening in this population and the NCI notes no reduction in mortality in women until 15 years after the start of screening when this group would be over 50. The NIH consensus statement from January 1997 does not universally recommend mammography for women in their forties but suggests that each woman should decide for herself based on her history and how she values the risks and benefits. The ACS, American College of Obstetrics and Gynecology (ACOG) and the American Medical Association (AMA) all recommend mammography every 1 to 2 years and CBE yearly for this age group.

Discontinuing Screening

The age at which breast cancer screening can safely be discontinued is another area of debate. There is limited clinical trial information for women over 70 but mammography sensitivity does increase with age as does breast cancer risk. On the other hand, the benefits of early breast cancer detection are often not apparent for many years, and elderly women have a shorter life expectancy and a greater possibility of dying from other causes before being able to experience the benefits of early breast cancer treatment. The USPTF and the CTF suggest routine mammography could stop at age 70. For reasonably healthy women over the age of 70 mammograms could be recommended on the basis of expert opinion and clinical experience according to the NCI and the USPTF. The ACS does not place an older age limit on its recommendations.

Table 13-6

Summary of Breast Cancer Screening Guidelines

ORGANIZATION	MAMMOGRAM	CLINICAL BREAST EXAM (CBE)	BREAST SELF-EXAM
National Institutes of Health Consensus Panel	**Ages 40–49**—Available data do not warrant a single recommendation. **Ages 50–69**—Annual	—	—
U.S. Preventive Services Task Force	**Ages 40–49**—Recommendations cannot be made on current evidence (C). **Ages 50–69**—Every 1–2 yr (A) **Ages 70–74**—Limited and conflicting evidence of benefit **Age 75 and older**—no evidence of benefit	**Ages 40–49**—Recommendation cannot be made on current evidence (C). **Ages 50–69**—May be done every 1–2 yr with mammogram insufficient evidence to recommend annual CBE alone (C)	Insufficient evidence to recommend for or against (C)
Canadian Task Force	**Ages 50–59**—Annual **Age less than 50**—Recommends against	**Ages 50–69**—Annual	
American Academy of Family Physicians	**Ages 40–49**—Counsel about potential benefits. **Ages 50–69**—Offer every 1–2 yr.	**Ages 40–49**—Counsel about potential benefits. **Ages 50–69**—Offer every 1–2 yr.	
American College of Radiology	**Asymptomatic women over the age of 40**—Annual **High-risk women younger than 40 yr**—May benefit from mammogram	Annual, although scientifically unproven	Monthly, although scientifically unproven
American College of Obstetricians and Gynecologists	**Ages 40–49**—Every 1–2 yr. **Age 50 and older**—Annual	**Age 40 and older**—Annual	Recommend teaching
American College of Surgeons and American Cancer Society	**Age 40 and older**—Annual	**Ages 20–39**—Every 3 yr **Age 40 and older**—Annual	**Ages 20–39**—Monthly **Age 40 and older**—Monthly

A = There is sufficient evidence to support the recommendation that the condition be specifically considered in a periodic health examination.
C = There is insufficient evidence to recommend for or against the inclusion of the condition in a periodic health examination, but recommendations may be made on other grounds.

Breast self-examination instruction and use are not recommended by either the VSPSTF or the CTF based on insufficient evidence for its effectiveness. The NCI considers BSE a supplement to but not a substitute for CBE and mammography due to limited evidence of value and does not suggest inclusion or exclusion of the exam in screening for breast cancer. The ACS and ACOG recommend routine instruction in BSE and the AAFP is reviewing its recommendations.

Follow-up of Positive Tests

BREAST LUMP

When a patient or clinician discovers a breast lump, an organized approach should be used to determine as quickly as possible whether the lump represents a breast cancer. A careful history and examination are the starting points. The history should establish how long the lump has been present, and whether it has changed in any way. A history of previous breast biopsy showing atypical hyperplasia, lobular carcinoma in situ or DCIS increases the likelihood of breast cancer, as does a history of carcinoma or of radiation treatment for Hodgkin's disease during childhood. Women with a strong family history are at greater risk of breast cancer. This risk also increases with age. Women in their 70s have breast cancer incidence rates that are 12 times higher than rates for women in their 30s. The absence of any of these risks on history does not rule out breast cancer, since most women in whom breast cancer is diagnosed have no identifiable risk factors. Conversely, most breast lumps turn out to be benign, even those occurring in women with common risk factors. The presence or absence of pain is not a good marker for the presence of breast cancer. While most breast cancers are painless, discomfort may be present, so the presence of pain or tenderness should not delay investigation.

Physical examination by a skilled clinician can provide valuable information. Benign lumps, such as those due to cysts or fibroadenomas, are smooth, well demarcated, and relatively mobile. Malignant masses are less smooth and less mobile, with poorly defined margins. Rubbery plaques that blend into surrounding tissues are usually benign zones of fibroglandular change. The latter will change if examined at different points in the menstrual cycle. Paget's disease of the nipple, when present, suggests an underlying breast cancer. This condition may resemble a benign dermatitis. The skin may be moist and eczematous, or dry and psoriatic, and is usually accompanied by some thickening of the underlying nipple or areola. The patient may report burning or itching. Biopsy is indicated if the condition fails to respond rapidly to topical treatment.

Physical examination will usually reveal a benign process as the cause of the lump. The most common of these are fibroadenoma, fibrocystic change, and benign cysts. Fibroadenomas and cysts feel very similar on palpation. Both are round, circumscribed, firm, and fairly moveable. Cysts may be tender, and the patient may report pain in the area. While cysts can be soft, they also can be quite hard when their fluid is under tension. Fibrocystic changes are usually accompanied by cyclical breast pain, which usually begins soon after ovulation, and intensifies until menses begins. The pain is often accompanied by a burning sensation, and may radiate to the shoulder or arm. Examination often reveals symmetric changes in both breasts, occurring most often in the upper outer quadrants. The affected tissue appears to blend into the more normal breast tissue without a clear line of demarcation, unlike malignancies, which have a discrete shape but an irregular and somewhat ill-defined border.

If red flags are present in the history, or if the physical examination reveals a discrete mass (even if it appears to be a benign mass) a breast imaging procedure should be ordered. The clinician needs to remember that failure to diagnose breast cancer is a leading cause of malpractice claims.

Mammography is the imaging procedure of choice for women over the age of 35. The mammogram can often clarify the nature of the lump, and can also provide information about the remainder of the breast and the opposite breast. Optimal imaging should therefore include two views of each breast with spot compression and magnification views of any abnormal area and of the area in question. Unfortunately, the sensitivity of mammography for a woman with a palpable breast tumor is rather low (only 82% in some studies). A normal mammogram therefore must not be considered to exclude a cancer, especially if cancer is suspected on clinical grounds.

Because younger women have more mammographically dense breasts, the procedure is less likely to give useful information. Breast ultrasound, in the hands of an experienced operator, can reliably differentiate cystic from solid lesions, and can therefore be helpful for younger women.

Fine needle aspiration (FNA) is a valuable adjunct to clinical evaluation and breast imaging. It can establish whether a lump is solid or cystic. If the tumor is solid, cells may be obtained for cytologic examination. FNA is a simple office procedure, and is virtually painless. When clear, straw-colored or gray-green fluid is obtained, and the mass disappears completely, the diagnosis is simple cyst. There is no need to send the fluid for cytology, since it is invariably normal. Bloody fluid, however, may indicate the presence of carcinoma with a cystic component, and this fluid should be sent for cytological evaluation. If no fluid is obtained, or a mass persists after fluid withdrawal, the same needle may be used to obtain a specimen for cytology. With an experienced operator and a pathologist experienced in cytology, FNA has a high accuracy rate (Table 13-7).

The combination of physical examination, mammography, and FNA has been referred to as the "triple test." The combination is highly sensitive (see Table 13-7). When all three indicate

Table 13-7

Accuracy of the Triple Test and Its Components

	SENSITIVITY	SPECIFICITY
Physical examination	89.0%	60.0%
Mammography	89.0%	73.0%
Fine-needle aspiration	93.0%	97.0%
Any one positive	100.0%	57.3%
All three positive	78.2%	98.4%

SOURCE: Kaufman et al.

benign disease, the probability of breast cancer is extremely low, and further investigation is unnecessary, although some physicians may feel it is prudent to follow such patients with periodic reexaminations. For younger women, ultrasound may be substituted for mammography in the triple test, with equivalent high sensitivity. As a refinement, each component of the triple test may be assigned 1, 2, or 3 points for a benign, suspicious, or malignant result. When this was done for a series of 259 women being evaluated for a breast mass, all patients with a score of 4 or less had benign lesions, whereas all those with scores of 6 or more had malignant disease.

Thermography and light scanning (a variation on transillumination also known as "diaphanoscopy") lack sensitivity and specificity, and have no role in screening or investigation of breast lumps. Magnetic resonance imaging may eventually play an important role. It is cumbersome, slow, and expensive, and should currently be used only in the context of a research project.

If any doubt remains at this point about whether a lump is benign or malignant, a core biopsy or open biopsy of the mass should be performed. The choice will depend on the experience, expertise, and preference of the examiner. Core biopsy is less invasive, but slightly less sensitive, especially for small lesions. In one study of 150 biopsies of palpable lumps, sensitivity was 89% overall, increasing to 94% for lesions over 2.5 cm diameter. For small, difficult to palpate lesions, stereotactic or ultrasound guided needle core biopsy can provide precise localization, with sensitivities ranging from 81% to 98.4% in different studies.

Since the presence of a breast lump can be a source of great anxiety to the patient, the workup should be accomplished as expeditiously as possible, with good communication and cooperation among the various clinicians. Good communication between patient and clinician can diminish immediate anxiety, and can lead to improved well being many months later. Full and sympathetic explanations, with time and encouragement of questions are important at each step of the process.

POSITIVE MAMMOGRAM

As with breast lumps detected by examination, radiographic abnormalities detected on screening mammography can be a source of anxiety for women. Any such abnormality therefore deserves a careful workup, including history and physical examination, further radiographic studies, and possibly needle aspiration or biopsy. The history and physical examination should follow the approach outlined above for the evaluation of a palpable breast lump. High quality diagnostic mammograms should be ordered to better define the extent and location of the abnormalities seen on the screening mammogram. Magnification and spot compression views are useful. Since both sensitivity and specificity of mammograms are highly dependent on the quality of the facility and its personnel, it is important to ensure that quality assurance standards are maintained. Previous films should be obtained if possible to see if there have been changes over time. The radiologist should be encouraged to provide a precise description of the abnormal features visualized as well as an estimate of the level of suspicion of cancer that they imply. The American College

of Radiology has suggested a standard classification scheme for mammograms, in which each finding is categorized into one of five grades (Table 13-8).

When there is any doubt, a second experienced radiologist should be consulted. Ultrasound examination can also be helpful in differentiating simple cysts from complex cysts or solid masses. Simple cysts can be drained under ultrasonic guidance, thus both diagnosing and treating the abnormality. Further workup will depend on the level of abnormality. The following suggestions assume that no red flags have been raised in the history and physical examination, and that the only abnormal finding is from a screening mammogram.

Category II abnormalities require no further investigation. Patients may not be reassured by the fact that the abnormality appears benign. Women have been shown to have persistent anxiety for as long as 18 months after receiving news of mammographic abnormalities. The clinician's skill in counseling and fully answering questions and concerns is critically important in these circumstances.

Category III abnormalities may be followed up by periodic mammography and clinical examination, since the probability of a malignancy is very small. In one follow up study of 543 such abnormalities, 3 patients eventually required biopsy, 2 of these were benign, and the other showed DCIS. While there are no studies to define optimal surveillance intervals,

Table 13-8

Mammogram Classification

I.	Negative
II.	Benign finding
III.	Probably benign
IV.	Suspicious abnormality
V.	Highly suggestive of malignant neoplasm

timing recommendations can be based upon our knowledge of tumor doubling time. Most breast cancers will show a change within 1 year, and very few remain stable for more than 2 years. This suggests that follow up examination at 6 and 12 months, with annual re-evaluations for the following 2–3 years should suffice. Women should be involved in making this decision after a full discussion of the risks, and an explanation that it is not possible to provide complete assurance that such an abnormality is benign. Some women may be uncomfortable with this approach and prefer to undergo immediate FNA or needle localization and open biopsy.

Category IV abnormalities usually require image-guided fine-needle or core biopsy. Fine needle aspiration and cytology (FNAC) under ultrasound guidance is minimally traumatic, and can give reliable information if perfomed by a skilled operator and the results are interpreted by an experienced cytologist. The technique has several limitations. Ultrasound does not allow visualization of very small carcinomas or those that appear as only microcalcifications on mammograms. FNAC cannot distinguish between invasive cancer and DCIS. Inadequate samples occur in up to 38% of attempts, although this problem decreases with increasing operator experience. FNAC sensitivity ranges from 68% to 93% and specificity from 88% to 100%. Core biopsy does not require special cytologic expertise, and may give a more definitive result. Sensitivities have ranged from 85% to 98%. Adverse effects, such as syncope, minor bleeding, hematoma, or infection are rare with either of these techniques.

Category V abnormalities should be excised, although excision can be preceded by image-guided needle biopsy in centers where this procedure has been proved to have high accuracy. The intact pathology specimen should be examined radiographically to confirm that all mammographic abnormalities have been removed.

Recommendations to Clinicians

HOW TO IMPROVE COMPLIANCE WITH RECOMMENDATIONS

It is clear that many women do not receive regular screening for breast cancer. This lack of screening occurs even when expert groups agree that the breast cancer prevention maneuver is beneficial and cost effective such as annual or biennial mammograms for women over 50. A telephone survey performed by the Centers for Disease Control and Prevention (CDC) in 1996–97 revealed that only 71% of women over 40 with medical insurance, and 46% of women with no insurance had received a mammogram during the prior 2 years. While these numbers represent an increase from those reported in similar studies 6 years earlier, the rates for uninsured women still fall short of the year 2000 goals which call for 60% of women over 50 to have received a mammogram within the preceding 2 years.

Physicians are more likely to recommend screening tests if they perceive them to be reliable, beneficial, and worth their costs to the patient. Other physician characteristics associated with performance of interventions are a group practice setting, HMO or IPA affiliation, and recent medical school graduation (lower rates of mammography recommendation are found in middle-aged physicians in solo practice). The higher rates among HMO physicians may be related to performance improvement feedback and other efforts by HMOs to make physicians aware of their compliance with guidelines.

Patients do not report cost as a barrier as much as physicians do. Patients do, however, perceive their physician's recommendation as a strong determinant of whether or not they will obtain a mammogram. The length of the patient-clinician relationship and the clinician's knowledge of the patient's socioeconomic circumstances and fears of the procedure also influence clinicians' recommendations. Patients' lack of knowledge about the need for mammography and concerns about the pain associated with it can be significant barriers.

Practice characteristics that influence prevention compliance include the medical record organization. Computer-generated or nurse-generated reminders affixed to the patient's chart at the time of a visit have positively correlated with performance of prevention interventions. Flow sheets and agreed upon practice standards have also been studied, but without reminders have not been as effective in generating compliance.

Health system barriers include the issue of reimbursement. Medicare coverage for mammograms in its first year had little impact on rates of mammography but as noted under physician issues, HMO association may have a favorable impact. Having multiple clinicians and requiring the need for a clinician to order tests may also decrease compliance with mammography recommendations.

The U.S. population is mobile and this sociocultural phenomenon accounts for some discontinous care and perhaps a lack of preventive health measures. Lack of health insurance also has been postulated as contributing towards poor mammography compliance.

With all these influences on the rate of screening mammography what can be done to increase its rate? First, clinicians must have access to rational analysis of the evidence that supports mammography screening through continuing education and must also be aware of their influence on patients' behavior by how they present the pros and cons of screening. If patients are to take part in the decision there must be patient education tools to explain the risks and merits in an unbiased, understandable manner that takes into account the patients' quality of life choices. Clinicians' offices must have medical record systems that provide reminders at the time of any visit that a mammo-

gram is due and a place to record test results as well as a system for appropriate management of the results. On the health policy level the government will need to continue to provide support for those with no insurance to obtain clinical breast exams and mammograms as has been done in the Centers for Disease Control and Prevention-funded National Breast and Cervical Cancer Early Detection Program. Performance improvement programs should be maintained that give feedback to clinicians regarding their successes and compliance rates with agreed upon prevention intervention.

HOW TO COUNSEL A PATIENT AND MAKE RECOMMENDATIONS

Clearly there is much uncertainty about the benefits and accompanying risks for many of the strategies being promoted for reduction of breast cancer risks. Clinicians counseling women must therefore be clear about these uncertainties, and the trade-offs involved. Clinicians must then honor women's personal choices and resist the urge to push their own preferences and biases. The record to date of the American medical establishment in providing this type of accurate, unbiased information about breast cancer is poor. American women in their 40s overestimate their personal risk of dying of breast cancer within the next 10 years by more than 20-fold, and the benefits of mammography by more than 100-fold. Clinicians can present a balanced approach, and incorporate patients preferences into cancer prevention by using a variety of strategies that change based on the availability of good evidence for benefit. Strong recommendations should be made only for interventions with a proven benefit and an acceptable risk. Even for these interventions, clinicians must be prepared to discuss potential benefits and harms, elicit patients values and preferences, and recognize the patient's right to decide how to proceed.

PREVENTIVE STRATEGIES SUPPORTED BY GOOD EVIDENCE

Mammography, with or without an accompanying breast exam by a skilled clinician, has been shown by several studies to reduce breast cancer mortality in women between 50 and 70 years of age. Clinicians should therefore encourage women in this age group to have regular mammograms and breast examinations. Encouragement by a trusted clinician is regularly cited by women as a powerful influence when deciding whether or not to have a mammorgram, and simply providing advice and reminders to do so will be effective with many women. If a woman in this age group is reluctant to have a mammogram or breast examination, it is important to explore her concerns and attempt to address them if possible. Many women find mammograms unpleasant and uncomfortable. For these women, sharing the information that trials of biennial mammography have had results that are very similar to trials using annual mammograms can be very helpful. Patients may agree to suffer the discomfort of a mammogram every 2 years—a distinct improvement over refusing to have a mammogram at all. Patients who absolutely refuse mammograms should be offered a clinical breast exam, particularly since the Canadian NBSS found no difference in cancer mortality rates for women screened with breast exam alone versus mammography plus breast exam.

Regular exercise is associated with lower breast cancer rates, and has additional benefits in prevention of coronary heart disease, hypertension, obesity, and diabetes. Based on this good evidence, clinicians should encourage regular exercise for their female patients. The "readiness for change" model provides a good framework for tailoring the recommendation to each patient's situation. Women in the "precontemplative" phase can be told of the multiple benefits of regular exercise. For women who have reached the "contemplation" phase but have not yet taken action, an exploration of the woman's perceptions of potential benefits and barriers can be helpful. Women in the "action" phase should be congratulated and encouraged to continue.

DEALING WITH INTERVENTIONS OF UNCERTAIN BENEFIT

None of the other breast cancer prevention strategies addressed in this chapter are supported by the solid evidence available for mammography for women in their 50s and for regular exercise. Breast self-examination and mammography for women under 50 allow discovery of smaller tumors, and tamoxifen leads to the development of fewer breast cancers, at least initially, among high-risk women. Unfortunately, none of these have been conclusively shown to reduce breast cancer mortality, and they all carry the potential for harmful or unpleasant results. The evidence for effectiveness of dietary modification is even weaker. Because of this uncertainty, it is totally inappropriate for clinicians to pressure women to adopt any of these potentially helpful practices. The clinician's proper role in these cases, is to present the evidence clearly to the patient, and allow each woman to make her own decision. This suggestion has been mocked by those who ask how a woman can be expected to make such a decision when experts cannot agree on the interpretation of the various studies, even after much debate. This argument completely misses the point. There is no expectation that a woman should restrict herself to scientific logic in this process. Since the scientists cannot provide unequivocal answers, it is quite appropriate for a woman to use other, more personal means to make her own decision. She may be strongly influenced by fears about cancer or about the procedures involved, by stories from friends or family members about their experiences with cancer or with prevention, by concerns about the financial burdens involved with some of the strategies, or simply by a tendency to procrastinate. Any of these, or any other factor which she finds important is fair game. The clinician's role is to provide unbiased information, answer questions, attempt to be certain that the woman understands the issues involved, and to then support her in her decision.

In presenting numerical information about risks to patients, the concepts of "Number Needed to Treat (NNT)" or "Number Needed to Harm (NNH)" can be very helpful. The NNT, as the name implies, is an estimate of the number of patients who would need to have a preventive strategy in order to achieve one additional beneficial outcome. The NNT can be calculated from a randomized trial by taking the inverse of the difference between the proportion of patients in the intervention group who have a particular outcome event and the proportion in the control group who have a similar event. For example, the NNT for a mammogram trial would be calculated as:

> NNT = 1/(the rate of breast cancer deaths in the control group minus the rate of breast cancer deaths in the group offered regular mammograms).

For women under 50, this NNT is 2,500 (assuming annual screening throughout the 40s). By contrast, the NNT for women aged 50–69 receiving regular mammography is 270. For adverse effects (such as false positives), we can calculate a number needed to harm (NNH), in exactly the same way. A woman who has 10 annual mammograms has a 30%–50% chance of having at least one false positive report. Thus the NNH is between 2 and 3.

As an alternative, potential risks and benefits can be presented in terms of a hypothetical large group of similar women. For example, the data on risks and benefits of a single mammogram for a woman under the age of 50 can be summarized as "If 10,000 such women have a mammogram, 640 of them will be told that the test is abnormal; 1280 additional follow up tests of some sort will be performed on these 640 women, including 150 breast biopsies. Seventeen of the women will turn out to have invasive breast cancer, and one may have her death from breast cancer prevented." Whenever possible, it is important to present such material as whole numbers, rather than as rates or proportions, which are more difficult for patients (and clinicians) to understand. Pictorial representations of these data may be helpful as well. When men considering the decision about whether to have PSA screening had additional information presented in one of these formats, they became significantly less interested in having the test. Surprisingly, no studies of the effects of offering this type of informed choice to women have been done.

Common Errors

FAILURE TO BIOPSY IF THE MAMMOGRAM IS NEGATIVE

An unfortunate by-product of the hype surrounding screening mammography has been an overestimation by clinicians and patients of the ability of this test to diagnose cancer when it is present (sensitivity). In fact, the sensitivity of a mammogram is so low that up to 20% to 30% of cancers may be missed. Studies in which both CBE and mammography were used to screen for breast cancer have consistently found that many of the cancers discovered by examination were not apparent on the mammogram. This is particularly true for women under 50. While the sensitivity of mammography has improved, it is still not high enough to exclude cancer in a lump that is felt by a clinician to be suspicious, and a fine needle aspiration or a biopsy should be performed on all such suspicious lumps.

PERFORMING BRCA TESTING

As noted above, BRCA testing raises a host of difficult issues, requiring careful patient counseling and informed consent. Clinicians may be tempted to order BRCA testing for a patient with a family history of breast cancer, but these urges should be resisted. Patients wishing to be tested should be encouraged to enroll in a clinical study where the issues of ethical testing, confidentiality, and informed consent can be dealt with in depth.

FAILURE TO CONSIDER THE PSYCHOSOCIAL CONSEQUENCES OF PREVENTIVE INTERVENTIONS

The intense focus on breast cancer prevention in this country has left women feeling excessively vulnerable to the disease. The resulting anxiety may take extreme forms for some women. These anxieties are heightened by positive test results, particularly for women who have not been prepared for the high probability that a positive test may occur, and the low predictive value if it does. There have been reports of suicides following receipt of a positive mammogram report. Clinicians also tend to underestimate their patients remaining concerns after a positive test has been shown to be false positive. In one study, women were contacted 3 months after a negative workup following a mammogram that was initially interpreted as "high suspicion of malignancy." Even though these women had known for 3 months that they did not have breast cancer, 26% reported that worries about breast cancer still had a negative effect on their mood, and 17% reported that these worries continued to affect their functioning. Clinicians counseling women about breast cancer prevention must warn them of the possibility of false positive tests, move as quickly as possible in the investigation of positives when they occur, and continue to be open to discussions about concerns and anxieties, even among women whose positive screening tests have been shown to be false positives.

LOSING SIGHT OF THE WHOLE PATIENT

In caring for women, it is important that clinicians avoid the trap of viewing a woman's health from the sole perspective of breast disease. Given our culture's overemphasis on the risks of breast cancer in women, it is easy to lose sight of the many other significant health problems for which women are at risk. Keeping this broader perspective is particularly important when preventive interventions are considered. Advice about HRT and alcohol consumption provide two examples of situations in which an analysis of risks involving breast cancer alone would lead to the opposite conclusions from an analysis looking at overall health. A clinician using risks of breast cancer alone would advise women to abstain completely from alcohol, since even moderate alcohol intake is associated with an increased breast cancer risk. A more holistic clinician would note that mortality rates for women with moderate alcohol intake (<0.9 drinks per day) are actually less than mortality rates for teetotalers. In the case of HRT, a small increase in breast cancer risk is balanced by a much larger decrease in the risk of osteoporosis and a possible benefit for cardiovascular disease.

TEACHING BSE TO WOMEN UNDER THE AGE OF 30

The value of BSE in women aged 40 or older is unknown, and is still being investigated. In younger women, breast cancer rates are much lower, and rates of benign conditions such as fibroadenoma and breast cysts are much higher. Thus, the possibility that BSE will lead to benefit in these women is quite remote, and the chance for harm resulting from false positives and their subsequent investigation is much higher. Opportunities for prevention in young women should not be wasted, but the opportunity should be used to discuss exercise, smoking cessation, or other issues likely to make a real difference in the woman's health and longevity.

Emerging Approaches to Breast Cancer Prevention

Genetic Testing

In the past decade, our understanding of cancer at the molecular and genetic level has grown immensely. The two breast cancer genes currently known (BRCA1&2) are likely to be only the first of many such genes. The soon to be completed Human Genome Project is likely to escalate the pace of these discoveries even more. Unfortunately, genetic testing is unlikely to be a useful strategy for the majority of women. Genetic testing would be useful if it could either identify a group of women whose risk was so low that they could ignore the possibility of breast cancer completely or if it could direct a subset of women to participate in effective early detection or preventive interventions. Breast cancer is a multifactorial disease, and it is unlikely that the majority of cases are due to specific inherited mutations. Thus, genetic testing is unlikely ever to be able to identify a group of very low risk women. On the other hand, as noted in our discussion of BRCA testing, it is not clear that women identified as high risk have received benefits from this knowledge.

Risk Factor Modification

As noted in the section on primary prevention, much uncertainty remains about the role of lifestyle factors in breast cancer. Ongoing

research efforts may well clarify this picture in the future. One such trial, the Women's Health Initiative (WHI) is a multi-method endeavor to assess the effects of HRT and dietary modification on risks of breast cancer, heart disease, osteoporosis, and colorectal cancer. As a part of this study, 64,500 postmenopausal women will be enrolled in a randomized trial, and 100,000 additional women will be studied in an observational study over an 8- to 12-year period. Quality of life, social support, symptoms, and sexuality will all be included among the assessed outcomes.

Chemoprevention

The recently reported trials of chemoprevention with tamoxifen will soon be followed by a number of similar trials. Three studies of tamoxifen are currently under way in Europe. While smaller than the recently reported U.S. study, they will provide longer follow up and include a more diverse group of women. They may be able to provide additional information about risks and benefits of this approach, allowing women to be more informed before they decide whether or not to start this drug. In the U.S., the STAR trial will provide a randomized comparison of tamoxifen versus raloxifen as chemopreventive agents. We can expect a number of other anti-estrogenic compounds to be tested as well. Whether any will provide greater benefits or lower risks than tamoxifen remains to be seen.

Screening Tests

Increasing technical proficiency holds out the promise for mammography units which can detect ever-smaller lesions. This increase in sensitivity may well be accompanied by a decrease in specificity, with a greater number of benign lesions being questioned and biopsied. The rate of detection of DCIS is likely to continue to grow with this new technology, leading to more biopsies, lumpectomies, and mastectomies. Other imaging techniques (such as ultrasound or MRI) are increasingly used in the investigation of suspicious breast lumps or mammographic abnormalities. None has been shown as yet to be as effective as mammography in early cancer detection. Any claims for effectiveness of such new technology would need to be supported by long-term randomized trials, such as the ones which have demonstrated the effectiveness of mammograms for women aged 50–70.

With all of our current knowledge of breast cancer and its prevention, there still exist major areas of controversy, uncertainty, and disagreement. The possible future developments outlined above have the potential to increase this uncertainty even more. There is therefore clear need for women to be aggressive in their efforts to obtain good information and to make their own decisions, incorporating their own beliefs and values. Those counseling women about breast cancer prevention will need to remain knowledgeable and up to date about the issues, and sensitive to women's preferences and values.

Bibliography

Andersson I, Janzon L: Reduced breast cancer mortality in women under age 50: updated results from the Malmo Mammographic Screening Program. *Journal of the National Cancer Institute Monographs* 63–67, 1997.

Baines CJ, Miller AB: Mammography versus clinical examination of the breasts. [Review]. *Journal of the National Cancer Institute Monographs*, 125–129, 1997.

Baines CJ: Reflections on breast self-examination [editorial; comment]. *J Natl Cancer Inst* 89:339–340, 1997.

Beam CA, Layde PM, Sullivan DC: Variability in the interpretation of screening mammograms by U.S. radiologists: Findings from a national sample. *Arch Intern Med* 156:209–213, 1996.

Black WC, Nease RF Jr, Tosteson AN: Perceptions of breast cancer risk and screening effectiveness in women younger than 50 years of age. *J Natl Cancer Inst* 87:720–731, 1995.

Brown J, Bryan S, Warren R: Mammography screening: an incremental cost effectiveness analysis of double versus single reading of mammograms. *BMJ* 312:809–812, 1996.

Brown ML, Houn F, Sickles EA, Kessler LG: Screening mammography in community practice: positive predictive value of abnormal findings and yield of follow-up diagnostic procedures. *Am J Roentgenol* 165:1373–1377, 1995.

Canadian Association of Radiation Oncologists, The Steering Committee on Clinical Practice Guidelines for the Care and Treatment of Breast Cancer. The management of ductal carcinoma in situ (DCIS). *Can Med Assoc J* 158(Suppl.3):S24–S34, 1998.

Centers for Disease Control and Prevention: Self-reported use of mammography and insurance status among women aged > or = 40 years—United States 1991–1992 and 1996–1997. *JAMA* 280(22): 1900–1901, 1998.

Chu KC, Tarone RE, Kessler LG, et al: Recent trends in U.S. breast cancer incidence, survival, and mortality rates. *J Natl Cancer Inst* 88:1571–1579, 1996.

Collaborative Group on Hormonal Factors in Breast Cancer: Breast cancer and hormonal replacement therapy: collaborative reanalysis of data from 51 epidemiologic studies of 52,705 women with breast cancer and 108,411 women without breast cancer. *Lancet* 350(9084): 1047–1059, 1997.

Collaborative Group on Hormonal Factors in Breast Cancer: Breast cancer and hormonal contraceptives: collaborative reanalysis of individual data on 53,297 women with breast cancer and 100,239 women without breast cancer from 54 epidemiological studies. *Lancet* 347(9017):1713–1727, 1996.

Costanza ME, Stoddard AM, Zapka JG, Gaw V, Barth R: Physician compliance with mammography guidelines: barriers and enhancers. *J Am Board Fam Pract* 5(2):143–152, 1992.

Eeles R, Cole T, Taylor R, Lunt P, Baum M: Prophylactic mastectomy for genetic predisposition to breast cancer: the proband's story. *Clin Oncol* 8(4):222–225, 1996.

Elmore JG, Barton MB, Moceri VM, Polk S, Arena PJ, Fletcher SW: Ten-year risk of false positive screening mammograms and clinical breast examinations [see comments]. *N Engl J Med* 338:1089–1096, 1998.

Epstein SA, Lin TH, Audrain J, Stefanek M, Rimer B, Lerman C: Excessive breast self-examination among first-degree relatives of newly diagnosed breast cancer patients. High-Risk Breast Cancer Consortium. *Psychosomatics* 38(3):253–261, 1997.

Ernster VL, Barclay MS, Kerlikowske K, Grady D, Henderson C: Incidence of and treatment for Ductal Carcinoma in Situ of the Breast. *JAMA* 275(12): 913–918, 1996.

Feuer EJ, Wun LM, Boring CC, et al: The lifetime risk of developing breast cancer. *J Natl Cancer Inst* 85(11):892–897, 1993.

Fisher B, et al: Tamoxifen for prevention of breast cancer: Report of the National Surgical Adjuvant Breast and Bowel Project. *J Natl Cancer Inst* 90: 1371–1388, 1998.

Freudenheim JL, Marshall JR, Vena JE, Laughlin R, Brasure JR, Swanson MK, et al: Premenopausal breast cancer risk and intake of vegetables, fruits, and related nutrients. *J Natl Cancer Inst* 88:340–348, 1996.

Frisell J, Lidbrink E: The Stockholm Mammographic Screening Trial: Risks and benefits in age group 40–49 years. *J Natl Cancer Inst Monogr* 49–51, 1997.

Gammon MD, John EM, Britton JA: Recreational and occupational physical activities and risk of breast cancer [Review] [107 refs]. *J Natl Cancer Inst* 90: 100–117, 1998.

Grann VR, Panageas KS, Whang W, Antman KH, Neugut AI: Decision analysis of prophylactic mastectomy and oophorectomy in BRCA1-positive or BRCA2-positive patients. *J Clin Oncol* 16(3):979–985, 1998.

Harris J, Hellman S: Natural History of Breast Cancer. Lippincott-Raven, 1996.

Hartmann LC, Schaid DJ, Woods JE, Crotty TP, Myers JL, Arnold PG, et al: Efficacy of bilateral prophylactic mastectomy in women with a family history of breast cancer. *N Engl J Med* 340:77–84, 1999.

Harvey BJ, Miller AB, Baines CJ, Corey PN: Effect of breast self-examination techniques on the risk of death from breast cancer [see comments]. *Can Med Assoc J* 157:1205–1212, 1997.

Hendrick RE, Smith RA, Rutledge JH 3rd, Smart CR: Benefit of screening mammography in women aged 40–49: a new meta-analysis of randomized controlled trials. *J Natl Cancer Inst Monogr* 87–92, 1997.

Holman CD, English DR, Milne E, Winter MG: Meta-analysis of alcohol and all cause mortality: a validation of NHMRC recommendations. *Med J Aust* 164(3):141–145, 1996.

Hoskins KF, Stopfer JE, Calzone KA, Merajver DS, Rebbeck TR, Garber JE, et al: Assessment and counseling for women with a family history of breast cancer. A guide for clinicians. *JAMA* 273(7): 577–585, 1995.

Hulka BS, Stark AT: Breast cancer: cause and prevention. [Review]. *Lancet* 346:883–887, 1995.

Hunter DJ, Spiegelman D, Adami HO, Beeson L, van den Brandt PA, Folsom AR, et al: Cohort studies of fat intake and the risk of breast cancer—a pooled analysis. *N Engl J Med* 334:356–361, 1996.

Kaufman Z, Shpitz B, Shapiro M, Rona R, Lew S, Dinbar A: Triple approach in the diagnosis of dominant breast masses: combined physical examination, mammography, and fine-needle aspiration. *J Surg Oncol* 56:254–257, 1994.

Kerlikowske C, Grady D, Barclay J, Sickles E, Ernster V: Likelihood Ratios for Modern Screening Mammography. *JAMA* 276:39–43, 1996.

Kerlikowske K, Grady D, Barclay J, Sickles EA, Ernster V: Effect of age, breast density, and family history on the sensitivity of first screening mammography. *JAMA* 276:33–38, 1996.

La Vecchia C, Negri E, Franceschi S, Decarli A, Giacosa A, Lipworth L: Olive oil, other dietary fats, and the risk of breast cancer (Italy). *Cancer Causes Control* 6:545–550, 1995.

Landis SH, Murray T, Bolden S, et al: Cancer Statistics. *Cancer J Clin* 48(1):6–29, 1998.

Lerman C, Trock B, Rimer BK, Boyce A, Jepson C, Engstrom PF: Psychological and behavioral implications of abnormal mammograms. *Ann Intern Med* 114:657–661, 1991.

Longnecker MP: Alcoholic beverage consumption in relation to risk of breast cancer: meta-analysis and review. *Cancer Causes Control* 5(1):73–82, 1994.

Lynch HT, Lemon SJ, Durham C, Tinley ST, Connolly C, Fynch JF, et al: A descriptive study of BRCA1 testing and reactions to disclosure of test results. *Cancer* 79(11):2219–2228, 1997.

Madigan MP, Ziegler RG, Benichou J, Hoover RN: Proportion of breast cancer cases in the United States explained by well-established risk factors. *J Natl Cancer Inst* 87(22):1681–1685, 1995.

Martin-Moreno JM, Willett WC, Gorgojo L, Banegas JR, Rodriguez-Artalejo F, Fernandez-Rodriguez JC, et al: Dietary fat, olive oil intake and breast cancer risk. *Intl J Cancer* 58:774–780, 1994.

Mathews KA, Shumaker SA, Bowen DJ, Langer RD, Hunt JR, Kaplan RM, et al: Women's health initiative: Why now? What is it? What's new? *Am Psychol* 52(2):101–116, 1997.

McQuay HJ, Moore RA: Using numerical results from systematic reviews in clinical practice. *Ann Intern Med* 126:712–720, 1997.

Morimoto T, Komaki K, Mori T, et al: The quality of mass screening for breast cancer by physical examination. *Surg Today* 23:200–204, 1993.

Mushlin AI, Kouides RW, Shapiro DE: Estimating the accuracy of screening mammography: a meta-analysis. *Am J Prev Med* 14(2):143–153, 1998.

Newcomb PA, Weiss NS, Storer BE, Scholes D, Young BE, Voigt LF: Breast self-examination in relation to the occurrence of advanced breast cancer. *J Natl Cancer Inst* 83:260–265, 1991.

NIH Consensus Statement: Breast cancer screening for women ages 40–49. *J Natl Cancer Inst* 89:1015–1020, 1997.

Pommier RF, Schmidt WA, Shih RL, Alexander PW, Vetto JT: Accurate evaluation of palpable breast masses by the triple test score. *Arch Surg* 133(9):930–934, 1998.

Prentice RL: Measurement error and results from analytic epidemiology: dietary fat and breast cancer. *J Natl Cancer Inst* 88:1738–1747, 1996.

Pritchard KI: Is tamoxifen effective in prevention of breast cancer? *Lancet* 352(9122):80–81, 1998.

Rohan TE, Howe GR, Friedenreich CM, Jain M, Miller AB: Dietary fiber, vitamins A, C, and E, and risk of breast cancer: a cohort study. *Cancer Causes Control* 4:29–37, 1993.

Rosenberg L, Metzger LS, Palmer JR: Alcohol Consumption and Risk of Breast Cancer: a review of the epidemiologic evidence. *Epidemiol Rev* 15(1):133, 1993.

Schrag D, Kuntz KM, Garber JE, Weeks JC: Decision analysis: Effects of Prophylactic Mastectomy and Oophorectomy on Life Expectancy among Women with BRCA1 or BRCA2 Mutations. *N Engl J Med* 336(20):1464–1471, 1997.

Semiglazov VF, Moiseenko VM, Protsenko SA, Bavli IL, Orlov AA, Ivanova OA, et al: Preliminary results of the Russia (St. Petersburg)/WHO program for the evaluation of the effectiveness of breast self-examination. *Vopr Onkol* 42(4):49–55, 1996.

Thomas DB, Gao DL, Self SG, Allison CJ, Tao Y, Mahloch J, et al: Randomized trial of breast self-examination in Shanghai: methodology and preliminary results. *J Natl Cancer Inst* 89(5):355–365, 1997.

U.S. Preventive Services Task Force. Guide to Clinical Preventive Services, 2d ed. Baltimore, MD, Williams & Wilkins, 1996.

Vetto JT, Pommier RF, Schmidt WA, Eppich H, Alexander PW: Diagnosis of palpable breast lesions in younger women by the modified triple test is accurate and cost-effective. *Arch Surg* 131:967–972. discussion 972–974, 1996.

Walker AR, Walker BF, Stelma S: Is breast cancer avoidable? Could dietary changes help? [Review]. [78 refs] *Intl J Food Sci Nutr* 46:373–381, 1995.

Weil JG, Hawker JI: Positive findings of mammography may lead to suicide. *BMJ* 314(7082):754–755, 1997.

Willett WC, Hunter DJ, Stampfer MJ, Colditz G, Manson JE, Spiegelman D, et al: Dietary fat and fiber in relation to risk of breast cancer: An 8-year follow-up. *JAMA* 268:2037–2044, 1992.

Wolf A, Nasser JF, Wolf AM, Schorling JB: The Impact of Informed Consent on Patient Interest in Prostate-Specific Antigen Screening. *Arch Intern Med* 156:1333–1336, 1996.

Chapter

14

Prostate Cancer

Introduction

How Common Is Prostate Cancer?

Prostate cancer is the most common cancer in men, comprising 29% of all cancers in American men (excluding basal and squamous cell skin cancers) in 1999. It is the second most common cause of cancer mortality among men, responsible for 13% of male cancer deaths and exceeded only by lung cancer, which causes 31% of cancer deaths in men. In 1999 estimates predict 179,000 new cases of prostate cancer and 37,000 deaths. Prostate cancer will develop in one of every six men living to age 80. The incidence of prostate cancer increases markedly with age.

Table 14-1 describes the proportion of U.S. men in three different age groups who will get prostate cancer. Prostate cancer will develop in less than 2% of men between the ages of 40 and 59 years versus close to 15% of men between the ages of 60 and 79. Table 14-1 also illustrates that 86% of men who get prostate cancer do so after the age of 60 years.

TIME TRENDS

The age-adjusted prostate cancer incidence rate increased in the United States from 1973 to 1992, with sharp increases from 1987 to 1992 (from 105/100,000 in 1987 to 195/100,000 in 1992). Between 1992 and 1995, the rate declined to 140/100,000. These trends probably indicate a better rate of detection through improved prostate cancer screening beginning in the late 1980s. Screening may have detected a pool of asymptomatic prostate cancers, exhausting this pool by the early 1990s. During the same time period (1992 to1995), the age-adjusted prostate cancer mortality rate declined from 24 to 20 per 100,000.

RACIAL/ETHNIC DIFFERENCES

There are marked racial/ethnic differences in the United States for prostate cancer incidence and mortality (Table 14-2). African American men have the highest incidence rates and mortality rates, whereas American Indians have the lowest incidence rates and Asians/Pacific Islanders have the lowest mortality rates for prostate cancer. The reasons for these differences are unknown.

INTERNATIONAL COMPARISONS

Worldwide statistics also demonstrate the significance of prostate cancer: there are close to 400,000 new cases and 165,000 deaths attributed to prostate cancer each year. The incidence in

Table 14-1

Proportion of Men in Whom Prostate Cancer Develops at Certain Ages

AGE	% IN WHOM PROSTATE CANCER DEVELOPS
Birth to 39 years	<0.0001
40 to 59 years	1.83
60 to 79 years	14.79
Birth to death	17.00

SOURCE: From Landis et al., 1999.

developed countries tends to be higher than in developing countries (Table 14-3), in part owing to improved rates of screening and detection of asymptomatic prostate cancers in developing countries. The mortality rates by country show less marked differences, providing evidence that many of the asymptomatic prostate cancers detected by screening do not cause death (a subject that will be discussed more under Natural History of Prostate Cancer). For instance, the prostate cancer incidence in North America is 92.4/100,000, and in China it is 1.1/100,000; the mortality rates in these two countries are 18.5/100,000 and 0.7/100,000, respectively (Parker et al., 1999).

Risk Factors

As just described, age and race are two risk factors for prostate cancer; older men and African American men are at higher risk. Family history of prostate cancer also is a risk factor, and one form of hereditary prostate cancer has been associated with earlier age at onset and possibly more aggressive tumors (Gronberg, 1997). There is some evidence that farmers, mechanics, sheet metal workers, and workers exposed to cad-

Table 14-2

Prostate Cancer Incidence and Mortality Rates for U.S. Men, 1990–1995

	INCIDENCE PER 100,000 MEN[a]	MORTALITY PER 100,000 MEN[a]
Caucasians	150.3	24.1
African Americans	224.3	55.0
Asians/Pacific Islanders	82.2	10.9
American Indians	46.4	14.2
Hispanics	104.4	16.8

[a] Age adjusted.
SOURCE: From Landis et al., 1999.

mium and rubber manufacturing may have higher risks of prostate cancer (Carter et al., 1989). There is conflicting evidence about the risk of vasectomy in prostate cancer, with one cohort study finding a 1.56 relative risk for men who had vasectomies (Giovannocci et al., 1993). Benign prostatic hyperplasia does not appear to be a prostate cancer risk. There are, therefore, no firmly established, modifiable risk factors for prostate cancer (with the possible exception of vasectomy). This leaves us without a strategy for primary prevention of prostate cancer.

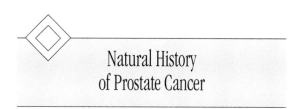

Natural History of Prostate Cancer

Table 14-3

Prostate Cancer Incidence by Country or World Region

COUNTRY/REGION	INCIDENCE PER 100,000 POPULATION
North America	92.4
Australia	49.7
Caribbean	42.4
Western Europe	39.6
Southern Africa	31.0
Tropical South America	28.1
Central America	24.8
Southern Europe	16.9
Japan	8.5
Western Asia	7.1
China	1.1

SOURCE: From Parker, et al., 1999.

The natural history of prostate cancer varies, spanning the spectrum from very slow growing and indolent to rapidly progressing and aggressive. The stages of prostate cancer are listed in Table 14-4 along with the 5-year survival rates for each stage. The time for progression from one stage to another varies considerably. Most men with prostate cancer do not die of the disease or suffer markedly from it. Latent, microscopic disease exists in approximately 30% of men age 50 years or older and in over 50% of men age 80 years or older; most cases are asymptomatic. In one study of a cohort of Swedish men with prostate cancer, after 12 years 10% had died from prostate cancer, and 56% had died from other causes (Johansson,

Table 14-4

Prostate Cancer Stages and Survival Rates

STAGE	DESCRIPTION	5-YR SURVIVAL
A	Nonpalpable	87%
A1	Well differentiated or three or fewer foci	
A2	Poorly differentiated or more than three foci	
B	Palpable, confined to the gland	81%
B1	<1.5 cm and one lobe	
B2	>1.5 cm or involving more than one lobe	
C	Local extension beyond the capsule	64%
D	Metastatic spread	30%
D1	Lymph node involvement only below aortic bifurcation	
D2	Lymph node involvement above the aortic bifurcation or distant metastasis to other sites	

SOURCE: From Mettlin et al., 1993.

1997). Slavin and colleagues (1995) have examined epidemiologic data and conclude that a 50-year-old man has a 42% chance that histologic signs of prostate cancer will develop, a 9.5% risk of experiencing clinical symptoms of prostate cancer, and a 2.9% chance of dying from the disease.

Wasson and colleagues (1993) studied 144 articles on prostate cancer and estimated that the annual risk of metastasis from untreated prostate cancer is low. Only 1.7% of such cancers metastasized, and the annual risk of death was 0.9%. Symptoms of prostate cancer include urinary hesitancy, poor urine stream, nocturia, and dribbling. These symptoms, however, are nonspecific—they are present in many men who have benign prostatic hyperplasia, urethral stricture, and other conditions. Metastasis of prostate cancer is most commonly to the liver, bone, lungs, and lymph nodes. Metastatic disease is frequently first detected because of bone pain.

Treatment of Prostate Cancer and Its Effectiveness

Treatment for prostate cancer includes prostatectomy, radiation therapy, hormone therapy, chemotherapy, and a combination of these methods. Hormone therapy is used because growth of prostate cells depends on testosterone. There are three types: orchiectomy to remove the source of testosterone; administration of diethylstilbesterol or luteinizing hormone-releasing hormone analogues to lower testosterone levels, and therapy with anti-androgens to block androgen uptake and receptor binding. There is no consensus as to which therapy is best. In 1990, 27% of stage B tumors were treated with prostatectomy, 41% with radiation, 9% with hormone therapy, 6% with combination therapy, and 17% with no therapy (Mettlin et al., 1993). Prostatectomy is used more frequently for stages B and C; radiation therapy for stages A, B, and C; and hormone therapy for stages C and D. Chemotherapy is not frequently used.

At present there is no direct evidence that treatment of prostate cancer results in improved outcomes. Support for therapy comes mainly from observational, uncontrolled reports. Several large clinical trials are in progress, with results expected in the next 5 to 10 years. The side effects of therapy can be significant. Prostatectomy results in urinary incontinence in up to 27%, impotence stemming from erectile dysfunction in 20% to 85%, as well as other complications (Table 14-5). Radiation therapy is also associated with significant morbidity (Table 14-5). Because of the lack of evidence for effectiveness of treatment and the side effects of treatment, no treatment is the preferred option for stage A and is also frequently chosen by patients with stage B.

Table 14-5

Complications of Prostate Cancer Treatments

TREATMENT AND COMPLICATION	%
Prostatectomy	
Impotence	20–85
Incontinence	1–27
Urethral stricture	10–18
Thromboembolism	2–30
Death	0.6
Radiation	
Gastrointestinal complications	3–67
Impotence	40–67
Urethral or bladder complications	3–17
Anorectal complications	2–23

SOURCE: From Woolf, 1995

Secondary Prevention

Screening Tests

There are three screening tests currently available for the early detection of prostate cancer: digital rectal examination (DRE), serum prostate-specific antigen (PSA), and transrectal ultrasound (TRUS).

DIGITAL RECTAL EXAMINATION

DRE is the oldest method of detecting prostate cancer. The DRE is relatively easy to perform and has no major complications. It has limited value, however, in that the clinician can examine only the posterior and lateral sides of the gland. Moreover, stage A tumors are nonpalpable. Several reviews have listed the sensitivity of DRE at 55% to 68%, with a positive predictive value of 6% to 33% (USPSTF, 1996; Ferrini and Wolf, 1998).

SERUM PROSTATE-SPECIFIC ANTIGEN

The serum tumor marker PSA is the most studied screening test to date. With a cutoff of 4.0 mg/dL, the test has a reported sensitivity of 29% to 80%. It appears to have a higher sensitivity for tumors that have characteristics associated with progressive disease. The positive predictive value is 28% to 35%. Prostatitis and benign prostatic hyperplasia can cause a false-positive PSA test. A DRE appears not to affect the test. There have been a number of studies using variations of the PSA test in attempts to decrease the number of false-positive results. The PSA test in conjunction with a DRE (both needing to abnormal) increases the positive predictive value to 49%. This result, however, still calls for biopsy in 18% of those screened (Catalona et al., 1994).

Other methods under investigation to improve the specificity and positive predictive value of PSA testing include calculating PSA density by dividing the PSA level by the prostate gland volume, as measured by TRUS; measuring PSA velocity as a rate of change in the PSA year to year; using age-adjusted reference levels and cutoffs; and measuring the free PSA ratio. The free PSA ratio is the ratio of free to complex PSA (prostate cancer being associated more frequently with a ratio of less than 25%). The future of these different methods as either primary screening tools or secondary confirmatory tests is unclear.

TRANSRECTAL ULTRASOUND

Ultrasound has limited utility as a screening test because of lack of acceptability on the part of patients and high cost. The sensitivity of TRUS as a screening tool is 57% to 68%, with a 5% to 31% positive predictive value. It is considered a useful tool for follow-up of abnormal DRE or PSA screening tests, not as a first-line screening test.

Follow-up of Abnormal Test Results

The confirmatory tests available to follow up abnormal DRE or PSA tests are TRUS and needle biopsy. There are no generally accepted guidelines as to when to perform either test. A nodule found on DRE will generally be submitted for biopsy. An abnormal DRE along with an elevated PSA level will also usually result in biopsy. An elevated PSA level in conjunction with a normal DRE may be grounds for another PSA test, an ultrasound and biopsy, or an ultrasound test with biopsy of suspicious masses. Transrectal needle biopsy is the usual method of biopsy. It has a low complication rate but can cause infection (0.3% to 5% of patients), sepsis (0.6%), and bleeding (0.1%) (USPSTF, 1996).

Evidence That Screening and Early Treatment Improves or Does Not Improve Outcomes

Since there is no evidence that prostate cancer treatment improves outcomes, it follows that screening and early treatment also lacks proof of effectiveness. There are several large clinical trials in progress studying this issue, and results are expected in 5 to 10 years. There is, however, indirect evidence that the increased screening that took place in the early 1990s might have had some effect, because prostate cancer mortality declined 11.2% between 1991 and 1995 (Smart, 1997). This improvement occurred uniformly across the country, even though screening rates varied, indicating that some other variable might be the cause.

Screening detects cancers in earlier stages, but this does not necessarily translate into improved outcomes if treatment is not effective. Collins and Barry (1996) point out that medicine faced a similar situation several decades ago with regard to lung cancer screening, which eventually proved to be of no benefit. Since evidence for effectiveness of prostate cancer screening does not exist, there are no data to assist in deciding at what age to start screening, at what age to stop, or even the appropriate frequency of screening.

Screening Recommendations

Formerly there were major disagreements in recommendations regarding prostate cancer screening, but these disagreements have abated markedly since 1997. Before then the American Cancer Society (ACS) recommended annual DRE and PSA for men age 50 years and older who have at least a 10-year life expectancy, and earlier screening for African American men and those with two or more first-degree relatives with prostate cancer. In 1997 the ACS changed their recommendation by stating that the PSA test and DRE should be offered annually and that men should be given information on the benefits and risks of screening. The American Urological Association agrees with the ACS position. The American College of Physicians and the American Academy of Family Physicians recommend providing information to men to help them make a decision based on their personal situation and preferences. The U.S. Preventive Services Task Force, the Canadian Task Force on the Periodic Health Examination, and the American College of Preventive Medicine recommend against routine screening.

Recommendations to Clinicians

Be Familiar with the Data

Clinicians should stay abreast of the prostate cancer-screening debate and informed about evidence regarding treatment and screening as it develops; they should be prepared to discuss this topic with their male patients. Clinicians should attempt to remain factual and unbiased as they present information to patients and discuss options with them.

Make Available Unbiased and Factual Information

Printed material that presents facts about known benefits and harmful effects of screening can assist clinicians to present an unbiased view of both sides of the screening debate. Hahn and Roberts (1993) have prepared a fact sheet for this purpose.

Assess the Patient's Preferences

Just as health professionals presented with the same information on prostate cancer screening cannot agree on recommendations, patients are also likely to have differences of opinion based on their own life circumstances, family histories, beliefs about screening, and preferences for treatment. Clinicians can assist patients to decide about screening by discussing with them the options for follow-up and treatment should a screening test result be positive.

Patients Who Have Positive Test Results

It is common for men to appear in a clinician's office with positive PSA test results in hand, having received a screening test in the office of another professional, at a community health fair, or through a cancer screening program. This can be an uncomfortable situation because of the medicolegal imperative to follow up on positive test results. Here again the clinician needs to discuss, without bias, all the options available, including repeating the test after a set time to see if any change has occurred. Family history and the PSA level obtained are factors that can influence the decision. Higher PSA values are of more concern than borderline or marginally high results.

Be Familiar with the Treatment Preferences of Consulting Specialists

As was discussed in the section on prostate cancer treatment, there are several treatment options available and a lack of consensus as to which is best. Clinicians should be aware of the preferences of their consultant urologists and oncologist so that patients can be advised about the likely treatment should prostate cancer be discovered.

Common Errors

Ordering Prostate-specific Antigen Tests Without Patients' Consent

The PSA test has been added to some routine chemistry panels and is at times ordered as a screening test without discussion with the patient and without his approval. Because of the rate of false-positives, the medicolegal imperatives to follow up positive tests, the potential side effects of diagnostic tests and treatment, and the unproven benefit of treatment, these practices are inappropriate.

Letting Personal Biases Influence Information Provided to Patients

Clinicians have personal opinions and biases, just as everyone else does. A clinician's personal experience with cancer or an experience with a patient who died from prostate cancer can influence perceptions about screening. Clinicians need to remember that there is a bias in such observations. Patients with aggressive cancers are highly visible and elicit sympathy and a desire to help, while patients who have subclinical cancers, with nothing to gain from diagnosis and treatment, are not appreciated, and iatrogenic complications of these cases tend to be overlooked. The only way to avoid letting such experiences unduly influence recommendations to patients is to present the known benefits and risks factually.

Believing That Digital Rectal Examination Affects Prostate-specific Antigen Results

Even though DRE and PSA screening have no proven benefit, many clinicians recommend and perform these tests. It is a common misconcep-

tion that DRE can elevate the PSA level. Clinicians will often have patients return for PSA testing if DRE has been performed recently. As discussed earlier, this is unnecessary.

Emerging Trends

Studies of Effectiveness of Prostate Cancer Screening

The only resolution to the lack of consensus regarding prostate cancer screening will be the results from clinical trials. Several are now being conducted, but results will not be available for 5 to 10 years.

Studies of Prostate Cancer Treatment Options

Which treatments work best for different stages of disease is not now known. Much of the treatment provided is based on less than optimal scientific evidence. Future clinical trials will provide information on the different therapies and combinations and will help guide more informed decision-making. New cancer treatments, such as immunotherapies and chemotherapies, will be developed and tried.

Improved Accuracy of Testing

As more experience is gained with PSA tests and the options previously discussed to increase PSA predictive value, screening will become more accurate. It is likely that a two-step screening process will evolve, with the first step being more sensitive, to avoid missing cancer, and the second step more specific, to avoid unnecessary biopsies and treatment of those with disease that is unlikely to progress.

New Surgical Procedures

Neurovascular-bundle-sparing radical prostatectomy is a new procedure with lower rates of postoperative impotence. It is likely that technological improvements and improvements in techniques will help lower the incidence of treatment complications and shift the cost-benefit analysis of treatment options.

Genetics

Research on the human genome will possibly uncover more genetic loci of prostate cancer susceptibility. This will have implications for screening and will create ethical dilemmas, just as have occurred with breast cancer gene screening. Along with the dilemmas will come the future promise of gene therapy.

Bibliography

Adolfsson J: Deferred treatment of low grade stage T3 prostate cancer without distant metastasis. *J Urol* 149:326–329, 1993.

Benson MC, Whang IS, Pantuck A, et al: Prostatic specific antigen density: a means of distinguishing benign prostatic hypertrophy and prostate cancer. *J Urol* 1476:815–816, 1992.

Bretton PR: Prostate specific antigen and digital rectal examination in screening for prostate cancer: A community-based study. *South Med J* 87:720–723, 1994.

Cantor SB, Spann SJ, Volk RJ, et al: Prostate cancer screening: A decision analysis. *J Fam Pract* 41:33–41, 1995.

Carter BS, Carter HB, Isaacs JT, et al: Epidemiological evidence regarding predisposing factors to prostate cancer. *Prostate* 16:187–197, 1990.

Catalona WJ, Partin AW, Slawin KM, Brawer MK: Use of the percentage of free prostate-specific antigen to enhance differentiation of prostate cancer from benign prostatic disease. *JAMA* 279:1542–1547, 1998.

Catalona WJ, Richie JP, Ahmann FR, et al: Comparison of digital rectal examination and serum prostate specific antigen in the early detection of prostate cancer: Results of a multi-center clinical trial of 6,630 men. *J Urol* 151:1283–1290, 1994.

Catalona WJ, Smith DS, Wolfert RL, Wang TJ: Evaluation of percentage of free serum prostate-specific antigen to improve specificity of prostate cancer screening. *JAMA* 274:1214–1220, 1995.

Chodak GW, Thisted RA, Gerber GS, et al: Results of conservative management of clinically localized prostate cancer. *N Engl J Med* 330:242–248, 1994.

Coley CM, Barry MJ, Fleming C, et al: Early detection of prostate cancer. II. Estimating the risks, benefits and costs. *Ann Intern Med* 126:468–479, 1997.

Collins MM, Barry MJ: Controversies in prostate cancer screening: Analogies to the early lung cancer screening debate. *JAMA* 276:1976–1979, 1996.

Ferrini R, Woolf SH: American College of Preventive Medicine Practice policy: Screening for prostate cancer in American men. *Am J Prev Med* 15:81–84, 1998.

Flood AB, Wennberg JE, Nease RF, et al: The importance of patient preferences in the decision to screen for prostate cancer. *J Gen Intern Med* 11: 342–349, 1996.

Gann PH, Hennekens CH, Stampfer MJ: A prospective evaluation of plasma prostate-specific antigen for detection of prostate cancer. *JAMA* 273:289–294, 1995.

Gerber GS, Thompson IM, Thisted R, Chodak GW: Disease-specific survival following routine prostate cancer screening by digital rectal examination. *JAMA* 269:61–64, 1993.

Giatto S, Bonardi R, Mazzotta A, et al: Comparing two modalities for screening for prostate cancer: Digital rectal exam plus transrectal ultrasound versus prostate-specific antigen. *Tumor* 81:225–229, 1995.

Giovannucci E, Ascherio A, Rimm EB, Colditz GA, et al: A prospective cohort study of vasectomy and prostate cancer in U.S. men. *JAMA* 269:873–877, 1993.

Gronberg H, Isaacs SD, Smith JR, et al: Characteristics of prostate cancer in families potentially linked to the hereditary prostate cancer 1 (*HPC1*) locus. *JAMA* 278:1251–1255, 1997.

Haas GP, Sakr WA: Epidemiology of prostate cancer. *Cancer J Clin* 47:273–278, 1997.

Hahn DL, Roberts RG: PSA screening for asymptomatic prostate cancer: truth in advertising. *J Fam Pract* 37:432–436, 1993.

Higashihara E, Nutahara K, Kojima M, et al: Significance of serum free prostate specific antigen in the screening of prostate cancer. *J Urol* 156:1964–1968, 1996.

Humphrey PA, Keetch CW, Smith DS, Catalona WJ: Prospective characterization of pathologic features of prostate carcinomas detected via serum prostate specific antigen based screening. *J Urol* 155:816–820, 1996.

Johansson JE, Holmberg L, Johansson S, et al: Fifteen-year survival in prostate cancer: A prospective population-based trial in Sweden. *JAMA* 277:467–471, 1997.

Krahn MD, Mahoney JE, Eckman, MH, et al: Screening for prostate cancer: A decision-analytic view. *JAMA* 262:773–780, 1994.

Labrie F, Candas B, Cusan L, et al: Diagnosis of advanced or noncurable prostate cancer can be practically eliminated by prostate-specific antigen. *Urology* 47:212–217, 1996.

Landis SH, Murray T, Bolden S, Wingo PA: Cancer statistics, 1999. *CA Cancer J Clin* 49:8–31, 1999.

Mettlin C, Jones GW, Murphy GP: Trends in prostate cancer care in the United States, 1974–1990: Observations from the patient care evaluation studies of the American College of Surgeons Commission on Cancer. *CA Cancer J Clin* 43:83–91, 1993.

Mettlin C, Murphy GP, Lee F, et al: Characteristics of prostate cancer detected in the American Cancer Society National Prostate Cancer Detection Project. *J Urol* 152:1737–1740, 1994.

Morgan TO, McLeod DG, Leifer ES, et al: Prospective use of free prostate-specific antigen to avoid repeat biopsies in men with elevated total prostate specific antigen. *Urology* 48:76–80, 1996.

Murphy GP, Natarajan N, Pointes JE, et al: Evaluation and comparison of two new prostate carcinoma markers. *Cancer* 78:809–818, 1996.

Oesterling JE, Jacobsen SJ, Chute CG, et al: Serum prostate specific antigen in a community-based population of healthy men: Establishment of age-specific reference ranges. *JAMA* 270:860–864, 1993.

Parker DM, Pisani PP, Ferlay J: Global cancer statistics. *CA Cancer J Clin* 49:33–64, 1999.

Reissigl A, Klocker H, Pointner J, et al: Usefulness of the ratio of free total prostate specific antigen in addition to total PSA levels in prostate cancer screening. *Urology* 48:62–66, 1996.

Scaletscky R, Koch MO, Eckstein CW, et al: Tumor volume and stage in carcinoma of the prostate detected by elevations in prostate specific antigen. *J Urol* 152:129–131, 1994.

Slawin KM, Ohori M, Dillioglugil O, Scardino PT: Screening for prostate cancer: An analysis of the early experience. *CA Cancer J Clin* 45:134–147, 1995.

Smart CR: The results of prostate carcinoma screening in the U.S. as reflected in the surveillance, epidemiology and end results program. *Cancer* 80:1835–1844, 1997.

Smith DS, Catalona WJ, Herschman JD: Longitudinal screening for prostate cancer with prostate-specific antigen. *JAMA* 276:1309–1315, 1996.

US Preventive Services Task Force: Screening for Prostate Cancer, in *Guide to Clinical Preventive Services*, 2d ed. Baltimore, Williams & Wilkins, 1996.

Warner J, Whitmore WF Jr: Expectant management of clinically localized prostate cancer. *J Urol* 152:1757–1760, 1994.

Wasson JH, Cushman CC, Bruskewitz RC, et al: A structured literature review of treatment for localized prostate cancer. *Arch Fam Med* 2:487–493, 1993. [Erratum, *Arch Fam Med* 2:1030, 1993.]

Wolf AMD, Nasser JF, Wolf AM, Schorling JB: The impact of informed consent on patient interest in prostate-specific antigen screening. *Arch Intern Med* 156:1333–1336, 1996.

Woolf SH: Screening for prostate cancer with prostate-specific antigen: An examination of the evidence. *N Engl J Med* 333:1401–1405, 1995.

Marvin Moe Bell

Chapter
15

Colon Cancer

Introduction

Incidence and Trends

Colorectal (hereinafter referred to as colon) cancer is the third most commonly diagnosed cancer in the United States and trails only lung cancer in number of deaths caused. Roughly 131,000 new cases of colon cancer were diagnosed in 1998, and 57,000 Americans died from the disease. Colon cancer affects men and women equally. The lifetime risk of being diagnosed with colon cancer in the United States is approximately 6%, and the lifetime risk of dying from the disease is 2.6%. Both incidence and mortality rates of colon cancer are highest in African Americans, moderate in Caucasians, and lowest in Asians, Pacific Islanders, and Hispanics

315

(Table 15-1). Among Caucasians, the incidence and mortality rates were fairly constant from 1950 through 1984 but have been declining steadily since 1985. Among African Americans, incidence and mortality rates increased though the 1980s but began to decline in the early 1990s.

Geographical Differences

There are regional differences in colon cancer rates within the United States, with the highest rate in the northeast. However, much greater variation in the incidence of colon cancer occurs in different regions of the world. Low-risk areas generally are found in developing countries and the tropics, including South America, equatorial Africa, southwest Asia, and India. The disease is ten times more common in high-risk areas that include northwest Europe, New Zealand, and North America. Between 1992 and 1995, the male age-adjusted disease rate per 100,000 was 16.0 in the United States, compared with 27.9 in Ireland and 6.8 in Japan. Migrants from areas of low incidence who move to areas of high incidence rapidly show higher rates of colon cancer. This finding was noted, for example, in Puerto Rican, Chinese, and Japanese immigrants to the United States.

Risk Factors

Geographic differences in colon cancer incidence and the fact that disease rates increase rapidly after age 50 make country of birth and advanced age strong risk factors for colon cancer. In the United States one of 114 men between the ages of 40 and 59 will contract colon cancer. This rate increases to one of every 24 between ages 60 and 79. Persons at highest risk have familial syndromes (polyposis or hereditary nonpolyposis colorectal cancer) or long-standing ulcerative colitis. Other strong risk factors for the disease include a history of colon cancer or adenomas in a first-degree relative and a personal history of large adenomatous polyps or cancer of the colon, endometrium, breast, or ovary.

Diets high in red meat and saturated fats and low in fiber appear to be important risk factors that help explain the geographic variation in colon cancer rates; in countries where per capita meat consumption is high, colon cancer rates are high. Frequent bouts of constipation during the previous 10 years were associated with a relative risk for cancer of 4.4 in one case-control study. Other, more modest risk factors include obesity, alcohol intake, cigarette smoking, cholecystectomy, and, possibly, tall stature.

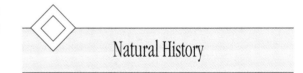

Natural History

Most colon cancers arise within adenomatous polyps. Although fewer than 5% of polyps will

Table 15-1

SEER Incidence and Mortality Rates and Trends, 1990–1995

	INCIDENCE[a]	ANNUAL CHANGE	MORTALITY[a]	ANNUAL CHANGE
African Americans	51.8	−1.8%	23.3	−0.8%
Caucasians	45.4	−2.6%	17.6	−1.8%
Asians/Pacific Islanders	41.4	−2.1%	11.2	−0.3%
Hispanics	32.4	−3.1%	10.5	−1.3%

[a] Rates are per 100,000 and age adjusted to the 1970 U.S. standard population.

undergo malignant transformation, the risk is much higher in dysplastic, villous, and large polyps. Cancers typically develop at the tip of adenomatous polyps and are often cured through polypectomy in the early stages. The transition from polyp to malignancy takes from 10 to 15 years. Without treatment, colon cancer will invade the bowel wall, spread to regional lymph nodes, and metastasize to the liver, throughout the abdominal cavity, and often to the lungs and bones. Death will occur, often as the result of bowel hemorrhage or obstruction or from generalized wasting and metastatic complications.

Persons diagnosed early in the course of the disease clearly have better survival rates than those with advanced colon cancer. The estimated 5-year survival rate, for example, improves from 6% in persons with distant metastases to 60% in persons with regional spread to 91% in those with local disease. The primary therapy for colon cancer is surgical resection. Many persons with local disease are cured by surgery. Patients with stage III colon cancer (spread to regional lymph nodes) appear to have better disease-free and overall survival rates when treated with 5-fluorouracil and levamisole after surgery compared with surgery alone. Even patients with a single isolated focus of liver or lung metastasis have a 25% chance of cure if the metastasis is removed.

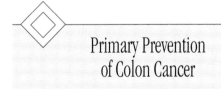

Primary Prevention of Colon Cancer

Diet

FIBER

Burkitt hypothesized that high-fiber diets prevent colon cancer after observing that African natives had high fecal bulk and very low colon cancer rates. The theory suggests that the pro-

tective effect is due to dilution of carcinogens in the bulkier stool and reduced contact due to rapid transit times. Human studies are limited owing to the difficulty of obtaining accurate long-term dietary intake information, and results regarding the protective effect of fiber have been mixed. Pooled data from 13 case-control studies, however, found a clear benefit associated with higher fiber intake, and it is possible that one-third of colon cancers could be prevented if Americans increased their fiber intake from foods by 13 g/day, representing a 70% increase in dietary fiber. Increased fiber intake has not yet been proved effective in a controlled trial, however.

FRUITS AND VEGETABLES

Fruits and vegetables contain numerous potential anticarcinogenic substances, such as antioxidant vitamins C and E, carotenoids, selenium, and flavonoids. Vegetarian groups, such as Seventh Day Adventists, have lower rates of colon cancer than nonvegetarians, even after controlling for other variables, such as geographic location. Human studies on dietary fruits and vegetables more consistently show protective effects, in fact, than studies on dietary fiber. A huge prospective study recently found that American men in the highest quintile of vegetable and grain consumers had a 25% lower risk of colon cancer compared with those in the lowest quintile. Risk reduction was even greater (38%) between the two quintiles of women.

FAT AND RED MEAT

Consumption of saturated fat is positively correlated with incidence of colon cancer, while monounsaturated fats may have a protective effect. Countries with a high incidence of colon cancer have diets with 40% of calories from fat, compared with less than half as much fat in countries with a low incidence of the disease. Red meat intake is a strong independent risk factor for colon cancer as well.

Exercise

Many studies have found that physical activity reduces the risk of colon cancer, although some of the studies found that this held true only for men. Both occupational and recreational activities appear to be important. Exercise seems to minimize the development of adenomas as well as cancers. It is hypothesized that the protective effect is due to increased colonic motility stimulated by physical activity.

Aspirin/ Nonsteroidal Anti-inflammatory Drugs

After rodents are exposed to carcinogens, nonsteroidal anti-inflammatory drugs (NSAIDs) lessen the development of colon tumors. In humans, several observational studies early in the 1990s raised hopes that regular aspirin or NSAID use could lower the risk of colon cancer. Nine studies found that self-selected aspirin or NSAID use decreased the incidence of colon cancer versus one study that found an increased incidence. The Physician's Health Study, the first large, prospective, controlled study of aspirin and colon cancer failed to find an association. Neither the randomized clinical trial nor the prospective cohort analysis showed an association between aspirin use and the incidence of colon cancer. Although low doses of aspirin were used and the study was of relatively short duration, the routine use of aspirin for prevention of colon cancer cannot be recommended at the present time. The discrepancy between observational studies and the randomized trial may be due to a greater importance of confounding by indication (factors that influence the choice to use medications on a regular basis) than was previously recognized. That is, those inclined to regularly take aspirin or NSAIDs may have had lower colon cancer risks for some other reason that was associated with their use of medication

Postmenopausal Hormones

Several studies have suggested that hormone use may reduce the risk of adenomas and colon cancers for postmenopausal women. The Nurses Health Study, a large, prospective, cohort study, found that the risk of colon cancer was lowered by 35% in hormone users compared with those who never used hormones. Risk was reduced 30% for women who stopped hormones within 5 years, but no risk reduction was found when hormones had been stopped for more than 5 years. Critics point out that postmenopausal women taking hormones have been thought to be at lower risk for a wide variety of conditions. Unfortunately, all of these nonrandomized studies suffer from confounding by indication, because women who choose to take hormone replacement are different in many ways from women who choose not to take hormone replacement.

Summary

The best recipe for primary prevention of colon cancer is probably a common-sense healthy lifestyle, including a diet rich in fruits, vegetables, and grains, with moderate amounts of red meat and fat. Regular exercise, avoidance of tobacco, and moderation in alcohol consumption round out the prevention menu.

Secondary Prevention

Screening Tests

The most commonly recommended screening tests for detecting colon cancer in asymptomatic people are the digital rectal examination (DRE), fecal occult blood testing (FOBT), and sigmoidoscopy. Colonoscopy and barium enema were generally used as diagnostic studies in the past but are more typically being suggested as screening options by some groups. Comparisons of characteristics of the screening tests for colon cancer are summarized in Table 15-2.

DIGITAL RECTAL EXAMINATION

Although it is inexpensive and easy to perform, the DRE has limited value in screening for colon cancer because the examiner's finger can reach only 7 to 8 cm. Polyps can be soft and nonpalpable. Thus, fewer than one-tenth of colon cancers are palpable on DRE. There are no studies to document the specificity of rectal exams for the detection of colon cancer.

FECAL OCCULT BLOOD TESTING

FOBT generally involves the collection of two samples from three consecutive stools, placed on a guaiac-impregnated card and tested to determine the presence or absence of blood. Traditionally, test reagent is applied to dried (nonrehydrated) stool specimens. The sensitivity reported for FOBT in detecting colon cancer among asymptomatic persons has ranged widely, from 26% to 92%. Large population studies using repeated FOBT over time have found the sensitivity of nonrehydrated stool samples to range from 72% to 78% for the detec-

tion of cancer. Tests can be false-negative when antioxidants like ascorbic acid interfere with the test reagent, and some colon cancers may not bleed or bleed only intermittently.

The specificity reported has ranged from 90% to 99%. False-positive tests can result from ingestion of foods containing peroxidases (Table 15-3), and bleeding often occurs in the context of nonmalignant conditions, such as hemorrhoids, diverticulosis, peptic ulcer disease, or gastritis. Rehydration of stool samples before testing slightly increases the sensitivity but at the cost of many more false-positive results. When population screening is performed, from 2% to 4% of persons tested will show positive results for blood. Since there is a low incidence of colon cancer among the asymptomatic population, most of these positive stool samples will be falsely positive. Thus, the positive predictive value of FOBT for persons over age 50 is only 2% to 11% for the presence of colon cancer, and 20% to 30% for adenomas.

FOBT is inexpensive, well accepted by patients, and virtually free of risk. The disadvantages include a greatly reduced sensitivity for detection of adenomatous polyps, because polyps are less likely to bleed than cancers. In addition, owing to false-positive tests, it is estimated that six to 10 people will undergo colonoscopy or barium enema for each cancer detected. Rehydration of slides will improve

Table 15-2

Comparison of Screening Tests for Colon Cancer

SCREENING TEST	COST	COMPLEXITY	RISK	EVIDENCE OF EFFECTIVENESS
FOBT	Low	Low	Low	Strongest
Sigmoidoscopy	Intermediate	Intermediate	Intermediate	Intermediate
DCBE	High	High	Intermediate	Weak
Colonoscopy	Highest	Highest	Highest	Weak

ABBREVIATIONS: Fecal occult blood test; double-contrast barium enema.

Table 15-3

Foods High in Peroxidase

Broccoli	Cucumbers
Turnips	French beans
Rare red meat	Lemon rind
Cauliflower	Cantaloupe
Artichokes	Red radish
Parsley	Zucchini

sensitivity, but 17 to 50 patients will still require a total colon examination for each cancer detected. It is important to instruct patients on the proper method of performing FOBT. They need to avoid red meat, vitamin C medications, iron tablets, nonsteroidal anti-inflammatory drugs, and high-peroxidase foods (Table 15-3) for 3 days before testing. Testing of specimens should be performed within 6 days of collection, and a single positive smear is considered to be a positive result. Some patients have difficulty collecting specimens, and special stool-collection devices are available to assist.

SIGMOIDOSCOPY

Sigmoidoscopy involves direct visualization of the rectum and distal colon to look for adenomas and colon cancers. Rigid scopes, 25 cm in length, have largely been replaced by flexible fiber-optic scopes that are generally 60 cm in length. Fiber-optic scopes can facilitate examination of more of the colon and are more comfortable for patients. Rigid sigmoidoscopy makes visible the distal 20 cm of the colon, to the rectosigmoid junction. The 60-cm flexible scope makes visible the entire sigmoid colon 80% of the time. Sigmoidoscopy will detect most cancers and large polyps within reach of the instrument—only 25% to 30% of colon cancers for the rigid instrument and 40% to 65% of all cancers for a 65-cm sigmoidoscope. In addition, sigmoidoscopy makes it possible to diagnose adenomatous polyps in as many as 75% of persons.

Sigmoidoscopy has the advantage over FOBT of detecting large adenomatous polyps that may not bleed and provides an opportunity to prevent the development of colon cancer by removing these polyps.

Sigmoidoscopy does result in some false-negative exam results, since barium enema studies after sigmoidoscopy have found lesions within reach of the sigmoidoscope that were not seen. False-positive findings also occur with sigmoidoscopy, mainly polyps that have a low chance of malignant transformation. There is ongoing debate about the need for colonoscopy in people found to have small polyps on sigmoidoscopy. In one study of 4,490 patients who underwent sigmoidoscopy, 9% were found to have neoplastic polyps. Of these patients, 44% had small tubular adenomas (less than 5 mm). None of the group with small tubular polyps who underwent colonoscopy was found to have advanced proximal polyps. Retrospective studies have suggested that there is a low long-term risk of proximal colon cancers among persons found to have polyps smaller than 1 cm in the distal colon. Unfortunately, despite existing recommendations to perform screening sigmoidoscopy, screening rates have been very low. Problems include an unpleasant preparation for the test with enemas or laxatives and discomfort caused by the procedure itself. The procedure is costly, and complications are rare but potentially serious, including perforation and prolonged bleeding.

BARIUM ENEMA

The barium enema, popularly referred to as the "lower GI," uses barium contrast dye to outline the walls of the colon for radiographic imaging. Using a double-contrast (or air) technique versus a single-contrast technique, the accuracy improves to approximate that of colonoscopy. The double-contrast barium enema (DCBE) has an estimated sensitivity ranging from 80% to 95% for detecting colon cancers and a specificity of roughly 90%. Barium enema is generally more expensive than sigmoidoscopy but costs less and has a lower risk than colonoscopy. The preparation and discomfort are similar to those for sigmoidoscopy. Patients receive 300 to 500 mrem of radiation in the course of a barium enema, which is slightly more than the dose from mammography. Complications are rare but have included bowel perforation and anaphylactic reactions to older rubber enema insertion tips.

COLONOSCOPY

Colonoscopy is the fiber-optic visualization of the entire colon. It requires a bowel-cleansing preparation similar to that for barium enema and generally calls for intravenous sedation and use of a hospital suite. It is the most expensive of the tests by far, but procedure-related discomfort is eliminated by the use of anesthesia. The complication rates from anesthesia and the procedure itself are much higher than those associated with other screening tests. It is estimated that 95% of colon cancers are within reach of the scope, and the sensitivity of detecting cancers within reach is 75% to 95%.

Evidence That Screening Reduces Mortality Rates

Although persons with early-stage colon cancer clearly have longer survival times than those with advanced disease, the extent to which lead time and length bias account for differences in survival is difficult to measure. A number of studies have looked at the effectiveness of FOBT and sigmoidoscopy in reducing colon cancer mortality rates; they are described later herein. Since they are less frequently used tests, very little evidence exists regarding colonoscopy or barium enema for screening. There are no studies of the effect of DRE on colon cancer mortality rates. The evidence for FOBT and sigmoidoscopy is summarized here.

FECAL OCCULT BLOOD TESTING

Several large prospective clinical trials were started during the 1970s and 1980s to examine the effects of screening FOBT on colon cancer mortality rates. The Minnesota Colon Cancer Control Study randomized 46,551 volunteers over the age of 50 to receive annual FOBT versus usual care. Stool samples in the study group were rehydrated before testing, and colonoscopy was performed on those persons testing positive for blood. The group screened annually with FOBT had a 33% reduction in mortality rates from colon cancer over the 13-year trial compared with the control group.

A study of FOBT screening in Denmark randomized 62,000 members of a community aged 45 to 75 to receive FOBT every other year versus usual care. Stool samples were not rehydrated before testing. Screened participants had an 18% reduction in colon cancer mortality rates over the 10-year study period compared with the control population. A similar study in Great Britain, using FOBT screening every other year, found a 16% reduction in mortality rates from colon cancer.

A good deal of debate followed the Minnesota study regarding the extent of mortality rate reduction that could be attributed to chance selection for colonoscopy stemming from a screening method (rehydrated FOBT) that had a high false-positive rate. Various authors have argued that anywhere from 16% to 50% of the mortality rate reduction can be accounted for by chance selection. In any case, the three large, randomized, prospective studies have proved that screening programs using FOBT do prevent deaths from colon cancer. In addition, annual screening may save twice as many lives as screening every other year.

SIGMOIDOSCOPY

No direct evidence from randomized, prospective, clinical trials exists yet to support sigmoidoscopy screening for colon cancer.

Instead, policymakers rely on a variety of indirect evidence. A case-control study from Kaiser-Permanente in Oakland, California, compared 261 patients who died of colon cancer arising in the distal 20 cm of the colon with 868 age- and sex-matched controls. Only 9% of the case patients had undergone rigid sigmoidoscopy versus 24% of the control group, suggesting a 60% reduction in risk of death for cancers within reach of the sigmoidoscope. It is important to note that this study found no protective association of rigid sigmoidoscopy and more proximal colon cancers, thus lowering the chance that hidden biases accounted for the protective effect found for the distal cancers.

A smaller case-control study found an 80% reduction in risk of death from colon cancer in subjects screened with sigmoidoscopy, with the benefit also limited to cancers within reach of the sigmoidoscope. Most of the older studies on sigmoidoscopy screening suffered from design limitations that make the results less useful, such as lack of randomization or controls. Until randomized, prospective study results are available, however, the bulk of indirect evidence suggests a reduction in mortality rates when screening sigmoidoscopy is offered.

Recommendations of Major Groups

AVERAGE-RISK INDIVIDUALS

In 1996, the U.S. Preventive Services Task Force recommended screening all persons starting at age of 50 for colon cancer. Both annual FOBT and periodic sigmoidoscopy were endorsed as effective. No suggestions were offered, however, regarding which test is preferable, whether the combined tests are better than one, whether to rehydrate the FOBT, the frequency of sigmoidoscopy, or the age at which to stop screening. Colonoscopy, barium enema, and DRE were not recommended.

The American Cancer Society (ACS) released updated guidelines for colon cancer screening in 1997. The ACS advocates screening starting by age 50 with *either* annual FOBT and sigmoidoscopy every 5 years or a total colon examination (colonoscopy every 10 years or DCBE every 5 to 10 years). DRE is recommended every 5 to 10 years at the time of sigmoidoscopy or total colon examination. (See Table 15-4 for complete ACS recommendations.)

The Agency for Health Care Policy Research (AHCPR) convened an interdisciplinary task force to develop guidelines for colon cancer screening. The American Gastroenterological Association published this task force's screening recommendations in 1997, along with an extensive review of the literature and a simulation model to estimate the benefits and complications of each screening strategy. Except for an option of either annual FOBT or sigmoidoscopy every 5 years, the recommendations are almost identical to those of the ACS and are endorsed by the American College of Gastroenterology, the American College of Colon and Rectal Surgeons, the American Society for Gastrointestinal Endoscopy, and others.

The American College of Physicians' (ACP) guidelines from 1995 recommended a menu of screening options based on patients' preferences and local resources, including sigmoidoscopy, colonoscopy, or air-contrast barium enema repeated at 10-year intervals. The ACP guidelines support annual FOBT for persons declining the other screening methods. Unlike the other organizations, the ACP suggested an upper age limit, stating that little benefit would be gained by screening past age 70 for persons who had been screened up to that age.

In 1994, the Canadian Task Force on the Periodic Health Examination failed to find evidence sufficient to endorse screening for colon cancer in asymptomatic, low-risk individuals. The American College of Radiology suggests barium enema every 3 to 5 years as an acceptable alternative to periodic sigmoidoscopy. The American Academy of Family Practice updated their *Summary of Recommendations for Periodic Health*

Table 15-4

American Cancer Society (ACS) Guidelines for Screening and Surveillance for Early Detection of Colorectal Polyps and Cancers[a]

RISK CATEGORY	RECOMMENDATION[b]	WHEN TO BEGIN	INTERVAL
Average risk			
All people 50 years or older who are not in the categories listed here	One of the following: FOBT plus flexible sigmoidoscopy or TCE[c,d]	Age 50 Age 50	FOBT every year and flexible sigmoidoscopy every 5 yr Colonoscopy every 10 yr or DCBE every 5–10 yr
Moderate Risk			
People with single, small (<1 cm) adenomatous polyps	Colonoscopy	At time of initial polyp diagnosis	TCE within 3 yr after initial polyp removal; if normal, as per average-risk recommendations
People with large (>1 cm) or multiple adenomatous polyps of any size	Colonoscopy	At time of initial polyp diagnosis	TCE within 3 yr after initial polyp removal; if normal, TCE every 5 yr
Personal history of curative-intent resection of colorectal cancer	TCE[e]	Within 1 yr after resection	If normal, TCE in 3 yr; if still normal, TCE every 5 yr
Colorectal cancer or adenomatous polyps in first-degree relative younger than 60 yr or in two or more first-degree relatives of any age	TCE	Age 4 or 10 yr earlier than the age of the youngest affected family member in the family, whichever is earlier	Every 5 yr
Colorectal cancer in other relatives (not including earlier categories)	As per average-risk recommendations: may consider beginning screening before age 50		
High risk			
Family history of familial adenomatous polyposis	Early surveillance with endoscopy, counseling to consider genetic testing, and referral to a specialty center	Puberty	If genetic test positive or polyposis confirmed, consider colectomy; otherwise, endoscopy every 1–2 yr

(Continued)

Table 15-4

American Cancer Society (ACS) Guidelines for Screening and Surveillance for Early Detection of Colorectal Polyps and Cancers[a]
(Continued)

RISK CATEGORY	RECOMMENDATION[b]	WHEN TO BEGIN	INTERVAL
Family history of hereditary non-polyposis colon cancer	Colonoscopy and counseling to consider genetic testing	Age 21	If genetic test positive or if patient has not had genetic testing, colonoscopy every 2 yr until age 40 yr, then every year
Inflammatory bowel disease	Colonoscopies with biopsies for dysplasia	8 yr after the start of pancolitis: 12–15 yr after the start of left-sided colitis	Every 1–2 yr

[a] Approximately 70% to 80% of cases are in average-risk individuals, approximately 15% to 20% are in moderate-risk individuals, and 5% to 10% are in high-risk individuals.

[b] Digital rectal examination should be done at the time of each sigmoidoscopy, colonoscopy, or DCBE.

[c] Annual FOBT has been shown to reduce mortality rates from colorectal cancer, so it is preferable to not screening; however, the ACS recommends that annual FOBT be accompanied by flexible sigmoidoscopy to further reduce the risk of colorectal cancer mortality.

[d] TCE includes either colonoscopy or DCBE. The choice of procedure should depend on the medical status of the patient and the relative quality of the medical examinations available in a specific community. Flexible sigmoidoscopy should be performed in those instances in which the rectosigmoid colon is not easily visible by DCBE. DCBE would be performed when the entire colon has not been adequately evaluated by colonoscopy.

[e] This assumes that a perioperative TCE was done.

ABBREVIATIONS: DCBE, double-contrast barium enema; FOBT, fecal occult blood testing; TCE, total colon examination.

Examination in 1997. Colon cancer screening was advocated for persons aged 50 and older, with a menu of choices that includes annual FOBT and periodic sigmoidoscopy, colonoscopy, or barium enema.

After intensive lobbying by the American College of Gastroenterology and other specialty organizations, the Balanced Budget Act of 1997 approved payment for certain colon cancer screening tests for Medicare patients over the age of 50. Average-risk patients can undergo annual FOBT ordered by their clinicians and flexible sigmoidoscopy every 4 years. Barium enema was not included but may be reimbursed if the attending clinician certifies that the screening potential for a given individual equals or exceeds the screening potential for sigmoidoscopy. In summary, while most organizations recommend some form of screening for colon cancer starting at age 50, there is lack of agreement on the preferred test and frequency.

HIGH-RISK INDIVIDUALS

The ACS includes detailed recommendations for types of screening, age to begin screening, and suggested intervals of screening for eight categories of moderate- and high-risk individuals (Table 15-4). For example, if a person has a first-degree relative younger than age 60 with colon cancer or adenomatous polyps, or two or more first-degree relatives of any age, he or she should have a total colon exam at age 40 or at an age 10 years younger than the youngest affected person in the family. The test should be repeated every 5 years. The AHCPR task force guidelines list very similar recommendations for six of the higher-risk groups.

The Balanced Budget Act of 1997 defined individuals at high risk for colon cancer to include those with a personal history of adenomatous polyps, colon cancer, or inflammatory bowel disease. Also included were those with a first-degree relative who has a history of colon cancer or adenomatous polyp or a history of familial adenomatous polyposis or hereditary nonpolyposis colon cancer. The act approved payment for screening colonoscopy up to every 2 years for these high-risk persons. Barium enema was not included but may be reimbursed if the attending physician certifies that the screening potential for a given high-risk individual equals or exceeds the screening potential for a colonoscopy.

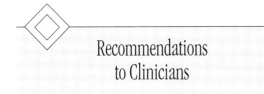

Recommendations to Clinicians

Clinicians must sort through the variety of recommendations listed to provide very specific advice to individuals, each with unique experiences, expectations, and value systems. There is a good deal of uncertainty in the recommendations, with a tendency to give a menu of acceptable options. A high priority should be placed on educating individuals about the types of screening tests available and the pros and cons of each. A practical suggestion is that the foundation of screening for average-risk individuals should be annual FOBT starting at age 50. It is the simplest, safest, least expensive, and most established of the strategies in terms of lowering the death rate from colon cancer. Patients should be instructed to follow the diet instructions carefully and should understand the implications of a positive result and the further

testing that will be required. Non-rehydrated samples should provide adequate sensitivity without the big increase in false-positive results that would occur using rehydrated samples.

Sigmoidoscopy is a screening method that should be discussed with average-risk patients. Offering the test every 5 to 10 years in addition to annual FOBT may be a reasonable approach that would balance the high costs and patients' dislike of the test with the presumed benefit in lowering colon cancer mortality rates. Studies on the degree of additional reduction in colon cancer mortality rates that could be achieved by supplementing FOBT with sigmoidoscopy and on the optimal frequency of sigmoidoscopy are needed. Within our current health care system, it is unlikely that high rates of compliance with sigmoidoscopy will be achieved. Creative approaches, such as reduced insurance premiums after a negative result on sigmoidoscopy, could be considered.

It is difficult to assess the appropriate age at which to stop screening. The incidence of colon cancer increases rapidly and steadily after age 50. The chance that individuals over age 70 with colon cancer will die of other conditions increases even more, however, as do the chances of complications from the screening process. As stated by the ACP, there is probably little benefit to be gained by widespread screening after age 70. This should remain an individual choice, and otherwise healthy individuals over age 70 should make an informed decision. Meanwhile, clinicians should target their efforts at those "golden years for cancer screening" between ages 50 and 70.

For low-risk individuals, the role of barium enema and colonoscopy in screening remains unclear. Until further evidence is available, the high cost and effort involved will preclude widespread population screening using these methods. Identification of high-risk individuals should be a high priority for clinicians. Public education programs would be helpful as well. Once such persons are identified, more intensive and earlier screening should take place. Clinicians can refer to the ACS or AHCPR guidelines for specific recommendations and come up with a plan agreeable to the person at risk.

Common Errors

Common errors made by clinicians include failure to provide dietary instructions before FOBT, failure to correctly assess colon cancer risk based on age and numbers of family members with colon cancer, failure to recognize that inflammatory bowel disease is a high-risk condition, and failure to ask about familial polyposis and hereditary cancers. Perhaps the most common error is performing an FOBT during a DRE as part of a physical examination, when the patient has not taken proper dietary precautions before the exam, and then considering this single FOBT to be an adequate colon cancer screening test. Clinicians can improve their own compliance with colon cancer screening and that of their patients by developing office-based systems that are prevention oriented. These include computer-assisted reminders, posted screening guidelines, and the involvement of other clinic staff.

Emerging Approaches to Prevention

Better Fecal Tests

A key to improving the secondary prevention of colon cancer will be the development of more sensitive and more specific screening tests using stool or blood specimens. For example, colon

cancers can lose protein into stool by a different mechanism of action than the loss of blood. Fecal protein loss, as measured using α_1 antitrypsin, has been proposed as a way to improve the sensitivity of stool testing for colon cancers. Ongoing studies on new screening tests and their effectiveness are needed.

Emerging Techniques

Less invasive and more comfortable ways to image the colon will likely improve screening and the diagnostic workup of positive screening results in the future. "Virtual colonoscopy," for example, is a radiographic technique that uses thin-section computed tomography scanning to generate three-dimensional images of the colon after air insufflation with a rectal tube. Scanning equipment available in 1997 used 4-mm imaging slices and was very effective in detecting large-mass lesions. A study of virtual colonoscopy before regularly scheduled colonoscopy found 100% sensitivity and 82% specificity for the detection of polyps larger than 5 mm in size. Improvements in equipment and further studies will likely add this technique to the list of options for colon cancer screening.

Genetic Testing

Exciting advances in the molecular biology of colon cancer may allow testing for stool or blood markers that will identify an individual as being at high risk for sporadic forms of colon cancer. These high-risk individuals, who would not be considered high risk under current guidelines, could then benefit from DCBE or colonoscopy screening. Molecular markers may have a role in evaluating qualitatively the degree of dysplasia of a person's colonic mucosa. This could help a patient with inflammatory bowel disease make a more informed decision on whether and when to undergo preventive surgery. Molecular biology research findings will need to be incorporated into clinically useful tests, which must be studied for effectiveness.

Genetic mapping, which is progressing at a rapid pace, will allow for much more accurate assessment of risk in persons with family histories of adenomatous polyps or colon cancers. Genetic markers, such as mismatch repair genes, glutathione transferase isoenzymes, acetylator status, and phospholipase A2 expression, are expected to give more precise estimates of an individual's risk for colon cancer. The benefits of genetic screening must be evaluated and guidelines for rational use developed.

Dietary Intervention

Efforts to show a benefit of specific diets in colon cancer prevention will continue. If these results are positive, attempts to raise public and medical professional awareness of the benefits of low-fat, high-fiber diets in primary prevention of colon cancer will be equally important. Public health programs could take an active role in this area. The combination of primary prevention with screening has tremendous potential to reduce the burden of colon cancer in the United States.

References

American Academy of Family Practice: *Summary of Recommendations for Periodic Health Examination: General Population Guidelines*, 1997. (http://www.aafp.org/policy/camp/app-d_c.html)

American Cancer Society: Guidelines for screening and surveillance for early detection of colorectal polyps and cancer: Update 1997. *CA Cancer J Clin* 47:154–160, 1997.

Atkin W, Morson B, Cuzick J: Long-term risk of colorectal cancer after excision of rectosigmoid adenomas. *N Engl J Med* 326:658–662, 1992.

Burt R: Cohorts with familial disposition for colon cancers in chemoprevention trials. *J Cell Biochem* 25(Suppl):131–135, 1996.

Canadian Task Force on the Periodic Health Examination: *Canadian Guide to Clinical Preventive Health Care*. Ottawa, Canadian Communication Group, 1994, pp 797–809.

Chu K, Chow W, Hankey B, Ries L: Temporal patterns in colorectal cancer incidence, survival, and mortality from 1950 through 1990. *J Natl Cancer Inst* 86(13):997–1006, 1994.

Ferrucci J: Screening for colon cancer: Programs of the American College of Radiology. *Am J Radiol* 160:999–1003, 1993.

Giovannucci E, Rimm E, Stampfer M, et al: Intake of fat, meat, and fiber in relation to risk of colon cancer in men. *Cancer Res* 54:2390, 1994.

Gnauck R, Macrae FA, Fleisher M: How to perform the fecal occult blood test. *CA Cancer J Clin* 34:134–146, 1984.

Grodstein F, Martinez M, Platz E, et al: Postmenopausal hormone use and risk for colorectal cancer and adenoma. *Ann Intern Med* 128(9):705–712, 1998.

Guide to Clinical Preventive Services, Report of the US Preventive Services Task Force, 2d ed. Alexandria, Virginia: International Medical Publishing, Inc., 1996.

Howe G, Benito E, Castelleto R, et al: Dietary intake of fiber and decreased risk of cancers of the colon and rectum: Evidence from the combined analysis of 13 case-controlled studies. *J Natl Cancer Inst* 84:1887, 1992.

Jacobs E, White E: Constipation, laxative use, and colon cancer among middle-aged adults. *Epidemiology* 9:385–391, 1998.

Kronberg O, Fenger C, Olsen J, et al: Randomised study of screening for colorectal cancer with faecal-occult-blood test. *Lancet* 348:1467–1471, 1996.

Landis SH, Murray T, Wingo PA, Bolden S: Cancer statistics 1998. *CA Cancer J Clin* 48:6–29, 1998.

Mandel J, Bond J, Church T, et al: Reducing mortality from colorectal cancer by screening for fecal occult blood: Minnesota Colon Cancer Control Study. *N Engl J Med* 328:1365–1371, 1993.

Moran A, Robinson M, Lawson N, et al: Fecal alpha 1-antitrypsin detection of colorectal neoplasia. *Dig Dis Sci* 40(12):2522–2525, 1995.

Naus N, Khandelwal M, Rowe W, et al: Prospective comparison of virtual colonoscopy to conventional colonoscopy in the detection of polyps. *Gastrointest Endose* program/abstract issue 45(4), 1997.

Newcomb P, Norfleet R, Storer B, et al: Screening sigmoidoscopy and colorectal cancer mortality. *J Natl Cancer Inst* 84:1572–1575, 1992.

Ries L, Miller B, Hankey B, et al: *SEER Cancer Statistics Review 1973–1991.* NIH publication no 94–2789. Bethesda, National Cancer Institute, 1994.

Sandler R: Epidemiology and risk factors for colorectal cancer. *Gastroenterol Clin North Am* 25:717–735, 1996.

Selby J, Friedman G, Quesenberry C, Weiss N: A case-control study of screening sigmoidoscopy and mortality from colorectal cancer. *N Engl J Med* 326:653–657, 1992.

Sturmer T, Glynn R, Lee I, et al: Aspirin use and colorectal cancer: Post trial follow-up data from the physicians' health study. *Ann Intern Med* 128:713–720, 1998.

Thun M, Calle E, Namboodiri M, et al: Risk factors for fatal colon cancer in a large prospective study. *J Natl Cancer Inst* 84:1491, 1992.

Wallace M, Kemp J, Trnka Y, et al: Is colonoscopy indicated for small adenomas found by screening flexible sigmoidoscopy? *Ann Intern Med* 129:273–278, 1998.

Winawer S, Fletcher R, Miller L, et al: Colorectal cancer screening: Clinical guidelines and rationale. *Gastroenterology* 112:594–642, 1997.

Wingo P, Ries L, Rosenberg H, et al: Cancer incidence and mortality, 1973–1995, a report card for the U.S. *Cancer* 82:1197–1207, 1998.

Randal J. Thomas
James K. Crager
Jeffrey L. Bush
James L. Arter

Chapter
16

Cardiovascular Disease

Live sensibly—among a thousand people only one dies a natural death; the rest succumb to irrational modes of living.

Maimonides, 1135–1204

Introduction

Cardiovascular disease (CVD) is the leading cause of death and disability in the United States, accounting for approximately $135 billion in health care expenditures per year and 40% of all deaths of adults. Because of its effect on health, CVD is a prime target for preventive medicine efforts. Prevention efforts are thought to explain approximately half of the marked decline over the past 30 years in coronary heart disease mortality (49% reduction) and stroke mortality (58% reduction). Despite these gains, however, CVD continues to be one of the leading health problems in the United States. Prevention efforts have yielded improvements in patient outcomes but are still lacking in many critical ways.

Definitions

CVD includes a wide array of clinical manifestations. For the purposes of this chapter, discussion is limited to three of the most common types of CVD—coronary heart disease (CHD), cerebrovascular disease (CBVD), and peripheral arterial, or peripheral vascular disease (PVD).

CORONARY HEART DISEASE

CHD involves atherosclerosis of the coronary arteries, usually leading to at least one of the following three clinical manifestations.

ANGINA PECTORIS Angina pectoris is the syndrome resulting from a brief episode of myocardial ischemia characterized by sudden chest pressure, often radiating to the shoulders or jaw and usually lasting less than 15 minutes. It also can be identified through ST depression on an electrocardiogram (ECG) at rest or during exercise.

MYOCARDIAL INFARCTION Myocardial infarction (MI) is the condition of acute myocardial necrosis caused by sustained myocardial ischemia. The diagnosis of MI generally is made in the presence of at least two of the following three factors: abnormal ECG (classic findings are ST elevation or new pathologic Q waves), abnormal cardiac enzyme levels, and sustained chest pressure that lasts for more than 15 minutes.

SUDDEN CARDIAC DEATH Sudden cardiac death generally is defined as a death that occurs within 24 hours of the sudden onset of cardiovascular symptoms to which no other cause of death can be ascribed.

CEREBROVASCULAR DISEASE

CBVD is the process characterized by cerebral ischemia caused by abrupt interruption of the normal blood supply to the brain. This interruption can be either short term, a transient ischemic attack (TIA), or long term (a stroke). The ischemic episode can be caused by one or more of the following mechanisms: (1) intrinsic blockage of the blood vessels supplying the brain caused by such processes as atherosclerosis or arterial dissection, (2) blockage by an embolus from a distant site, usually in the heart or extracranial vessels, (3) a decrease in perfusion pressure to the brain either from a considerable and sustained decrease in blood pressure or an elevation in blood viscosity, or (4) rupture of an intracranial blood vessel. Although a TIA lasts for less than 24 hours, it does mean the person is at high risk for a subsequent stroke. Symptoms of a stroke may be permanent or may resolve entirely over a period of days to months.

PERIPHERAL VASCULAR DISEASE

PVD, or peripheral arterial disease, in the broadest definition is the process characterized by atherosclerosis of the abdominal aorta and arteries of the lower extremities. PVD usually is manifest by exertional weakness and pain in the lower extremities, commonly called *intermittent claudication*. Progression of PVD can lead to a more serious clinical syndrome known as *critical limb ischemia*, which is associated with high risk for skin ulceration, infection, and, ultimately, amputation of the lower extremities.

Association between Coronary Heart Disease, Cerebrovascular Disease, and Peripheral Vascular Disease

Because atherosclerosis is a systemic process, the association of CHD, CBVD, and PVD is strong, although not absolute. In one study, for example, investigators reported that approximately one-third of elderly participants with documented CHD had evidence of CBVD and PVD. Among participants with documented CBVD or PVD, approximately one-half had evidence of CHD. Results of autopsy studies suggest that the prevalence of CHD among persons with severe PVD may be even higher.

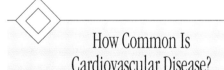

How Common Is Cardiovascular Disease?

MI and stroke are two of the most common manifestations of CVD. with An estimated 750,000 MIs and 700,000 strokes per year in the United States contribute to more than 1,000,000 deaths from CVD each year. The prevalence of CHD in the elderly population has been estimated to be nearly 25%, and the prevalence of symptomatic CBVD is estimated to be 6 to 10%. The prevalence of undetected, or silent, CHD is thought to be nearly as high as that of symptomatic disease. Sigurdsson, et al, for example, found that among the elderly adult population they studied, the prevalence of symptomatic MI was 7% and that of asymptomatic MI was 5%. Silent CBVD is more difficult to estimate, but authors of one review of published studies on silent CBVD found that asymptomatic carotid artery stenosis, one marker of CBVD, was present in 2 to 8% of the general adult populations studied.

PVD affects more than 5 million adults in the United States each year. Symptomatic PVD has been reported among 2% of persons younger than 60 years of age, 4% of those between 60 and 70 years, and 5% of those older than 70 years. PVD has been reported to occur among as many as 85% of persons with PVD. If this is true, the prevalence of PVD, both asymptomatic and symptomatic, may be as high as 15% among persons older than 55 years, making it one of the most prevalent forms of CVD among older adults.

Differences by Age, Sex, Race, Geographic Area, and Socioeconomic Status

The complex relation between the genetic and environmental influences on the development of CVD is illustrated by the marked variability in its occurrence by age, sex, race, geographic area, and socioeconomic status (SES). The prevalence of CHD, for example, increases significantly with age among both men and women, becoming the leading cause of death among men by 50 years of age and among women by 65 years.

Although rates of CVD have been reported to increase with increasing exposure to risk factors for CVD among a variety of racial and ethnic groups, there is variability in the incidence of CVD even after accounting for differences in the prevalence of risk factors for CVD among different groups. For example, African-Americans

have high rates of hypertension, diabetes, and obesity, but have rates of CHD that tend to be lower than those among non-Hispanic whites, particularly for men. Stroke rates, however, are significantly greater among African Americans than among Caucasians. Data on Hispanic Americans are scant and inconclusive, but a recent report suggests that Hispanic Americans, with higher rates of diabetes and obesity have higher rates of CHD than do non-Hispanic whites. The reasons behind these conflicting reports are unclear but may have to do with differences in the prevalence, detection, and management of risk factors for CVD. They also might be explained by socioeconomic and psychosocial factors.

Considerable geographic variability in rates of CVD occurs throughout the world, even among industrialized nations. Data from 1991 show that rates for both mortality from CVD and all-cause mortality are intermediate among U.S. adult men and women compared with rates in other countries. The highest rates of CVD are reported in eastern European countries, including the former Soviet Union, where deaths from CVD are nearly twice as common as in the United States. The lowest reported rates of CVD are in France and Japan, where the death rate of CVD is approximately half that in the United States (Table 16-1).

The dramatic decline in rates of CVD in the United States during the past three decades also has occurred in most other industrialized nations. Exceptions to these trends have been in countries of eastern Europe, Spain, and the United Kingdom, where little improvement or considerable worsening in rates of CVD have been observed. Worsening rates of CVD around the world are probably influenced by the adoption of unhealthful lifestyles, as reported among Japanese immigrants to the United States.

Geographic differences are likely explained in part by variability in lifestyle-related risk factors for CVD. For example, countries with high rates of CVD tend to have high rates of obesity, physical inactivity, diets high in saturated fat,

Table 16-1

Death Rates from Cardiovascular Disease in Selected Countries, 1991

Poland	934
Romania	829
Ireland	627
England	539
United States	487
Australia	477
China	446
Canada	387
Spain	321
Mexico	290
France	258
Japan	238

Rates per 100,000 population.
SOURCE: From National Heart, Lung, and Blood Institute, 1994.

and cigarette smoking. Although cigarette smoking is prevalent in Japan, physical activity, dietary habits, and obesity rates are more positive than in countries with higher rates of CVD. The so-called "French paradox" refers to the low rates of CVD in France despite relatively high rates of cigarette smoking and intake of saturated fat. The paradox may be explained in part by the relatively large consumption of wine per capita in France but also may be due to relatively low rates of physical inactivity and obesity.

Considerable variability in rates of CVD also is seen in the United States. The highest age-adjusted mortality rate for CVD is reported in the southeastern states (more than 288 deaths from CVD per 100,000 population). The lowest rates are reported in the Pacific northwest and intermountain western states (201 to 240 CVD deaths per 100,000 population).

Consistent differences in cardiovascular health by SES have been reported for the past three decades. Whether the measure for SES is education level, income, or job classification, numerous studies have documented that persons of lower SES are at significantly greater risk for CVD than those of higher SES, even after adjustment for differences in risk factors for CVD. A number of factors probably contribute to the relation between low SES and risk for CVD, including (1) limitations in access to and use of health care systems, (2) occupational and environmental health hazard exposure, and (3) relative lack of social networking and support.

Time Trends

CORONARY HEART DISEASE

A remarkable drop in mortality from CVD has been observed in the United States over the past 30 or more years (Figure 16-1). This decline has been observed among African-Americans and Caucasians of both sexes but has been particularly dramatic among men of both races (Figure 16-2). The decline has been caused by reductions in both the incidence and the case fatality rate of MI. Hunink, et al (1997) estimated that the underlying mechanisms for declining incidence and case fatality rates of CHD have to do with reduction in the prevalence of risk factors for CVD, which has accounted for approximately half of the decline, and medical and surgical care, which has helped produce the other improvements.

CEREBROVASCULAR DISEASE

The decline in CBVD has been significant among men and women, African-American and Caucasian, but it has been particularly dramatic among African-Americans. Between 1950 and 1990, stroke mortality among African-Americans decreased approximately 60% (Figure 16-3). Although stroke mortality among African-Americans remains higher than among Caucasians, the difference has narrowed markedly over the past 40 years. It is curious that stroke mortality began

Figure 16-1

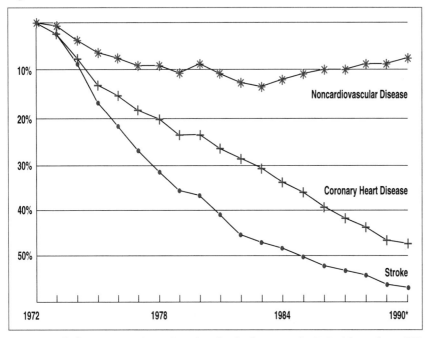

Percentage decline in non-CVD, CHD, and stroke death rates in the United States from 1972 to 1990, adjusted for age. (Reproduced from the Fifth Report of the Joint National Committee on Detection, Evaluation, and Treatment of High Blood Pressure.)

to decline in the 1950s and 1960s, even before widespread therapy for hypertension was administered. Recent evidence suggests that mortality rates for CBVD may have increased to levels previously seen in 1970. The worsening statistics for CBVD may be caused in part by a recent decline in the percentage of persons with hypertension who are aware of their condition and are treated appropriately (Table 16-2). The principal driving force behind the failure in CBVD prevention, however, is probably the success observed in CHD prevention. That is, the

improved survival rates among persons with MI have produced an increasing pool of persons who are at high risk for future cerebrovascular events. Shifting demographic characteristics in the United States toward longer life expectancy and an increasing elderly population undoubtedly have had an effect on rates of CBVD.

PERIPHERAL VASCULAR DISEASE

Data that can help identify trends in the occurrence of PVD in the United States over the

Figure 16-2

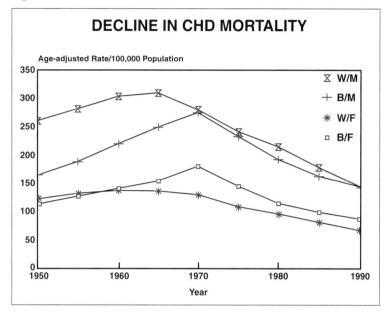

Age-adjusted CHD mortality rates by race and sex from 1950 to 1990. B/M, black males; W/M, white males; B/F, black females; W/F, white females. (Reproduced from the Fifth Report of the Joint National Committee on Detection, Evaluation, and Treatment of High Blood Pressure.)

past 30 years are scant. In addition to a deficiency in the quantity of longitudinal data collected on PVD during recent decades, there have been qualitative problems in data collection. Newer methods of detection of PVD have more than likely helped find more persons with PVD at earlier stages of the disease than was the case in previous years, when detection was based primarily on symptoms. Use of these newer diagnostic methods has led to different, more objective defining criteria. Table 16-3 presents one suggested diagnostic schema. With

these factors in mind, it would be expected that the prevalence of PVD in the general population would be greater today than in the past three decades. Published reports contradict this assumption, however. A study from Iceland showed that the incidence of PVD decreased sharply between 1968 and 1986 and that the decline in PVD began even before the decline began in rates of CHD for Iceland. Approximately one-half of the decline in PVD was attributed to decreases in smoking and cholesterol levels.

Figure 16-3

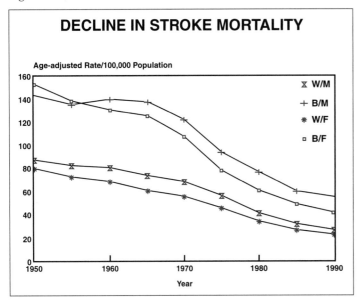

Age-adjusted stroke mortality rates by race and sex from 1950 to 1990. B/M, black males; W/M, white males; B/F, black females; W/F, white females. (Reproduced from the Fifth Report of the Joint National Committee on Detection, Evaluation, and Treatment of High Blood Pressure.)

Table 16-2

Trends in Awareness, Treatment, and Control of High Blood Pressure among U.S. Adults, 1976–1994

	1976–1980	1988–1991	1991–1994
Awareness	51	73	68
Treatment	31	55	54
Control	10	29	27

Values are percentage of adults with hypertension.
SOURCE: Modified from the Sixth Report of the Joint National Committee on Prevention, Detection, Evaluation, and Treatment of High Blood Pressure.

Table 16-3

Suggested Diagnostic Criteria for Peripheral Arterial Disease

GRADE	CATEGORY	5-YEAR SURVIVAL RATE (%)	CLINICAL FINDINGS	ANKLE-BRACHIAL INDEX	OTHER FINDINGS
0	0	>95	Asymptomatic	0.90–1.30	Normal exercise test result[a]
	1	80	Mild claudication	0.70–0.89	Completes test, posttest ankle BP <50 mm Hg, but <25 mm Hg below brachial BP
I	2	70	Moderate claudication	0.40–0.69	—
	3	55	Severe claudication	0.30–0.39	Cannot finish exercise, posttest ankle BP <50 mm Hg
II	4	40	Rest pain	<0.30	Rest ankle BP <40 mm Hg
	5	≤40	Minor tissue loss, focal gangrene, non-healing ulcer	<0.30	Rest ankle BP <60 mm Hg Toe BP <40 mm Hg
III	6	≤40	Major tissue loss, above metatarsal level, foot not salvageable	<0.30	Same as category 5

[a] Exercise on treadmill for 5 min at 2 mph and 12% incline.

ABBREVIATION: BP, blood pressure.

Adapted from Rutherford et al., 1986, McKenna et al., 1991 and McDermott et al., 1994.

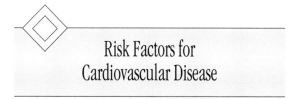

Risk Factors for Cardiovascular Disease

In the late 1950s a small group of researchers began to dispel the myth that CVD was a natural part of the aging process. Stamler, et al, helped identify several factors, including high levels of dietary fat and cholesterol, cigarette smoking, hypertension, and a sedentary lifestyle, predictive of higher risk for CVD. Numerous other potential risk factors for CVD were explored by other investigators. A report by Hopkins and Williams in 1981 suggested 246 potential risk factors that had been associated with CVD in the medical literature to that date. Since their report was published, numerous other risk factors have been found associated with CVD. A list of the most important risk factors and their relative weights is shown in Table 16-4, as identified by the panel from the 27th Bethesda Conference on Matching the Intensity of Risk Factor Management with the Hazard for Coronary Disease Events. The important risk factors for CVD and their responsiveness to therapy are as follows.

Table 16-4

Risk Factors, Strength of Association with Cardiovascular Disease (CVD) and Response to Therapy

RISK FACTOR	ASSOCIATION WITH CVD FROM EPIDEMIOLOGIC STUDIES	ASSOCIATION WITH CVD FROM CLINICAL TRIALS	RESPONSE TO NONDRUG THERAPY	RESPONSE TO DRUG THERAPY
RISK FACTORS FOR WHICH TREATMENT REDUCES CVD RISK				
Smoking	+++	++	+++	++
LDL cholesterol	+++	+++	++	+++
Saturated fat	+++	++	++	—
Hypertension	+++	+++	+	+++
Left ventricular hypertrophy	+++	+ (stroke)	—	++
Thrombogenic factors	+++ (fibrinogen)	+++ (aspirin, warfarin)	+	+++ (aspirin, warfarin)
Atrial fibrillation	+++ (stroke)	—	—	+++ (warfarin)
RISK FACTORS FOR WHICH TREATMENT IS LIKELY TO REDUCE CVD RISK				
Diabetes mellitus	+++	+	++	+++
Physical inactivity	+++	++	++	—
HDL cholesterol	+++	+	++	+
Obesity	+++	—	++	+
RISK FACTORS FOR WHICH TREATMENT MAY REDUCE CVD RISK				
Estrogen deficiency (women)	+++	—	—	++
Psychosocial factors	++	+	+	—
Triglycerides; small, dense, LDL	++	++	++	+++
Lipoprotein (a)	+	—	—	+
Homocysteine	++	—	++	++
Oxidative stress	++	—	++ (vitamin E, C)	—
Alcohol intake (Direct in cerebrovascular disease) (Inverse in coronary heart disease)	++	—	++	—
RISK FACTORS FOR WHICH TREATMENT IS UNLIKELY TO REDUCE CVD RISK				
Age	+++	—	—	—
Male sex	+++	—	—	—
Socioeconomic status (low)	+++	—	—	—
Family history of premature CVD	+++	—	—	—

KEY: —, no clear evidence or not applicable to factors; +, weak evidence; ++, moderately strong evidence, +++, very strong, consistent evidence.

SOURCE: Modified with permission from Pearson and Fuster.

Risk Factors for Which Treatment Reduces Risk for Cardiovascular Disease

CIGARETTE SMOKING

Incontrovertible evidence has been collected over the past 50 years that cigarette smoking is a leading cause of CVD. It is estimated that more than 400,000 deaths each year are attributable to cigarette smoking, making it the most deadly correctable risk factor identified to date. The relation between cigarette smoking and CVD is linear; that is, risk for CVD increases with each cigarette smoked. The danger of cigarette smoking to the cardiovascular system is particularly severe when other risk factors are present, such as hypertension, hypercholesterolemia, or diabetes. Results of numerous studies have suggested that exposure to secondhand smoke, or passive smoking, significantly increases risk for CVD, contributing to an estimated 40,000 deaths per year in the United States.

Cigarette smoking appears to increase risk for CVD by increasing thrombogenicity, directly damaging the endothelium of the arterial wall, and increasing platelet aggregability and fibrinogen level. Cigarette smoking probably increases risk for CVD through other mechanisms as well. Smoking, for example, has been associated with decreases in levels of high-density lipoprotein (HDL) cholesterol and increases in plasma catecholamine levels, the latter probably part of the reason smokers are at elevated risk for sudden cardiac death.

CHOLESTEROL

The relation between cholesterol level and CHD is graded, continuous, and strong, as documented extensively with research performed throughout the world over the past 40 years. A person with a total serum cholesterol level > 264 mg/dL has a risk for CHD approximately 15 times that of a person with a total cholesterol level < 167 mg/dL. Cholesterol probably plays an important role in the development of CBVD

and PVD, although studies generally show it to be a weaker risk indicator for these disorders than for CHD.

LOW-DENSITY LIPOPROTEIN CHOLESTEROL

Low-density lipoprotein (LDL) cholesterol in particular is thought to be a critical component of the development of atherosclerosis and is an important risk factor for morbidity and mortality from CVD. Other lipid components of the blood, such as HDL cholesterol, triglycerides, and lipoprotein (a), also have important roles in atherogenesis, but none has been studied as extensively, nor do any appear as strong or as correctable as LDL cholesterol. Although the *quantity* of LDL has been the focus of much attention in cardiovascular research and clinical activities, the *quality* of LDL is emerging as an important determinant of atherogenesis. The size of the LDL particle and its susceptibility to oxidation help determine its atherogenic potential. Smaller, more dense LDL particles are thought to be more atherogenic than larger particles, in part because the smaller particles are more prone to oxidation. Once it is oxidized, LDL becomes more likely to bind to and damage endothelial cells in the arterial wall, promoting the atherogenic process. The actual quantity and quality of LDL cholesterol in the blood are determined by multiple genetic and environmental factors.

Lifestyle-related factors, including intake dietary fat, physical activity, obesity, and cigarette smoking, exert a particularly strong influence on the atherogenic potential of the LDL particle. Thus, adoption of optimal lifestyle habits appears to improve risk for CVD in part through the positive effect on quantity of LDL, particle size, and oxidative potential. A variety of drugs have been shown to lower the quantity of LDL cholesterol (the statin group of lipid lowering drugs), whereas others may improve LDL particle size (niacin and gemfibrozil) or reduce the oxidative potential of LDL (vitamin E, vitamin C, selenium). Ranges for total and LDL cholesterol have been described on the basis of risk for CVD from epidemiologic and clinical trial data by the National Cholesterol Education Program Adult Treatment Panel II. An LDL cholesterol level of $\geq$ 160 mg/dL is considered a high-risk factor. An LDL cholesterol level of $\leq$ 130 mg/dL is considered desirable for persons without CVD. Among persons with CVD the desirable level of LDL cholesterol is $\leq$ 100 mg/dL.

HIGH SATURATED FAT, HIGH CHOLESTEROL DIET

Dietary saturated fat and, to a lesser degree, dietary cholesterol are associated with serum cholesterol concentration and its related risk for CVD. Both saturated fat and cholesterol intake may influence risk for CVD in ways that are independent of their lipid effects (increases in thrombogenicity and blood pressure levels). Interventions to lower saturated fat and cholesterol intake have been shown to lower risk for CVD. Polyunsaturated and monounsaturated fats generally have beneficial effects on lipids and risk for CVD when used in moderation.

HYPERTENSION

Hypertension has a graded, continuous, and strong association with risk for development of CVD. This relation has been documented for both systolic and diastolic blood pressures and varies somewhat by race and sex. Women, for example, have lower risk for CVD events for a given level of blood pressure than do men. African-American men have a lower risk for CHD but a higher risk for CBVD than do Caucasian men for any given blood pressure level.

LEFT VENTRICULAR HYPERTROPHY

Left ventricular hypertrophy, a thickening of the left ventricular wall that often occurs in per-

sons with hypertension because of the chronic adaptations of the heart to increased blood pressure and blood volume, has been identified as a strong predictor of both CHD and CBVD. Reversal of left ventricular hypertrophy and a subsequent reduction in risk for CVD can occur as hypertension is controlled. Left ventricular hypertrophy can be detected with an ECG, but detection by means of echocardiographic techniques is more accurate.

THROMBOGENIC FACTORS

Because of their critical role in atherogenesis and acute arterial thrombosis, thrombogenic factors have emerged as important risk factors for CVD. Fibrinogen increases risk for CVD by promoting hemostasis and complex atherosclerotic plaque formation. (See section of Cardiovascular Disease Natural History.) Plasminogen activator inhibitor-1 may increase risk for acute CVD events by inhibiting native fibrinolytic factors. Increased intrinsic activity of these native fibrinolytic factors, such as tissue plasminogen activator (tPA), may protect against acute CVD. Fibrinolytic agents such as tPA and streptokinase have been found to be useful treatments for improving survival after acute MI and stroke. There is some evidence that certain interventions, such as physical activity and smoking cessation, may improve the relative balance of these factors, but no clear recommendations can be made at present. Use of agents with antiplatelet (aspirin) or anticoagulant (warfarin) activity has been associated with reduced risk for CHD. Use of warfarin reduces risk for stroke among persons with atrial fibrillation.

ATRIAL FIBRILLATION

Atrial fibrillation has long been associated with increased risk for stroke among persons with rheumatic mitral valve disease. It also has been associated with a fivefold increase for stroke among persons with nonvalvular atrial fibrillation ("lone" atrial fibrillation). It is estimated that one-third of all ischemic strokes among elderly persons are related to atrial fibrillation. This is an important factor given that the occurrence of atrial fibrillation increases with age, reaching approximately 35% among persons older than 80 years. The risk for stroke among persons with atrial fibrillation is particularly strong in the presence of any of the following characteristics: age greater than 75 years, female sex, hypertension, recent episode of congestive heart failure, diabetes mellitus, smoking, left atrial enlargement, mitral annular calcification, and left atrial thrombus. Numerous trials have documented reductions of more than 50% in the incidence of stroke among persons with nonvalvular atrial fibrillation receiving warfarin therapy. Risk for intracranial hemorrhage increases slightly with warfarin therapy when anticoagulation is within optimal range [international normalized ratio (INR) between 2.0 and 3.0], but the risk-to-benefit ratio still strongly favors warfarin therapy over aspirin or no anticoagulation therapy.

Risk Factors for Which Treatment Is Likely to Reduce Risk for Cardiovascular Disease Events

DIABETES MELLITUS

Diabetes has long been identified as a risk factor for the development of CVD, doubling the risk among men and tripling the risk among women. The risks associated with diabetes mellitus type II are particularly strong because a number of other risk factors for CVD (hypertension, hyperlipidemia, and obesity) tend to cluster among such persons. Hyperglycemia at the time of a CVD event may portend a worse prognosis, perhaps because an adverse (anaerobic) metabolic milieu may help extend an area of

ischemia. For further information on diabetes, see Chapter 17.

PHYSICAL INACTIVITY

The most prevalent correctable risk for CVD in the United States, occurring among approximately 60% of the U.S. population, is physical inactivity. It is estimated that 29 to 40% of all deaths of CHD are attributable to a sedentary lifestyle. Physical activity is thought to affect rates of CVD by improving several risk factors for CVD, including HDL cholesterol level, blood pressure, obesity, glucose metabolism, and possibly hemostatic factors. (See Section of Cardiovascular Disease Primary Prevention.)

HIGH-DENSITY LIPOPROTEIN CHOLESTEROL

HDL cholesterol level is inversely associated with risk for CVD. A 2 to 3% decrease in risk for CHD is associated with every 1% increase in HDL cholesterol concentration. The Adult Treatment Panel II cholesterol treatment guidelines classified an HDL level <35 mg/dL as a risk factor for CHD. Several lifestyle (smoking cessation, physical activity, and weight loss by obese persons) and drug interventions (niacin, fibrates, and statins) can increase HDL levels. Although some studies suggest indirectly that interventions to raise HDL may decrease risk for CHD, no large-scale studies have been performed to investigate this issue.

OBESITY

Obesity affects 30% of adults in the United States and is strongly associated with the occurrence of hypertension, diabetes, and lipid disorders. The American Heart Association considers obesity a major risk factor for CVD. Whether the risk for CVD associated with obesity is truly independent of other related risk factors is debatable. High levels of abdominal obesity, indicated by elevations in waist circumference or waist-to-hip ratio, may be the strongest weight-related predictor of CVD and its related risk factors.

Risk Factors for Which Treatment May Reduce Risk for Cardiovascular Disease Events

ESTROGEN DEFICIENCY

Estrogen replacement therapy in post-menopausal women was thought to reduce risk of CVD as much as 50%. The HERS study, however, showed no clear benefit of estrogen and progestin therapy on a five-year, or total, mortality for CVD among postmenopausal women randomized to the hormone replacement arm of the trial. Results of a large number of observational studies, however, strongly suggest a protective effect of estrogen on risk for CVD, particularly in the primary prevention of CVD events. The potential beneficial effects of estrogen on risk for CVD are probably in large part caused by its favorable effects on factors that help control atherogenesis, such as LDL cholesterol, HDL cholesterol, lipoprotein (a), fibrinogen, and arterial wall endothelial cells.

PSYCHOSOCIAL FACTORS

Hostility, depression, social isolation, and lower SES have been shown in a variety of studies to be associated with an increased risk for CVD. Part of this association may be caused by coexistent unhealthful lifestyle habits and poor adherence to medical treatment. Much of the association, however, is thought to be caused by real biochemical (adrenergic system) and metabolic (lipid, glucose, and blood pressure) changes that can occur with the chronic "stress" that typifies these adverse psychosocial factors. For example, patients who do not have a

spouse or confidant are three times more likely to die during the 6 months after MI than are patients who do have a spouse or confidant. There is some evidence that treatment aimed at hostility, depression, and social isolation may improve risk for CVD, but definitive recommendations await the final results of ongoing large-scale randomized studies.

TRIGLYCERIDES

Serum triglyceride concentration is an independent risk factor for CVD, but this risk is also a reflection of the role of triglycerides in the so-called syndrome X or atherogenic lipid profile. In this syndrome abdominal fat deposition and insulin resistance help set off a cascade of metabolic derangements that result in glucose intolerance, hypertension, and lipid disorders (high triglycerides, low HDL cholesterol, and small, dense LDL cholesterol particles). There also is an associated increase in thrombogenicity that further increases risk for CVD events. There are no published reports of clinical trials in which lowering of triglyceride levels, independent of other factors for an atherogenic lipid profile, decreases risk for CVD.

LIPOPROTEIN (a)

Lipoprotein (a) is a complex lipoprotein particle associated with increased risk for CVD, particularly among persons with high serum concentrations of LDL cholesterol. Elevated lipoprotein (a) level is a common disorder, occurring among 20% of persons with premature CHD. Its effect on risk for CVD may be caused by its close resemblance to plasminogen, which causes competitive inhibition of normal fibrinolysis. Levels of lipoprotein (a) are higher in African-Americans than in Caucasians and increase in women after menopause. Estrogen replacement therapy, anabolic steroids, niacin, and LDL apheresis may lower lipoprotein

(a) levels, but no definitive studies have been reported that show that lowering lipoprotein (a) results in improvement in risk for CVD.

HOMOCYSTEINE

Clearance of homocysteine, an amino acid, is another emerging risk factor for CVD. When homocysteine is not cleared appropriately because of either a genetic defect in its regulatory enzyme (cystathionine B-synthase) or a deficiency of folate, vitamin B6 or vitamin B12, homocysteine levels increase and promote atherogenesis by a mechanism that is still unclear. Hyperhomocysteinemia is a common condition, occurring in as much as 20% of the adult population. Its association with CVD is strong with a three- to 30-fold increase in risk for CVD among persons with the disorder. Homocysteine levels can be reduced in affected individuals with dietary supplements of folate, vitamin B6, and vitamin B12, but the effect of treatment on risk for CVD still is uncertain.

OXIDATIVE STRESS

Oxidation of LDL cholesterol particles increases the atherogenic potential of LDL by promoting endothelial damage and LDL uptake. Agents that impede LDL oxidation, including vitamin C, vitamin E, and β-carotene, have been associated with a reduced risk for CVD. Other factors that also might decrease oxidative stress include exercise training and selenium, estrogen, magnesium, and monounsaturated fats. Iron has been suggested as a promoter of LDL oxidation and a possible risk factor for CVD, but results of published reports are conflicting. The most promising evidence to date is for the antioxidant effects of vitamin C and vitamin E. In a randomized, controlled trial involving persons with CHD, vitamin E supplementation was associated with a 77% reduction in rate of nonfatal MI, although no clear improvement in total CVD mortality was found.

Risk Factors for Which Treatment Is Unlikely to Reduce Risk for Cardiovascular Disease Events

A number of strong but untreatable risk factors for CVD have been identified, including older age, male sex, and a family history of premature CVD (a CVD event before 55 years of age for a first-degree male relative or before 65 years of age for a first-degree female relative). Because some of the associations of these risk factors are likely to be explained by other, treatable risk factors for CVD (inheritance of lipid disorders in families, for example), it is possible that some of these unmodifiable risk factors might be altered by means of medical or lifestyle treatments. Short stature, baldness, earlobe crease, and ear canal hair have been identified as relatively weak, unmodifiable risk factors for CVD.

Relative Importance of Risk Factors for Coronary Heart Disease, Cerebrovascular Disease, and Peripheral Vascular Disease

Because the process of atherosclerosis is systemic, it would seem logical that risk factors known to accelerate the atherosclerotic process in one vascular bed (the heart) would also be associated with risk for atherosclerotic disease in another area (the brain). Whereas this is true for the most part, there are minor differences in the relative importance of the various risk factors for CVD in the development of CHD and CBVD. For example, cholesterol level is a strong predictor of CHD but is a relatively weak predictor of CBVD. This is probably because of the inclusion of nonatherosclerotic strokes (e.g., intracranial hemorrhage) in this category. Atrial fibrillation is a risk factor for CBVD but is not directly related to CHD or risk for CHD.

Natural History of Cardiovascular Disease

The process of atherogenesis begins early in life, perhaps as early as birth, when the interplay between genetics and environment begins. Small foci of smooth-muscle cells are found in the intima of arterial walls soon after birth and appear to track into adulthood as sights of future atherosclerotic lesions. Through years of interaction between environmental and genetic stressors on the arterial wall, a recurring cycle of arterial wall injury and repair occurs and leads to the formation of three specific atherosclerotic lesions—fatty streaks, fibrous plaques, and complicated lesions. Once an initial injury to the vessel wall takes place, either from a direct toxin (e.g., oxidized LDL cholesterol, infection, or tobacco constituents) or from direct trauma (e.g., hypertension), the initial steps in the atherosclerotic process begin.

Oxidized LDL cholesterol is taken up across the injured endothelium by macrophages, which transform into lipid-laden foam cells. These foam cells congregate into a soft, unstable lipid core that can rupture and cause further toxic injury to the surrounding endothelium. Various inflammatory responses such as platelet aggregation, thrombosis, and smooth-muscle cell proliferation repair the injured endothelium and produce a thin, unstable fibrous cap that covers the lipid core. With continuing exposure to endothelial toxins (risk factors for CVD), early atherosclerotic lesions advance to larger, more complicated ones as the cycle of intimal injury and repair continues. Acute occlusion of an arterial lumen can occur when the thin fibrous cap of a complicated lesion ruptures and exudes the underlying thrombogenic lipid core. If the resulting thrombosis is large enough to totally occlude the arterial lumen, ischemia and, even-

tually, infarction can develop and involve the downstream tissues.

Reductions in risk factors for CVD can improve risk for CVD by interrupting the injury—repair cycle and stabilizing the complicated lesion. Lipid-lowering therapy stabilizes the lesion by shrinking the underlying lipid core while promoting development of a more stable, thickened fibrous cap that is less prone to injury and rupture. Antiinflammatory agents and possibly some antibiotics are thought to diminish the inflammatory response in complicated lesions, stabilize the fibrous cap itself, and decrease the risk for rupture and subsequent thrombosis.

Because CHD, CBVD, and PVD are manifestations of a chronic condition (atherosclerosis), progression of the disease and recurrence of CVD events are the rule if no efforts are made to slow, stop, or reverse the process of atherosclerosis. Most patients with CHD survive their first MI (approximately 60% to 65%, including survivors of out-of-hospital cardiac arrest) but remain at risk for recurrent MI without preventive intervention. The death rate among survivors of MI who receive standard therapy is 3% to 5% 1 month after and 8% to 12% 6 months after MI.

Persons at low risk (1% risk for recurrent MI in the first year after MI) are those who have uncomplicated MI, one without significant left ventricular failure, complex ventricular arrhythmia, or inducible myocardial ischemia. Persons at high risk (10% risk for recurrent MI in the first year after MI) are those who have left ventricular failure, frequent complex ventricular arrhythmias, and severe inducible myocardial ischemia. Persons at moderate risk (approximately 5% risk for recurrent MI in the first year after MI) are those who have mild-to-moderate left ventricular impairment, ventricular arrhythmia, or myocardial ischemia.

Short-term disability after MI is not unusual, but substantial long-term disability occurs among only a minority of persons who experience MI. Approximately 85% of MI survivors who were employed before the MI return to at least part-time work during the first year after the MI.

Death rates from stroke are approximately 7.6% per year after a major stroke, and approximately 4.9% after a minor stroke. Among survivors of stroke, approximately 20% have severe disabilities that necessitate hospitalization, and another 40% to 50% have mild-to-moderate disabilities from their stroke. As many as 30% of stroke survivors may recuperate without long-term disability.

Once symptoms of CHD or CBVD are present, risk for subsequent CVD events increases significantly. In one study involving persons with angina pectoris, for example, the one-year incidence of death, MI, or hospitalization for CHD was 15%. Studies suggest that the annual risk for stroke following a TIA is 4% to 12%. The highest risk for stroke is during the first few months after a TIA. This is somewhat controversial because approximately 25% of what are believed to be TIAs are found at computed tomography (CT) or magnetic resonance imaging (MRI) to be actual strokes.

Primary Prevention of Cardiovascular Disease

Numerous reports have documented the feasibility of the primary prevention of CVD, defined as the application of interventions to reduce CVD events among persons in the general population who do not have symptoms. Most research has been conducted on the primary prevention of CHD, although there is a growing body of literature on the primary prevention of

CBVD. Limited data are available on the primary prevention of PVD.

Management of Risk Factors for Cardiovascular Disease

HYPERTENSION

Removal of risk factors for CVD should in theory slow or even reverse the damaging effects of the atherogenic cycle. Management of hypertension, for example, has been shown to improve risk for first time CHD and CBVD events. Among patients with hypertension who are given appropriate therapy, a reduction in CHD events of 10% to 15% has been observed by several investigators. One study that has shown even more significant benefits of hypertension treatment is the Systolic Hypertension in Elderly Project (SHEP). Investigators in SHEP found that among an otherwise healthy group of elderly persons with hypertension, treatment with a diuretic or β-blocking agent, or both resulted in a 27% reduction in CHD events and a 36% reduction in CBVD events.

LIPIDS AND LIPOPROTEINS

Lipid-lowering therapy has been shown to prevent CVD events (both MI and stroke) among patients without previously documented CVD. The West of Scotland Coronary Prevention Study showed that lipid-lowering therapy with pravastatin among persons with hypercholesterolemia resulted in a 31% reduction in CHD events (nonfatal MI and CHDs) and a 32% reduction in all CVD deaths. There was a reduction in CBVD events of approximately 30%, a finding that was somewhat surprising given the relatively weak association between cholesterol and risk for CBVD. Some investigators have theorized that the reduction in risk CBVD with pravastatin therapy (and therapy with other statins in other trials) is caused in part by the effect of lipid-lowering therapy on plaque stabilization, among other nonlipid effects of the drugs.

DIABETES

Aggressive management of diabetes has been shown to improve risk for microvascular complications of diabetes (retinopathy, nephropathy, and neuropathy), but until recently there has been no evidence that such treatment improves risk for CVD or life expectancy among persons with diabetes. The U.K. Prospective Diabetes Study did recently find that aggressive treatment of patients with diabetes by means of metformin significantly lowered mortality for CHD and CBVD in the population studied.

CIGARETTE SMOKING

Cigarette smoking clearly increases a person's risk for CVD. Avoidance of smoking has been reported in observational studies to be associated with a decreased risk for death of CVD. Risk for CVD also improves among smokers who successfully stop smoking. Within 3 to 5 years after smoking cessation most if not all of the atherogenic effects of smoking subside, and a person's risk for cardiovascular death returns to that of a nonsmoker. Risk for sudden cardiac death among smokers decreases within a short time after cessation of smoking. Smoking prevention and cessation are essential elements in the prevention of CVD (see Chapter 10).

Physical Activity

Studies suggesting that physical activity plays an important role in the primary prevention of CVD date back to early work by Paffenbarger, Morris, and others that documented reduced risk for CVD among workers who were most physically active compared with risk among those who were less active. These early findings have been

supported by those of more recent observational studies that show that risk for CVD is reduced with physical activity among men, women, and the elderly.

Although some studies have assessed the effect of work-related physical activity, the most recent, convincing, and consistent evidence supports the protective role of leisure-time physical activity in primary prevention of CVD. Any physical activity, whether during work or leisure time, can help reduce risk for morbidity and mortality due to CVD.

The work of Paffenbarger and others shows the relation between physical activity and reduction in risk for both CHD and CBVD is continuous and linear up to a level of 2000 to 2500 kcal/week (the equivalent of walking or jogging 20 to 25 miles per week), beyond which the benefits of exercise plateau. Persons who habitually engage in at least 2000 kcal/week of physical activity have 20 to 25% lower risk for CVD events than those who do not achieve that level of physical activity. There are a number of possible mechanisms for the cardiovascular benefits of exercise, including positive effects on lipid metabolism, glucose metabolism, blood pressure, and coagulation factors (Table 16-5).

Although risk for CVD has been shown to be lower among persons who habitually exercise, physical activity does not come without its own inherent risk for CVD. Risk for CVD events increases *during* a bout of exercise compared with risk at rest, probably because of increased risk for rupture of an atherosclerotic plaque as systolic blood pressure rises during a bout of exercise. Still, the absolute risk for a CVD event during exercise is extremely small among persons without symptoms in the general population.

Counseling a patient to begin an exercise training program involves a variety of steps that also are applicable in counseling persons to modify dietary habits and smoking. Once it is ascertained that a patient is sedentary and has no medical conditions that would preclude physical activity, the following steps are recom-

Table 16-5

Effect of Habitual Physical Activity on Important Cardiovascular Disease Risk Factors

FACTOR	REPORTED EFFECT OF HABITUAL PHYSICAL ACTIVITY
Serum lipids	Increase in HDL cholesterol
	Decrease in triglycerides, LDL cholesterol
	Improved LDL subfractions (less atherogenic)
	Possible improvement in apolipoprotein A
	No change in apolipoprotein B or lipoprotein (a)
Glucose metabolism	Decrease in incidence of diabetes mellitus, type II
	Increase in insulin sensitivity
Blood pressure	Decrease in incidence of hypertension
	Decrease in resting systolic and diastolic blood pressure
Clotting factors	Decrease in hemostatic factors (fibrinogen, factor VII, platelet aggregability
	Improvement in fibrinolytic factors (increased tissue plasminogen activator decreased plasminogen activator inhibitor-I).
Fat metabolism	Improved free fatty acid and total fat oxidative capacity

mended to help promote a consistent physical activity program—ask, assess, advise, assist.

Ask patients about their readiness to change exercise habits. This helps separate persons who are ready to change from those who are not ready to change. The latter group is unlikely to change habits on the basis of clinician recommendations alone. They should be given encouragement and basic information on the benefits of habitual physical activity and then be asked again during future clinical visits about their interest in becoming more physically active.

Assess the risk for CVD on the basis of the patient's risk factor profile, history, and physical examination findings. Persons with multiple risk factors for CVD, men older than 40 years of age, and women older than 50 years of age should consider undergoing an exercise stress test before initiating a vigorous exercise program to determine whether they are at increased risk for exercise-related cardiovascular events. (See section, Screening for Risk Factors for Cardiovascular Disease.) Patients' confidence in their ability to begin and maintain an exercise program,

degree of support from family or friends, and barriers to regular exercise (e.g., time, interest, weather) should be ascertained. Those who lack confidence or social support or have substantial barriers to exercise need additional follow-up intervention, encouragement, and training to help build their confidence and problem-solving skills.

Advise patients about an appropriate exercise program based on their interests and needs. The patient should generally begin with low-intensity activity for 10 to 15 minutes a day 3 to 5 days a week and build gradually to 30 to 60 minutes a day for 4 to 6 days a week. More frequent, shorter bouts of exercise (10 to 15 minutes three times a day) promote similar health benefits and may be more feasible for some persons. Low-to-moderate intensity can confer considerable health benefits and is preferable to high-intensity activity for most persons because patient compliance and enjoyment and risk for musculoskeletal injury are optimal with low-intensity activities. Patients should be encouraged to involve a friend or family member in their exercise program because social support is a strong predictor of maintenance of an exercise program.

Assist patients as needed by making written recommendations for the exercise program, prompting them to identify important barriers to exercise and ways to overcome them, and simply by asking about their progress at regular intervals (office visits, letters, or telephone calls).

Diet Counseling

All adults and children should be counseled to limit their dietary intake of fat and cholesterol and to limit their intake of saturated fat by emphasizing fruits, vegetables and grains. Adopting healthy dietary habits, as does any modification of health behaviors, requires patient interest, patient commitment, skill and confidence building, and proper follow-up and assessment. Three ways to eat less fat are to eat foods high in saturated fat less often, eat smaller portions of foods high in saturated fat, and substitute low-fat foods for those high in saturated fat. Table 16-6 lists foods to choose and foods to avoid.

Control of Other Risk Factors for Cardiovascular Disease

Avoidance or control of other risk factors for CVD has been shown to reduce future risk for CVD. In particular, smoking cessation has been associated with a significant reduction in risk for CVD, the risk returning to that of a nonsmoker within 5 to 10 years after smoking cessation. Maintenance of ideal body weight and body fat distribution also is associated with significantly improved CVD outcomes compared with those for persons with obesity and excessive abdominal fat deposition. Less is known about the long-term effects of weight loss among obese persons. It has been shown to promote consid-

Table 16-6

Dietary Advice for Cardiovascular Disease Reduction of Risk

FOODS TO CHOOSE	FOODS TO AVOID
Fruit	Pies, cookies, doughnuts, pastries
Vegetables	Fried meats
Soy products	Hamburger, meatloaf, beef burritos
Fish, baked, broiled, or grilled	Hot dogs
Poultry, skinless, baked, broiled, or grilled	Bologna, salami
Margarine, low-fat or fat-free	Bacon, sausage
Vegetable spray	Margarine
Olive or canola oil (sparingly)	Butter
Cheese, low-fat or fat-free	Cream cheese
Milk, skim or 1% fat	Lard, bacon fat, shortening
Mayonnaise, low-fat or fat-free	Whole milk, cream, half-and-half
Pretzels, air-popped popcorn, low-fat chips	Salad dressing, regular
Bagels, low-fat muffins	Potato chips, french fries
Bread, whole grain	Ice cream
Sherbet, fruit ice, low-fat frozen yogurt	
Nuts (sparingly)	

erable improvements in cardiovascular risk factors, even more than those associated with exercise training alone. Table 16-4 lists other important risk factors for CVD and the effect of therapy on the associated risk for CVD.

Screening for Risk Factors for Cardiovascular Disease

HYPERLIPIDEMIA

Screening recommendations for cholesterol abnormalities among adults were given in the Second Report of the Expert Panel on Detection, Evaluation, and Treatment of High Blood Cholesterol in Adults. Although there is some controversy about cholesterol screening tests for young adults and the elderly, the expert panel recommendations call for cholesterol screening for all adults older than 20 years of age at least every 5 years. The measurements should include total and HDL cholesterol initially followed by a complete fasting lipid profile if total cholesterol is not < 200 mg/dL or if HDL cholesterol is < 35 mg/dL (Figure 16-4). If LDL cholesterol level is > 130 mg/dL, appropriate dietary therapy should be initiated. If after 3 to 6 months of aggressive dietary therapy, LDL cholesterol remains elevated, drug treatment should be considered (Table 16-7). Because dietary modification can reduce LDL cholesterol an average of only 5 to 15% among most persons, combined drug and dietary therapy may be initiated for persons with severely elevated lipid levels.

The U.S. Preventive Services Task Force (USPSTF) recommends cholesterol screening for all men 35 to 65 years of age and women ages 45 to 65 years of age. They found insufficient evidence to recommend screening in other age groups but stated that screening might be justified for adolescents and young adults who have major risk factors for CHD (smoking, diabetes, hypertension, family history of premature CHD in a first-degree relative, family history of very high cholesterol level) and persons 65 to 75 years

of age with major risk factors for CHD (smoking, diabetes, hypertension).

Measurement of lipids and lipoproteins should only be performed by a laboratory that follows standardization procedures of the National Network Laboratories of the Centers for Disease Control and Prevention to minimize excessive laboratory error and variability. Total and HDL cholesterol levels can be drawn in the nonfasting state, but other lipoprotein measurements should be done after a fast of 8 to 12 hours. Care should be taken when interpreting lipid levels when factors are present that can transiently lower (acute illness) or raise (pregnancy) lipid levels. Serum should be used for measurement, although plasma cholesterol level, generally 3 to 5% lower than serum levels, also can be measured. Finger stick blood testing for total cholesterol, HDL cholesterol, and triglycerides is acceptable if performed with standardized equipment by well-trained staff.

HYPERTENSION

There is agreement among all authoritative groups that all adults and children should be periodically screened for hypertension. The Joint National Committee on Prevention, Detection, Evaluation, and Treatment of High Blood Pressure has published its sixth report and recommendations. Screening blood pressure measurements should be performed on adults older than 18 years of age according to the guidelines in Table 16-8.

Classification of normal and abnormal blood pressure readings are shown in Table 16-9. Adults with normal blood pressure readings should undergo repeat blood pressure measurements every 2 years, whereas those with abnormal readings need more frequent follow-up measurements and treatment as shown in Table 16-10. Treatment options include lifestyle modification (weight reduction and limitations on alcohol, sodium, and saturated fat) and pharmacologic therapy. Treatment should be

Figure 16-4

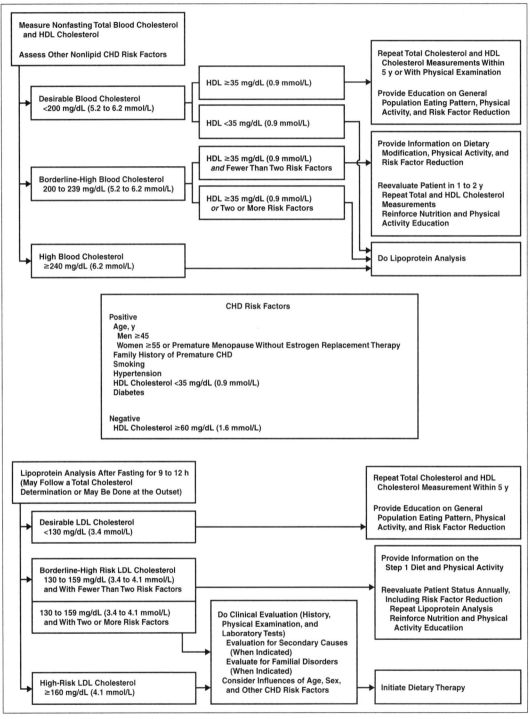

Recommendations for cholesterol screening among adults. (Modified with permission from the Second Report of the Expert Panel on Detection, Evaluation, and Treatment of High Blood Cholesterol in Adults.)

Table 16-7

Drug Therapy for Selected Lipid Abnormalities

LIPID ABNORMALITY	DRUG OPTION	EXAMPLE
Elevated LDL cholesterol	Nicotinic acid (NA)	NA (niacin)
	HMG Co-A reductase inhibitors (statins)	Atorvastatin, fluvastatin, lovastatin, pravastatin, simvastatin
	Bile acid resins (BAR)	Cholestyramine, colestipol, psyllium fiber
Elevated triglycerides	NA	NA (niacin)
	Fibrates	Fenofibrate, gemfibrozil
Elevated LDL and triglycerides	NA	NA (niacin)
	Statin	Atorvastatin (most potent)
	Combination therapy	NA + statin[a]
		NA + BAR
		NA + fibrate[b]
		Statin + fibrate
		Statin + BAR
		Statin + NA[a]

[a] Slightly increases risk for myositis and chemical hepatitis.
[b] Slightly increases risk for myositis; close monitoring recommended.
SOURCE: Modified from the Second Report of the Expert Panel on Detection, Evaluation, and Treatment of High Blood Cholesterol in Adults.

Table 16-8

Blood Pressure Screening Guidelines

1. Patients should be seated for at least 5 minutes and should refrain from smoking or drinking caffeinated products for the 30 minutes before the measurement.
2. The cuff used should be large enough so that the air bladder encircles at least 80% of the arm.
3. Because considerable measurement error can occur with different blood pressure measurement devices, measurements should ideally be taken with a mercury sphygmomanometer or other device that has been calibrated and validated.
4. The first appearance of sound (Korotkoff phase 1) is the value for systolic blood pressure, and the disappearance of sound (phase 5) is the value for diastolic blood pressure.
5. Two or more readings at least 2 minutes apart should be taken and averaged.

Table 16-9

Classification of Blood Pressure Levels for Adults as Recommended in The Sixth Report of the Joint National Committee on Detection, Evaluation, and Treatment of High Blood Pressure

BLOOD PRESSURE CATEGORY	SYSTOLIC BLOOD PRESSURE (MM HG)	DIASTOLIC BLOOD PRESSURE (MM HG)
Optimal	<120	<80
Normal	<130	<85
High normal	130–139	85–89
Stage 1 hypertension	140–159	90–99
Stage 2 hypertension	160–179	100–109
Stage 3 hypertension	≥180	≥110

Table 16-10

Recommendations for Follow-up Blood Pressure Measurements

INITIAL BLOOD PRESSURE (MM HG)	FOLLOW-UP RECOMMENDATIONS
<130/<85	Recheck in 2 yr
130–139/85–89	Recheck in 1 yr
140–159/90–99	Confirm within 2 mo
160–179/100–109	Evaluate within 1 mo
≥180/≥110	Evaluate immediately or within 1 wk depending on the clinical situation

This schedule should be modified according to the patient's other cardiovascular risk factors and underlying clinical disease.
SOURCE: Modified from The Sixth Report of the Joint National Committee on Prevention, Detection, Evaluation, and Treatment of High Blood Pressure.

recommended according to the patient's underlying risks (Table 16-11). Lifestyle modification should be recommended for most if not all patients with hypertension. For persons who need additional therapy, first-line pharmacologic therapies include diuretics and β-blocking agents because these agents have been shown in several large-scale studies to reduce risk for CVD. Treatment choices should be matched with patient characteristics to optimize treatment responses. For example, therapy with an angiotensin-converting enzyme (ACE) inhibitor is preferred in the care of diabetic persons with hypertension because these agents have blood pressure and renal protective effects for persons with diabetes.

DIABETES

The issue of screening for diabetes and the role of control of diabetes in the prevention of CVD are discussed in Chapter 17.

Other Issues in Primary Prevention of Cardiovascular Disease

Several other factors play important roles in the primary prevention of CVD. Aspirin therapy, for example, was reported in one randomized trial to reduce risk for first time heart attack among men. Observational data suggest that similar benefits probably occur for women who take aspirin. The effect of aspirin therapy on risk for first time stroke is less clear, however, although recently published results of an observational study suggest that aspirin may actually increase risk for stroke among elderly men and women. Because of associated bleeding complications, aspirin generally is contraindicated for use by persons with bleeding disorders and active peptic ulcer disease. Although aspirin shows

Table 16-11

Recommendations for Management of High Blood Pressure, According to Patient Risk Status

BLOOD PRESSURE STAGE (MM HG)	RISK GROUP A (NO RISK FACTORS, TOD, OR CCD)	RISK GROUP B (AT LEAST 1 RISK FACTOR, NO TOD, CCD, OR DIABETES	RISK GROUP C (TOD, CCD, OR DIABETES, WITH OR WITHOUT OTHER RISK FACTORS)
High normal (130–139/85–89)	Lifestyle modification	Lifestyle modification	Lifestyle modification and drug therapy
Stage 1 (140–149/90–199)	Lifestyle modification (up to 12 mo)	Lifestyle modification (up to 6 mo)	Lifestyle modification and drug therapy
Stages 2 and 3 (≥160/≥100)	Lifestyle modification and drug therapy	Lifestyle modification and drug therapy	Lifestyle modification and drug therapy

ABBREVIATIONS: TOD, target organ disease; CCD, clinical cardiovascular disease.
Diseases include left ventricular hypertrophy, angina pectoris, prior myocardial infarction, prior condition that necessitated coronary revascularization, heart failure, stroke, transient ischemic attack, nephropathy, peripheral arterial disease, or retinopathy.
SOURCE: Modified from The Sixth Report of the Joint National Committee on Prevention, Detection, Evaluation, and Treatment of High Blood Pressure.

promise as a primary preventive intervention, the long-term effects and risks are not fully understood, and routine use is not currently recommended.

Adjusted-dose warfarin therapy (to an INR of 2.0 to 3.0) has been shown significantly to reduce risk for stroke among persons with atrial fibrillation. Estrogen for postmenopausal women, folate, vitamin E, and vitamin C also show promise in the primary prevention of CVD, but their true role awaits the results of ongoing randomized clinical trials.

Community Interventions

There is ongoing debate about the cost effectiveness of primary prevention of CVD, particularly with regard to community-wide efforts to reduce risk factors for CVD and CVD events. Community-wide experiments have been implemented throughout the world, including the North Karelia Project, Stanford 5 Cities Project, the Minnesota Heart Health Project, and the Pawtucket Heart Health Project. All these pro-

jects include the following strategies: community mobilization, social marketing, school-based health education, work-site health promotion, screening and referral of those at high risk, education of health professionals and adults, and modification of physical environments to promote healthy lifestyle habits. Although expensive, these projects have produced modest improvements in a variety of risk factors for CVD, particularly cigarette smoking, dietary fat intake, high serum cholesterol level, and high blood pressure.

Secondary Prevention of Cardiovascular Disease

In traditional preventive cardiology the term *secondary prevention* refers to efforts aimed at preventing or slowing disease progression among persons with documented CVD. To adhere to a more precise use of the term in this chapter, however, *secondary prevention* is defined as efforts aimed at the detection and management of asymptomatic CVD.

Screening for Cardiovascular Disease

Several screening tests are available to detect asymptomatic CHD, CBVD, and PVD. In brief, the efficacy of each test depends largely on two factors: (1) the pretest likelihood that a given patient has the disease, and (2) the inherent sensitivity and specificity of the test. Exercise stress testing, for example, has a sensitivity of approximately 65% and a specificity of approximately 80% for detecting CHD compared with coronary angiography, considered the criterion standard. For a patient with a low pretest likelihood of having CHD, the positive predictive value of an exercise stress test also is quite low (approximately 15% to 25%). For a person at high risk, however, the positive predictive value is quite high (approximately 75% to 85%). The use of exercise stress testing to screen for CHD therefore should probably be reserved only for certain groups at high risk, in accordance with exercise stress testing guidelines from the American Heart Association, American College of Cardiology, and others.

CORONARY HEART DISEASE

Other more accurate screening tests for detection of CHD are available but generally at increased cost and risk to the patient. Nuclear stress imaging and stress echocardiography generally are more expensive and have modestly better sensitivity and specificity than exercise stress testing alone, particularly for a patient with an abnormal baseline ECG. These tests can be performed with pharmacologic stressing agents (dipyridamole, dobutamine, and adenosine) for persons who cannot exercise. Newer testing modalities hold promise for the accurate identification of asymptomatic CVD, including electron beam CT, MRI, and positron emission tomography (PET). The use of CHD screening tests is likely to improve the identification and management of CHD and reduce risk for death and disability from CHD, although data on the subject are somewhat limited.

The USPSTF takes the following position: (1) There is insufficient evidence to recommend for or against screening for asymptomatic CHD. (2) There is reason to recommend against screening those with low risk for CHD. (3) Screening can be recommended for the care of middle-aged and older men and women at high risk if it will influence treatment decisions, such as use of aspirin or lipid-lowering agents. (4) Stress ECGs are more accurate that resting ECGs, but are more expensive.

CEREBROVASCULAR DISEASE

Direct identification of asymptomatic CBVD is somewhat difficult given the relative inaccessibility of the intracranial vessels to tests other than invasive angiography, the criterion standard. Carotid ultrasonography, on the other hand, is an accurate, relatively low-risk, and low-cost screening test that can be used to ascertain whether a patient has severe carotid artery atherosclerosis, placing them at very high risk for a TIA or stroke. A one-time screening program of carotid ultrasonography for elderly men at high risk (history of CHD, PVD, or presence of a carotid bruit) is probably cost efficient (approximately $35,000 per quality of life year gained), but a one-time screening program for elderly men at lower risk is too expensive for practical use (approximately $53,000 per quality of life year gained). Listening for a carotid bruit is a simple, low-cost method of identifying severe carotid atherosclerosis, although the sensitivity of this maneuver is relatively low. Trials in which persons with asymptomatic carotid atherosclerosis were treated with surgical endarterectomy have produced mixed results. Most recent findings suggest that at least among men with severe carotid stenosis (>80%), surgical therapy may reduce risk for stroke and reduce the overall death rate. The USPSTF finds insufficient evidence to recommend for or against screening for asymptomatic CBVD; it states, however, that screening might be useful for persons older than 60 years of age who are at high risk.

Peripheral Vascular Disease

Screening for asymptomatic PVD can be done with moderate accuracy in a clinician's office by means of first eliciting signs that suggest the presence of PVD, such as foot sores or lack of pulses in the feet. Unfortunately, these signs generally are present only in severe PVD. Identification of PVD can be more accurate and timely with calculation of ankle-to-brachial blood pressure index (ABI). Systolic blood pressure in the ankle is measured with a Doppler probe and divided by systolic blood pressure in the brachial artery. The lower the ABI the greater is the likelihood of serious PVD and the greater is the risk for CVD mortality. The ABI is normally between 0.90 and 1.30, considered mildly low between 0.70 and 0.89, moderately low between 0.40 and 0.69, and severely abnormal if less than 0.40. Although among a large number of persons with PVD, the disease is asymptomatic, abnormal ABI measurements generally correlate well with patient symptoms of intermittent claudication. A number of other screening tests can be performed in a specialized vascular laboratory to identify the presence of PVD, including a variety of ultrasonic and plethysmographic measurements. Angiography is invasive, expensive, and risky, but remains the criterion standard for evaluation of PVD.

Data are lacking regarding the potential benefit in long-term CVD outcomes of screening and management of asymptomatic PVD. Although surgical revascularization of the peripheral arteries does lead to improvement in symptoms and limb salvage for many persons with PVD, the USPSTF recommends against routine screening for PVD.

Tertiary Prevention of Cardiovascular Disease

The prevention or delay of disease progression among persons with symptomatic CVD (tertiary prevention) involves techniques to properly quantify and appropriately modify factors that increase a person's risk for recurrent CVD events.

Special Testing

Once a clinical diagnosis of symptomatic CVD has been made (MI, angina, TIA, stroke, or intermittent claudication), a variety of tests can help quantify a person's risk for future CVD events. Risk stratification of CHD depends largely on traditional risk factors for CVD and the following four clinical factors associated with poor prognosis: (1) inducible myocardial ischemia, (2) left ventricular dysfunction, (3) high-grade ventricular arrhythmia, and (4) impaired functional capacity. Persons without any of the four factors are at low risk for recurrent CHD events (<1% during the subsequent year). Persons with all four factors are at extremely high risk for a recurrent event and usually need revascularization therapy to improve the overall prognosis. Exercise testing, with or without imaging, is a standard test used for accurate assessment of the four factors for persons with symptomatic CHD. Nuclear and echocardiographic imaging techniques allow more accurate assessment of ventricular function and extent of coronary ischemia. Coronary angiography is the criterion standard for identifying coronary atherosclerosis that is amenable to revascularization techniques.

For CBVD, carotid ultrasonography remains the primary diagnostic and prognostic tool, although angiography occasionally is used to identify intracranial disease or clarify carotid artery disease. CT and MRI of the head help quantify the amount and location of brain injury after a stroke, although this information generally is apparent at physical examination.

With PVD, findings at clinical examination (sores, absent pulses) and the ABI are strong prognostic factors for future CVD outcomes. Several tests can help ascertain whether a revascularization procedure is appropriate for a certain patient. Some of these tests are invasive, such as angiography, and some are noninvasive, such as ultrasonography and plethysmography.

Risk Factor Modification

Modification of risk factors for CVD has been shown to improve risk for CVD among affected persons. Figure 16-5 shows the recommendations from the American Heart Association Secondary Prevention Panel for risk factor modification and other interventions in the care of persons with symptomatic CVD. Because of the higher rates of CVD events among persons with symptomatic CVD, the effect and therefore the cost-efficiency of risk factor modification generally is much greater among persons with CVD than among persons without disease. The relative risk reduction for both groups is similar, but the absolute risk reduction is greater among persons with disease because their absolute risk for CVD events is greater than that of persons without disease. In primary prevention studies of lipid-lowering therapy, for example, approximately 40 persons with hyperlipidemia must be treated for every CHD event (nonfatal MI or death) prevented. In tertiary prevention studies, one CHD event is prevented for every 13 persons treated.

LIPID-LOWERING THERAPY

A growing body of evidence shows that lipid-lowering therapy with statin drugs can reduce risk for CHD, CVD, and probably PVD among persons with documented CVD. These benefits occur even among persons with normal levels of cholesterol at the time of the initial CVD event. The stabilizing effect of statin therapy on the atherosclerotic plaque probably explains much of the improvement in rates of CVD in these studies. On the basis of the growing body of evidence to support aggressive lipid-lowering treatment of persons with CVD, the Second Adult Treatment Panel Report recommended that the LDL cholesterol goal among such persons should be < 100 mg/dL.

SMOKING CESSATION AND DIET

Smoking cessation among persons with documented CVD reduces risk for future CVD events by 50% or more and generally helps improve symptoms related to CVD. Risk for sudden cardiac death also improves soon after smoking cessation occurs.

Dietary therapy to reduce risk for CHD has long been recommended to patients with CHD. Diets that have been shown to have the greatest effect on tertiary CHD prevention are diets low in saturated fats and diets relatively high in monounsaturated and polyunsaturated fats (Mediterranean-type diet). Pritikin, Ornish, and others have promoted the use of a vegetarian diet very low in saturated fat (10% of total calories). Following this type of diet results in substantial improvement in risk factors for CVD, symptoms, and disease progression among the relatively small group of persons with CHD who can adhere to the strict regimen. More modest reductions in saturated fat (approximately 30% of total calories from fat, 5% to 10% less than the U.S. average), as recommended by the American Heart Association, bring about equally modest lipid-lowering effects and have not been shown systematically to lower risk for recurrent CHD in large-scale studies. A Mediterranean-type diet (emphasis on a low saturated fat diet of fruits, vegetables, fish, nuts, whole grains, and olive or rapeseed oil) has been shown to greatly improve risk factors for CVD and CHD

Figure 16-5

Guide to Comprehensive Risk Reduction **for Patients With Coronary and Other Vascular Disease**	
Risk Intervention	**Recommendations**

Smoking:
  Goal
  complete cessation
	Strongly encourage patient and family to stop smoking.
	Provide counseling, nicotine replacement, and formal cessation programs as appropriate.

Lipid management:
  Primary goal
  LDL<100 mg/dL
  Secondary goals
  HDL>35 mg/dL;
  TG<200 mg/dL
	Start AHA Step II Diet in all patients: ≤30% fat, <7% saturated fat, <200 mg/d cholesterol.
	
	Assess fasting lipid profile. In post-MI patients, lipid profile may take 4 to 6 weeks to stabilize. Add drug therapy according to the following guide:
	
	See detailed guide below.

Physical activity:
  Minimum goal
  30 minutes 3 to 4
  times per week
	Assess risk, preferably with exercise test, to guide prescription.
	Encourage minimum of 30 to 60 minutes of moderate-intensity activity 3 or 4 times weekly (walking, jogging, cycling, or other aerobic activity) supplemented by an increase in daily lifestyle activities (e.g., walking breaks at work, using stairs, gardening, household work). Maximum benefit 5 to 6 hours a week.
	Advise medically supervised programs for moderate- to high-risk patients.

Weight management:	Start intensive diet and appropriate physical activity intervention, as outlined above, in patients >120% of ideal weight for height. Particularly emphasize need for weight loss in patients with hypertension, elevated triglycerides, or elevated glucose levels.
Antiplatelet agents/ anticoagulants:	Start aspirin 80 to 325 mg/d if not contraindicated. Manage warfarin to international normalized ratio=2 to 3.5 for post-MI patients not able to take aspirin.
ACE inhibitors post-MI:	Start early post-MI in stable high-risk patients (anterior MI, previous MI, Killip class II [S₃ gallop, rales, radiographic CHF]). Continue indefinitely for all with LV dysfunction (ejection fraction ≤ 40%) or symptoms of failure. Use as needed to manage blood pressure or symptoms in all other patients.
Beta-blockers:	Start in high-risk post-MI patients (arrhythmia, LV dysfunction, inducible ischemia) at 5 to 28 days. Continue 6 months minimum. Observe usual contraindications. Use as needed to manage angina, rhythm, or blood pressure in all other patients.
Estrogens:	Consider estrogen replacement in all postmenopausal women. Individualize recommendation consistent with other health risks.

Blood pressure control:
  Goal
  ≤140/90 mm Hg
	Initiate lifestyle modification—weight control, physical activity, alcohol moderation, and moderate sodium restriction—in all patients with blood pressure >140 mm Hg systolic or 90 mm Hg diastolic.
	Add blood pressure medication, individualized to other patient requirements and characteristics (i.e., age, race, need for drugs with specific benefits) if blood pressure is not less than 140 mm Hg systolic or 90 mm Hg diastolic in 3 months **or** if *initial* blood pressure is >160 mm Hg systolic or 100 mm Hg diastolic.

Lipid management detailed guide:

LDL<100 mg/dL	LDL 100 to 130 mg/dL	LDL>130 mg/dL	HDL<35 mg/dL
No drug therapy	Consider adding drug therapy to diet, as follows:	Add drug therapy to diet, as follows:	Emphasize weight management and physical activity. Advise smoking cessation. If needed to achieve LDL goals, consider niacin, statin, fibrate.
	Suggested drug therapy		

TG <200 mg/dL	TG 200 to 400 mg/dL	TG >400 mg/dL
Statin Resin Niacin	Statin Niacin	Consider combined drug therapy (niacin, fibrate, statin)

If LDL goal not achieved, consider combination therapy.

ACE indicates angiotensin-converting enzyme; MI, myocardial infarction; TG, triglycerides; and LV, left ventricular.

Guide to comprehensive risk reduction for patients with CVD, from the American Heart Association Consensus Panel Statement on preventing heart attack and death, Smith SC, et al (1995), used with permission.

recurrence among patients with preexisting CHD and generally rates high in acceptability and compliance in the general population.

Data are scarce regarding the effects of dietary therapy on persons with symptomatic CBVD or PVD. It seems likely, however, that dietary therapy, by lowering a variety of risk factors for CVD, should help slow the progression of CBVD and PVD, just as it has been shown to do among persons with CHD.

EXERCISE

Results of numerous studies show that exercise training is associated with improved functional capacity and a 25% reduction in mortality among persons with symptomatic CHD. The role of exercise training among patients with CBVD in preventing recurrent events is not well studied, although exercise can be safe when prescribed appropriately and can modestly improve the functional capacity of survivors of stroke. A regular program of interval walking (a cycle of walking to the point of severe claudication symptoms, followed by a brief rest until the symptoms resolve, and then resumption of walking) can improve functional capacity as much as 200% among persons with symptomatic PVD. No results have been published on the effect of exercise training on rates of recurrent CVD or death among patients with PVD.

HYPERTENSION THERAPY, β-BLOCKERS, ASPIRIN

Data are scarce concerning persons with PVD, but antihypertensive therapy does promote tertiary prevention among persons with CHD and CBVD. Studies are particularly strong regarding the use of β-blocking agents in reduction of recurrent events among persons with CHD. Recent studies suggest that the use of aspirin and possibly ACE inhibitors may reduce the risk for recurrent events among persons with CHD.

DIABETES CONTROL

Aggressive control of diabetes would logically seem to improve CVD-related outcomes among persons with CVD, but there are no data from large-scale studies. No data have been published regarding the effect of weight reduction on CVD outcomes among obese persons with symptomatic CVD, although logic would dictate that reduction of weight and central obesity would reduce other related risk factors for CVD and thereby reduce risk for recurrent CVD events.

ESTROGEN

In longitudinal studies, estrogen therapy generally has been found to be associated with reduced rates of recurrent CHD events. One randomized controlled trial found, however, that combination therapy with estrogen and progestin did not significantly improve long-term outcomes among postmenopausal women with CHD. Likewise, the role of antioxidant agents (e.g., vitamin E, vitamin C, selenium), although promising, is still unclear in the tertiary prevention of CVD.

Advice to Clinicians

Primary care clinicians should emphasize primary prevention of CVD to all patients. Primary prevention includes screening for and managing hypertension and high cholesterol, counseling to prevent tobacco use, promoting physical activity, counseling about healthful diets, and discussing hormone replacement with peri- and postmenopausal women. Table 16-12 lists the recommendations by the USPSTF for primary prevention of CVD for each age group. Table 16-13 lists primary prevention recommendations

Table 16-12

USPSTF Recommended Primary Prevention of Cardiovascular Disease by Age Group

Age Group (yr)	Screening Criterion	Counseling	Chemoprophylaxis
Birth to 10 yr	Blood pressure, height, weight	Engage in regular physical activity Limit fat and cholesterol intake Maintain calorie balance	—
11–24 yr	Blood pressure, height, weight	Avoid tobacco Engage in regular physical activity Limit fat and cholesterol intake Maintain calorie balance	—
25–64 yr	Blood pressure height, weight total blood cholesterol (men 35–64 yr, women 45–64 yr)	Stop using tobacco Engage in regular physical activity Limit fat and cholesterol intake Maintain calorie balance	Discuss estrogen prophylaxis with peri- and postmenopausal women
65 and older	Blood pressure, height, weight	Stop using tobacco Engage in regular physical activity Limit fat and cholesterol intake Maintain calorie balance	Discuss estrogen prophylaxis with peri- and postmenopausal women

Abbreviation: USPSTF, U.S. Preventive Services Task Force.

Table 16-13

American Heart Association Recommendations for Primary Prevention

Risk Factor	Recommendation
Cigarette smoking	Counseling recommended for all age groups
Hypertension	Goal: blood pressure of 140/90 mm Hg or less, consistently Lifestyle modification should be tried initially Drug therapy recommended for severe hypertension or uncontrolled mild-to-moderate hypertension
Serum cholesterol	Desirable: total cholesterol <200 mg/dL, LDL 130 mg/dL Borderline high: total cholesterol 200–239 mg/dL, LDL 130–159 mg/dL High: total cholesterol ≥240 mg/dL, LDL ≥160 mg/dL
Diabetes	Strict control of blood glucose Strict control of other cardiovascular disease risk factors
Physical inactivity	Physical activity recommended for all persons free of contraindications 30 min on most days of the week Include aerobic, strengthening, and flexibility exercises

Source: Grundy SM, Balady GJ, Criqui MH, et al. Primary prevention of coronary heart disease: Guidance from Framingham. A statement for healthcare professionals from the AHA Task Force on Risk Reduction. Circulation 1998;97:1876–1887.

from the American Heart Association task force on risk reduction. The second area of emphasis is tertiary prevention among those with symptomatic CVD, as described in Figure 16-5. Secondary prevention, or screening for asymptomatic CVD should be reserved mainly for persons at high risk for CVD when the results will influence treatment decisions. Screening of persons with occupations that involve public safety, such as airline pilots and truck drivers, also might be considered.

Common Errors

Despite the growing body of evidence that shows the significant benefits of preventive cardiology services, it is clear that only a minority of eligible persons receive the appropriate level of these services. This appears to be the case for a number of preventive cardiology treatments, including use of aspirin, β-blocking agents, lipid-lowering dietary and drug therapy, and cardiac rehabilitation services.

Failure to Emphasize Primary Prevention to All Patients

Because CVD usually becomes clinically apparent in middle and old age, it is common for clinicians not to emphasize CVD prevention to children and young adults. Counseling about a healthful diet and regular physical activities often is overlooked. Smoking is the most common cause of preventable death in the United States, yet clinicians often do not ask patients about their smoking status. Children, adolescents, and young adults often do not receive smoking prevention messages from clinicians. Those who do smoke often are not encouraged to stop. When clinicians do counsel patients to stop smoking, they often do not recommend the most effective cessation methods (see Chapter 10). Official recommendations regarding the screening and management of hypertension and hypercholesterolemia frequently are not applied.

Failure to Implement Tertiary Preventive Interventions

Tertiary preventive interventions frequently are not performed. Many patients with symptomatic CVD, even those who have had an MI, do not receive indicated treatments such as antiplatelet agents, β-blockers, and ACE inhibitors.

Emerging Trends

Genetic Research

Research is uncovering potential ways to improve the identification and management of CVD. Trials of gene therapy are underway for treatment of persons with homozygous familial hypercholesterolemia, a condition characterized by a lack of LDL receptors in the liver, severe elevations in LDL cholesterol serum concentrations, and high risk for death from MI at very young ages. Work also continues on the genetic links to apolipoproteins and their link to atherogenesis.

The pathophysiologic study and management of hypertension are advancing on several fronts. One area of interest is the growing understanding of the role of ACE genes in the development and control of hypertension in a sociodemographic variety of patient populations. Unraveling the genetic basis of other disorders, such as obesity and diabetes, has been proven to be complex, although ongoing work with intrinsic markers such as leptin may help elucidate its apparent links with obesity and CHD.

Infectious Agents

Organisms that may promote atherogenesis have been identified. They include *Chlamydia pneumoniae*, a common respiratory pathogen; *Helicobacter pylori*, a causative agent in peptic ulcer disease, and cytomegalovirus, a relatively common cause of viral infections. Early studies involving long-term use of antibiotics to treat persons with positive titers for *C. pneumoniae* are promising; large-scale studies in this area are ongoing. Some investigators have suggested that the marked increase in the use of antibiotics during the past four decades accounts for part of the dramatic improvement in CVD mortality in most developed countries during the same time.

Arterial Revascularization

Revascularization therapies are advancing at a rapid pace. As our understanding of the injury and repair mechanisms involved in atherosclerosis expands, so does our understanding of the roles of nitric oxide, endothelial cell activity, platelet alloantigens, and angiogenesis in the management of atherosclerotic diseases. This has led to new experimental therapies (coronary angiogenesis) and to improvements in older therapies (e.g., the use of intravascular stenting and platelet alloantigen [IIb/IIIa] blockers to prevent restenosis after coronary angioplasty). This area will continue to expand and improve the array of interventions available to persons with CHD, CBVD, and PVD.

Risk Factor Reduction Research

The role of newly discovered risk factors and the effects of modifying them will be clarified by further research and clinical trials. Estrogen replacement, modification of psychosocial factors, the use of antioxidants, and the lowering of triglycerides, lipoprotein (a) and homocysteine all are areas in which research may lead to preventive interventions in CVD.

Bibliography

Albers FW, Sherman DG, Gress DR, et al: Stroke prevention in nonvalvular atrial fibrillation: A review of prospective randomized trials. *Ann Neurol* 30: 511–518, 1991.

Aronow WS, Ahn C: Prevalence of coexistence of coronary artery disease, peripheral arterial disease, and atherothrombotic brain infarction in men and women ≥62 years of age. *Am J Cardiol* 74:64–65, 1994.

Broderick J, Brott T, Kothari R, et al: The greater Cincinnati/northern Kentucky stroke study: Preliminary first-ever and total incidence rates of stroke among blacks. *Stroke* 29:415–421, 1998.

Clarke R, Daly L, Robinson K, et al: Hyperhomocysteinemia: An independent risk factor for vascular disease. *N Engl J Med* 324:1149–1155, 1991.

Coronary heart disease attributable to sedentary lifestyle: Selected states, 1988. *JAMA* 264:1390–1391, 1991.

de Lorgeril M, Renaud S, Mamelle N, et al: Mediterranean alpha-linoleic acid-rich diet in secondary prevention of coronary heart disease. *Lancet* 343: 1454–1459, 1994.

Eckel RH, Krauss RM, for the AHA Nutrition Committee: American Heart Association call to action: Obesity as a major risk factor for coronary heart disease. *Circulation* 97:2099–2100, 1998.

Executive Committee for the Asymptomatic Carotid Atherosclerosis Study: Endarterectomy for asymptomatic carotid artery stenosis. *JAMA* 273:1421–1428, 1995.

Fletcher GF: How to implement physical activity in primary and secondary prevention: A statement for healthcare professionals from the Task Force on Risk Reduction, American Heart Association. *Circulation* 96:355–357, 1997.

Folsom AR: Physical activity and incidence of coronary heart disease in middle-aged women and men. *Med Sci Sports Exerc* 29:901–909, 1997.

Gibbons RJ, Balady GJ, Beasley JW, et al: ACC/AHA guidelines for exercise testing: executive summary. *Circulation* 96:345–354, 1997.

Gillum RF: Trends in acute myocardial infarction and coronary heart disease death in the United States. *J Am Coll Cardiol* 23:1273–1277, 1993.

Glantz SA, Parmley WW. Passive smoking and heart disease. Mechanisms and risk. *JAMA* 273:1047–1053, 1995.

Goff DC, Nichaman MZ, Chan W, et al: Greater incidence of hospitalized myocardial infarction among Mexican Americans than non-Hispanic whites: The Corpus Christi Heart Project, 1988–1992. *Circulation* 95:1433–1440, 1997.

Gordon DJ, Probstfield JL, Garrison RJ, et al: High-density lipoprotein cholesterol and cardiovascular disease: Four prospective American studies. *Circulation* 79:8–15, 1989.

Hennekens CH: Increasing burden of cardiovascular disease: Current knowledge and future directions for research on risk factors. *Circulation* 97:1095–1102, 1998.

Hertzer NR: The natural history of peripheral vascular disease: Implications for its management. *Circulation* 83(Suppl I):I-12–19, 1991.

Higgins M, Thom T: Trends in stroke risk factors in the United States. *Ann Epidemiol* 3:550–554, 1993.

Hill AB: Should patients be screened for asymptomatic carotid artery stenosis? *Can J Surg* 41:208–213, 1998.

Hopkins PN, Williams RR: A survey of 246 suggested coronary risk factors. *Atherosclerosis* 40:1–52, 1981.

Hunink MGM, Goldman L, Tosteson ANA, et al: The recent decline in mortality from coronary heart disease, 1980–90: The effect of secular trends in risk factors and treatment. *JAMA* 277:535–542, 1997.

Kannel WB, McGee DL. Diabetes and cardiovascular disease: The Framingham Study. *JAMA* 241:2035–2038, 1979.

Kottke TE, Brekke ML, Solberg LI: Making "time" for preventive services. *Mayo Clin Proc* 68:785–791, 1993.

Kronmal RA, Hart RG, Manolio TA, et al: Aspirin use and incident stroke in the Cardiovascular Health Study. CHS Collaborative Research Group. *Stroke* 29:887–894, 1998.

Krumholz HM, Radford MJ, Wang Y, et al: National use and effectiveness of β-blockers for the treatment of elderly patients after acute myocardial infarction. National Cooperative Cardiovascular Project. *JAMA* 280:623–629, 1998.

Lantz PM, House JS, Lepkowski JM, et al: Socioeconomic factors, health behaviors, and mortality: Results from a nationally representative prospective study of U.S. adults. *JAMA* 279:1703–1708, 1998.

Marmot MG, Syme SL, Kagan A, et al: Epidemiologic studies of CHD and stroke in Japanese men living in Japan, Hawaii and California: Prevalence of coronary and hypertensive heart disease and associated risk factors. *Am J Epidemiol* 102:514, 1975.

McDermott MM, Feinglass J, Slavensky R, et al: The ankle-brachial index as a predictor of survival in patients with peripheral vascular disease. *J Gen Intern Med* 9:445–449, 1994.

McKenna M, Wolfson S, Kuller: The ratio of ankle and arm arterial pressure as an independent predictor of mortality. *Atherosclerosis* 87:119–128, 1991.

Morris JN, Kagan A, Pattison DC, et al: Incidence and prediction of ischaemic heart disease in London busmen. *Lancet* 2:553–559, 1966.

Moye LA, Davis BR, Hawkins CM, et al: Conclusions and implications of the systolic hypertension in the elderly program. *Clin Exp Hypertens* 15:911–924, 1993.

National Heart, Lung, and Blood Institute: *The Fifth Report of the Joint National Committee on Detection, Evaluation, and Treatment of High Blood Pressure*, NIH publication no. 93-1088. Washington, DC, US Department of Health and Human Services, 1993.

National Heart, Lung, and Blood Institute: *Report of the Task Force on Research in Epidemiology and Prevention of Cardiovascular Diseases.* Washington, DC: US Department of Health and Human Services, 1994.

Neaton J, Wentworth D, Sherwin R, et al: Comparison of 10 year coronary and cerebrovascular disease mortality rates by hypertensive status for black and non-black men screened in the Multiple Risk Factor Intervention Trial (MRFIT) (abstr.). *Circulation* 80 Suppl II:II-300, 1989.

O'Connor GT, Buring JE, Yusuf S, et al: An overview of randomized trials of rehabilitation with exercise after myocardial infarction. *Circulation* 80:234–244, 1989.

Oparil S: Cardiovascular health at the crossroads: outlook for the 21st century. *Circulation* 91:1304, 1995.

Ornish D, Brown SE, Scherwitz LW, et al: Can lifestyle changes reverse coronary heart disease? The Lifestyle Heart Trial. *Lancet* 336:129, 1990.

Paffenbarger RS JR, Hale WE: Work activity and coronary heart mortality. *N Engl J Med* 292:545–550, 1975.

Pasternak RC, Grundy SM, Levy D, Thompson PD: Task force 3: Spectrum of risk factors for coronary heart disease. *J Am Coll Cardiol* 27:978–990, 1996.

Pearson TA, Fuster V: Executive summary: 27th Bethesda Conference: Matching the intensity of risk factor management with the hazard for coronary disease events. *J Am Coll Cardiol* 27:961–963, 1996.

Rexrode KM, Carey VJ, Hennekens CH, et al: Abdominal adiposity and coronary heart disease in women. *JAMA* 280:1843–1848, 1998.

Ross R: The pathogenesis of atherosclerosis: An update. *N Engl J Med* 314:488–500, 1986.

Rutherford RB, Flanigan DP, Guptka SK: Suggested standards for reports dealing with lower extremity ischemia. *J Vasc Surg* 4:80–94, 1986.

Sacks FM, Pfeffer MA, Moye LA, et al: The effect of pravastatin on coronary events after myocardial infarction in patients with average cholesterol levels. *N Engl J Med* 335:1001–1009, 1996.

Scandinavian Simvastatin Survival Study Group: Randomized trial of cholesterol lowering in 4444 patients with coronary heart disease: The Scandinavian Simvastatin Survival Study (4S). *Lancet* 344: 1383–1389, 1994.

Scanu AM, Lawn RM, Berg K. Lipoprotein (a) and atherosclerosis. *Ann Intern Med* 115:209–218, 1991.

Shea S, Basch CE. A review of five major community-based cardiovascular disease prevention programs, II: Intervention strategies, evaluation methods, and results. *Am J Health Promotion* 4:279–287, 1990.

Shepherd J, Cobbe SM, Ford I, et al: Prevention of coronary heart disease with pravastatin in men with hypercholesterolemia. *N Engl J Med* 333:1301–1307, 1995.

Sixth Report of the Joint National Committee on Prevention, Detection, Evaluation, and Treatment of High Blood Pressure. *Arch Intern Med* 157:2413–2446, 1997.

Smith SC Jr, Blair SN, Criqui MH, et al: Preventing heart attack and death in patients with coronary disease. *Circulation* 92:2–4, 1995.

Steering Committee for the Physician's Health Study Research Group. Physician's Health Study: Aspirin and primary prevention of coronary heart disease. *N Engl J Med* 321:129–135, 1989.

Stephens NG, Parsons A, Schofield PM, et al: Randomised controlled trial of vitamin E in patients with coronary disease: Cambridge Heart Antioxidant Study. *Lancet* 347:781–786, 1996.

Summary of the second report of the National Cholesterol Education Program (NCEP) Expert Panel on Detection, Evaluation, and Treatment of High Blood Cholesterol in Adults (Adult Treatment Panel II). *JAMA* 269:3015–3023, 1993.

UK Prospective Diabetes Study (UKPDS) Group: Effect of intensive blood-glucose control with metformin on complications in overweight patients with type 2 diabetes (UKPDS 34). *Lancet* 352:854–865, 1998.

US Department of Health and Human Services: *Morbidity and Mortality Chartbook on Cardiovascular, Lung,, and Blood Diseases 1990.* Bethesda, MD: National Institutes of Health, National Heart, Lung, and Blood Institute, 1990.

Wolf PA, Dawber TR, Thomas HE, et al: Epidemiologic assessment of chronic atrial fibrillation and the risk of stroke: The Framingham study. *Neurology* 28:973–977, 1978.

Jeff Susman
Lynn Helseth

Chapter

17

Diabetes

**Recommendations to Clinicians Regarding
  Tertiary Prevention**
   American Diabetes Association
     Recommendations
   American College of Physicians
     Recommendations
   American Academy of Family Physicians
     Recommendations
   World Health Organization Recommendations
   Centers for Disease Control and Prevention
     Recommendations
   Quality-monitoring Measures
   Practical Management Tips
     Increasing Patient Adherence
     Improving the Provision of Services
**Other Preventive Services of Particular
  Importance in Patients with Type 2 Diabetes**
   Primary Prevention
     Immunizations
       INFLUENZA VACCINE
       PNEUMOCOCCAL VACCINE
     Smoking Cessation and Osteoporosis
     Prevention

   Secondary Prevention
     Tuberculosis
     Dental/Oral Disease
     Depression
     Asymptomatic Bacteriuria
     and Vaginitis
Common Errors
   Not Counseling Patients Regarding Diet,
     Exercise, and Weight Control
   Not Comprehensively Treating Patients
     with Diabetes
   Not Aggressively Controlling Other
     Cardiovascular Risk Factors
   Not Implementing Other Prevention
     Interventions
   Failure to Consider the Patient's Personal
     Circumstances
Emerging Trends
   Primary Prevention
   Secondary Prevention
   Tertiary Prevention and Treatment

Introduction

Definitions of Types 1 and 2 Diabetes

Diabetes mellitus is a complex disease affecting many systems and causing changes in protein, lipid, and carbohydrate metabolism. It is identified by inappropriate hyperglycemia. Diagnosis can be made by detecting any of the following signs on more than one occasion in well patients who are not on medications known to temporarily alter blood glucose:

1. Fasting plasma glucose level ≥126 mg/dL after 8 hours of fasting
2. Random plasma glucose (nonfasting) ≥200 mg/dL with symptoms of diabetes (polyuria, polydipsia, visual blurring)

3. Glucose tolerance test (75 g glucose) with 2-hour values ≥200 mg/dL in individuals without recent carbohydrate restriction

Table 17-1 summarizes the diagnostic criteria for diabetes and impaired glucose tolerance.

There are many types of diabetes mellitus. In addition to the most common types (1, 2, and gestational diabetes), others may result from endocrinopathies, pancreatic disorders, and medications. Type 1 diabetes mellitus includes all forms of diabetes that are primarily due to pancreatic β-cell destruction or a primary defect in β-cell function; patients with type 1 diabetes are predisposed to ketoacidosis. Type 2 diabetes, the focus of this chapter, results from insulin resistance, with inadequate insulin secretion. Individuals with type 2 diabetes generally do not need insulin treatment to survive, unlike those with type 1. While it may be difficult to

Table 17-1

Diabetes Criteria

PARAMETER	IMPAIRED GLUCOSE METABOLISM	DIABETES
Fasting plasma glucose (mg/dL)	$\geq$110 and <126	$\geq$126
2-h plasma glucose (after 75 g glucose)	$\geq$140 and <200	$\geq$200
Random plasma glucose (+ symptoms of diabetes)	—	$\geq$200

SOURCE: From the American Diabetes Association, 1998.

determine a patient's type of diabetes, the primary goal regardless of classification is to treat the hyperglycemia and prevent the onset or progression of complications.

Epidemiology of Type 2 Diabetes

The prevalence of diagnosed diabetes in 1988 to 1994 was estimated to be 5.1% for U.S. adults $\geq$20 years of age and of undiagnosed diabetes, 2.7%. This equates to approximately 16 million people. Another 15 million people may have impaired glucose tolerance. Of those with diabetes, 90% to 95% have type 2 diabetes mellitus. While some studies suggest that more women have diabetes than men (1.1 to 1.4 times as prevalent), others show no significant difference in prevalence by gender. Prevalence rates for non-Hispanic blacks and Mexican-Americans are 1.6 and 1.9 times, respectively, the rate for non-Hispanic whites (Table 17-2). Native Americans (as studied in Arizona, Oklahoma, and the Dakotas) have very high prevalence rates, ranging from 33% to 72% of adults between 45 and 74 years of age. Surveys from the World Health Organization (WHO) indicate that the overall prevalence of diabetes (types 1 and 2) ranges from less than 3% in some developing countries to 50% among certain southwestern Native American tribes.

Table 17-2

Prevalence of Diabetes and Impaired Fasting Glucose in the U.S. Population Age 40 to 74 Years

Diabetes	
Caucasians	11.2%
African-Americans	18.2%
Mexican-Americans	20.3%
Impaired fasting glucose	
Caucasians	9.5%
African-Americans	9.4%
Mexican-Americans	12.2%

SOURCE: From Harris et al., 1998.

In the United States, the prevalence of diabetes dramatically increases with age, from 1.7% in 20- to 39-year olds to 19% in persons 60 to 74 years old (Table 17-3). In comparing diabetic and nondiabetic populations, people with type 2 diabetes have less education and lower income levels, even after adjusting for age. They are also less likely to be employed. Other risk factors for type 2 diabetes in addition to age, minority ethnicity, and lower socioeconomic status are listed in Table 17-4. Recent trends in the United States show an increase in the prevalence of type 2 diabetes. Using the

Table 17-3

Prevalence of Diabetes in the U.S. Population by Age

Men	(%)	Women	(%)
Age (yr)		Age (yr)	
20–39	1.6	20–39	1.7
40–49	6.8	40–49	6.1
50–59	12.9	50–59	12.4
60–74	20.2	60–74	17.9

Source: From Harris et al., 1998.

1997 American Diabetes Association (ADA) diagnostic criteria, the prevalence of diabetes (diagnosed plus undiagnosed) in the U.S. population aged 40 to 74 years increased from 8.9% in 1976 to 1980 to 12.3% in 1988 to 1994. Diabetes is a common disease.

Visits to primary care physicians make up approximately 80% of all office visits for diabetes. The cost of all diabetes care (types 1 and 2) in 1992 was more than 90 billion dollars (about one-half direct medical costs and one-half indirect costs) and has been estimated to make up 12% of U.S. health care expenditures.

Natural History of Type 2 Diabetes

Type 2 diabetes generally begins with a state of impaired glucose tolerance (or impaired fasting glucose). Impaired glucose tolerance (IGT) is defined as a 2-hour plasma glucose level of ≥140 mg/dL and <200 mg/dL during an oral glucose tolerance test or as a fasting plasma glucose level of ≥110 mg/dL and <126 mg/dL. Characteristics associated with progression from IGT to type 2 diabetes include age up to 40 years (after which increasing age has a beneficial effect), higher fasting and postprandial plasma glucose levels, higher fasting serum insulin levels, and lower postprandial insulin levels. Obesity is not predictive after adjustment for glucose and insulin levels.

Mortality Rates

Type 2 diabetes results in an average of 5 to 10 years of lost life. Diabetes-related death rates are shown in Table 17-5. From 1990 to 1995,

Table 17-4

Risk Factors for Type 2 Diabetes

Obesity (≥20% over desired body weight or body mass index ≥27 kg/m^2)
Family history of diabetes (parents or siblings with diabetes)
Race/ethnicity (e.g., African-Americans, Hispanics, Native Americans, Asian-Americans, Pacific Islanders)
Age ≥45 yr
Sedentary lifestyle
Previous diagnosis of impaired fasting glucose or impaired glucose tolerance
Hypertension (blood pressure ≥140/90 mm Hg)
High-density lipoprotein cholesterol level ≤35 mg per dL (≤0.90 mmol per L) or a triglyceride level ≥250 mg per dL (≥2.82 mmol per L)
History of gestational diabetes or delivery of baby with a birth weight of 9 lb (4 kg) or more

Source: From the American Diabetes Association, 1998.

Table 17-5

Diabetes-related Deaths in 1995 (age adjusted per 100,000)

Overall rate	40
African-Americans	76
Native Americans/Alaskan Natives	63
Mexican-Americans	57
Hispanics	63

SOURCE: From the National Center for Health Statistics: *Healthy People 2000 Review, 1997.* Hyattsville, MD, Public Health Service, 1997.

for all groups, diabetes-related deaths have increased. Adjusted for age and sex, the all-cause mortality rate in individuals with diabetes is twice the mortality rate in those without diabetes. Fifty-five percent of deaths in people with type 1 or 2 diabetes is caused by coronary heart disease (CHD). Other significant underlying causes of death are malignant neoplasms (10%) and cerebrovascular disease (9%).

Rates of End-organ Damage

The macrovascular complications of diabetes include cerebrovascular, cardiovascular, and peripheral vascular disease. Microvascular complications include retinopathy, nephropathy, and neuropathy.

CARDIOVASCULAR DISEASE

Individuals with type 2 diabetes or impaired glucose tolerance have a 1.7 to sixfold higher risk of heart disease than those without diabetes. Patients with type 2 diabetes have as high a risk of myocardial infarction (MI) as nondiabetic patients who have had a previous MI. The 1976 to 1980 second National Health and Nutrition Examination Survey (NHANES II) found that people with type 2 diabetes are 1.6 times as likely to have hypertension as people with normal glucose tolerance. They have a mean cho-

lesterol level of 232 mg/dL compared with 208 mg/dL for individuals without diabetes. In the 10-year follow-up of NHANES II, there was a 2.5-fold higher risk of stroke in subjects with diabetes than in subjects without diabetes.

Peripheral pulse deficits, suggestive of peripheral vascular disease, are two to three times as prevalent in people with type 2 diabetes as in those with normal glucose tolerance. The presence of peripheral vascular disease increases a patient's risk of lower-extremity amputation. Lower-extremity amputations, as a complication of diabetes, were present in 0.9% of people with diabetes in 1995.

NEUROPATHY

Neuropathic complications, defined as sensory symptoms and defects in the hands and feet, affect 30 to 40% of people with type 2 diabetes—four times the percentage of individuals without diabetes. Patients with loss of feeling are at high risk of neuropathic ulcers, infections, and lower-extremity amputations. Neuropathic complications of diabetes also take the form of autonomic and focal neuropathy.

RETINOPATHY

Diabetic retinopathy accounts for 10% of new cases of blindness in the United States. In 1994, 0.2% of people with diabetes had diabetes-related blindness. Retinopathy may be present in 39% of men and 35% of women at the time of diagnosis with type 2 diabetes. Retinopathy begins as retinal exudates and hemorrhages and progresses to arterial proliferation. Proliferative retinopathy, if untreated, can lead to retinal detachment and blindness. More severe retinal lesions at the time of diabetes diagnosis have been associated with poorer visual acuity in men. According to the Wisconsin Epidemiologic Study of Diabetic Retinopathy, 55% of patients with type 2 diabetes have evidence of retinopathy within 15 years of onset of diabetes.

370

NEPHROPATHY

Diabetic nephropathy accounts for 35% of all end-stage renal disease (ESRD) in the United States. In 1993, 0.2% of people with diabetes had ESRD. Chronic renal failure develops within 10 years in 11% of patients with type 2 diabetes and persistent proteinuria, and proteinuria develops in roughly 50% of patients with type 2 diabetes within 20 years of diabetes onset.

ACUTE METABOLIC DISORDERS

Diabetic ketoacidosis is rarely seen in patients with type 2 diabetes. Hyperosmolar nonketotic coma with type 2 diabetes occurs almost exclusively in patients over the age of 65 years and accounts for 0.4% of hospitalizations. Although hypoglycemia accounts for only 2% of all diabetic hospitalizations, hypoglycemic events may cause encephalopathy, significant psychologic distress, limitation of activities, and unwillingness to comply with recommendations for tighter glycemic control.

Primary Prevention of Type 2 Diabetes

The ideal goal in terms of any disease is primary prevention. Significant evidence supports the effectiveness of primary prevention of type 2 diabetes mellitus with increased physical activity irrespective of body mass index (BMI). Weight control over time is also associated with a lower incidence of type 2 diabetes. Less robust data implicate the role of nutritional factors and smoking. Unfortunately, no large randomized, controlled trial in the United States has investigated these last two issues, although several are underway.

Physical Activity

A number of studies have investigated the association of physical activity with insulin resistance or the development of type 2 diabetes. Helmrich and colleagues (1991) studied 5990 male college alumni and found that for each 500 kcal increment in energy expenditure, the adjusted risk of type 2 diabetes was reduced by 6%. These findings persisted after correcting for obesity, and the protective effect of physical activity was highest in those at greatest risk. Likewise, the Nurses' Health Study of 121,700 women (Colditz and Coakley, 1997) found an inverse relationship between the onset of type 2 diabetes and physical activity independent of BMI.

The Physician's Health Study followed 21,271 male physicians between the ages of 40 and 84 who were initially free of diabetes. During more than 100,000 person-years of follow-up, type 2 diabetes developed in 285 individuals. Men who exercised vigorously at least once per week had an age-adjusted relative risk of type 2 diabetes of 0.64, and this risk declined with higher rates of exercise. This finding persisted after adjustment for BMI, smoking, hypertension, and other coronary risk factors. Risk reduction was particularly evident in those patients who were most obese.

The Insulin Resistance Atherosclerosis Study (Mayer-Davis et al, 1998) explored the relationship of nonvigorous physical activity to insulin sensitivity, as measured by an intravenous glucose tolerance test, in a cross-sectional investigation of 1467 individuals of diverse ethnic background. Persons who participated in vigorous exercise five or more times weekly had significantly greater insulin sensitivity than those who rarely or never engaged in vigorous exercise. Moreover, even those persons who participated in regular, nonvigorous physical activity demonstrated enhanced insulin sensitivity.

The Pitt County Study looked at the association of physical activity with the development of type 2 diabetes in a working class African-American population (James et al., 1998). The study showed that moderately active subjects were one-third as likely as inactive individuals to suffer type 2 diabetes. These findings suggest that even regular nonvigorous exercise, such as walking, might prevent or forestall the onset of type 2 diabetes. Taken as a whole, these studies strongly suggest that, at a minimum, regular exercise can forestall the development of overt type 2 diabetes.

While evidence does show that exercise is effective in delaying or preventing type 2 diabetes, we know little about how to motivate the two-thirds of Americans who lead sedentary lifestyles to become more active. Investigations of the application of the readiness for change model and self-efficacy theory and the influence of physician counseling and community involvement are needed.

Diet and Weight Control

The association of diet, obesity, and weight gain with the development of type 2 diabetes has also been studied extensively. As noted earlier, exercise appears to have a particularly powerful role in preventing type 2 diabetes in those who are overweight. The Nurses' Health Study showed a direct relationship between BMI and the risk of type 2 diabetes. Moreover, patients who gain the most weight from age 18 to midlife are at the greatest risk. This finding mirrors the results of the U.S. NHANES study, which showed that the prevalence of impaired glucose tolerance (IGT) was 23% in individuals whose weight increased by 50% compared with 6% in those whose weight increased by <5% after age 25 years. Weight loss has also been shown to enhance insulin sensitivity.

Work from Finland and Sweden has shown that weight reduction in patients with newly diagnosed type 2 diabetes or IGT is associated with better metabolic control and less use of antidiabetic medications (Eriksson and Lind-

garde F, 1991). Likewise, a 6-year study of 530 subjects with IGT in DaQing, China, showed a reduction in the progression from IGT to type 2 diabetes in groups who were given dietary advice and/or who increased their exercise levels (Pan, 1994). A short-term study has shown improved insulin sensitivity in patients consuming a diet high in monounsaturated fats, and there is active research looking at the effect of trivalent chromium on the development of type 2 diabetes.

Smoking Cessation

Several studies suggest that smoking is independently associated with high plasma insulin levels and reduced insulin sensitivity. The Nurses' Health Study has established a dose-response trend between the incidence of type 2 diabetes and the amount of smoking (Colditz and Coakley, 1997). The relative risk of type 2 diabetes was 1.42 among women smoking 25 or more cigarettes per day compared with nonsmokers. These findings suggest that smoking cessation may improve insulin sensitivity, prevent IGT, and forestall type 2 diabetes.

Current Studies

Ideally, data from randomized, controlled trials (RCTs) would support primary prevention of type 2 diabetes. The Diabetes Prevention Program began recruitment of patients in 1996 with the intention of enrolling four thousand individuals with impaired glucose tolerance; more than 50% represent high-risk ethnic groups, including Native Americans, Hispanics and African-Americans. Patients are being randomized to four arms: intensive lifestyle modification, usual lifestyle modification with metformin and a troglitazone placebo, usual lifestyle modification with troglitazone and a metformin placebo, and usual lifestyle modification with both troglitazone and metformin placebos. Patients will be followed for an average of 4½ years. The trial is scheduled to conclude in 2002.

Community Interventions

There is no evidence at this time that community-wide interventions can affect the prevalence of type 2 diabetes. It is reasonable that community norms regarding diet, activity levels, and perceived desirable weight might have an effect, but no longitudinal community-wide trials of such interventions have yet been conducted.

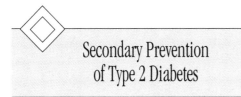

Secondary Prevention of Type 2 Diabetes

What Screening Tests Are Available?

The diagnosis of diabetes is outlined in the introduction. It does not require an oral glucose tolerance test (OGTT), although the OGTT is often used as the gold standard by which the

sensitivities and specificities for other screening tests are measured (Table 17-6). Positive predictive values for screening tests will be highest in high-risk populations. Urinalysis is not used as a diabetes-screening test because of its lower sensitivity. While the Hemoglobin A_{1c} (glycosylation of A_{1c} subfraction of hemoglobin) has been explored as a screening test, it is not currently recommended because of the large variation in test characteristics.

While screening capillary whole blood with a blood glucose meter is not recommended by any group, obtaining a result ≥110 mg/dL should warrant additional testing. Clinicians need to remember that plasma glucose values are 10 to 15% higher than capillary whole blood glucose values. The tests shown in Table 17-6 are comparable in terms of price; they are all about $10, except for the glycosylated hemoglobin test, which is about $25.

Does Early Detection of Asymptomatic Diabetes Lead to Better Outcomes?

There is no direct evidence that shows that screening for type 2 diabetes leads to improved

Table 17-6
Sensitivity and Specificity of Diagnostic Tests for Diabetes Mellitus[a]

TEST	SENSITIVITY (%)	SPECIFICITY (%)
FPG ≥140 mg/dL (7.8 mmol/L)	21–75	99
FPG ≥126 mg/dL (7.0 mmol/L)[b]	25–91	96–100
Random PG ≥140 mg/dL (7.8 mmol/L)	45	86
Random capillary blood glucose[c]	81–82	78–80
Urine dipstick, semiquantitative ≥ a "trace positive"	23–64	98–99
Urine quantitative assay in high-risk populations	81	98
Glycosylated hemoglobin or albumin	15–93	84–99

[a] Compared with the oral glucose tolerance test.
[b] Finch CF, Zimmet PZ, Alberti KG: Determining diabetes prevalence: a rational basis for the use of fasting plasma glucose concentrations? *Diabetes Med* 7(7):603–610, 1990.
[c] Optimum cutoff point increases with age: 115 mg/dL at age 30 to 140 mg/dL for age 75. Engelgau MM, Thompson TJ, Smith PJ et al: Screening for diabetes mellitus in adults: The utility of random capillary blood glucose measurements. *Diabetes Care* 18(4):463–466, 1995.
ABBREVIATIONS: FPG, fasting plasma glucose; PG, plasma glucose.

outcomes. There are more data that link the duration and severity of hyperglycemia with microvascular complications. In theory, therefore, early detection of diabetes could improve outcomes. Screening may be justified in high-risk populations.

Screening Recommendations

Many recommendations regarding screening were developed before the most recent data became available linking risk factor modification with improved outcomes. The American College of Physicians (ACP) and the American Academy of Family Physicians (AAFP) have recommended against routine screening for diabetes in asymptomatic patients, although each of these organizations concluded that screening is reasonable among high-risk individuals, such as older obese persons or those with a strong family history. It is important to note that although the classic initial symptoms of diabetes are polyuria, polydipsia, and polyphagia, they are not present in the majority of patients at diagnosis. Other symptoms and signs associated with diabetes include weight loss, fatigue, frequent infections, pruritus, vision changes, numbness or tingling of the extremities, sexual impotence, periodontal disease, constipation, cystitis, and nocturia. Many patients are asymptomatic at the time of diagnosis, however.

The U.S. Preventive Services Task Force (USPSTF) suggests that there is insufficient evidence to recommend for or against routine screening for type 2 diabetes in nonpregnant adults. They also suggest that although there has been no proven benefit of early detection for any group, the clinician may decide to screen high-risk patients because of the increased positive predictive value of the tests in these groups and because of the potential benefits of minimizing asymptomatic hyperglycemia through diet and exercise. The USPSTF recommends fasting plasma glucose as the screening test of choice. Frequency of screening is left to the cli-

nician's discretion.

The ADA recommends screening all individuals at age 45 years and older. If test results are normal, the test should be repeated at 3-year intervals. Testing should be done at a younger age or more frequently in individuals who are obese, have a first-degree relative with diabetes, are members of a high-risk ethnic population, have been diagnosed with gestational diabetes or have delivered a baby weighing more than 9 pounds, are hypertensive, have a high-density lipoprotein (HDL) cholesterol level ≤35 mg/dL and/or a triglyceride level ≥250 mg/dL, or who have had IGT or impaired fasting glucose (IFG) on previous testing (Table 17-4).

Workup of Positive Screening Tests

Patients with a positive diabetes screening test should be evaluated by a history and a second test. The history should focus on the presence of diabetes symptoms and any possible secondary forms of diabetes, such as pancreatic disease, Cushing's syndrome, and such medications as oral contraceptives, thiazide diuretics, β blockers, and nicotinic acid. If type 2 diabetes is confirmed, a complete workup and management plan should be implemented, as described in a later section. Those with IGT or IFG can be advised regarding diet and exercise and reevaluated periodically.

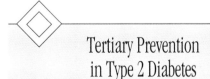

Tertiary Prevention in Type 2 Diabetes

Factors to Consider When Initiating Therapy

The goals for the management of type 2 diabetes include elimination of symptoms of the disease, avoidance of acute complications, and prevention of development or progression of complications (tertiary prevention). This section reviews the evidence linking better glycemic control with improved outcomes and other important interventions in the prevention of the complications of type 2 diabetes (Table 17-7). Evidence supports many of these strategies on a population level, while the benefits and harms for an individual patient may vary substantially. When evaluating a particular proposed therapy it is important to consider the following issues.

STRENGTH OF EVIDENCE SUPPORTING THE INTERVENTIONS

The data supporting physical activity as a primary preventive measure for type 2 diabetes are based largely on observational and cross-sectional data. A large RCT is now underway. Stronger, more consistent evidence about an intervention should bolster its use more widely. Likewise, evidence gained from RCTs of patients with type 2 diabetes would be more convincing than similar studies in patients with type 1 diabetes.

Table 17-7

Management of Type 2 Diabetes Patients to Minimize Complications

Methods for lowering blood glucose levels
    Exercise therapy
    Diet therapy
    Oral agent therapy (see Table 17-10)
    Insulin therapy (see Table 17-11)
Methods for lessening cardiovascular risk
    and risk factors
        Smoking cessation program
        Diet therapy
        Exercise therapy
        Aspirin (81 to 325 mg/d)
        Hormone replacement therapy
        Antihypertensive agents
        Lipid-lowering agents

MAGNITUDE AND FREQUENCY OF BENEFIT(S) IN TERMS MEANINGFUL TO PATIENTS

Many investigations report intermediate outcomes or benefits that are unquantifiable by patients, such as improvements in nerve conduction velocity, a change in serum creatinine, or decrease in serum cholesterol. Of more meaning to patients are functional and quality-of-life measures, such as the need for dialysis or the incidence of myocardial infarction. Moreover, most of the literature expresses benefits in relative rather than absolute terms and does not place these findings in a meaningful context. For example, the risk of MI during a 10-year follow-up may be reduced from 20% to 10%. This reduction might be expressed as a relative 50% decrease in MI or an absolute risk reduction of 10%. Perhaps most meaningful, however, would be to discuss this benefit in terms of the median complication-free interval, years of life gained, or absolute reduction of MI in a given population of patients (i.e., a decrease from 85 to 42 fatal and 212 to 139 in nonfatal MIs in a population of 2345 individuals with type 2 diabetes).

MAGNITUDE AND FREQUENCY OF HARM(S) IN TERMS MEANINGFUL TO PATIENTS

Likewise, the harm of therapies should be adequately explored. For example, intensive glycemic control may increase the incidence of weight gain and hypoglycemic episodes. Ideally, a balance sheet would present benefits and harms in terms meaningful to patients. Unfortunately, such information is difficult to collate and is sometimes contradictory.

COST AND SAVINGS OF TREATMENT

For many patients and health plans, costs and savings remain important factors. The recent U.K Prospective Diabetes Study (UKPDS 33) data (1998) failed to find differences in the aggregate endpoints among three drugs (chlorpropamide, glibenclamide, and insulin). On the basis of cost, one of these agents might be preferred. Indeed, insulin is significantly cheaper than the newer antidiabetic agents. Cost-effective analyses have been performed for relatively few interventions.

PATIENT PREFERENCES

Ultimately, many patients will have significant preferences in terms of therapy or be willing to make their own tradeoffs between benefits and harms. For example, many might prefer an oral agent over injectable insulin.

PATIENT CO-MORBID CONDITIONS, LIFE EXPECTANCY, AND MITIGATING CIRCUMSTANCES

The benefits from tighter glycemic control accrue over years. A patient who is older or has severe co-morbid conditions may not live long enough to reap the rewards of improved glycemic control. There may be a different magnitude of benefit depending on the patient's initial health status. A 42-year old with an HbA_{1C} of 13 and no other medical problems could expect significant benefits from improved glycemic control. A frail 85-year old with an HbA_{1C} of 7.4 and several medical co-morbid conditions may benefit only marginally from tighter control and have a greater risk of complications, such as hypoglycemia, that might precipitate a hip fracture.

SOCIAL AND MEDICAL SUPPORT

Many therapies require significant personal, family, and community resources. Intensive control of blood sugar necessitates substantial support from medical professionals and family members.

ADHERENCE ISSUES

A given therapy might be ideal (such as several daily injections), but the real-world ef-

fectiveness could be diminished by lack of adherence or barriers to care or access. Many patients with type 2 diabetes use several medications (e.g., aspirin, an oral agent, an antihypertensive drug, and an antihyperlipidemic agent), and follow a diet and exercise plan. While all of these therapies could individually prove effective, taken together, they may become overwhelming. Thus, it is very important to carefully assess the benefits and harms of a given intervention in a broad context. The following section will concentrate on efficacy data, recognizing that an individual patient's preferences and circumstances will often guide decision-making.

Acute Complications

Most of the literature focuses on the incidence or prevalence of acute complications, but few trials have tested specific interventions aimed at minimizing these problems even though each has a significant effect on quality of life. Educational interventions directed at preventing uncontrolled hyperglycemia, profound hypoglycemia, weight changes, infections, and foot problems would seem prudent and carry few associated harms.

HYPOGLYCEMIA AND HYPERGLYCEMIA

Much attention is focused on the longer-term microvascular and macrovascular complications of diabetes, but short-term harms are also important to consider. Perhaps the most common of these issues is hypoglycema. In the UKPDS 33 (1998), more serious hypoglycemic episodes were associated with substantial use of health care resources and decreased quality of life. Particularly at risk were patients without symptoms associated with hypoglycemia (nonwarning hypoglycemia or hypoglycemic unawareness). Such patients may be at risk of profound hypoglycemia, accidents, seizures, and other related complications. It is important to counsel patients about the prevention and treatment of hypoglycemia and potential influences on glycemic control (such as exercise and illness).

Hyperglycemia is associated with osmotic diuresis, electrolyte disturbances, dehydration, infection, and symptoms of polyuria, polydipsia, and polyphagia. These issues can be bothersome and diminish the patient's quality of life. Severe hyperglycemia can bring about diabetic ketoacidosis and hyperosmolar coma, both of which carry a significant risk of death. At a minimum, therapy should target control of symptoms related to hyperglycemia and prevention of more acute complications. Blurred vision is associated with flux in blood sugar and changes in lens hydration. Such alterations can be irksome and influence the ability to drive and participate in occupational and recreational activities. More stable glycemic control can prevent these problems.

CHANGES IN WEIGHT

Weight loss and associated metabolic derangements can be significant in uncontrolled diabetes. Weight gain often accompanies tight control of blood sugar, particularly for those patients on insulin. This weight gain can lead to further glucose intolerance and the need for increased therapy. The UKPDS suggests, however, that weight gain is not a necessary outcome for patients seeking improved metabolic control.

INFECTIONS

Patients with diabetes are prone to infections, ranging from influenza and pneumonia to cellulitis. Particularly common are diabetic foot problems, including infections, which can lead to prolonged morbidity and amputations. This topic is discussed below in more detail.

FOOT PROBLEMS

The feet are particularly vulnerable to acute problems because of diabetes-related neurovascular compromise and increased susceptibility to infection. Neuropathy and macrovascular and microvascular changes in the extremities make proper foot care a priority. Standards for routine foot care have been established by the ADA based on whether the patient is at high or low risk of having foot ulcers. Patients at high risk include those with vascular disease or loss of protective sensation and those who have had ulcers.

Patients at high risk should receive regular care by a clinician with experience in treating diabetic foot problems. This care should include regular inspection of the feet and care of nails and calluses. Protective sensation is measured by the ability to feel a 10-g monofilament. The monofilament is attached at a right angle to a thin handle. The examiner holds the handle between the thumb and forefinger and places the monofilament tip against the skin. Pressure is gradually increased, as if the examiner were trying to press the filament into the skin until the filament bends. The patient is asked if he or she feels the pressure of the monofilament. If protective sensation is lost, patients should be instructed to wear athletic shoes or shoes that are custom-molded.

Low-risk patients should receive guidance in preventive foot care and foot inspections from their clinicians. Education for both low- and high-risk patients should include information about foot hygiene, proper shoes and socks, avoiding foot trauma, smoking cessation, and the need for immediate treatment of infections and ulcers.

Glycemic Control

The Diabetes Control and Complications Trial (DCCT, 1993) conclusively established the efficacy of improved glycemic control in minimizing the incidence of certain complications in patients with type 1 diabetes. Even as this chapter was first being written, comparable data for patients with type 2 diabetes were scanty. Fortunately, the recent reports of the UKPDS provide parallel data in this population.

The UKPDS was an RCT of intensive blood glucose control in 3867 newly diagnosed patients with type 2 diabetes. Patients were randomized to intensive control or conventional treatment. Within the intensive control group, patients were assigned either a sulfonylurea (glipizide, chlorpropamide, or glibenclamide) or insulin, and subgroups of overweight patients received metformin. Three outcomes were assessed: diabetes-related complications, diabetes-related mortality, and all-cause mortality. For 10 years, the average HbA_{1C} was 7.0% in the intensive group compared with 7.9% in the conventional group. Compared with the conventional group, the intensive group had an 11% lower rate of diabetes-related complications, including a significant 25% risk reduction in microvascular complications. There was also a 10% lower diabetes-related death rate and a 6% lower all-cause mortality rate, but these results were not statistically significant. The median complication-free interval was 1.3 years longer in the intensive group.

Patients in the intensive group had more hypoglycemic episodes and greater weight gain. Insulin use was associated with more frequent hypoglycemic events, but the agents were otherwise comparable. The analysis of metformin use in overweight patients suggests that this agent is more effective than other agents at decreasing the rate of diabetes-related endpoints, all-cause mortality, and stroke in diet-controlled patients. In combination with a sulfonylurea, metformin was associated with an increased risk of diabetes-related death, but this finding may have been due to selection bias. Other benefits of intensive control in the UKPDS included a 16%

reduction in myocardial events, a 21% lowering of the rate of retinopathy progression, and a 34% reduction in albuminuria progression.

A study in Japan (Ohkubo et al., 1995) looked at the benefit of several injections daily of insulin versus conventional insulin therapy in type 2 diabetics. The intensive control group experienced delayed onset and progression of microvascular complications and fewer macrovascular complications, with no increase in hypoglycemic episodes or weight gain. Studies to date show no clear threshold for complications above euglycemia. Suggested goals cited by the ADA for glycemic control of patients with type 2 diabetes are the same as for individuals with type 1 diabetes: a preprandial blood glucose level of 80 to 120 mg/dL (4.4 to 6.7 mmol/L), a bedtime blood glucose level of 100 to 140 mg/dL (5.5 to 7.8 mmol/L), and HbA_{1C} levels less than 7%. These data are consistent with findings from the best clinical trials of type 2 diabetes. Nonetheless, the particular goal set for glucose control in individual patients is dependent on a number of factors (Tables 17-8 and 17-9).

A Markov decision model (based on the DCCT data) suggests that patients with earlier onset of type 2 diabetes will benefit most from tighter glucose control (Vijan, Hofer, Haywood 1997). The probability model also suggests substantially greater benefit for those patients going from poor to moderate control as opposed to

Table 17-8

Ideal Goals for Glycemic Control for Type 2 Diabetes

	GOAL	ACTION NEEDED
Preprandial capillary glucose (mg/dL)	80–120	<80 >140
Bedtime capillary glucose (mg/dL)	110–140	<100 >160
HbA_{1C} (%)	<7	>8

SOURCE: American Diabetes Association, 1998.

Table 17-9
Patient Characteristics Affecting Goals for Glycemic Control

> Relative contraindications to goal of normalization of blood glucose levels
> > Repeated severe hypoglycemia
> > Major mental disorder
> > > Severe manic or depressive disorders
> > > Schizophrenia
> > > Substance abuse
> > > Eating disorders
> > > Severe personality disorders
> > Lack of financial resources
> > Severe family or environmental instability
> Indications for moderating treatment goals
> > Patient expectations and priorities
> > Previous poor experience with rigorous self-care regimens
> > Social support problems
> > Advanced age or isolation
> > Unavailability of medical support resources
> > Unacceptable weight gain
> > Other environmental, intellectual, emotional, or physical limitations

SOURCE: Adapted from Lorenz RA, et al, 1996.

patients moving from moderate to tight control. It was concluded that targeting 20% of patients would yield 80% of preventable patient-time spent blind. Unfortunately, another model using different assumptions predicts slightly different outcomes, underscoring the challenges of applying modeling efforts to practice.

The best method to achieve glucose control is open to debate, with each therapeutic method (diet, exercise, and use of medical treatments, including oral agents and insulin) having its own sets of benefits and harms (Tables 17-10 and 17-11). The clinician should be alert to possible hypoglycemic episodes that could interfere with compliance associated with insulin, sulfonylurea, and repaglinide therapy. Metformin, acarbose, and troglitazone do not cause hypoglycemia in and of themselves, though metformin and acarbose may be associated with

adverse gastrointestinal side effects influencing food intake and absorption. Weight gain, in particular, is associated with insulin, sulfonylurea, and troglitazone therapy. Liver disease is connected to metformin and troglitazone treatment. Metformin is contraindicated in patients with elevated creatinine, congestive heart failure, and chronic obstructive pulmonary disease.

Based on current information, there are no convincing data of the superior effectiveness of one agent over another. The UKPDS raises important questions about the role of metformin by itself and in combination with sulfonylureas and about whether obese and nonobese patients should be treated differently. At this time individual therapeutic decisions should be based on a careful review of the patient's circumstances and preferences. Whatever approach is taken, the goals of therapy should be negoti-

Table 17-10

Oral Agent Therapy for Glycemic Control

CLASS/GENERIC NAME (AND RELATIVE COST)[a]	BRAND NAME	DURATION OF ACTION (HR)	MECHANISM OF ACTION	SIDE EFFECTS/PRECAUTIONS
First-generation sulfonylureas ($)			Stimulates insulin secretion.	Weight gain
Tolbutamide	Orinase	6–12		Hypoglycemia; fever or disulfiram/flushing reaction. Avoid use in those with significant liver or renal impairment.
Chlorpropamide	Diabinese	Up to 60		
Acetohexamide	Dymelor	12–18		
Tolzamide	Tolinase, Ronase	12–24		
Second-generation sulfonylureas ($–$$)			Stimulates insulin secretion.	Weight gain, hypoglycemia. Avoid use in those with significant liver or renal impairment.
Glipizide	Glucotrol	Up to 24		
Glipizide GITS	Glucotrol	24		
Glyburide	Diabeta, Micronase	Up to 24		
Micronized glyburide	Amaryl	24		
Non-sulfonylureas				
Troglitazone ($$$$)	Rezulin	24	Improves insulin action in muscle; may reduce liver glucose production; lowers triglycerides and increases HDL.	Liver failure—check bilirubin and LFTs; hypoglycemia; weight gain
Metformin ($$)	Glucophage	8–12	Reduces hepatic glucose production and may increase muscle glucose utilization; decrease triglycerides and increases HDL.	Diarrhea, nausea, lactic acidosis. Avoid use if serum creatinine >1.5 mg/dL and those with CHF and COPD.
Acarbose ($$)	Precose	3–4	Delays intestinal absorption of carbohydrates and lowers peak postprandial glucose levels.	Flatuence, cramps, diarrhea
Repaglinide ($$$)	Prandin	3–4	Stimulates insulin secretion.	Use with caution in patients with decreased hepatic function; may be used alone or with metformin.

[a] In general, $ = $20 or less; $$ = $20–50; $$$ = $50–100; and $$$$ = more than $100.

ABBREVIATIONS: HDL, high-density lipoprotein; LFT, liver function test; CHF, congestive heart failure; COPD, chronic obstructive pulmonary disease.

Table 17-11

Insulin Therapy for Glycemic Control

TYPE OF HUMAN INSULIN[a]	ONSET	PEAK (HR)	DURATION (HR)
Lispro	5–15 min	0.5–1.5	2–4
Regular	30–60 min	2–3	3–6
NPH	2–4 hr	4–10	10–16
Lente	3–4 hr	4–12	12–18
Ultralente	6–10 hr	12	18–20

[a] Animal insulin is slower and longer-acting.
SOURCE: American Board of Family Practice, *Diabetes mellitus reference guide.* 6th ed. Lexington, KY, 1997.

ated, and increases or changes in treatment methods must be made when these targets are not met.

To summarize, our best studies to date suggest that improved glycemic control limits microvascular complications and does not increase the incidence of macrovascular complications, but it is often accompanied by the risk of additional weight gain and more frequent and severe hypoglycemic episodes. In addition, no differences in overall mortality rates have been established firmly, and data to support the effectiveness of intense glycemic control are scanty outside the research setting. For example, studies evaluating therapy of patients with type 2 diabetes in community practices and varied health systems have been unable to achieve ideal glycemic control and have resulted in significantly increased resource use in some cases. In other settings, continuous quality-improvement efforts have yielded more positive results, and most patients, particularly those who have the worst glycemic control, made substantial improvements in HbA_{1C}.

Self-Monitoring of Blood Glucose and Use of the HbA_{1C}

While self-monitoring of blood glucose (SMBG) and testing for HbA_{1C} are widely recommended

as tools for improved diabetes care, little evidence links them with improved outcomes. Nonetheless, it can be argued that SMBG and the use of HbA_{1C} may be foundations for successful treatment. First, more intensive therapy is guided by home blood glucose readings. In controlled trials, this has meant checking blood sugars several times daily, including regular nocturnal measurements. Second, SMBG can provide confirmation of hypoglycemia, guide meal consumption and exercise, and prompt preventive measures. SMBG also gives patients an important self-management tool and empowers them in assuming control of their disease. Nonetheless, it must be acknowledged that clear evidence linking SMBG to improved outcomes in broad, unselected populations is lacking. Still, the selective use of SMBG in those patients seeking tight or improved blood sugar control appears reasonable. The monitoring of glycemic control with HbA_{1C}, in and of itself, is only weakly associated with clinical outcomes, but as part of an overall strategy to enhance glycemic control (which is clearly linked to outcomes), the use of HbA_{1C} can be recommended.

Macrovascular Complications

Macrovascular complications include MI, stroke, peripheral vascular disease, and sudden death due to cardiovascular disease (CVD). One cohort study of 361,662 men showed a three times higher adjusted risk of CVD death in the group with diabetes than in those without diabetes. In both groups, serum cholesterol, systolic blood pressure, and smoking were significant predictors of CVD mortality, but the mortality rates of men with diabetes and multiple risk factors were far greater. Cardiovascular risk factors (including smoking, hyperlipidemia, and hypertension) can be modified, and controlled trials provide evidence that doing so results in benefits. The use of aspirin is also strongly supported, but the role of hormone replacement therapy (HRT) in women is uncertain. Nutritional therapy may help in the attainment of glycemic control and the treatment of hyperlipidemia and hypertension. Exercise may also help promote euglycemia and improve hyperlipidemia.

SMOKING CESSATION

Smoking cessation is particularly important, not only to decrease cardiovascular risk but also because of the other complications that arise in the context of smoking coupled with diabetes, including peripheral vascular and renal disease. Evidence from RCTs suggests that primary care clinicians can be effective in helping their patients stop smoking by providing brief counseling and nicotine replacement therapy (see Chapter 10). All patients with type 2 diabetes should be strongly counseled to quit smoking and offered proven strategies to support cessation. This will engender benefits not only in preventing macrovascular complications but also in mitigating all other smoking-related morbidity and mortality factors described in Chapter 10.

CORRECTING HYPERLIPIDEMIA

Hyperlipidemia confers substantial additional risk of CVD in patients with type 2 diabetes. Characteristic changes in lipids associated with

diabetes are a reduction in HDLs and an elevation in triglycerides. Chapter 16 describes the elevated risks of hyperlipemia for cardiovascular disease and the benefits of treatment.

Several studies have shown that cholesterol reduction by medication (pravastatin or simvastatin) results in a decrease in subsequent major cardiovascular events in patients with diabetes who have had MIs. Primary prevention trial data are not available on lipid lowering in patients with type 2 diabetes without clinical coronary disease, however. Given our current knowledge, it appears reasonable to offer treatment with a statin to individuals with elevated total serum cholesterol, low-density lipoprotein (LDL), or non-HDL cholesterol or reduced levels of HDL. The combination of statins plus fibric acid derivatives may be more effective, especially in many patients with highly elevated triglycerides. There appears to be a higher risk of myopathy, however, and careful monitoring is warranted.

Appropriate dietary and exercise therapy and correction of other risk factors should also be considered. Minimum and ideal goals of therapy are largely consensus based: lower than 200 and 170 mg/dL for total cholesterol, 130 and 100 mg/dL for LDL, and 160 and 130 mg/dL for non-HDL cholesterol, respectively.

CONTROLLING HYPERTENSION

Approximately 40% of 45-year old patients with type 2 diabetes and 60% of those age 75 years have hypertension. The UKPDS 38 (1998) investigated whether tight control of blood pressure prevented macro- and microvascular complications. This RCT achieved a mean blood pressure in the control group of 154/87—while avoiding the use of a β blocker or angiotensin-converting enzyme inhibitor (ACEI)—versus 144/82 in the treatment group, with captopril or atenolol as the active agents. While all-cause mortality rates were not significantly reduced, a number of macro- and microvascular outcomes were significantly ameliorated, including stroke, diabetes endpoints overall, diabetes-related death, microvascular disease, and visual deterioration. Myocardial infarctions, peripheral vascular disease, and amputations were all decreased, but insignificantly. When all macrovascular diseases were combined, those in the tighter control group saw a 34% decline in complications. These reductions were of a magnitude similar to that seen in other large prospective studies of hypertension control and more substantial than that seen with improved glycemic control.

In a separate study comparing the results with captopril and atenolol, no significant differences were found in micro- or macrovascular endpoints. These results suggest that absolute blood pressure control may be more important in influencing the development and progression of nephropathy than the agent chosen to control it. Significantly more patients remained on captopril than atenolol (78% versus 65%). Cost-effectiveness analysis suggests that tight control of blood pressure substantially lowers costs and has a cost-effectiveness ratio similar to other accepted interventions.

A similar investigation in the United States, the Appropriate Blood Pressure Control in Type 2 Diabetes (ABCD) Trial, should be reporting its final results soon. Measures to enhance compliance, such as a teaching program, have been shown to have a favorable impact on the incidence of cardiac and cerebrovascular events. On the basis of these studies, an ACEI or β blocker should be administered to control blood pressure to a goal of approximately 130 to 140/80 to 85 mm Hg. Measures to enhance long-term adherence should be instituted.

USING ASPIRIN

The Early Treatment of Diabetic Retinopathy Study (1992), a large RCT, and the Antiplatelet Trialists' Collaboration (1994), a meta-analysis, suggest that aspirin lessens the incidence of cardiovascular endpoints in patients with type 2 diabetes, without an increased likelihood of side effects, including retinal or vitreous hemorrhage. Aspirin appeared to lower the risk of MI by approximately 15% to 30% and the risk of death by approximately 15%. The specific appropriate dose of aspirin is unclear and should be between 81 mg and 325 mg/d. Enteric-coated aspirin can significantly mitigate the risk of gastrointestinal bleeding.

HORMONE REPLACEMENT THERAPY, ESTROGEN, REPLACEMENT, AND OSTEOPOROSIS PREVENTION

The potential benefits of HRT include reduction of osteoporosis and its complications and a decrease in CVD. The prevalence of osteoporosis may be higher in patients with type 2 diabetes, though it is the subject of controversy. Risk factors for falls and fractures, such as orthostatic hypotension, peripheral neuropathy, and visual impairment, are clearly present in many patients. There are no additional harms derived from vitamin D and calcium therapies for most patients with type 2 diabetes. Estrogen replacement has a salutary effect on osteoporosis and appears to have minimal effect on diabetes itself. The most important potential benefit of estrogen replacement is the reduction in CHD. Multiple RCTs provide data concerning HRT in patients without diabetes, but primarily observational studies have investigated populations with type 2 diabetes. If HRT is used, triglyceride and lipid levels should be followed closely. On the basis of incomplete information, patients should be informed of the potential benefits and harms of HRT.

Weight Loss

The majority of patients with type 2 diabetes are overweight. Even modest improvements in weight (10- to 20-pound weight losses) are associated with improved glycemic control and lessen hyperlipidemia and hypertension. Unfortunately, long-term weight loss is difficult to sustain. No single diet is effective for every patient, and meal planning should be individualized to the patient's preferences and requirements. Given the moderate association with improved intermediate outcomes and the challenges of sustaining long-term lifestyle changes, patients should be encouraged to approach weight control and dietary changes in a modest and endurable fashion.

EXERCISE

Regular aerobic exercise could well have a favorable effect on glycemic control, glucose tolerance, weight loss, hypertension, cardiovascular fitness, and quality of life. Effects are particularly evident with regular, more vigorous programs of physical activity and indicate a training effect. Patients with absolute insulin deficiency are less likely to improve. Benefits appear to wane as rapidly as 3 days after ceasing an exercise program.

Most experts suggest a thorough physical examination targeting the presence of retinopathy, neuropathy, and vascular disease, which may influence the exercise prescription. Many would advocate a pre-exercise noninvasive evaluation for coronary artery disease, given the higher prevalence of occult cardiac problems in patients with diabetes. Exercise associated with Valsalva-type maneuvers may cause larger blood pressure increases and could precipitate retinal hemorrhage in patients with proliferative retinopathy. Such patients should also avoid shear forces and head trauma. Scant evidence exists concerning exercise and nephropathy. While protein excretion increases acutely in proportion to the level of physical activity, there does not appear to be a greater risk of progression of nephropathy. Wearing appropriate shoes is important, particularly for patients with neuropathy and peripheral vascular disease. Finally, patients should monitor blood sugar levels more closely and understand how to treat hypoglycemia. While exercise is heralded as a cornerstone of diabetes therapy, its longer term benefits are largely supported by short-term observational studies.

Microvascular Complications

RETINOPATHY AND BLINDNESS

Twelve thousand Americans with diabetes become blind each year. Up to 21% of patients with type 2 diabetes have retinopathy at the time of diagnosis, and as many as 10% become blind as the result of retinopathy, cataracts, retinal detachment, and vitreous hemorrhage. The UKPDS and Kumamoto Trial (Ohkubo 1995) have provided clear evidence from RCTs that improved glycemic control diminishes the development and progression of retinopathy and the need for photocoagulation. With a reduction in the HbA_{1C} value from a level of 11% to one of 7%, the lifetime rise of development of retinopathy can be lowered by approximately 7.6% in a 45-year old, as opposed to <0.5% in a 75-year old. Moreover, there is good evidence that even modest improvements in HbA_{1C} are associated with significant reductions in the lifetime risk of blindness. The presence of hypertension is an additional risk factor for retinopathy in diabetes.

The Euclid study (Chaturvedi et al., 1998) recently showed that the use of lisonopril slows the progression of retinopathy in patients with type 1 diabetes. The applicability of this finding to patients with type 2 diabetes remains unknown. The relative importance of using an ACEI, as opposed to simply controlling blood pressure, is also unclear. The UKPDS suggests that control of hypertension may be the mediating effect.

Retinopathy can be detected by funduscopic examination. It is possible for primary care clinicians to perform accurate dilated fundus examinations, but many will choose to allow a qualified eye specialist to conduct this test. Regular ophthalmologic care is cost-effective and can prevent visual loss. RCTs have shown that laser therapy can prevent visual loss due to diabetic retinopathy. Many changes related to retinopathy can be asymptomatic. Thus, given the high burden of eye problems, which are often asymptomatic and amenable to therapies accepted by many patients, routine visual screening by a qualified practitioner is reasonable. Most authorities recommend yearly screening.

NEPHROPATHY AND RENAL FAILURE

Diabetic nephropathy is the leading cause of ESRD, and approximately 20% of patients with type 2 diabetes will suffer chronic renal failure. More than 10% of patients with type 2 diabetes will die of complications associated with nephropathy. RCTs have established that glycemic control and hypertension are independent risk factors for nephropathy. The typical urine dipstick test will detect albumin levels of more than 300 mg, but microalbuminuria is defined as albumin levels between 50 and 300 mg, and these must be detected via specific testing. RCTs show that ACEIs slow the decline of the glomerular filtration rate in patients with nephropathy, decrease the amount of proteinuria, and lessen the progression from microalbuminuria to overt proteinuria. One RCT has shown similar effects in normotensive, normoalbuminuric patients with type 2 diabetes.

Data clearly showing a reduced incidence of chronic renal failure or need for dialysis are largely indirect. Nonetheless, current recommendations to screen for microalbuminuria yearly and to treat patients who have abnormal results with an ACEI seem reasonable. How frequently such tests should be performed and the added value of more exhaustive renal evaluation (e.g., 24-hour urine collection) in asymptomatic patients are unclear. Trials, including the UKPDS and Kumamoto, also suggest that blood pressure should be controlled to 130/85 mm Hg or less. Protein restriction has not been well studied in patients with nephropathy and type 2 diabetes and is difficult to achieve in practice.

PERIPHERAL NEUROPATHY

Peripheral neuropathy is prevalent in about half of patients with type 2 diabetes after 15 years. Improved glycemic control can slow the development and progression of neuropathy. Early detection of neuropathy can diminish admissions related to foot ulcers and amputations. Screening for neuropathy with a monofilament test along with education of patients have been shown to minimize foot ulcers and possibly amputations. No clear data demonstrate the possible benefit of typical sensory testing, but referral to a multidisciplinary care team specializing in foot care has been shown to enhance outcomes. Orthotics and prompt treatment of structural abnormalities and infections are recommended on the basis of expert opinion. It is also felt that glycemic control may lessen the effect of neuropathy.

AUTONOMIC NEUROPATHY

Autonomic neuropathy is another common cause of disability in patients with type 2 diabetes; it encompasses gastroparesis, diabetes-related bowel problems, orthostatic hypotension, and erectile dysfunction. While each of these complications can be detected by a variety of tests, the advantages of screening are unproved. The DCCT found that intensive diabetes therapy can slow the development of abnormal physiologic parameters of autonomic function. Regular inquiry about symptoms and exercising caution in adding medications, which can aggravate these problems, are reasonable approaches on the basis of expert opinion.

FOOT PROBLEMS, LIMB LOSS

Diabetic patients are at risk of foot problems and limb loss not only because of peripheral neuropathy but also as the result of circulatory and immune system defects. As noted, case finding of foot problems can be an effective preventive measure. The physical examination should emphasize careful visual inspection and monofilament testing. Any foot infections or ulcers on the foot of a diabetic patient need immediate care, including debridement, broad-spectrum antibiotics, and avoidance of mechanical stress on the affected site through bed rest, special shoes, shoe inserts, or full-contact casts.

SEXUAL FUNCTION

Diabetes affects both male and female sexual function. The best cohort studies available suggest that libido usually remains intact in patients with type 2 diabetes, but the increased burden of disease management can influence body concept and self-esteem, and other co-morbid conditions and complications of diabetes can greatly influence sexuality. Decreased vaginal lubrication is seen in women with diabetes. Erectile dysfunction is a common consequence of autonomic problems and vascular disease in men. Whether vasocongestive problems are present in women is not known. Patients can be asked about these complications and offered advice on artificial lubricants, penile prosthesis, and medical therapy for erectile dysfunction.

Diabetes and Pregnancy

Gestational diabetes and pregnancy in women with type 2 diabetes are discussed in Chapter 9. To prevent the risks of birth defects and adverse outcomes associated with diabetes in the early stages of pregnancy, it is important to maintain periconception glucose control in women with type 2 diabetes who are trying to become pregnant. Early detection and control of gestational diabetes (impaired glucose control resulting from the pregnancy and not present at conception) are vital in preventing macrosomia and its risks.

Patient Education

Patients with diabetes should be educated about a number of topics: diet; exercise; SMBG, including use of monitors and Lancers and when to test; medication use and/or insulin injection; foot care; and response to high or low SMBG values. Patient education responsibilities can be shared with nurses, dieticians, and certified diabetes educators. Patient education programs have favorably influenced the health status and clinical outcomes of patients with type 2 diabetes. Programs integrating clinical care with patient education appear to be particularly effective. Even though they are associated with increased knowledge on the part of the patient, isolated educational programs have failed to show improved clinical outcomes.

Recommendations to Clinicians Regarding Tertiary Prevention

American Diabetes Association Recommendations

Tables 17-12 and 17-13, from the 1998 ADA "Standards of Medical Care for Patients with Diabetes Mellitus," list the recommendations for initial and routine care for diabetics. The ADA also suggests specifically screening for smoking as a cardiovascular risk factor. The ADA endorses aspirin therapy (at a dose of 81 to 325 mg/day) in patients at high risk of cardiovascular disease (i.e., any patients with evidence of large-vessel disease or family history of CHD, those who smoke cigarettes or are obese, or those with hypertension, microalbuminuria or macroalbuminuria, or hyperlipidemia). The ADA favors palpation of lower-extremity pulses and use of the monofilament exam to detect loss of protection sensation.

American College of Physicians Recommendations

The ACP recommendations agree with those of the ADA. In addition, the ACP emphasizes that

Table 17-12
Components of the Initial Visit

Medical history	Foot examination
Symptoms, laboratory results related to	Skin examination
diagnosis	Neurological examination
Nutritional assessment, weight history	Oral examination
Previous and present treatment plans	Sexual maturation (if peripubertal)
Medications	Laboratory evaluation
Medical nutrition therapy	Fasting plasma glucose (optional)
Self-management training	Glycohemoglobin
Self-monitoring of blood glucose results	Fasting lipid profile
Current treatment plan	Serum creatinine
Exercise history	Urinalysis
Acute complications	Urine culture (if indicated)
History of infections	Thyroid function tests (if indicated)
Chronic diabetic complications	Electrocardiogram (adults)
Medication history	Management plan
Family history	Short- and long-term goals
Coronary heart disease risk factors	Medications
Psychosocial/economic factors	Medical nutrition therapy
Physical examination	Lifestyle changes
Height and weight	Self-management education
Blood pressure	Monitoring instructions
Ophthalmoscopic examination	Annual referral to eye specialist
Thyroid palpation	Specialty consultations (as indicated)
Cardiac examination	Agreement on continuing support/follow-up
Evaluation of pulses	

SOURCE: American Diabetes Association, 1998.

oral medications should not be used as a substitute for diet and exercise. For diabetic retinopathy, the ACP suggestions agree with those of the ADA, with one addition. If "skilled reading of seven-field stereoscopic photographs is available and reveals no retinopathy at the initial screen (shortly after the diagnosis of diabetes), then the next screening examination does not need to be for 4 years" unless the patient has persistently elevated glucose levels or proteinuria. Subsequent screening (after 4 years), using either stereophotography or dilated ophthalmoscopy, should be done annually.

American Academy of Family Physicians Recommendations

The AAFP recommendations for the routine care of nephropathy, retinopathy, and the foot are consistent with those of the ADA. In addition to the guidelines of the ADA, the AAFP also proposes an initial fasting urine test for glucose and acetone. The AAFP favors foot examinations at every visit only for patients specifically at risk of foot problems, such as those over age 40 years, cigarette smokers, those with diabetes of 10 or more years' duration, and those who report foot

Table 17-13

Components of the Continuing Care Visit

Contact frequency	Laboratory evaluation
Daily for initiation of insulin or change in	Glycohemoglobin
regimen	Quarterly if treatment changes of patient
Weekly for initiation of oral glucose-lowering	are not meeting goals
agent(s) or change in regimen	Twice per year if stable
Routine visits	Fasting plasma glucose (optional)
Quarterly for patients who are not meeting	Fasting lipid profile annually
goals	Urinalysis for protein annually
Semiannually for other patients	Microalbumin measurement annually (if
Medical history	urinalysis gives negative results for protein)
Assess treatment regimen	Review of management plan
Frequency/severity of hypo-hyperglycemia	Evaluate each visit
Self-monitoring of blood glucose results	Short- and long-term goals
Patient regimen adjustments	Medications
Adherence problems	Glycemia
Lifestyle changes	Frequency/severity of hypoglycemia
Symptoms of complications	Self-monitoring of blood glucose results
Other medical illnesses	Complications
Medications	Control of dyslipidemia
Psychosocial issues	Blood pressure
Physical examination	Weight
Physical examination annually	Medical nutrition therapy
Dilated eye examination annually	Exercise regimen
Every regular visit	Adherence to self-management training
Weight	Follow-up of referrals
Blood pressure	Psychosocial adjustment
Previous abnormalities on the physical	Evaluate annually
examination	Knowledge of diabetes
Foot examination	Self-management skills

SOURCE: American Diabetes Association, 1998.

problems or intermittent claudication. A glyco-hemoglobin measurement is recommended every 3 to 4 months regardless of the level of glycemic control. The AAFP also suggests that it is important to limit the amount of information the patient receives at any one time, because overwhelming the patient with information can contribute to poor compliance.

World Health Organization Recommendations

WHO recommendations are also generally consistent with those of the ADA. The WHO suggests, however, that if no retinopathy is present, it might be safe to wait 4 years until further retinal examination. The WHO proposes annual urinary albumin measurements until age 70 only and recommends that the routine foot examination include inspection of the skin, hair, and nails; grading of vibratory sensation on the dorsum of the great toe; and grading of ankle reflexes. The WHO specifically endorses the assessment of cardiovascular autonomic neuropathy before a patient undergoes general anesthesia, since the presence of this abnormality increases the risk of death from general anesthesia.

Centers for Disease Control and Prevention Recommendations

The recommendations of the Centers for Disease Control and Prevention (CDC) are generally consistent with those of the ADA. In addition to proposing that the primary physician perform an oral exam, they suggest that the physician instruct the patient to see a dentist every 6 months. The CDC recommends that the comprehensive annual screening examination of the patient's feet (which is recommended by the ADA) also include tests of temperature sensation, pinprick and pressure sensation, distal vibratory sensation, and position sense.

Quality-monitoring Measures

The National Committee for Quality Assurance (NCQA) has announced six measures, the reporting of which was voluntary in 1999 and will become mandatory for NCQA participants in 2000. This report assesses whether a diabetic patient's HbA_{1C} was tested within the past year, if the patient's HbA_{1C} level is controlled, if a lipid profile was taken, how well lipid levels are controlled, whether patients underwent a dilated-eye exam within the past year, and whether kidney disease is appropriately monitored.

The Health Care Financing Administration has proposed a number of "accountability" and "quality improvement" measures to be used in the Diabetes Quality Improvement Project. These measures examine the percentage of patients receiving more than one glycohemoglobin test in a year, a nephropathy assessment, a lipid profile once in 2 years, a periodic dilated-eye exam, and an annual documented foot exam, including a risk assessment. They will also examine the percentages of patients in various categories of glucose control (by glycohemoglobin level) and the distribution of LDL and blood pressure values.

Practical Management Tips

INCREASING PATIENT ADHERENCE

Many clinicians would list patient nonadherence as one of the most common barriers to better diabetes care. Clinicians should not assume, however, that patients whom they judge to be nonadherent will not change their behaviors. Studies have shown that physicians are not very accurate in predicting which patients will be more successful at diabetes management. Furthermore, patients who respond positively to educational interventions may do so because of unexpected conversion experiences rather than from following a model of predictable stages of change. Because of the unpredictability of patients' adherence to self-management procedures, providers should continually encourage their patients to make lifestyle changes and improve their self-management, regardless of the perceived level of adherence.

SMBG has many benefits for the patient with diabetes. Not only is it an excellent patient education tool and an aid in making adjustments in diet, exercise, and medications to achieve better glycemic control, but it also allows the patient to feel more in control of his or her treatment. Even patients who are not routinely doing SMBG should periodically check blood sugar levels throughout the day and at 3 A.M. to detect hypo- and hyperglycemic swings that may cause weight gain or symptoms. The patient-held record of blood glucose levels can also contain information about the patient's medications, recent lab results, and health care team. Increasing a patient's feeling of control over diabetes and its treatment can enhance their long-term adherence.

It is important to set specific therapy goals— failing to set such goals limits the effectiveness of therapy. Many patients will be unwilling to switch to insulin, and with these patients, providers need to emphasize the target glucose control ranges and set time limits for achieving them. It is important to be as specific as possible when negotiating behavioral changes, such as using the patient's normal daily activities to cue home blood glucose measurements and planning specific exercise activities. Patient education has been shown to improve glycemic control, especially in newly diagnosed patients, and might lower the risk of complications. Unfortunately, there is a lack of evidence for the long-term benefits of education, and some data suggest that the physiological improvements are temporary. Continuing education may be a key to success.

Participation in support groups can also strengthen patients' compliance with self-care recommendations and provide valuable information about diabetes management. Clinicians may want to monitor the information patients receive to be sure that it is not inappropriate. Family support is also important, especially that of the person who is responsible for meal preparation. While family support is important, it must be provided judiciously and with concern for the patient's autonomy. One study reports that help with diet and medication given by family members to older adults with diabetes is twice as likely to be unwelcome as not.

In managing a chronic disease such as diabetes, the clinician should try to change from a prescriptive style to a collaborative style of interaction. Enlisting the patient's participation in the decision-making process during an office visit is likely to improve adherence to self-care plans. On the other hand, one focus group study exploring the experiences of 17 women with type 2 diabetes who were judged to be exemplars of good diabetes management showed that even exemplary patients may not be ready to accept a collaborative, highly responsible role in diabetes management until they have gained experience with their disease (Ellison et al., 1988).

IMPROVING THE PROVISION OF SERVICES

Patient self-monitoring systems, medical record flowcharts, and office-based patient reminder systems can all be used to improve diabetes care. Clinic routines, such as having a nurse or aide remove the patient's shoes and socks, can be a major factor in determining whether the physician conducts a foot exam. Having the patient remove his or her shoes and socks at every clinic visit may also increase the patient's awareness of the important of monitoring feet, regardless of whether the provider does a thorough foot exam during that particular visit.

Other Preventive Services of Particular Importance in Patients with Type 2 Diabetes

The guide to clinical preventive services of the USPSTF provides a comprehensive and up-to-date overview of prevention issues important to any individual. Patients with diabetes deserve comprehensive preventive services, not just attention focused on avoiding complications of their disease. Indeed, the absolute risks of such problems as breast and cervical cancer remain high and merit consideration. This section highlights specific preventive services particularly germane to individuals with diabetes.

Primary Prevention

IMMUNIZATIONS

INFLUENZA VACCINE   On the basis of a large number of quasi-experimental studies, influenza vaccination should be offered to all individuals with diabetes mellitus. The magnitude of benefit can be expected to be greater in elders with diabetes or other independent risk factors, such as chronic pulmonary disease. Yearly immunization is recommended.

PNEUMOCOCCAL VACCINE   Data from observational studies support the offering of pneumococcal vaccination to patients with diabetes. The benefit of immunization can be expected to be greatest in those with other chronic diseases and those who are likely to be able to mount a sufficient immune response. Chapter 19 contains more detailed information on both influenza and pneumococcal immunizations.

SMOKING CESSATION AND OSTEOPOROSIS PREVENTION

These interventions have already been discussed and are mentioned again here because of their importance to those with diabetes. Chapters 10 and 18 discuss these issues in more depth.

Secondary Prevention

TUBERCULOSIS

Major authorities, including the USPSTF and the CDC, recommend screening asymptomatic high-risk individuals—including patients with diabetes—for tuberculosis at an interval left to the discretion of the clinician. The Mantoux test should be used.

DENTAL/ORAL DISEASE

Diabetes predisposes individuals to oral and dental disorders. Up to 95% of patients with diabetes have periodontal disease. Improved glycemic control is associated with decreased severity and incidence of periodontal disease in uncontrolled, observational studies. Patients with very poor glycemic control may have a higher incidence of caries. Data linking specific screening strategies to improved outcomes is lacking. Nonetheless, yearly dental examinations coupled with routine dental care at home would be reasonable based on expert opinion, with more frequent attention focused on patients with poor glycemic control.

DEPRESSION

The prevalence of depression is approximately threefold higher in patients with diabetes compared with individuals without this disease. A subgroup of patients with diabetes may be at greater risk of depression (e.g., those with major complications), but comprehensive longitudinal studies are not available. While no major authorities recommend routine screening for depression in patients with diabetes, clinicians should remain alert for clinical signs and symptoms of depression, given its high prevalence, known morbidity, and response to treatment.

ASYMPTOMATIC BACTERIURIA AND VAGINITIS

Although diabetes predisposes individuals to asymptomatic bacteriuria and urinary tract infection and vaginitis, there is insufficient evidence to recommend specific screening procedures. Treatment of asymptomatic bacteriuria is effective initially, but bacteriuria recurs in more than two-thirds of patients. The association of bacteriuria and renal damage is unproved in this population, and, for this reason, the efficacy of screening remains unclear. Yeast vaginitis is also more common in patients with diabetes and should be considered in the differential diagnosis of urinary tract infections.

Common Errors

Many studies have shown that routine diabetes care often does not meet recommended standards. Some of the most common errors are cited here.

Not Counseling Patients Regarding Diet, Exercise, and Weight Control

All patients should receive a clinician's advice regarding a healthy diet, exercise, and weight control. This is especially true for those who are at risk of type 2 diabetes because of family history, weight, or other risk factors. Clinicians often do not provide this advice or do not provide it effectively.

Not Comprehensively Treating Patients with Diabetes

Clinicians perform poorly in terms of nearly every recommended diabetic intervention, including regular eye exams, regular foot exams, monitoring kidney function, and checking HbA_{1C} levels.

Not Aggressively Controlling Other Cardiovascular Risk Factors

Clinicians often do not anticipate the risk of cardiovascular disease caused by diabetes in concert with other risk factors, such as hypertension, hyperlipidemia, and smoking. This leads to inadequate attempts to alleviate those additional risk factors.

Not Implementing Other Prevention Interventions

Patients with diabetes should receive the full array of recommended prevention interventions, just like any other patient. The time and effort needed to treat diabetes can distract clinicians from considering what other services are indicated, such as immunizations and cancer screens.

Failure to Consider the Patient's Personal Circumstances

As described earlier in this chapter, there are many contingencies that need to be considered and discussed with each patient when developing treatment goals and plans. Failure to do so can lead to poor adherence to treatment. Moreover, aggressive attempts to achieve intensive diabetes control can lead to hypoglycemia and its complications in patients who have personal, social, and economic situations that interfere with regular food intake if these issues are not considered.

Emerging Trends

Primary Prevention

The results of the Diabetes Prevention Program should be available around 2002. Other controlled trials may provide further data supporting primary prevention of type 2 diabetes in the form of information about the potential of exercise, diet, and weight control in diabetes prevention. Behavioral research will assist the clinician in learning how to persuade patients to change their behavior and adopt healthful lifestyles to prevent diabetes.

Secondary Prevention

Type 2 diabetes mellitus is a disease of insulin resistance, which appears to be mediated by environmental, lifestyle, and genetic factors. There is approximately 90% concordance for type 2 diabetes mellitus between twins. Two genes have been discovered to be associated with type 2 diabetes mellitus in young patients [maturity-onset diabetes of the young (MODY)]. With the rapid advances of the human genome project, the genetic basis for other forms of type 2 diabetes may be discovered and effective prevention, screening, and treatment strategies developed. Future studies should help define the accuracy of the screening tests in use today and assist in setting cutoffs that provide the best combination of predictive values. The future use of HbA_{1C} as a screening tool is likely to grow as more experience is gained with it and standardization improves.

Tertiary Prevention and Treatment

Many new medications are in the development stage. New insulin sensitizers in the thiazolidinedione family (such as troglitazone) have recently been approved and released by the Food and Drug Administration (FDA) or are in Phase III trials. These include englitazone, rosiglitazone, and pioglitazone. Rapid-release bromocriptine is being administered to obese patients and appears to reduce blood sugars and postprandial triglyceridemia. Repaglinide, an agent unrelated to current oral medications, has now received FDA approval. It promises to be a rapidly acting drug that could be used preprandially. Other medications are being explored

that delay carbohydrate absorption, increase insulin release, delay glucose absorption, modify glucose and lipid metabolism, treat diabetic neuropathy, and minimize microvascular complications. Even new forms of insulin—from aerosolized to rectally administered—are under investigation.

Insulin delivery and measurement systems continue to be enhanced. Insulin pumps are becoming more reliable, and implantable insulin pumps have compared favorably with multiple daily injections in RCTs. Noninvasive means of blood sugar monitoring using spectroscopy, radio wave impedance, and interstitial fluid analysis being developed. A practical, affordable closed-loop system (one that automatically and accurately adjusts therapy on the basis of blood sugar) may be forthcoming.

Bibliography

American Board of Family Practice: *Diabetes Mellitus Reference Guide.* Lexington, KY, American Board of Family Practice, 1997.

American College of Physicians, American Diabetes Association, and American Academy of Ophthalmology. Screening guidelines for diabetic retinopathy. *Ann Intern Med* 116:683–685, 1992.

American Diabetes Association: Standards of medical care for patients with diabetes mellitus. *Diabetes Care* 21:S23, 1998.

Antiplatelet Trialists' Collaboration. Collaborative overview of randomised trials of antiplatelet therapy—I: Prevention of death, myocardial infarction, and stroke by prolonged antiplatelet therapy in various categories of patients. Antiplatelet Trialists' Collaboration [see comments] [published erratum appears in BMJ Jun 11;308(6943):1540] 1994. BMJ 308:81–106, 1994.

Brown SA: Meta-analysis of diabetes patient education research: Variations in intervention effects across studies. *Res Nurs Health* 15:402, 1992.

Centers for Disease Control: *The Prevention and Treatment of Complications of Diabetes Mellitus.* Atlanta, GA, Division of Diabetes Translation, Department of Health and Human Services, 1991.

Chaturvedi N, Sjolie AK, Stephenson JM, et al: Effect of lisinopril on progression of retinopathy in normotensive people with type 1 diabetes. The EUCLID Study Group. EURODIAB controlled trial of lisinopril in insulin-dependent diabetes mellitus. *Lancet* 351:28, 1998.

Colditz GA, Coakley E: Weight, weight gain, activity, and major illnesses: The Nurses' Health Study. *Int J Sports Med* 18:S162, 1997.

Diabetes Control and Complications Trial Research Group: The effect of intensive treatment of diabetes on the development and progression of long-term complications in insulin-dependent diabetes mellitus. *N Engl J Med* 329:977, 1993.

ETDRS Investigators. Aspirin effects on mortality and morbidity in patients with diabetes mellitus: Early Treatment Diabetic Retinopathy Study. Report 14. *JAMA* 268:1292, 1992.

Ellison GC, Rayman KM: Exemplars' experience of self-managing type 2 diabetes. *Diabetes Educ* 24: 325, 1998.

Eriksson KF, Lindgarde F: Prevention of type 2 (non-insulin-dependent) diabetes mellitus by diet and physical exercise: The 6-year Malmö feasibility study. *Diabetologia* 34:891, 1991.

Expert Committee on the Diagnosis and Classification of Diabetes Mellitus: Report of the Expert Committee on the Diagnosis and Classification of Diabetes Mellitus. *Diabetes Care* 20:1183, 1997.

Haffner SM: Management of dyslipidemia in adults with diabetes. *Diabetes Care* 21:160–178, 1998.

Harris MI, Flegal KM, Cowie CC, et al: Prevalence of diabetes, impaired fasting glucose and impaired glucose tolerance in U.S. adults. *Diabetes Care* 21: 518, 1998.

Hayward RA, Manning WG, Kaplan SH, Wagner EH, Greenfield S: Starting insulin therapy in patients with type 2 diabetes: Effectiveness, complications, and resource utilization. *JAMA* 278:1663–1669, 1997.

Heinonen OP, Huttunen JK, Manninen V, et al: The Helsinki Heart Study: Coronary heart disease incidence during an extended follow-up. *J Intern Med* 235:41–49, 1994.

Helmrich SP, Ragland DR, Leung RW, Paffenbarger RS: Physical activity and reduced occurrence of non-insulin-dependent diabetes mellitus. *N Engl J Med* 325:147–152, 1991.

Henry RR, Genuth S: Forum One: Current recommendations about intensification of metabolic control in non-insulin-dependent diabetes mellitus. *Ann Intern Med* 124:175–177, 1996.

Ivy JL: Role of exercise training in the prevention and treatment of insulin resistance and non-insulin-dependent diabetes mellitus. *Sports Med* 24:321–336, 1997.

James SA, Jamjoum L, Raghunathan TE, Strogatz DS, Furth ED, Khazanie PG: Physical activity and NIDDM in African-Americans: The Pitt County Study. *Diabetes Care* 21:555–562, 1998.

Klonoff DC: Noninvasive blood glucose monitoring. *Clin Diabetes* 16:43–45, 1998.

Leichter SB: Traditional versus corporate influence on diabetes care in managed health organizations: Risks and opportunities. *Clin Diabetes* 16:46–48, 1998.

Levin JA, Muzyka BC, Glick M: Dental management of patients with diabetes mellitus. *Compendium* 17(1):82–90, 1996.

Lorenz RA, Bubb J, Davis D, et al: Changing behavior: Practical lessons from the diabetes control and complications trial. *Diabetes Care* 19:648–652, 1996.

Manson JE, Nathan DM, Krolewski AS, Stampfer MJ, Willett WC, Hennekens CH: A prospective study of exercise and incidence of diabetes among U.S. male physicians. *JAMA* 268:63–67, 1992

Mayer-Davis EJ, D'Agostino R Jr, Karter AJ, et al: Intensity and amount of physical activity in relation to insulin sensitivity: The Insulin Resistance Atherosclerosis Study. *JAMA* 279:669–674, 1998.

Moss S, Klein R, Klein B: Cause-specific mortality in a population-based study of diabetes. *Am J Public Health* 81:1158–1162, 1991.

Mudaliar SR, Henry RR: Strategies for preventing type II diabetes: What can be done to stem the epidemic? *Postgrad Med* 101:181–186, 1997.

National Diabetes Data Group: *Diabetes in America*, NIH publication no 95-1468. Bethesda, National Institutes of Health, National Institute of Diabetes and Digestive and Kidney Diseases, U.S. Department of Health and Human Services, 1995.

National Institute of Diabetes and Digestive and Kidney Diseases: *Diabetes Prevention Program, Fact Sheet.* Bethesda, National Institutes of Health, 1996.

O'Connor PJ, Crabtree BF, Yanoshik K: Differences between diabetic patients who do and do not respond to a diabetes care intervention: A qualitative analysis. *Fam Med* 29:424–428, 1997.

Ohkubo Y, Kishikawa H, Araki E, et al: Intensive insulin therapy prevents the progression of diabetic microvascular complications in Japanese patients with non-insulin dependent diabetes mellitus: A randomized prospective 6-year study. *Diabetes Res Clin Prac* 28:103–117, 1995.

Pan XR, Li GW, Hu YH, et al.: Effects of diet in preventing NIDDM in people with impaired glucose tolerance—the Da-Qing IGT and diabetes study. *Diabetes Care* 20:537–544, 1997.

Ravid M, Brosh D, Levi Z, Bar-Dayan Y, Ravid D, Rachmani R: Use of enalapril to attenuate decline in renal function in normotensive, normoalbuminuric patients with type 2 diabetes mellitus: A randomized, controlled trial. *Ann Intern Med* 128:982–988, 1998.

Ravid M, Lang R, Lishner M: Long-term renoprotective effect of angiotensin-converting enzyme inhibition in non-insulin-dependent diabetes mellitus: A 7-year follow-up study. *Arch Intern Med* 156:286–289, 1996.

Sacks FM, Pfeffer MA, Moye LA, et al: The effect of pravastatin on coronary events after myocardial infarction in patients with average cholesterol levels: Cholesterol and Recurrent Events Trial investigators. *N Engl J Med* 335:1001–1009, 1996.

Scandinavian Simvastatin Survival Study Group: Randomized trial of cholesterol lowering in 4444 patients with coronary heart disease: The Scandinavian Simvastatin Survival Study (4S). *Lancet* 344:1383–1389, 1994.

Stout RW: Hyperinsulinemia and atherosclerosis. *Diabetes* 45:S45–S46, 1996.

UK Prospective Diabetes Study Group: Cost effectiveness analysis of improved blood pressure control in hypertensive patients with type 2 diabetes (UKPDS 40). *BMJ* 317:720–726, 1998.

UK Prospective Diabetes Study Group: Effect of intensive blood-glucose control with metformin on complications in overweight patients with type 2 diabetes (UKPDS 34). *Lancet* 352:854–865, 1998.

UK Prospective Diabetes Study Group, Intensive blood-glucose control with sulphonylureas or insulin compared with conventional treatment and risk of complications in patients with type 2 diabetes (UKPDS 33). *Lancet* 352:837–853, 1998.

UK Prospective Diabetes Study Group: Tight blood pressure control and risk of macrovascular and microvascular complications in type 2 diabetes (UKPDS 38). *BMJ* 317:703–713, 1998.

U.S. Preventive Services Task Force: Screening for diabetes mellitus, in *Guide to Clinical Preventive Services: Report of the U.S. Preventive Services Task Force.* Baltimore, Williams & Wilkins, 1996, pp. 193–208.

Vijan S, Hofer TP, Hayward RA: Estimated benefits of glycemic control in microvascular complications in type 2 diabetes. *Ann Intern Med* 127(9):788–794, 1997.

Vijan S, Stevens DL, Herman WH, Funnell MM, Standiford CJ: Screening, prevention, counseling, and treatment for the complications of type II diabetes mellitus: Putting evidence into practice. *J Gen Intern Med* 12:567–580, 1997.

World Health Organization: *Prevention of Diabetes Mellitus: Report of a WHO Study Group.* Geneva, World Health Organization, 1994.

Zoorob RJ, Hagen MD: Guidelines on the care of diabetic nephropathy, retinopathy and foot disease. *Am Fam Physician* 56:2021–2028, 2033–2034, 1997.

Fred E. Heidrich

Osteoporosis

Introduction

Definition

Osteoporosis, or porous bone, is a clinical syndrome in which bone density (BD) is decreased and fractures occur after trauma that would not harm normal bone. In osteoporosis, bone mineralization (the ratio of mineral to collagen) is generally normal, but the total quantity of bone tissue is reduced, and there are disturbances of bone microarchitecture. The World Health Organization (WHO) has defined osteoporosis based on BD comparisons with young, normal persons. By this system, individuals with a BD more than 2.5 standard deviations (SDs) below the comparison mean are considered to have osteoporosis, whereas those between 1 and 2.5 SDs below the comparison mean have osteopenia. A third category is called "established osteoporosis," which refers to osteoporotic BD with a previous associated fracture. The WHO criteria are defined for Caucasian women. There are no generally accepted criteria for women of other races or for men. The WHO definition is useful for epidemiologic purposes, but its reliance on BD data limits its clinical usefulness. The occurrence of characteristic fractures, such as spinal compression fractures and hip or distal radius fractures, in low-trauma situations often serves to indicate the presence of osteoporosis without measurement of BD.

Bone Physiology

Bone is a metabolically active tissue, with bone turnover controlled by the action of osteoblasts, which lay down new bone, and osteoclasts, which absorb bone. These cells work in tandem in a cyclic fashion at sites called bone-remodeling units. The remodeling cycle starts with osteoclastic resorption of bone, leaving a microscopic cavity. Osteoblasts then enter the cavity to lay down bone matrix protein, which is subsequently calcified. This sequence takes place over 3 to 6 months. Remodeling allows for repair of microfractures of bony pedicles and plates, which can result from repeated stresses. Remodeling also provides a way for the body to make calcium "deposits and withdrawals"—critical to bone's function as the stabilizer of serum calcium levels.

Bone tissue can be divided into two types: trabecular and cortical. Trabecular (also called spongy or cancellous) bone tissue is more metabolically active than the more dense cortical (also called dense or compact) bone and hence shows changes attributable to osteoporosis more quickly. Bones have a mix of both tissue types, but many bones have a predominance of one type. Trabecular bone comprises the majority of vertebral bodies and is also found in the ends of long bones. It resists compressive loads well and is four times lighter than cortical bone. Cortical bone, the majority tissue of the long bones, is better structured to withstand bending and twisting.

BD increases during childhood and reaches a peak in the twenties or early thirties. Trabecular BD peak is achieved earlier in life than is cortical BD. On average, men have bones that are denser than those of women, and African-Americans have greater BD than Caucasians. Two goals of osteoporosis prevention, which apply to both genders and all races, are to promote a high peak BD and to delay or minimize the decline in density that follows the peak.

Prevalence and Incidence of Osteoporosis

In the United States, approximately 1.5 million fractures annually are caused by osteoporosis. Hip, vertebral, and wrist fractures are the most common. Among Caucasian women, 40% will sustain an osteoporotic wrist, hip, or vertebral fracture in their lifetimes; the corresponding figure for men is 13%. Estimates of the financial impact of osteoporosis in the United States range from $10 to $20 billion, with hip fractures the major source. Factors influencing fracture rates are described herein.

AGE EFFECTS

The single most important predictor of low BD and fractures is age. Using the WHO criteria cited earlier, the proportion of Caucasian women who have osteoporosis in their sixth decade of life (ages 50 to 59) is 15%, in the seventh decade is 22%, in the eighth decade is 39%, and at older ages is 70% (Figure 18-1). Fracture rates show a similar pattern, especially for hip and vertebral fractures. In women, hip fracture rates double each decade after age 50, to a rate of 3% per year at age 85. Among men, the rapid increase with age begins about 10 years later until the fracture rate reaches 1.9% per year by age 85. Because osteoporotic fractures increase markedly at the end of life, delaying the onset of osteoporosis by 5 to 6 years could result in a halving of the fracture incidence.

ETHNIC/RACIAL DIFFERENCES

Studies of ethnic and racial factors in osteoporosis are complicated by confounding issues, including activity levels, economic factors, and longevity. Age-adjusted studies in women show hip fracture rates for Caucasians about 2.5 to 4.5 times higher than for African-Americans or Asian-Americans. Among men, Caucasians have rates 1.4 to 2.2 times higher than African-Americans or Asian-Americans. Much less data are available for Hispanics, but rates are similar to those for African-Americans and Asian-Americans. BD studies among Asians and Hispanics have shown values intermediate between African-Americans and Caucasians. The relatively low fracture rates among Asian-Americans may be related to bone geometry (shorter hip axis) more than to BD.

GENDER DIFFERENCES

Osteoporotic fractures are seen much more frequently in women than in men. The greater numbers of women surviving into an age of risk is surely a factor, as is lower BD in women

Figure 18-1

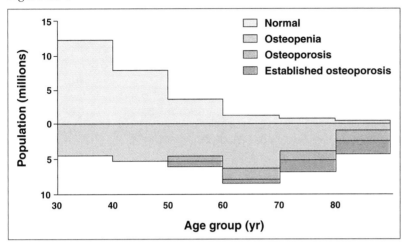

Proportion of caucasian women in the U.S. with abnormal bone density. (Reproduced with permission, from Melton LJ III: How many women have osteoporosis now? *J Bone Miner Res* 10:175, 1995.)

compared with men, both at the time of peak density and in old age. Among African-Americans the ratio of hip fractures in women (adjusted for age) is 1.2 to 1.8 times that seen in men. In other races there is a two- to threefold higher rate among women.

SOCIOECONOMIC AND GEOGRAPHIC DIFFERENCES

Hip fracture rates vary remarkably from country to country. While some of the variation can be explained on the basis of race and age, other factors found to play a role include latitude (more fractures in the southern United States), water quality (harder water, less fractures; fluoridated water, more fractures), poverty (more fractures), and urbanization (more fractures in rural areas).

TIME TRENDS

Osteoporosis is becoming a health problem of increasing importance as the population ages. For example, in Rochester, Minnesota, the incidence of hip fracture has increased thirtyfold from 1930 to 1990. During the same time period the proportion of the population over age 65 has increased from 5 to 11%. The disproportionate rise in hip fracture rates reflects the exponential increase in rates for the oldest. At present, the lifetime risk of hip fracture in Caucasian women is 17.5%, with a mean age of occurrence of about 80 years. Considering the continued aging of the U.S. population, the number of fractures will increase two- to threefold by 2050 if no further preventive efforts are undertaken.

RISK FACTORS

In addition to the factors already mentioned, a variety of other risk factors for osteoporosis have been identified. Some of them can be modified and, for this reason, are suitable targets for preventive intervention. Others are not subject to change but can be used to pinpoint persons for whom other efforts are particularly indicated (Table 18-1).

Table 18-1
Risk Factors for Osteoporosis

MODIFIABLE	NONMODIFIABLE
Low calcium intake	Gender (female)
Hormone-deficiency	Age
states	Race (Caucasian)
Thinness	Poverty
Inactive lifestyle	Living in rural area
Smoking	Family history
Heavy alcohol use	Chronic disease
Medications	Renal failure
Corticosteroids	Liver failure
Anticonvulsants	Hyperthyroidism
Heparin	Hyperparathyroidism
Methotrexate	Rheumatoid arthritis
L-Thyroxine	Cushing syndrome
Depoprovera	Malabsorption
	Type 1 diabetes

HEREDITY Beyond the effects of race, habits, and geography, twin studies and other epidemiologic evidence indicate increased risk among those with relatives with osteoporosis. For example, women whose mothers had a hip fracture are at about twice the risk of hip fracture, even after adjusting for BD. Two genes have been identified that may play a role–coding for a collagen polypeptide and vitamin D receptor—but much remains to be learned.

GONADAL HORMONE DEFICIENCY STATES Menopause, ovariectomy, andropause, orchiectomy, extremes of athleticism, anorexia nervosa, and stress all have been linked to hormone deficiency states and to increased risk of osteoporosis.

LOW CALCIUM INTAKE Many, but certainly not all, studies have shown a low calcium intake to be associated with lower BD. Possible reasons for inconsistency among the studies include confounding factors (such as activity and genetics) that may be associated with calcium intake. The amount of calcium needed to protect the bones is greater than that consumed by the majority of Americans.

THINNESS One definition of thinness is a weight <90% of weight at age 25, which is associated with a 2.5-fold increased risk, but lifelong thinness is also likely a risk factor. Weight gain after age 25 has been reported as a protective factor. Several mechanisms have been implicated: adipose tissue metabolically increases postmenopausal estrone levels by conversion from androstenedione, fatty tissue provides padding to absorb the impact from trauma, and increased body mass increases the weight-bearing stresses on bone. In addition, excessive thinness may be an indicator of general poor health. It has also been speculated that obese people may have a lower risk of falls because of lower levels of activity.

INACTIVE LIFESTYLE Bone responds to weight-bearing exercise by becoming more dense and loses density with inactivity. A minimum level of exercise to promote bone health has not been defined. If the National Institutes of Health "Healthy People 2000" guideline of 30 minutes per day, 6 days per week of light to moderate exercise is used as a criterion, more than three-fourths of middle-aged women get insufficient exercise and are at risk of osteoporosis and fractures. Increasing exercise as a means of reducing the risk of osteoporosis is discussed in more detail later in this chapter.

TOBACCO USE Smoking is particularly a factor in older women. In English women of at least age 85, 19% of smokers and 12% of nonsmokers have sustained a hip fracture. Adjustments for confounding factors, such as thinness and lack of exercise, suggest an independent effect of smoking.

ALCOHOLISM Alcohol excess increases the chance of falls and other injuries leading to fractures. The effect of alcohol on BD is not well understood. It does suppress bone formation, and alcoholic men have been found to have markedly decreased BD, but a number of confounding factors (smoking, exercise, liver disease, hypogonadism, malabsorption) may be the primary cause. Moderate intakes of alcohol have been found to be associated with a modest increase in BD, so to protect against osteoporosis one should counsel against excessive intake rather than discouraging all intake.

BONE-THINNING DRUGS Corticosteroids, anticonvulsants, heparin, methotrexate, depo-medroxyprogesterone acetate, and excessive doses of L-thyroxin have all been associated with decreased BD. Thiazide use, on the other hand, has been protective of BD in most studies because it reduces urinary excretion of calcium.

CHRONIC DISEASES Renal or hepatic failure, hyperthyroidism, hyperparathyroidism, rheumatoid arthritis, Cushing syndrome, and gastrointestinal malabsorption are the most common chronic diseases associated with osteoporosis. Those with type 1 diabetes have more porous bones than controls, perhaps owing to microvascular effects. Those with type 2 diabetes do not appear to be at increased risk and, probably because of obesity, actually have a decreased risk of osteoporosis.

FALLS While they are not directly related to osteoporosis, falls do commonly cause fractures in people with osteoporosis. Disturbances of vision, balance, coordination, cognition, or strength all contribute to falls.

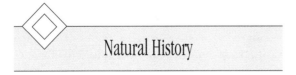

Natural History

The most common manifestations of osteoporosis are fractures of the proximal femur, vertebral crush fractures, and distal radius fractures. Other common fractures caused by osteoporosis include metatarsal, proximal humerus, rib, toe, proximal tibia, patella, and pelvic fractures. Death from osteoporosis is often considered to be associated with fractures, but reduced BD is a marker for increased risk of death independent of the occurrence of fractures. For each SD decrease in BD, the risk of death increases by 20% among elderly women followed for 3 years.

Morbidity and Mortality of Hip Fractures

Hip fracture is the fourth most common reason for hospital admission in geriatric patients, after heart disease, pneumonia, and osteoarthritis. There is an excess risk of death after hip fracture of 10 to 20%, mostly in the first 6 months after fracture. The mortality is higher in men than in women and increases with age. The 1-year mortality rate after hip fracture is about 20% at age 65, but it increases to 50% by age 90. While some of the deaths are related to the trauma that produced the fracture or to the treatment of the fracture, the majority of deaths are related to the underlying frailty of the patient. Patients who survive the fracture often have a decreased level of independence. Among patients who were ambulating without assistance before fracturing their hips, about one-half lose that independence, and about one-quarter require long-term institutional care.

Hip fracture is one of the most common reasons for loss of independence, comparable to stroke. Ferrucci and colleagues (1997) reported on hospitalizations related to new onset of severe disability, defined as needing help with three or more of the six basic activities of daily living (ADL). For patients who went from being independent in all ADLs to being severely disabled, hip fractures had occurred in 11.1%, second only to stroke (16.4%) as a cause of disability. Of those already needing help in one or two ADLs who then became severely disabled, hip fracture was the most commonly associated condition (8%), with stroke second (5.8%).

Morbidity and Mortality of Vertebral Fractures

Most vertebral crush fractures have subclinical symptoms; only about 35% of fractures seen in radiographic surveys had previously come to the patient's attention. Of those that manifest in clinical symptoms, the average length of symptoms, primarily back pain, is 10 days, but it is not uncommon for patients to experience discomfort for weeks to months. About one in five such clinically apparent fractures results in hospitalization. There is about a 20% increase in mortality risk during the 5 years after a clinical vertebral crush fracture, but unlike the situation for hip fractures, the increased death rate is distributed rather evenly throughout that 5-year period.

Morbidity and Mortality of Colles Fractures

Fracture of the distal radius (Colles fracture) is a marker of increased risk for other fractures, but it is not associated with an increased risk of death. Some disability in use of the affected arm is commonly seen 6 months after the fracture.

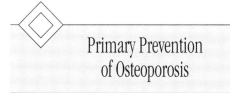

Primary Prevention of Osteoporosis

BD is highest in the second and third decades of life. Primary prevention of osteoporosis involves maximizing the peak BD and minimizing its decline with aging. Prevention of osteoporosis should be included in health maintenance for patients of all ages. Key aspects of primary pre-

vention include exercise, calcium intake, hormonal replacement therapy, and risk factor modification.

Exercise

Bone, as a metabolically active tissue, responds to demands placed upon it by increasing in density. Weight-bearing exercise has been correlated with enhanced BD in numerous cross-sectional studies looking at groups ranging from athletes to frail nursing home residents, although interventional studies have shown mixed results. Conversely, conditions with unusually low demands on bone, including bed rest, paralysis, and the weightlessness of space travel, are associated with declines in BD.

Lack of weight bearing is a more substantial risk factor than lack of exercise per se. While a person on total bed rest can lose 40% of bone mineral in 1 year, professional athletes have gains of only a few percentage points over average. For an average middle-aged patient, gain in BD from a yearlong program of exercise can be lost during 1 week of bed rest. The gains in BD with exercise are likely greatest in young people and diminish with age. Bone gains from exercise are greatest during the initial months and plateau despite continued exercise.

While exercise is generally held to be beneficial for bone, it has not been found to be sufficient to prevent osteoporosis. In women it appears that hormonal factors are more important determinants of BD than exercise. For example, young women who exercise to the point of becoming amenorrheic or oligomenorrheic have lower BD than their counterparts who maintain regular menstruation. Postmenopausal runners not on hormonal replacement lose bone mass compared with premenopausal women.

The amount of exercise needed to promote BD change is unknown. Just 30 to 60 minutes of weight-bearing exercise three times a week is commonly advised for adults as a minimum for bone health, but this is largely based on cardio-vascular considerations. The type and amount of exercise must be tailored to the patient's condition, but weight bearing is important and balance training may be as well. While swimming is excellent cardiovascular exercise, it does not promote increased skeletal strength. Walking is often suggested as a readily accomplished, acceptable form of exercise for many, but other weight-bearing activities that may have more appeal include dancing, sports, running, weight lifting, and exercise on a variety of in-home machines. Walking with a backpack is sometimes suggested as a way to increase weight bearing, but the possibility of inducing spinal compression fractures must be kept in mind in making this suggestion to the elderly.

Walking for exercise and even time spent standing are associated with a lower risk of hip fracture in the elderly. Such findings could simply reflect exercise as an indicator of overall better health, however. In addition to BD changes, exercise may prevent fractures by improving coordination, thus making falls less likely, or by building muscle strength, which would improve protective actions taken in the event of a fall. Fall prevention could be considered primary prevention of fractures, but because the target group of such efforts is generally the frail elderly, who are already likely to have osteoporosis, such efforts are considered in the category of tertiary prevention.

Risks of an exercise program include injury due to inappropriate exercise or equipment. An occasional excuse to avoid exercise is the concern that calcium losses in sweat will lead to bone loss. The calcium loss through sweat during a 10-km run is about 20 mg, which can be made up by consuming one tablespoon of milk. In conclusion, the benefits of exercise for *BD* are modest but not negligible. Benefits not related to BD make exercise a particularly important aspect of preventive care of the whole patient. The advantage of an exercise intervention program in *fracture prevention* has been difficult to establish, in part because a larger sample size is needed to show a benefit for fractures than is needed for BD benefits but also because the effects are likely modest and compliance is limited. Exercise is thus commonly recommended as a fundamental part of osteoporosis prevention despite the paucity of definitive intervention studies with patient-oriented evidence, and it cannot be relied upon to the exclusion of other preventive efforts for osteoporosis.

Calcium

Calcium, in the form of the phosphate salt, is crucial to the mechanical rigidity of bone. The nutritional requirements for calcium (see Table 18-2) are greatest during childhood, when there is rapid growth, and during the senior years. Calcium absorption is quite efficient in childhood; more than 40% of calcium taken in the form of cow's milk is absorbed (human milk is even better absorbed). Adolescents often are deficient in their intake of calcium-containing foods, however. Teenage girls in the United States are among the worst—only 15% consume the recommended daily allowance. In the senior years low-calcium absorption and low-calcium intake are problems. Inadequate vitamin D (see below), estrogen, and gastric acid and duodenal mucosal atrophy, with a resulting decrease in vitamin D receptors and lactase, combine to limit the absorption of calcium. Nutritional surveys indicate that three-fourths of elderly women consume less than 800 mg of calcium daily.

FOOD SOURCES OF CALCIUM

Even though calcium is found in a variety of foods, adequate intake is difficult to attain if dairy products (or calcium-fortified beverages) are not consumed. For example, almost six half-cup servings of broccoli are needed to provide the same amount of calcium as a glass of milk. For some patients who avoid milk, calcium-forti-

Table 18-2

Recommended Daily Calcium and Vitamin D Intake

GROUP	CALCIUM (MG/DAY)	VITAMIN D (IU/DAY)
1994 National Institutes of Health		
Children		
1–5 yr	800	
6–10 yr	1000	
11–adult	1500	
Women		
Pregnant or nursing	1500	
25–50 yr	1000	
50–65 yr		
On estrogen	1000	
Not on estrogen	1500	
Older than 65 yr	1500	
Men		
25–65 yr	1000	
Over 65 yr	1500	
1997 National Academy of Sciences		
Age		
1–3	500	200
4–8	800	200
9–18	1300	200
19–50	1000	200
51–70	1200	400
Over 70	1200	600

fied fruit drinks are a good substitute, providing more bioavailable calcium than an equal volume of milk. Powdered milk can also be added to foods, such as hot cereal or mashed potatoes, as long as lactose intolerance is not the cause of milk avoidance.

Many adults, especially African-Americans, report an intolerance of lactose, the principal sugar of dairy products. They experience gaseousness or diarrhea within hours of consumption. Most such persons can tolerate small, more frequent servings to provide adequate calcium. Yogurt, which contains lactase enzyme to process the lactose, and aged cheeses like Swiss and cheddar, which are low in lactose, are often tolerated. Yogurt has 300 to 400 mg calcium per cup, depending on fruit and milk solid content, and cheeses have about 150 mg per ounce.

CALCIUM SUPPLEMENTS

Food sources of calcium are often preferred, but supplemental sources are sometimes needed to achieve adequate intakes. Calcium carbonate, which is 40% calcium by weight, is an inexpensive, common supplement. For patients with achlorhydria or intolerance of calcium carbonate (because of bloating, constipation, or flatulence), other salts, such as citrate or gluconate, can be used. The amount of calcium given at one time should not exceed 500 mg, since any excess is not well absorbed. Calcium is best absorbed without competing foodstuffs in the intestine, but the carbonate salt depends on adequate gastric acidity for absorption. For this reason, it is preferable to give patients with hypochlorhydria calcium carbonate with food. Contrary to common opinion, the majority of elderly people have adequate gastric acidity, even without the stimulation of food.

Intakes of calcium within the stated guidelines appear to be quite safe. Milk-alkali syndrome, from the combination of calcium and antacids, is associated with a considerably higher intake—more than 4 g per day of calcium. Even among patients with a history of calcium-containing renal stones, supplementation appears to be safe; checking the urinary calcium levels of such individuals while they are on supplements may be a sensible precaution.

EVIDENCE THAT CALCIUM SUPPLEMENTATION PREVENTS OSTEOPOROSIS-RELATED FRACTURES

Studies of calcium supplementation for the primary prevention of fractures have shown positive results in both average- and high-risk groups. Dawson-Hughes and associates (1997) reported a 3-year, double-blind, randomized, controlled trial of 500 mg supplemental calcium (as the citrate maleate salt) and 563 to 768 IU vitamin D in 389 persons more than 65 years old, with a mean age of 71. All of the subjects were healthy, ambulatory, and lived at home. The subjects' baseline calcium intake was low, about 700 mg, so the supplementation could be considered medically indicated. The rate of nonvertebral fractures was 5.9% in the group receiving calcium and vitamin D and 12.9% in the control group ($P = 0.02$). The number needed to treat (NNT) to prevent one fracture over a 3-year period is 14. It is worth noting that the BD changes observed during the trial were quite modest, emphasizing the importance of studying clinically significant endpoints. Rates of falling were not different between the two groups.

Chapuy and co-workers (1994) studied a more frail population, also in a randomized controlled trial. Subjects were 3270 ambulatory women with a mean age of 84 who were residing in nursing homes or housing complexes for the elderly. They had a mean baseline calcium intake of 510 mg, and active treatment was 1200 mg calcium and 800 IU vitamin D. The study lasted 3 years. Nonvertebral fractures occurred in 21.7% of the actively treated group and 27.3% of the controls. The NNT to prevent one fracture over a 3-year period is 18. Looking specifically at hip fractures, 15.8% of the controls and 11.6% of those on supplements had hip fractures (NNT = 24). Similarly to the other study cited, the changes reported in BD were not as significant as changes in fracture rates.

Vitamin D

Vitamin D plays an important role in absorption of calcium from the intestine. It also promotes osteoclast formation in bone. Production of the active form—1,25-dihydroxyvitamin D—is initiated from the action of sunlight on precursors in the skin, followed by two hydroxylation steps in the liver and kidney. This sequence is important clinically because the homebound, with limited sun exposure, and persons with diminished renal or hepatic function, such as is the case for many elderly, are often deficient in vitamin D. Even younger patients who get outside are sometimes lacking; among inpatients with no risk factors for vitamin D deficiency, 14% were found to be severely deficient in a study from Boston. The amount of sun exposure needed to produce adequate vitamin D varies considerably with latitude, season, skin pigmentation, and use of sunscreens. For example, in the northern United States (above 42 degrees, which includes Boston) the angle of sunlight during winter is such that no significant vitamin D production takes place in the skin from November through February.

The daily recommended intake of vitamin D is shown in Table 18-2. There are few natural sources of vitamin D (egg yolks, liver, cod liver oil, fatty fish), but fortified milk, with 400 IU/quart, is a common dietary source. Vitamin D status can be assessed by blood tests, usually by measuring serum 25-hydroxyvitamin D. Considering its low toxicity in recommended amounts and the need for ongoing surveillance if serum tests are used, most clinicians orally supplement those at risk whose dietary intake may be inadequate. Multiple vitamin preparations commonly contain 400 IU and are a readily available source of supplementation. The elderly and homebound should take 600 to 800 IU daily through a combination of dietary and supplemental sources.

Vitamin D alone does not appear to provide adequate fracture protection in the context of modest calcium intake. Lips et al. (1996) reported the results of a randomized, controlled trial of vitamin D, 400 IU, in 2578 persons with a mean age of 80. Most subjects were healthy and required no assistance to walk. Their mean daily calcium intake from dairy products was estimated at 868 mg. After 3.5 years of follow-up there was no difference in fracture rates.

Estrogen Replacement

Women experience osteoporosis more often than men for two main reasons: peak BD, which occurs in the twenties and thirties, is lower for women, and the rate of bone loss after the peak is particularly rapid for 5 to 10 years after menopause. Estrogen blocks the resorptive activity of osteoclasts through a complex series of events not fully understood. Without adequate estrogen, bone resorption outpaces formation, and BD declines. Natural and surgical menopause are the most common estrogen-deficient states, and extremes of exercise, stress, or weight loss sufficient to induce amenorrhea are also associated with bone thinning. Estrogen replacement is also effective for preservation of bone mass in postmenopausal women treated with corticosteroids as well as for premenopausal women who experience menstrual irregularities on corticosteroid therapy. Gonadal hormone replacement in women is called "hormonal replacement therapy" (HRT) when both estrogen and progesterone are given, and "estrogen replacement therapy" when just estrogen is given. For simplicity, the term HRT will be used throughout this chapter with the understanding that progesterone may or may not be included, as medically indicated.

EVIDENCE THAT ESTROGEN PREVENTS OSTEOPOROSIS AND OSTEOPOROSIS-RELATED FRACTURES

Cauley and colleagues (1995) reported the results of a cohort study of almost 10,000 women with an average age of 71 years. Among those who were current but short-term users of HRT (mean use, 3.5 years—starting, on average, in their late sixties), the risk of nonspinal fractures, compared with the risk in those who never used HRT, was 0.67 [95% confidence interval (95% CI), 0.49 to 0.92]. In contrast, for current long-term users (average use for 19.6 years), the relative risk was 0.60 (95% CI, 0.45 to 0.83). Women who were former users of HRT (for a mean of 14.6 years) did not have a demonstrable benefit compared with those who had never used HRT. The same data set can be analyzed in a different fashion, with less support for initiating HRT in the elderly. When the subgroup of current users of HRT who started more than 5 years after menopause was analyzed, benefit fell just short of statistical significance (relative risk, 0.75; 95% CI, 0.55 to 1.02).

In the randomized, controlled Postmenopausal Estrogen Progestin Intervention (PEPI) trial, 875 women aged 45 to 64 years received either placebo or a variety of HRT regimens for 3 years. Those who were aged 55 to 64 at entry gained 7.9% in spinal BD and 4.2% in hip density, while those aged 45 to 54 at entry gained

7.9 and 5.0%, respectively, (P <0.001 in all cases compared with placebo). In a cross-sectional study in a southern California retirement community (Schneider et al., 1997), which included women older than those in the PEPI study, current HRT users who started after age 65 (at a mean age of 68.8) had significantly increased BD compared with those who had never used HRT.

TIMING OF INITIATION, DURATION, AND DOSAGE

Estrogens are most beneficial to bone when taken at the beginning of deficiency, but they are also somewhat helpful when taken later. Some would argue that postponing HRT until age 70 is cost-effective, since the benefits to BD may be almost as great and the NNT less when women at greater risk are treated. This point of view is not well accepted, however, and most clinicians prefer to initiate estrogen soon after menopause, to accrue other benefits and to preserve BD. It is unlikely that density regained from therapy confers the same structural strength as density maintained by prevention. BD benefits are lost within a few years of stopping estrogen, so it is appropriate for fracture prevention to continue estrogen therapy indefinitely, as long as contraindications do not intervene.

A dosage of 0.625 mg of conjugated equine estrogens daily (or the equivalent of other products) is often recommended as the minimum necessary for BD maintenance. This dosage has been found to have a 96% response rate (proportion of women who do not lose bone mass), making it unnecessary to follow serial BD or resorption markers. In one randomized trial (Genant et al., 1997), a 0.3 mg dosage given daily with 1000 mg of calcium was effective in maintaining BD when compared with placebo, although the results were better for higher dosages. Thus, a 0.3 mg dosage may be adequate for bone preservation but may not be adequate for restoration of density in advanced

disease. While estrogen is most often given orally, transdermal and vaginal preparations are also effective in maintaining BD.

SIDE EFFECTS

Side effects of estrogen replacement therapy are listed in Table 18-3. The nuisances, often related to the progestational component, are commonly the cause of early cessation of therapy. They require careful explanation and support in the early stages of therapy and sometimes call for a change in the progestational agent or a reduction in dosage. Breast cancer risk with HRT is the subject of controversy, but one large meta-analysis found an increased incidence of about 30% after 5 or more years of use of HRT. Mortality rates from breast cancer, however, do not appear to be higher among HRT users. Endometrial cancer is increased eightfold in women on estrogen without progesterone, so it is very important that women who still have their uterus receive progesterone (or undergo periodic endometrial aspirations or transvaginal ultrasonography).

A minimum of 12 days per month of progesterone is advisable, and daily low-dosage therapy is becoming standard. Even when estrogen

Table 18-3

Risks and Side Effects of Estrogen Replacement Therapy

Withdrawal bleeding, bloating, needing to take medication
Endometrial cancer
Breast cancer
Thrombophlebitis and pulmonary embolism
Symptomatic gallstones
Possible increased ischemic heart disease (in women with preexisting coronary artery disease)

is administered with progesterone, the incidence of endometrial cancer may be slightly higher than the rate seen in women not taking estrogen; for this reason, it is important to be alert to that possibility in women who report unusual bleeding patterns. Thromboembolic disease, both pulmonary embolus and deep-vein thrombophlebitis, are increased about two- to threefold among HRT users, but they remain uncommon problems. Nonetheless, HRT is generally contraindicated in persons with a history of thromboembolic disease or who are at high risk for it. Other contraindications include suspected pregnancy, unexplained vaginal bleeding, and breast or endometrial cancer (although in those with a remote history, estrogen is sometimes used).

ADDITIONAL BENEFITS

In addition to the bone benefits described earlier, HRT has other proven and possible benefits, as listed in Table 18-4. Estrogen and coronary heart disease (CHD) are discussed in Chapter 16.

COMPLIANCE

Of women who receive a prescription for HRT, about one-third fail to fill the prescription, and about one-fourth of those who do start the medicine discontinue it within 1 year. Reasons include misunderstanding the personal risk of breast cancer and heart disease, poor awareness of the benefits of HRT, a desire to live as "naturally" as possible, and side effects. Starting HRT should be a decision shared between clinician and patient, with the patient fully informed about the balance of risks and benefits.

ALTERNATIVE HORMONAL APPROACHES

Selective estrogen receptor modulators (SERMs), also called "designer estrogen," offer a pattern of risks and benefits different from that of traditional HRT. Raloxifene is the only SERM that has Food and Drug Administration (FDA) approval for osteoporosis prevention. It appears to impart no increased risk of breast or uterine cancer and, in fact, may offer protection from breast cancer compared with no hormone use.

Table 18-4

Benefits of Hormone Replacement Therapy

ESTABLISHED	POSSIBLE
Reduces osteoporotic fractures	Decreases coronary artery disease events[a]
Improves lipid profile	Increases longevity
Lessens hot flushes	Improves mood
Reverses genitourinary atrophy	Prevents Alzheimer disease
	Prevents colon cancer
	Lessens osteoarthritis
	Improves skin thickness and appearance
	Builds muscle strength

[a] In women with established coronary artery disease, hormone replacement therapy may be harmful in the first year of therapy.

It does, however, have thromboembolic risks similar to HRT and does not help (and may worsen) hot flushes. BD studies show a benefit that is about one-half that of HRT. Raloxifene has positive effects on serum lipids, though less than those of HRT, especially for HDL cholesterol. Effects on cardiovascular disease rates remain to be determined. Raloxifene is therefore potentially useful for women with a history of breast cancer or with strong concerns about breast cancer, but long-term studies are still needed to clarify its role.

Tamoxifen is another SERM and is used in treating breast cancer. While it is not indicated primarily for prevention of osteoporosis, women taking tamoxifen for other reasons do gain BD benefits. Unlike raloxifene, tamoxifen stimulates uterine endometrium, increasing the risk of endometrial cancer.

Phytoestrogens are compounds found in legumes and other plants that have both agonist and antagonist actions on estrogen receptors. Soybeans represent the principal source at present. Their "natural" origin appeals to many patients, but there are conflicting, limited data regarding their efficacy in terms of preserving BD. It is a matter of opinion whether soy powder is more natural than yam extracts or pregnant mare urine, which are sources for commonly prescribed forms of HRT.

Bisphosphonates

The bisphosphonates in clinical use include alendronate, etidronate, and pamidronate, the first two as oral agents and the last as a parenteral agent. Bisphosphonates bind avidly to bone remodeling sites, disrupting osteoclastic resorption activity. In addition, several bisphosphonates negatively affect osteoclast differentiation. Alendronate and other bisphosphonates are chiefly used as tertiary prevention agents and will be discussed in more detail later, but alendronate has also been approved for primary prevention. It is particularly useful for men and

in situations where estrogen is contraindicated or not tolerated. Patients who receive glucocorticoid treatment in dosages as low as 6 mg of prednisone daily, or the equivalent, show rapid bone loss over the first several months; for this reason, they have been the focus of numerous prevention trials. Many of these trials have used etidronate or alendronate, both of which appear to be effective at reducing bone losses. Excessive dosages of some bisphosphonates can slow remodeling to the extent that microfractures are not repaired and osteomalacia ensues. This concern, combined with their long half-life in bone and relative lack of long-term studies, makes bisphosphonates less favored than estrogen for primary prevention of osteoporosis. Osteomalacia has not been seen, however, with the usually recommended dosages of alendronate, and its comparable efficacy to that of estrogen makes it a good second choice for prevention.

For prevention, alendronate is given at a dosage of 5 mg daily. Further information about its administration is given in the section on tertiary prevention. The effect of bisphosphonates diminishes soon after the drug is discontinued. While the chemical has a long half-life in the hydroxyapatite crystal of bone, its effect on osteoclasts depends on fluid rather than crystal concentrations. Thus, to be useful preventive agents, bisphosphonates likely must be given for many years, if not indefinitely, but no long-term studies (comparable to those for HRT) are yet available.

EVIDENCE THAT ALENDRONATE PREVENTS OSTEOPOROSIS

PERIMENOPAUSAL USE Alendronate, in a dosage of 2.5 to 5 mg per day, was found in a randomized trial of 1609 postmenopausal women age 45 to 59 (Hosking et al., 1998) to produce increased BD in both the hip and spine. The gains were most dramatic after 1 year but carried through into the second year of this trial, which is planned to continue for 6 years. The gains seen with the 5 mg dosage were somewhat greater than those of the 2.5 mg dosage, but they were 1 to 2% less than those seen for HRT, a therapy to which some of the patients were randomized. For example, after 2 years, vertebral BD diminished by 1.8% in the placebo group but increased by 2.3% in the 2.5 mg alendronate group and by 3.5% in the 5 mg group. The two HRT groups (given European-type and American HRT) gained 5.1 and 4.0%, respectively. Side effects of alendronate, HRT, and placebo were similar, with the exception of the expected urogenital effects (bleeding) of HRT. The clinically more relevant outcome of fractures was too uncommon an event in this age group to be assessed.

CORTICOSTEROID USE In a randomized controlled trial of 477 men and women, ages 17 to 83, taking glucocorticoids (at least 7.5 mg of prednisone daily) for a variety of reasons, Saag et al. (1998) reported that those on alendronate gained BD, whereas those on placebo lost density over a 48-week follow-up. A 10 mg daily dosage was marginally more effective than 5 mg. Alendronate appeared to be effective in those recently started on glucocorticoids as well as those who had been long-term users. The alendronate group had fewer fractures, but this finding was not statistically significant, and the study was not designed to be large enough to find a difference in fracture rates.

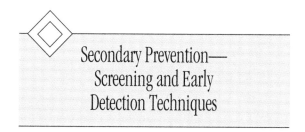

Secondary Prevention— Screening and Early Detection Techniques

A variety of strategies have been proposed and used to identify individuals at risk of fracture before the occurrence of a fracture. Three general categories of such screening tools exist: measurement of BD or other energy-absorption characteristics, measurement of biochemical markers of bone turnover in urine or serum, and assessment by historical risk factors. These three categories are reviewed, and strategies using combinations of the three are described.

Bone Densitometry

INSTRUMENTS AVAILABLE

BD determinations are most commonly made by measuring the absorption of photons or x-rays. Measurement of ultrasound attenuation and the speed of sound in bone is emerging as an alternate technology, which may give information both about the density of bone and its microstructural integrity. A wide variety of techniques and devices are available and are listed in Table 18-5.

Dual-energy x-ray absorptiometry (DXA) is the clinical standard because of its precision, accuracy, moderate cost, and low radiation exposure. DXA is typically applied to the femoral neck and lumbar vertebral bodies and thus measures directly the areas of primary clinical interest. A new application for this technique, called peripheral DXA, uses less expensive and smaller machines but is limited to peripheral sites, such as the hand.

Bone ultrasound is a promising new technology that measures the attenuation of ultrasound waves and the speed of their transmission. No ionizing radiation is involved, and relatively small devices are available, which may be feasible for individual practices. Measurement can be done only peripherally, typically at the heel. This technique can measure qualities of bone in addition to density, which is a potential advantage in fracture prediction. Bauer et al. (1997) reported that the predictive value of ultrasound for hip fracture was comparable to that of DXA among 6189 elderly white community-dwelling women followed for 2 years. The precision of

Table 18-5

Bone Densitometry Technology Available

NAME	TYPICAL SITES	ADVANTAGES/DISADVANTAGES
Dual-energy x-ray absorptiometry (DXA)	Femoral neck, lumbar bodies	Most precise and accurate method available, low radiation dose
Peripheral DXA	Hand, wrist	Less expensive, less precise, limited to peripheral sites
Single-photon absorptiometry	Wrist, heel	Less expensive, less precise, limited to peripheral sites
Dual-photon absorptiometry	Hip, spine, wrist	Not as accurate as DXA, takes more time to perform
Quantitative computed tomography (QCT)	Spine, radius	Higher radiation dose, cannot measure femur
Radiographic absorptiometry	Hand	Uses standard x-ray equipment, less accuracy
Bone ultrasound	Heel	Limited to peripheral sites, accuracy not determined

ultrasound was less than that of DXA, which is a disadvantage, particularly if serial measurements are contemplated.

SENSITIVITY, SPECIFICITY, AND PREDICTIVE VALUES OF BONE DENSITOMETRY

Like any laboratory test, bone densitometry has limitations as a predictor of who will sustain fractures. BD measurements are limited by variations among machines and manufacturers, patient positioning variability, artifactual structures (nearby osteophytes or vascular calcification), and differing predictive abilities depending on the site measured and the site of fracture predicted. Even with the most precise technique, DXA studies done a few minutes apart in the same patients not infrequently show 3% to 6% differences, an amount comparable to natural losses over many years or therapeutic gains of 2 to 3 years. Even if BD could be perfectly assessed, it is but one of many factors that are involved in fracture risk. Other considerations are listed in Table 18-6. Despite the limitations, BD measurement, particularly of hip and spine, is better than any other method at predicting who will sustain an osteoporotic fracture.

FOR THE ELDERLY The predictive ability of bone densitometry at age 70 is superior to that of blood pressure for stroke or serum cholesterol for cardiovascular disease. BD correlates best with fracture risk where the site of measurement is the same as the site of fracture, for example, hip fractures are best predicted by measurements at the hip. But there is also a significant correlation of BD at one site and fracture at another site. Considering multiple sites, for each 1 SD decrease in BD there is approximately a twofold increase in fracture risk; for a measurement of hip density, the risk of hip fracture increases 2.6 times for each SD below average. By comparison, each SD increase in serum cholesterol is associated with an increase of 1.2 to 1.5 times in CHD risk, and each SD increase in diastolic blood pressure increases stroke risk by 1.3 to 2.2 times (depending on the patient's age). Expressed in common clinical terms, for a 70-year old woman at average risk of fracture,

Table 18-6

Limitations of Bone Densitometry in Predicting Fractures

Rapidity of change: A single bone density (BD) determination gives information about a single point in time. Two patients with equal BDs at the same age would have quite different fracture risks if one is losing bone rapidly and the other is losing slowly or not at all.

Bone macrostructure: If two bones have equal density, the one with the largest diameter is least likely to break. Similarly, a patient with a long hip axis (distance from the greater trochanter to the acetabulum) is more prone to fracture than a patient with equal BD but a shorter axis.

Bone microstructure: Trabecular bone is composed of interlocking plates and bridges. If connections between these structures are lost, the bone is weakened. Simply making the structures larger, while increasing BD, does not make bone stronger if the structures do not reconnect. Similarly, microfractures of the delicate bridges may not affect the density but can lessen strength.

Protective factors: Soft tissues absorb impact in a fall and lessen the force on bone. Both natural padding (adipose and muscle) and artificial pads have been found to lower fracture rates. Similarly, improvements in muscle strength and coordination can lessen the likelihood of trauma leading to fracture.

Falls commonly precede fractures. Debilitating disease or medications that affect alertness can affect fracture risk independently of bone density. Similarly, risk-taking behaviors (wearing high-heeled or otherwise unstable shoes, refusing to use indicated ambulation assists, crawling over bed rails) increase fracture likelihood.

BD determination that she is 1 SD below the mean for her age (Z-score of −1, see later discussion on BD interpretation) has a sensitivity of 37%, a specificity of 88%, and a positive predictive value of 36% for hip fracture at some time in the future.

FOR THE PERIMENOPAUSAL YEARS The use of BD measurements for perimenopausal women has not been as thoroughly studied—prospective studies of a risk occurring several decades after a measurement are obviously very difficult. One would expect that the relationship of BD to risk of fracture is attenuated by a longer time interval until fracture. Assuming a 2.0 relative risk of hip fracture per 1 SD decrease in BD for femoral neck measurements in a 50-year old woman, Cummings and Black (1995) calculated that such women in the 10th percentile of BD would have a 21% lifetime risk of sustaining a hip fracture. Women of average density have a 14% risk, and those in the 90th percentile have a 9% risk. Con-

sidering the relatively small difference in risk between the two extremes, BD determinations are not recommended as part of routine perimenopausal care but can occasionally be useful (see later discussion on clinical utility).

Interpretation of Bone Density Measurements

Bone densitometry results are usually reported as both an absolute number (grams per square centimeter) and on two standardized scales that compare the individual to persons of the same age (the Z-score) and to young (25- to 30-year old) individuals (the T-score). Both the Z- and T-scores are expressed as the number of SDs above or below the mean. For example, a T-score of −1 means that the individual has a BD that is one SD below the mean for young people (corresponding to the WHO cutoff point for osteopenia). A Z-score of −1 indicates a BD 1

SD below the mean for individuals the same age as the person tested and generally means a lower absolute density than the same T-score value.

BD can be measured at many sites, but it is often determined at either the hip or the vertebral body. In older women, using the latter site creates difficulties because osteophytes and vascular calcification can artifactually raise the reported value. In fact, in one longitudinal study of BD in elderly women (mean age, 77 years), spine density actually increased during the 1-year follow-up, likely because of such artifacts. Thus, the hip is the preferred site of measurement, as long as there is no orthopedic appliance present. The spine, however, does show change most rapidly, and, for this reason, it is the preferred site if the goal of densitometry is to follow time trends. Machines of different manufacturers use different standards, and so caution must be used in comparing absolute numbers from two tests in the same individual. WHO criteria are often used to summarize BD measurements. The clinician receives reports citing "moderate osteopenia" or "osteoporosis" as the summary evaluation. Such phrases are of limited utility, especially with reference to the elderly. Since the WHO criteria are set with regard to young persons, the majority of elderly patients show "abnormal" results.

Clinicians unfamiliar with densitometry often ask whether they should pay more attention to the T-score or the Z-score. The answer depends on the question asked at the time the test is ordered. The T-score gives an idea of the nature of the patient's skeleton compared with those of young healthy people. Just as fracture risk increases with age, T-scores decrease with age (in almost everyone), reflecting the advancement of bony fragility. If you want to know how your patient is faring compared with younger people, use the T-score to give that information. The Z-score assesses the patient compared with others of the same age. All 80-year olds have a high risk of fracture, but some have preserved their BD better than others. If you want to assess whether your patient is at higher or lower risk than someone of comparable age, the Z-score will help. This author uses the T-score to be honest about the risk and the Z-score as a "pat on the back" for someone who is looking for reassurance that their efforts toward good health are paying off. The Z-score is also quite helpful in subdividing the elderly into those at unusual risk and those with lesser risk (see later discussion on clinical utility of densitometry).

Alternative Risk-assessment Tools

BONE MARKERS

Biochemical tests of bone resorption (e.g., pyridinolines and N and C telopeptides) and bone formation (e.g., bone-specific alkaline phosphatase, osteocalcin) are often employed in research studies to measure bone turnover and the effects of treatments in groups of people. They indicate changes sooner than BD changes can be seen and may predict future rates of change. Diurnal and laboratory variability limits the usefulness of such markers in individual patients. Significant correlation coefficients of marker values and BD changes are often reported and reflect a biologic relationship of the markers to bone physiology. However, test sensitivity, specificity, and, particularly, positive predictive value and likelihood ratios do not reach clinically useful values. In unusual situations these tests may be useful. For example, if a patient does not appear to be responding to an antiresorptive agent, a high level of resorption marker would corroborate the impression of treatment failure, a low level would indicate that the medication was active, and an intermediate value would not be helpful because of variability.

RISK FACTOR ASSESSMENTS

Assessments of risk factors for falls or for osteoporosis can be particularly useful to indicate areas for intervention, such as medication withdrawal or exercise programs. Risk factors alone have limited sensitivity and specificity for fracture prediction. They can be used to designate individuals likely to benefit from BD determination and, when combined with densitometry results, indicate populations at unusual risk. In the frail elderly, BD can help identify those at unusual risk of fracture to target aggressively with preventive efforts.

In a prospective study, Cummings and colleagues (1995) showed the potential utility of BD measurements in frail women about age 70 years (Figure 18-2). Subjects were divided by terciles of BD (the axis of the figure that runs up and toward the left) and into three risk groups (the axis that runs up and toward the right). The highest-risk group had five or more of the 15 factors listed in Figure 18-2 and included about 15% of the population. Each patient fits into one of the nine "boxes," or subgroups, depending on her BD and risk characteristics. Hip fracture rates were measured prospectively for each of the nine subgroups and are represented by the height of the rectangular columns. In the low- and medium-risk subgroups, fracture rates did not vary much among the terciles of BD. In other words, measuring BD in those women would not have contributed much information.

In the high-risk subgroups (at least five factors), however, there was a threefold difference

Figure 18-2

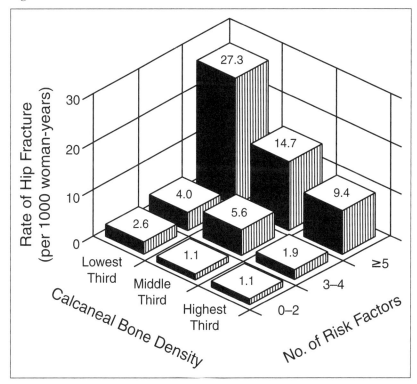

Hip fracture risk in women according to number of risk factors and bone density. (Reproduced with permission from Cummings SR, Nevitt MC, Browner WS et al: Risk factors for hip fracture in white women. *N Engl J Med* 332:767, 1995. Copyright © 1995, Massachusetts Medical Society. All rights reserved.)

in observed hip fracture rates between the lowest and highest tercile of BD, and those rates were higher than the rates of any of the other subgroups. One could conclude that all individuals in the high-risk subgroups should be subject to some intervention; however, those in the lowest tercile of BD (corresponding to a Z-score below −0.43) had a hip fracture rate of nearly 3% per year, and so they would likely gain the most from intervention.

Screening Recommendations

In spite of the widespread use and advocacy of osteoporosis screening, there is no evidence that screening and early detection improve outcomes. The treatments available for asymptomatic osteoporosis are the same as those recommended for primary prevention, further raising questions about the wisdom of screening rather than advocating for primary prevention. These reasons, plus the cost of BD testing and workup of positive tests, have led the U.S. Preventive Services Task Force to recommend against routine screening.

Clinical Utility of Bone Densitometry

Even though bone densitometry is not recommended for universal screening, it is unquestionably a useful tool in evaluating osteoporosis. It is important to realize its limitations before ordering the test. Age is an even more important factor in considering the risk of fracture. In groups of people with similar BD measurements, the aged are more likely to sustain fractures, the likely result of many factors, including a propensity to fall, falling to the side, and a diminished ability to remodel fatigue damage.

AID IN DIAGNOSIS

When the patient has evidence of osteoporosis, such as advancing kyphosis or a radiographic report of "demineralization," bone densitometry can help confirm or refute the diagnosis. When the clinician uses the test for this purpose, he or she must keep in mind the large proportion of elderly who have "abnormal" values on bone densitometry (Figure 18-1). Typical findings of osteoporosis in an elderly person do not require bone densitometry for confirmation.

AID IN DECISIONS REGARDING PREVENTION

In the perimenopausal years, HRT decisions usually hinge on heart and breast cancer risks, hot flushes, and personal preferences, but sometimes a tie-breaking factor is needed when the decision is not clear. As mentioned earlier, the risk difference between the 10th and 90th percentiles of perimenopausal density is not large, and one must be careful not to place too much importance on this measurement as a factor arguing for or against HRT. In women who are unable or unwilling to take HRT, but who are potential candidates for aggressive prevention based on family history or other considerations, BD may be of importance in deciding about bone-specific interventions, such as alendronate. In caring for elderly women, it is sometimes important to have an assessment of risk. A scoring tool based on Figure 18-2 can be used to guide decisions about obtaining BD measurements (Table 18-7). In patients who are not already on bone-sparing drugs, such as HRT or bisphosphonates, and who have scores of 5 or more after interventions to minimize the score, a BD measurement is obtained to help decide whether further intervention is best aimed at BD or at fall risk.

AID IN THERAPY DECISIONS

In general, therapy for osteoporosis is instituted with the confidence that the vast majority of people gradually accrue benefit over the course of several years and BD need not be followed. When using unconventional therapy

Table 18-7

A Hip Fracture Risk-Assessment Tool for Those Aged 65 Years or More

Score one point for each of the following 15 risk factors, if present

    Postmenopausal woman not on hormone replacement therapy or other clinically hypogonadal state[a]

    No walking for exercise[a]

    Unable to rise from chair without using arms[a]

    Currently uses long-acting benzodiazepines[a]

    Currently uses systemic corticosteroids[a]

    Currently uses anticonvulsants[a]

    Weight less than at age 25 yr (if pregnant at 25 use closest nonpregnant weight)[a]

    On feet ≤4 hr per day[a]

    Age ≥80 yr

    First-degree relative with history of hip fracture

    Height at age 25 yr >5′6″ (ignore this question for men)

    Resting pulse >80 beats per min

    Clinically diagnosed dementia

    Self-rated health fair or worse (scale of excellent, good, fair, poor, very poor)

    Has had a fracture since age 50 yr

Interpretation

    Women with ≥5 risk factors have approximately a 2% per yr risk of hip fracture over the next 3 yr.
      An aggressive approach to osteoporosis is warranted. Bone density determination may further
      stratify risk.

    Men have not been studied in this regard, but men with a high score are expected to be at increased
      risk of hip fracture.

[a] Modify these risk factors if possible and include in score only if not modified.

SOURCE: Modified from Cummings et al., 1995. Original risk factors were modified to make the score easier to administer during a health mainte-nance visit and to reflect other data on risk factors. The original study included only female subjects.

(such as low-dosage estrogen), BD determinations might be helpful. If serial determinations are needed, be aware that the precision of BD testing (1 to 6%) is similar to the average annual changes in BD (1 to 4%, the higher value for the spine for a few years after menopause) without therapy. Therefore, follow-up intervals of less than several years are likely to give specious results. In rapid-loss states (such as that induced by corticosteroids, where losses can be 12% in the first 6 months), however, a shorter follow-up interval may be useful.

AID IN COMPLIANCE

HRT has both poor initial acceptance and limited long-term compliance. Women who have been informed of their BD results are more likely to initiate HRT. It is interesting to note that women found to have normal BD are also more likely to start HRT than are those who do not have the test. The potential for such "false" decision-making could be considered a risk of the test, as could the heightened fear of falling that sometimes results.

ASSESSMENT OF THOSE AT UNUSUAL RISK

Patients with hyperparathyroidism being followed without surgery and patients on long-term corticosteroids are at high risk of osteoporosis. BD is useful if the results can potentially affect therapy. BD is not useful where no decision depends on the result—for example, in a perimenopausal woman who has already made a decision regarding HRT or in a patient who has had an osteoporotic fracture and is being started on therapy that would not be altered by the result.

Follow-up of Positive Screening Test Results

All screening tests are subject to false-positive and false-negative results. For densitometry, the steps to take after a result is obtained include confirming the result if it is from an instrument of low validity and evaluating the patient with low density to see whether a diagnosis other than osteoporosis is appropriate.

CONFIRMATION

BD results are most predictive when the site of interest from the standpoint of fracture prevention is the site measured. Hip fracture is the most important fracture to prevent and thus is often the site of greatest interest. If a peripheral site is chosen for screening for economic reasons or for convenience, a follow-up hip density study may be warranted if the initial results are in the midrange.

WORKUP

The differential diagnoses of osteoporosis are listed in Table 18-8. Many of these conditions can be excluded by history and physical examination. Standard laboratory evaluation of a

Table 18-8
Differential Diagnosis of Osteoporosis

Metastatic lesions
Malabsorption syndrome
Gonadal hormone deficiency
Excesses of cortisol, parathyroid hormone (PTH), or thyroxin
Alcoholism (particularly when osteoporosis occurs unexpectedly, such as in young people or middle-aged men)
Multiple myeloma
Immobilization
Renal or hepatic failure

patient with osteoporosis includes a complete blood count, calcium, phosphate, creatinine, and alkaline phosphatase. Substantial abnormalities in any of these tests should prompt an evaluation for an alternate cause of the bone disease, although alkaline phosphatase can be temporarily elevated in the context of healing osteoporotic fractures. Other tests that may be useful in guiding differential diagnosis in appropriate clinical circumstances include serum protein electrophoresis, 25-hydroxyvitamin D, liver function tests, thyroid-stimulating hormone, testosterone, parathormone, and 24-hour urinary calcium and free cortisol. Once the diagnosis of osteoporosis is confirmed, tertiary prevention should be implemented.

 Tertiary Prevention

Tertiary prevention refers to the preventive treatment of persons who have osteoporosis, including those who have already sustained one or more osteoporotic fractures. Prevention of future fractures begins with the basic elements of primary prevention, including calcium and vitamin D, weight-bearing exercise, and HRT. Additional possibilities include bisphosphonates at higher dosages than used in primary prevention, calcitonin, and aggressive fall/injury prevention, including hip padding. (See Table 18-9 for a summary of commonly used pharmacologic products.) The NNT of preventive efforts among patients who have sustained fractures is lower than for primary prevention, making efforts at tertiary prevention particularly important in population-based programs.

Calcium and Vitamin D

For the patient who has already sustained a fracture, the recommended calcium and vitamin D intake is the same as that for persons following the guidelines for primary prevention (Table 18-2). Such patients frequently are elderly and often institutionalized, particularly those who have sustained a hip fracture. In such patients a higher dose (800 IU) of vitamin D is appropriate. Calcium can be obtained either from diet or by supplementation, but the latter path is often followed to ensure adequate intake of calcium when overall food intake may be reduced. Calcium carbonate depends on gastric acidity for absorption, whereas other forms of calcium do not. The elderly generally have adequate gastric acidity to absorb calcium carbonate, which is the most economical form of calcium.

Calcium is best given in several small doses (less than 500 mg elemental calcium), with food. A common dosage is 500 mg of a chewable form of calcium carbonate (such as TUMS), which provides 200 mg of calcium. Two tablets are taken with each meal, along with a multivitamin pill (with 400 IU vitamin D) twice daily. Changing to one of the noncarbonate forms of calcium supplement may help constipation or gaseousness. Calcium is generally considered a necessary, though not sufficient, element of tertiary prevention. The use of calcium in tertiary prevention is supported by its efficacy in primary prevention; a randomized trial involving inadequate intake of calcium for persons with established osteoporosis would likely be ruled unethical.

Exercise

Exercise recommendations must be governed by considerations of the site of any fracture, its stage of healing, and co-morbid disability. The goal is to exert weight bearing over as much of the skeleton as possible. Bouncing a ball or lifting light weights can be beneficial for arm BD. Walking or more vigorous weight-bearing exercise is appropriate for leg BD in some patients, while for others pushing against the floor while seated in a wheelchair may be all that is practical. Spinal extension exercises to prevent

Table 18-9

Medications for Tertiary Prevention of Osteoporosis

Estrogen	0.3–0.625 mg/d	Take with or without progestins (see text).
Alendronate	10 mg daily	Take on empty stomach; follow with 8 oz of water. Sit upright 30 min.
Calcitonin	200 IU (1 spray) intranasal daily	Alternate nostrils one day to the next.

kyphosis and wedging of the anterior portions of the vertebral bodies have theoretical appeal but little evidence of efficacy. Walking with a backpack may increase the load on the spine and hips and result in BD gains, but that benefit must be weighed against the risk of compressive force causing a fracture in those who are quite frail. If extra weight is to be used, the patient should be particularly warned against sudden compression, such as that accompanying a misstep on an uneven surface. Exercise has benefits for the heart and sense of well-being in addition to bone benefits, but the bone benefits are at most modest. For this reason, exercise regimens should not be emphasized to the exclusion of other therapies. Fall-prevention aspects of exercise are mentioned later.

Hormone Replacement Therapy

Until recently, HRT for women was thought to be effective mainly for the perimenopausal years, and therapy was often stopped at about age 65. Evidence now indicates the importance of continuing therapy indefinitely and also has shown the value in starting therapy even quite late in life. The gains in BD seen when estrogen is started in women with established osteoporosis are similar to the gains seen with alendronate. Unlike the situation with alendronate, randomized, controlled trials of estrogen therapy, with fracture as the outcome, have not been reported among elderly women with osteoporosis. The recommended dosages and the patterns of use, including concomitant administration of progesterone, are similar to the recommendations for younger women. When initiating HRT in women over age 65, however, it is wise to start with lower dosages of estrogen for the first several months, to help the patient adjust to possible breast tenderness or other side effects.

As with calcium or other antiresorptive agents, the increase in BD from estrogen accrues over several years. Thus, the patient who continues to experience fractures during the initial phase of estrogen therapy should not be considered a treatment failure. Raloxifene may be an alternate estrogen for tertiary prevention in the elderly. Clinical trials in progress will answer this question in the near future. In men, testosterone is sometimes employed as a bone-sparing agent in advanced disease. This should be limited to situations where the serum testosterone has been found to be low and benefits appear to outweigh risks. The tertiary benefit of HRT is inferred based on the primary benefits for fractures and evidence of benefit in terms of BD gains in the elderly. Specific studies of fracture prevention among patients with established osteoporosis have not been reported.

Bisphosphonates

Alendronate is the FDA-approved bisphosphonate for the treatment of established osteoporosis. BD gains with alendronate are comparable to those from HRT, and fracture prevention is also of similar magnitude—about 50%. Whereas the fracture benefit from HRT is inferred from descriptive studies, the benefit from alendronate is confirmed by randomized trials. Gains in BD take place gradually over the course of several years of use. Alendronate accumulates in bone with a very long half-life and slow release into serum; there is thus a theoretical point in therapy, perhaps after 10 years, when adequate stores are built up in bone so that additional doses are not needed. At present, though, alendronate therapy is given for an indefinite period of time, pending further studies to clarify long-term risks as well as benefits.

In a randomized, controlled trial of 2027 women aged 55 to 81 years with established osteoporosis (at least one vertebral fracture), followed for 3 years, Black et al. (1996) reported that the rate of clinically apparent new vertebral fractures was 2.3% in the alendronate group and 5.0% in the placebo group (relative risk, 0.45; 95% CI, 0.27 to 0.72). For hip fracture, the corresponding data were 1.1% and 2.2%, with a relative risk of 0.49 (95% CI, 0.23 to 0.99). In this study, the dosage of alendronate used was 5 mg daily for the first 2 years; thereafter it was increased to 10 mg because of data showing greater BD gains at the higher dosages. A subsequently reported subgroup analysis showed that the risk reduction for vertebral fractures was consistent for those over and under 75 years of age and for those above and below the median of the group for BD. The NNT for 3 years to prevent one fracture is 35 for vertebral fracture, 22 for any fracture, and 91 for hip fracture.

In another study (Cummings et al., 1998) of 4432 women with low BD but no preexisting fracture, alendronate reduced clinical fractures by 36% (relative risk, 0.64; 95% CI, 0.50 to 0.82) among those with BD T-scores below −2.5. It did not have a significant effect on fractures among those with more moderate osteopenia (T-score between −1.6 and −2.5). In a post hoc analysis of the same data set, hip fracture risk was decreased by about 50% (95% CI, 0.18 to 0.97) among those with T-scores less than −2.5.

Alendronate can be considered the drug of first choice for men with established osteoporosis and second choice for women. HRT is generally preferred for women because of other benefits and lower cost. Side effects of alendronate in clinical trials have been minimal. Erosive esophagitis has been reported as one adverse effect; for this reason, major clinical trials have excluded patients with peptic disorders. Under those circumstances, there has been no increase in gastrointestinal side effects with alendronate. Osteomalacia has not been found to result from alendronate administration in the recommended dosages, but it remains a possible concern for use longer than current trials (about 5 years). Alendronate is contraindicated in the context of renal insufficiency (glomerular filtration rate of <35 ml/min) and should be avoided in pregnancy.

The FDA-approved dosage for alendronate therapy, 10 mg daily, is double the primary prevention dosage. The added benefit of the greater dosage is small: typical values of lumbar spine density gain after 3 years on 5 mg are 5% and on 10 mg are 7%, and the major study of fracture reduction used a combination of these dosages. For adequate absorption, alendronate should be taken on an empty stomach, and the patient should allow at least 30 minutes to elapse before eating. To avoid esophageal complications, alendronate should be taken with at least 8 ounces of water (not mineral water), and the patient must be instructed to remain upright for the next 30 minutes.

An alternate bisphosphonate, etidronate, is not FDA approved for osteoporosis but is often employed for this condition. It is not as well absorbed as alendronate. Unlike alendronate, continuous (daily) use of etidronate has led to osteomalacia; thus, it is given in a cyclic fashion. The strongest evidence of etidronate's efficacy is BD studies of patients on corticosteroids. The usual dose is 400 mg on an empty stomach (conveniently given at bedtime, since the restrictions on position for alendronate do not apply for etidronate). This dose is given for 2 weeks (14 consecutive days) every 3 months. Calcium particularly interferes with etidronate absorption—supplements and dairy products should be avoided within several hours of each dose.

Among bisphosphonates, alendronate is generally the agent of choice. In patients with esophageal contraindications or in whom the restriction about remaining upright and not eating for 30 minutes after each dose is troublesome, etidronate could be considered an alternate, though off-label, agent. The dosing schedule for etidronate can be confusing to many patients. A once-weekly dose of alendronate is being investigated and may be helpful for those whose lifestyle makes the drug difficult to take otherwise. A third bisphosphonate, pamidronate, has the advantage of administration every third month, but it is given intravenously. It may be particularly useful for patients with difficulties taking other agents, but further study is needed, and severe systemic reactions have occurred.

Calcitonin

Like estrogen and the bisphosphonates, calcitonin is an inhibitor of osteoclasts and thus decreases bone resorption. It is approved for treatment (or tertiary prevention) but not for primary prevention of osteoporosis. Until recently, the use of calcitonin was limited by the need for parenteral administration, but an intranasal form is now available. Both salmon and human calcitonins have been synthesized for pharmacologic use. The salmon form is somewhat more potent than the human type, although it is not clear if this difference is clinically significant.

The strongest peer-reviewed, published evidence of a benefit in preventing fractures derives from a 2-year randomized, controlled trial (Overgaard et al., 1992) of 208 healthy women aged 68 to 72 with osteoporosis (T-scores less than -2). They were randomized to receive placebo or three different doses (50, 100, 200 IU) of intranasal salmon calcitonin daily. Most of the fractures were changes in vertebral height seen on radiography, rather than clinical fractures. Combining such vertebral and other peripheral fractures, the women on calcitonin had about a third as many fractures as those on placebo. The expected dose response was not seen—fracture rates were similar in all three dosage groups, although the 200 IU group was the only group to have a significant increase in BD. A commonly used dosage, and the FDA-approved dosage for osteoporosis treatment, is 200 IU salmon calcitonin taken intranasally each day. This corresponds to one spray from a commercially available product. It is administered in alternate nostrils to minimize nasal irritation, which is a main side effect. Flushing is another side effect of the nasal preparation, though less so than with the parenteral preparation. It does not cause hypocalcemia.

The effects of calcitonin on BD are primarily seen in the first 2 years of therapy. Thereafter BD achieves a plateau. This finding has led some researchers to investigate a variety of cyclical ways of giving calcitonin, such as 2 months of every 3 or 3 months on and 3 months off, to allow bone formation to resume between courses of the drug. It is not yet clear that any of the cyclical regimens is superior to others or to daily use. Calcitonin is not approved for primary prevention of osteoporosis; studies in perimenopausal women have been limited and have sometimes involved subtherapeutic doses but have not been as convincing as those using other agents.

An interesting and sometimes useful additional action of calcitonin is its analgesic effect on bones. This effect appears to be independent of the effect on BD and may be the result of stimulation of endorphin release from the pituitary. In one randomized, controlled trial of calcitonin in acute vertebral compression fracture (Lyritis et al., 1997), one-half of patients receiving placebo remained bedridden at 4 weeks, whereas by 2 weeks all of the calcitonin-treated patients were walking. Less dramatic but nonetheless encouraging results have been reported in other studies.

The effects of calcitonin on BD are not as great as those of estrogen or alendronate. Fracture data, however, may not directly parallel density data. One report, available only as an abstract at this time, showed fracture prevention effects only slightly less strong than those of alendronate, although no direct comparisons are available. Therefore, calcitonin is considered third-line treatment for women, after estrogen and bisphosphonates, and second-line treatment for men. Calcitonin may have a uniquely useful role for the first 4 to 6 weeks after fracture; it may also have economic and clinical advantages if it precludes hospitalization.

Fluoride

Fluoride is unique among the drugs discussed so far: it is a stimulator of osteoblastic activity and thus has the potential to produce greater BD increases than the osteoclast inhibitors. Studies have shown that fluoride-treated patients experience a greater increase in BD, especially of the trabecular bone—trabecular bone density increases up to five times more than with bisphosphonates or estrogen. Unfortunately, the bone of fluoride-treated subjects is more brittle than normal, and the fracture rate can be higher compared with controls. Side effects, including gastritis and lower-extremity periarticular pain, also limit the usefulness of fluoride.

Fluoride is an excellent example of the importance of considering patient-oriented outcomes (fractures) rather than disease-oriented outcomes (BD) in assessing a therapy. Attempts are underway to identify a form of fluoride (slow release, various anions) or a dosage that can impart net beneficial effects. Combinations of fluoride with other agents are also being considered, to advantageously modify the bone remodeling cycle. So far these remain under investigation, and fluoride cannot be recommended outside the setting of clinical inquiry.

Fracture Prevention Through Fall Prevention and Hip Protectors

While much attention in osteoporosis prevention is paid to BD, the ultimate aim is to limit the likelihood of fractures. Preventing falls and minimizing their impact are two important approaches to fracture prevention. Such methods are clearly appropriate primary prevention strategies, but they are included in this section because they usually apply to the elderly population, in whom tertiary prevention is also common.

More than 90% of hip fractures occur during a fall. Annually about 30% of people over age 65 fall at least once, and about 6% of falls result in a fracture. Even noninjurious falls are a strong predictor of nursing home placement. Fall prevention in the elderly includes removing environmental hazards, minimizing medications that affect alertness or balance, encouraging appropriate ambulation and transfer assists, and promoting muscle strength and balance

(Table 18-10). Among predictors of who will fall, two of the stronger factors are agitation and dementia. Compliance with exercise programs and use of walkers and other assist devices is very challenging in these groups. In this situation, minimizing the shock of a fall, either by having more resilient flooring or by padding appropriate body areas, such as the greater trochanter, is sometimes the most reasonable approach. In clinical terms, it is important to pay attention to the person who has fallen even if no injury was sustained; the first fall can be a warning of more falls to come, one of which is likely to cause injury.

Studies of interventions to prevent falls have had mixed and modest results, however. Home-safety modifications have common-sense appeal and are often recommended, but experimental studies show little or no benefit. There is a lack of evidence about which home hazards are most important, and many patients refuse the suggested interventions. It is also unclear which forms of exercise are most beneficial to fracture prevention. While weight-bearing exercise is needed to improve BD, other forms of exercise aimed at improving balance, strength, endurance, protective reactions, or gait might be more important in limiting the effect of falls. Clearly, any exercise recommendation must take into account the physical limitations as well as the preferences of the patient. Some interventions, such as initiating new exercise programs, may cause falls or other injury.

Hip protectors or pads are designed to cover the greater trochanter of the femur, to disperse the impact of a fall to the side. They have shown remarkable success in preventing hip fracture; however, compliance with wearing the pads is difficult to achieve. Some clinicians have suggested football-type pads to accomplish the same end, but these are particularly troublesome to don and take off, making them unsuitable for a population with limited hand strength who need to urinate frequently. Geriatric-oriented hip protectors are available from the following Internet sites: http://www.ozemail.com.au/~hip-

Table 18-10

Fall-prevention Methods

Environmental
  Adequate lighting, particularly in areas traveled at night, such as from bedroom to bathroom,
    and for stairs
  Stairs with a sturdy handrail and nonskid tread.
  Toilet, bathtub, and shower safety: nonskid surface, grab bars
  Carpets with low pile, edges tacked down flat
  Scatter rugs that are skid-proof
  Avoiding clutter in walking areas—loose cords, misplaced toys, etc.
  Shoes with flat heels, nonskid soles, good fit
  Chair with adequate height and arm support
  Avoidance of excessively cool temperatures in home at night
Behavioral
  Ambulation assistance if needed
  Avoidance of bulky packages that obscure vision
  Use of eyeglasses; have them checked
  Taking time in standing up, especially after a big meal, to be sure of balance
Medications associated with increased risk of falls
  Polypharmacy (four or more prescription medicines)
  Sedatives/hypnotics
  Antipsychotics
  Antidepressants (including selective serotonin release inhibitors)
  Agents causing postural hypotension
  Alcohol

saver and http://www.safehip.com/prodinfo. htm.

While fall prevention appeals to common sense as a way to prevent fractures, the evidence is mixed. There is limited compliance with many interventions, and the possible injury-causing role of exercise raises concern for some programs. Limited success has been reported for fall-prevention programs, but none has shown a benefit in terms of fewer fractures. It is likely that successful programs to minimize the number of fractures by preventing falls will need to address several factors, probably some yet to be determined combination of exercise, medication use, and modifications of home hazards. The effects of programs appear to be short-lived, so the intervention needs to be sustainable. In some cases the best method may be aimed at moderating the result of the fall rather than the fall itself.

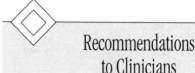

Recommendations to Clinicians

Approach to the Patient

It has long been held that prevention of osteoporosis is superior to treatment, and there is much to be said for that point of view. Surely it is preferable to prevent a first fracture than to act after the fracture has taken place. When preventive efforts are excessively expensive, entail risk, are difficult for patients to comply with, or are of marginal benefit, however, targeting efforts at high-risk groups, such as those with substantial osteopenia, becomes a reasonable option. The benefit of intervention is greatest in those groups at highest risk, such as the frail and elderly.

Efforts at prevention in low-risk groups, including most children and adolescents, premenopausal women, and men younger than 65, should include interventions of low risk, acceptable side effects and cost, and additional benefit to that involving bone. For example, exercise has many benefits besides BD increases and can be widely advocated and tailored to the condition of each patient. Similarly, smoking cessation, alcoholism counseling, and elimination of unnecessary medication have multiple potential benefits. Estrogen replacement therapy also imparts benefit in areas other than bone but at times can cause harm or discomfort.

Recommendations regarding HRT must take into account many factors. Because the effect of estrogens on bone diminishes rapidly upon cessation, and because the likelihood of fracture is low in women in their fifties and sixties, the actual benefit to fracture prevention in those age groups is small. In some patients postponing estrogen until fracture risk has increased with age is a reasonable option. Similarly, calcium supplementation is easily accomplished for some patients but is quite difficult for others. In the latter group, the NNT is smallest where the target group is at highest risk. Finally, such medications as bisphosphonates or calcitonin generally provide no non-bone benefit, entail substantial cost and/or risk, and are best reserved for high-risk situations. Identifying those high-risk situations is an area of great need in osteoporosis research. The current standard, bone densitometry, has limitations of predictive value, cost, and convenience, but it is nonetheless the best available tool. A combination of

risk scoring and targeted BD measurement is the most practical approach.

Table 18-11 gives suggestions for osteoporosis prevention that can be incorporated into routine health-maintenance patterns. Primary prevention advice should be provided to all age groups. A form can be used that addresses each of these areas, with questions specific to each age group. Positive responses by the patient should lead to specific verbal counsel by the clinician, supplemented by printed advice about such subjects as calcium intake and exercise. BD screening should be offered whenever it is important to a clinical decision. The elderly should be screened for modifiable risk and total risk (Table 18-7). Those patients whose risk remains high after addressing the modifiable risks should receive the most intense attention, including consideration of pharmacologic management. Table 18-12 compares the NNTs of common interventions in a variety of populations. Note that the lowest NNTs are found in the highest risk populations.

Unusual Risk Categories

Some patients have specific risk factors for osteoporosis that need special attention and treatment.

LONG-TERM USE OF CORTICOSTEROIDS

Corticosteroid use is a major risk factor for osteoporosis—patients receiving daily dosages as low as 6 mg of prednisone typically experience substantial declines in trabecular (such as vertebral) BD in the first 6 months, which is less severe thereafter. Both inhibition of osteoblasts and stimulation of osteoclasts occur in the context of corticosteroid therapy. Unlike other forms of osteoporosis, men and African-Americans are affected as often as women and Caucasians. Recommendations for those patients taking long-term corticosteroids are listed in Table 18-13.

Table 18-11

Health Maintenance Interventions for Osteoporosis

Primary prevention
  Advice to be included with all health maintenance visits
    Exercise—Weight-bearing exercise, minimum of 30 min three times weekly
    Calcium and vitamin D—see Table 18-2 for specific amounts
    Habits—avoidance of smoking and excessive alcohol
  Advice specific for certain groups
    Adolescent girls: avoidance of amenorrhea, eating disorders
    Perimenopausal and postmenopausal women: discussion of hormonal replacement therapy
    Elderly: Assessment of risk (see Table 18-7), discussion of fall prevention, review of unnecessary
      or potentially harmful medication.
    High-risk patients: HRT is usual first line. If side effects or contraindications, bisphosphonates for
      second line, calcitonin for third line. For men, bisphosphonates for first line, calcitonin for second
      line. Consider testosterone if patient is hypogonadal.
Secondary prevention
  Screening most useful in those not already on osteoclast inhibition therapy (hormonal replacement
    therapy, bisphosphonates, or calcitonin) who, based on risks or findings, would be candidates for
    therapy only if density is found to be low.
Tertiary prevention
  For those with existing fractures, continue primary efforts; also emphasize fall prevention, padding;
    consider bone density augmentation with estrogen, testosterone, bisphosphonates, calcitonin.

AMENORRHEIC ATHLETES

Premenopausal women who exercise to the point of oligomenorrhea (fewer than four periods per year) or amenorrhea rapidly lose BD, presumably because of hypoestrogenemia. Preferred management consists of decreasing exercise to eumenorrheic levels; replacement doses of estrogens (birth control pills or HRT) can be tried. A benefit of pharmacologic treatment in athletes is that the timing of menses can be controlled, but the efficacy of HRT on BD in younger women (including anorexics) is far from firmly established.

IMMOBILIZATION

Patients on bed rest or with other limitations of weight bearing, such as hemiplegic patients or patients who have had polio, need special attention. Particularly at risk are those who are to resume ambulation but will be at risk for falls, such as the hemiplegic patient returning to the community from a rehabilitation setting. Specific areas to emphasize include all of the primary prevention strategies, weight-bearing exercises for the involved skeletal areas if practical, protective padding for the hip where appropriate, and drug therapy aimed at increasing BD. Patients with osteoporosis who sustain fractures should be encouraged to avoid bed rest if at all possible. Calcitonin can be helpful in this context, particularly for patients with spinal compression fractures. The use of pharmacologic agents to stop resorption is controversial in such situations. With long-term immobility or paralysis, osteoclastic and osteoblastic actions reach a new steady state where further loss does not

Table 18-12

Number Needed to Treat (NNT) for Common Interventions[a]

FRACTURE TYPE	INTERVENTION	POPULATION[b]	NNT (3 YR)[c]	REFERENCE[d]
Hip	Hip padding	Nursing home patients (men and women)	7	Lauritzen et al., 1993
	Alendronate	Women with previous vertebral fracture	91	Black DM et al., 1996
Vertebral[e]	Alendronate	Women without previous fracture	100	FIT
	Raloxifene	Women without previous fracture	47	MORE
	Alendronate	Women with previous fracture	14	Black DM et al., 1996
	Calcitonin	Women with previous fracture	13	PROOF
	Raloxifene	Women with previous fracture	11	MORE
All except vertebral	Alendronate	Women with previous fracture	36	Black DM et al., 1996
	Calcium/vitamin D	Healthy men and women, mean age of 71	14	Dawson-Hughes et al., 1997

[a] Comparisons between studies must be viewed with caution because NNTs are quite sensitive to the risk of fracture in the population studied. Calcium and vitamin D were included in both control and medication groups in the studies of other medications, so the NNTs in those cases should be viewed as the marginal benefit in addition to calcium/vitamin D rather than as a direct comparison to the latter.

[b] All enrollees (except in the hip-pad study) had osteoporosis at entry.

[c] The studies cited were of varying length, so NNTs were normalized to 3 yr to permit comparison, assuming the NNT for 3 yr is equal to the NNT for x years times x/3. Most of these interventions have benefits that gradually accrue over 1 to 3 yr, but hip pads provide benefit immediately.

[d] References are to citations in the reference list. FIT, MORE, and PROOF references are to studies that so far have appeared only in meeting abstracts.

[e] The vertebral fractures were radiologically diagnosed and not necessarily clinically evident.

take place after the first few years. In such a situation it is not clear what the effect of reducing osteoclast action may be.

FRAIL FALLERS

Particularly at risk in this group are those with cognitive impairment—the usual safety devices may be ignored by the patient. In addition to environmental interventions to minimize the likelihood of falls (Table 18-10), consider hip protective padding and drug therapy for BD.

Common Errors

INADEQUATE PREPARATION OF THE PATIENT FOR HORMONE REPLACEMENT THERAPY

Long-term adherence to HRT is notoriously low. Factors include breast tenderness, fear of breast cancer, annoyance at spotting and bloating, and the inconvenience of taking medicine. It is important to carefully advise each patient about the reasons HRT is being recommended. A follow-up visit, in person or by phone, 1 to 3 months after starting therapy encourages further

Table 18-13

Recommendations to Minimize the Risk of Osteoporosis in Those Taking Corticosteroids

> Use the lowest effective steroid dose, topically when possible.
>
> Maintain adequate calcium and vitamin D in the diet or with supplements.
>
> Encourage physical activity, but within limits of safety.
>
> Replace gonadal hormones when deficient. Consider measuring the estradiol or testosterone level when there is a question of deficiency.
>
> Alendronate and etidronate each appears to be useful in preventing steroid-associated osteoporosis.

discussion and modification if needed. Progesterone is important for those patients who have a uterus, but earlier ideas that progesterone may also diminish the risk of breast cancer have been discarded. Progesterone need not be given for patients who have had a hysterectomy. Taking continuous low-dose progesterone can minimize withdrawal bleeding. Breast discomfort and bloating can sometimes be helped by changing to an alternate form of progesterone, such as from medroxyprogesterone to micronized progesterone or norethindrone. Less frequent dosing of estrogen can be achieved with transdermal products, although the indications for progesterone remain. Finally, women can be reassured that controlled studies have not shown increased weight gain with HRT.

MISINTERPRETATION OF BONE DENSITY STUDIES

The diagnosis of severe osteopenia has raised considerable concern on the part of some clinicians because of the initial adjective "severe." The concern warranted depends on the age of the patient. While "osteoporosis" refers to a BD

2.5 SDs below the mean for young people, "severe osteopenia" generally indicates a density 2 to 2.5 SD below this mean and so is of less consequence than osteoporosis. BD in the "severe osteopenia" range is a very common finding in the elderly, but it justifies particular consideration if it is diagnosed in persons under 60.

Interference by artifacts can lead to falsely high densitometry values. This is most commonly seen in vertebral studies, where osteophytes and arterial calcification can confound many BD measurement techniques. Orthopedic metallic hardware can also produce misleading values. In patients with spinal degenerative joint disease (DJD), the hip is generally the preferred site to measure density. For those techniques that permit it, viewing the image can help explain some anomalous values, which can then be ignored. Averaging over several sites (such as the first through the fourth lumbar vertebrae or the femoral neck and the greater trochanter) can also minimize the effect of artifacts. If one is using a technique that does not give an image of the site, it is worth considering confirmation of an unexpected result with DXA or quantitative computed tomography (QCT), methods that allow the nature of a potential artifact to be seen.

Variability of BD measurements makes interpretation of serial measurements difficult. A patient scanned by DXA, one of the most precise techniques available, who gets off the table and back on again (for experimental purposes) can often have a reading 1 to 2% different from the original; occasionally, differences up to 6% are seen. Since the losses of BD with aging are usually on the order of 0.5% to 1.0% per year, it can be impossible to distinguish a trend in density from the variability of the technique. A clinician trying to compare results obtained by different centers, with different techniques, or at different body sites is very likely to come to false conclusions. If BD is to be used to follow serial results, the same machine should be used at the same body site. Allow at least a couple of years to elapse between determinations. An exception might be the patient recently started on corticosteroids, in whom trabecular (such as vertebral) density can decline 6 to 12% in a year. In such a circumstance, however, one could question the clinical value of observing the decline rather than preemptively intervening.

OVERDIAGNOSIS OF "TREATMENT FAILURE"

The commonly available treatments for osteoporosis all affect BD by impeding the bone resorption phase of remodeling, but treatment must await the natural bone formation phase to have an effect. An effect on fracture rates is not seen until about 2 years after treatment initiation, although BD increases are apparent by 6 months. In addition, even the most effective agents decrease fracture risk by only about 50%. The patient who sustains a fracture while on therapy is thus not necessarily a "treatment failure," particularly during the first 2 years of therapy. Failure to recognize this fact can lead to unwarranted changes in medication to those with less evidence of benefit or greater risk or to misguided combinations of therapy. Medication side effects, rather than fractures, generally should guide changes in therapy. For the patient who sustains further fractures despite therapy, remember to consider environmental modifications to minimize the risk of fracture.

NEGLECTING TO CONSIDER HORMONE REPLACEMENT THERAPY FOR THE ELDERLY

Until recently, HRT was considered mainly in the context of perimenopausal counseling. Two findings are significant in that regard. First, the effect of HRT on fracture prevention is short-lived, so that HRT is most important during the time of life that most fractures occur, and, second, there is now evidence indicating that initiating HRT in patients over age 65 is effective in reducing fracture risk. Women who are on HRT should continue to use it until complications

dictate other decisions or until life expectancy is 1 to 2 years. HRT is generally the first line of therapy for any hormonally deficient woman at risk of osteoporosis.

OVERRELIANCE ON BONE MARKERS

Bone markers and urine or serum tests of bone remodeling rates are typically used in research to give early indications of the effects of therapy. In such situations, where large groups are being compared, the laboratory and biologic variability of the tests averages out and allows useful interpretations to be made. There is much less utility in terms of individual patients. In studies of the commonly used osteoporosis agents (except calcitonin), resorption markers are suppressed in the vast majority of recipients, which makes checking unnecessary. If medication adherence is in question, most clinicians prefer discussion with the patient to laboratory tests as a way to deal with the issue.

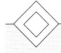

Emerging Trends

Screening

New ways of measuring BD are being developed to make testing less expensive and more readily available. Ultrasound assessments by machines dedicated to bone measurement have the appeal of ease of use and no radiation exposure. Ultrasound has the additional attraction that it may assess bone qualities of importance other than density—such as microstructural integrity. Peripheral measurements by photon techniques also show promise and are widely available. Further study is needed to define the clinical utility of these techniques.

Serum and urine markers of bone remodeling activity have the potential to guide osteoporosis prevention in several ways. A person with high turnover, or with excessive absorption compared with formation, is at higher risk of osteoporosis and could be targeted for specific interventions. The interventions could also be chosen based on the marker results. Finally, the effect of those interventions, in theory, can be followed by serial measurements of the markers. Unfortunately, currently available markers are not sufficiently accurate for such use. Finally, combinations of risk factor assessment, BD/bone quality measurement, and evaluation of bone dynamics through markers hold great promise for cost-effective and reliable guidance to intervention.

Pharmacologic Management

ESTROGENS

Raloxifene, the most recent agent to be approved for prevention of osteoporosis, is likely the first of a series of "designer" estrogens intended to treat osteoporosis. Studies of BD effects with raloxifene have shown positive results, and its role in fractures is promising. The effects on breast cancer and heart disease will need to be evaluated, to clarify the role of this and similar agents. Low-dosage estrogens, taken orally or via vaginal ring, both show promise as agents that may have benefit for bone without the need for progesterone to protect the uterus. Clarification of the cardioprotective effects and breast cancer risks of estrogen through randomized, controlled trials will be of great benefit in choosing among available osteoporosis therapies. The role of nutritional estrogens, such as those found in soy, remains to be clarified and may offer alternatives for patients who prefer to avoid pharmacologic treatment.

BISPHOSPHONATES

Alternate dosing patterns, such as once-weekly alendronate or pamidronate given every 3 months, promise to make these agents more convenient. Long-term follow-up is still needed to assess possible risks in starting these agents in young patients, and the total duration of therapy remains to be clarified. Recent work regarding a possible protective effect of clodronate against implantation of metastases suggests the prospect of added benefits from these agents.

COMBINATION THERAPY

Agents currently available for osteoporosis therapy all work by impeding osteoclasts. It is thus questionable whether combining two such agents will result in any additional benefit over either agent alone. A combination of agents could modify remodeling to such an extent that osteomalacia results. Promising work has been reported regarding the combination of HRT and etidronate, however. An additive effect was seen in this small study, and no osteomalacia was documented after 4 years of combination therapy. Further work is required, however, before combination therapy can be recommended. As already mentioned, it can be difficult to determine which patients have failed standard therapy and would be candidates for the combination, but presumably BD and marker values would prompt such a decision.

OTHER AGENTS

Agents that affect osteoblasts and thereby promote bone formation are needed to complement the osteoclast-affecting agents already available. Fluoride and parathyroid hormone (or synthetic fragments) are two such agents that continue to be studied. The safety and efficacy profiles of neither permit general use yet.

Population Management

A variety of public health campaigns, established by governmental agencies, managed care organizations, or special interest groups inform the public regarding nutrition and exercise, BD screening, and other aspects of bone health. Assessment tools, such as brief questionnaires and densitometers, show the promise of raising awareness of osteoporosis. The impact of such campaigns has yet to be determined. It is important that such initiatives have as their goal the patient's well-being rather than the dissemination of a particular technology or drug.

Bibliography

Bauer DC, Gluer CC, Cauley JA, et al: Broadband ultrasound attenuation predicts fractures strongly and independently of densitometry in older women. *Arch Intern Med* 157:629–634, 1997.

Black DM, Cummings SR, Karpf DB, et al: Randomised trial of effect of alendronate on risk of fracture in women with existing vertebral fractures. *Lancet* 348:1535–1541, 1996.

Browner WS, Seeley DG, Vogt TM, et al: Non-trauma mortality in elderly women with low bone mineral density. *Lancet* 338:355–358, 1991.

Campbell AJ, Robertson MC, Gardner MM, et al: Randomised controlled trial of a general practice programme of home based exercise to prevent falls in elderly women. *BMJ* 315:1065–1069, 1997.

Cauley JA, Seeley DG, Ensrud K, et al: Estrogen replacement therapy and fractures in older women. *Ann Intern Med* 122:9–16, 1995.

Chapuy MC, Arlot ME, Delmas PD, et al: Effect of calcium and cholecalciferol treatment for three years on hip fractures in elderly women. *BMJ* 308:1081–1082, 1994.

Collaborative Group on Hormonal Factors in Breast Cancer: Breast cancer and hormone replacement therapy: Collaborative reanalysis of data from 51 epidemiological studies of 52,705 women with breast cancer and 108,411 women without cancer. *Lancet* 350:1047–1059, 1997.

Cooper C, Melton LJ III: Magnitude and impact of osteoporosis and fractures, in Marcus R, Feldman D, Kelsey J (eds): *Osteoporosis.* San Diego, Academic Press, 1996, p 419.

Cummings SR, Black D: Bone mass measurements and risk of fracture in Caucasian women: A review of findings from prospective studies. *Am J Med* 98(Suppl 2A):24S–28S, 1995.

Cummings SR, Black DM, Thompson DE, et al: Effect of alendronate on risk of fracture in women with low bone density but without vertebral fractures. *JAMA* 280:2077–2082, 1998.

Cummings SR, Nevitt MC, Browner WS, et al: Risk factors for hip fracture in white women. *N Engl J Med* 332:767–773, 1995.

Dawson-Hughes B, Harris SS, Krall EA, et al: Effect of calcium and vitamin D supplementation on bone density in men and women 65 years of age or older. *N Engl J Med* 337:670–676, 1997.

Delmas PD, Bjarnason NH, Mitlak BH, et al: Effects of raloxifene on bone mineral density, serum cholesterol concentrations, and uterine endometrium in postmenopausal women. *N Engl J Med* 337:1641–1647, 1997.

Ferrucci L, Guralnik JM, Pahor M, et al: Hospital diagnoses, Medicare charges, and nursing home admissions in the year when older persons become severely disabled. *JAMA* 277:728–734, 1997.

Feskanich D, Willett WC, Stampfer MJ, et al: Protein consumption and bone fractures in women. *Am J Epidemiol* 143:472–479, 1996.

Genant HK, Lucas J, Weiss S, et al: Low-dose esterified estrogen therapy. *Arch Intern Med* 157:2609–2615, 1997.

Greenspan SL, Maitland LA, Myers ER, et al: Femoral bone loss progresses with age: A longitudinal study in women over age 65. *J Bone Miner Res* 9:1959–1965, 1994.

Hosking D, Chilvers CED, Christiansen C, et al: Prevention of bone loss with alendronate in postmenopausal women under 60 years of age. *N Engl J Med* 338:485–492, 1998.

Hulley S, Grady D, Bush T, et al: Randomized trial of estrogen plus progestin for secondary prevention of coronary heart disease in postmenopausal women. *JAMA* 280:605–613, 1998.

Hurwitz A, Brady DA, Schaal SE, et al: Gastric acidity in older adults. *JAMA* 278:659–662, 1997.

Kanis JA, Melton LJ III, Christiansen C, et al: The diagnosis of osteoporosis. *J Bone Miner Res* 9:1137–1141, 1994.

Lauritzen JB, Petersen MM, Lund B: Effect of external hip protectors on hip fractures. *Lancet* 341:11–13, 1993.

Law MR, Hackshaw AK: A meta-analysis of cigarette smoking, bone mineral density and risk of hip fracture: Recognition of a major effect. *BMJ* 315:841–846, 1997.

Lips P, Graafmans WC, Ooms ME, et al: Vitamin D supplementation and fracture incidence in elderly persons: A randomized, placebo-controlled clinical trial. *Ann Intern Med* 124:400–406, 1996.

Lyritis GP, Paspati I, Karachalios T, et al: Pain relief from nasal salmon calcitonin in osteoporotic vertebral crush fractures. *Acta Orthop Scand* 68(Suppl 275):112–114, 1997.

Maricic M: Early prevention vs late treatment for osteoporosis. *Arch Intern Med* 157:2545–2546, 1997.

Marshall D, Johnell O, Wedel H: Meta-analysis of how well measures of bone mineral density predict occurrence of osteoporotic fractures. *BMJ* 312: 1254–1259, 1996.

Melton LJ III, Therneau TM, Larson DR: Long-term trends in hip fracture prevalence: The influence of hip fracture incidence and survival. *Osteoporos Int* 8:68–74, 1998.

Overgaard K, Hansen MA, Jensen SB, et al: Effect of salcatonin given intranasally on bone mass and fracture rates in established osteoporosis: A dose-response study. *BMJ* 305:556–561, 1992.

PEPI Trial Writing Group: Effects of hormone therapy on bone mineral density. *JAMA* 276:1389–1396, 1996.

Province MA, Hadley EC, Hornbrook MC, et al: The effects of exercise on falls in elderly patients. *JAMA* 273:1341–1347, 1995.

Ray WA, Taylor JA, Meador KG, et al: A randomized trial of a consultation service to reduce falls in nursing homes. *JAMA* 278:557–562, 1997.

Rubin SM, Cummings SR: Results of bone densitometry affect women's decisions about taking measures to prevent fractures. *Ann Intern Med* 116: 990–995, 1992.

Saag KG, Emkey R, Schnitzer TJ, et al: Alendronate for the prevention and treatment of glucocorticoid-induced osteoporosis. *N Engl J Med* 339:292–299, 1998.

Schneider DL, Barrett-Connor EL, Morton DJ: Timing of postmenopausal estrogen for optimal bone mineral density: The Rancho Bernardo study. *JAMA* 277:543–547, 1997.

Seeley DG, Browner WS, Nevitt MC, et al: Which fractures are associated with low appendicular bone mass in elderly women? *Ann Intern Med* 115: 837–842, 1991.

Silverman SL, Greenwald M, Klein RA, et al: Effect of bone density information on decisions about hormone replacement therapy: A randomized trial. *Obstet Gynecol* 89:321–325, 1997.

Thomas MK, Lloyd-Jones DM, Thadhani RI: Hypovitaminosis D in medical inpatients. *N Engl J Med* 338: 777–783, 1998.

Villa ML, Nelson L: Race, ethnicity, and osteoporosis, in Marcus R, Feldman D, Kelsey J (eds): *Osteoporosis*. San Diego, Academic Press, 1996, p 435.

Wagner EH, LaCroix AZ, Grothaus L, et al: Preventing disability and falls in older adults: A population-based randomized trial. *Am J Public Health* 84: 1800–1806, 1994.

Wimalawansa SJ: A four-year randomized controlled trial of hormone replacement and bisphosphonate, alone or in combination, in women with postmenopausal osteoporosis. *Am J Med* 104:219–226, 1998.

Richard Kent Zimmerman
Ellen R. Ahwesh

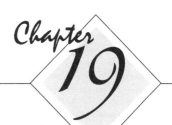

Chapter

19

Adult Vaccinations[1]

<table>
<tr><td>

Introduction

  Why Are Vaccination Rates So Low?

  Chapter Overview

Indications for Vaccination According to Age

  Influenza Vaccine

    Significance

    Recommendations

  Pneumococcal Vaccine

    Significance

    Recommendations

  Tetanus and Diphtheria Toxoids

    Significance

    Recommendations

  Measles, Mumps, and Rubella Vaccines

    Significance

    Recommendations

  Varicella Vaccine

    Significance

    Recommendations

  Age 50 Vaccination Check

Indications for Vaccination: High-Risk Medical Conditions

  Alcoholic Cirrhosis and Chronic Liver Disease

  Asplenia

</td><td>

Chronic Cardiac and Pulmonary Conditions and Diabetes Mellitus

Clotting Factor Deficiency

Immunocompromising Conditions

Renal Disease and Hemodialysis

Vaccination during Pregnancy

  Measles-Mumps-Rubella and Varicella Vaccines

  Yellow Fever Vaccine

  Influenza Vaccine

  Tetanus and Diphtheria Toxoids

Indications for Vaccination According to Occupational Risks

  Matriculation in a Post-High School Educational Program

  Health Care Workers

    Measles-Mumps-Rubella Vaccination

    Influenza Vaccination

    Hepatitis B Virus Vaccination

    Varicella Vaccination

  Public Safety Workers

  Veterinarians and Animal Handlers

    Rabies

    Plague

    Hepatitis A Virus

</td></tr>
</table>

[1] This chapter was adapted from an article, written as a component of the Teaching Immunization in Medical Education (TIME) Project. The TIME Project was supported by funding from the Centers for Disease Control and Prevention, National Immunization Program, through Cooperative Agreement U50/CCU300860-10 to the Association of Teachers of Preventive Medicine (ATPM).

Copyright © 1999 by the Association of Teachers of Preventive Medicine. The use of trade names and commercial sources is for identification purposes only and does not constitute endorsement by the U.S. Department of Health and Human Services, the U.S. Public Health Service, the Centers for Disease Control and Prevention, or the Association of Teachers of Preventive Medicine.

Introduction

Why Are Vaccination Rates So Low?

Adult vaccination saves lives and is cost effective. For example, each year an estimated 8260 adults die unnecessarily of influenza, and 19,200 adults die unnecessarily of pneumococcal infection (Table 19-1). A study of the cost effectiveness of vaccinating against influenza elderly adults who do not live in long-term care facilities found that vaccination resulted in reduced hospitalization for acute and chronic respiratory disease and congestive heart failure (CHF). The direct savings was $117 per person vaccinated per year. For persons 65 years of age and older, cost-effectiveness analyses show that pneumococcal vaccination saves $8.27 per person and adds 1.21 quality-adjusted days of life per person. Hepatitis B vaccination also has been found to be cost effective.

Despite the benefits of vaccination of adults and the availability of usage guidelines, vaccination rates remain low; in 1997 only 66 and 45% of persons 65 years of age or older reported receiving influenza and pneumococcal vaccines, respectively, in the preceding year. Influenza vaccination rates were lower for Hispanics (58%) and African-Americans (50%). Influenza vaccination rates also were lower for adults younger than 65 years of age with high-risk medical conditions and for persons below poverty level.

Why, when so many deaths and hospitalizations can be prevented with full compliance with adult vaccination recommendations, does the rate of vaccination remain so low? The National Vaccine Advisory Committee cited the following reasons for lack of vaccination of adults: (1) limited appreciation of the burden of vaccine-preventable diseases among adults; (2) doubts about the safety and efficacy of adult vaccines; (3) existence of different target groups for different vaccines, necessitating a selective rather than a universal approach; (4) too few

Table 19-1

Estimated Effect of Full Use of Vaccines Currently Recommended for Adults

DISEASE	ESTIMATED ANNUAL NO. OF DEATHS	ESTIMATED VACCINE EFFICACY (%)[a]	CURRENT VACCINE USE (%)[b]	NO. OF ADDITIONAL PREVENTABLE DEATHS PER YEAR
Influenza	20,000[c]	70	41	8260
Pneumococcal infection	40,000	60	20	19,200
Hepatitis B	5,000	90	10	4050
Tetanus-diphtheria	<25	99	40	<15
Measles, mumps, or rubella	<30	95	Variable	<30

[a] Indicates efficacy in immunocompetent adults. Among elderly and immunocompromised patients, estimated efficacy may be lower.
[b] Percentage of targeted groups who have been immunized according to current recommendations.
[c] Variable (range 0 to 40,000).
SOURCE: Adapted from Gardner P, Schaffner W. Immunization of adults. *N Engl J Med* 328:1252–1258, 1993, updated in National Vaccine Advisory Committee: Adult immunization. National Vaccine Program, Department of Health and Human Services, 1994, p 36.

programs, either public or private, to deliver adult vaccines; and (5) issues regarding payment for adult vaccination.

The limited appreciation by patients and clinicians in the Untied States of the burden of diseases preventable with adult vaccination may be caused in part by the greater incidence of and therefore attention to cardiovascular and neoplastic diseases. Even those aware of the burden of vaccine-preventable diseases may not know about recommendations for vaccination of older adolescents and adults, particularly those with certain medical, occupational, or lifestyle risks for vaccine-preventable diseases. Another factor is that many adults are unsure of their vaccination history. Many health care providers were not exposed to paradigms for adult vaccination during their training and thus may not evaluate the vaccination status of adult patients, particularly the status of patients with indications for vaccination based on lifestyle or occupational exposures.

Doubts about the safety and efficacy of adult vaccines cause many adults to be hesitant about

vaccination. Although serious adverse events caused by vaccination are rare, attention in the news media to rare adverse events increases public awareness that these events can occur and may decrease receptivity to vaccination.

Different target groups for different vaccines has necessitated a selective rather than a universal approach to adult vaccination. As a result, clinicians need to consider a variety of indications for vaccination with a variety of vaccines for patients encountered in a range of health care settings.

The shortage of programs to deliver adult vaccines contributes to a low rate of vaccination. For example, unless a hospital has developed a program to evaluate each adult patient's vaccination status at hospital discharge, many discharged patients miss this opportunity for vaccination. Patients of clinics and physician offices without programs for adult vaccination also may miss opportunities for vaccination at visits for acute or chronic health problems. Many medical offices may not stock certain adult vaccines, particularly hepatitis B vaccine, or may experience temporary shortages of influenza vaccine, which may lead to referral to public vaccine clinics. The cumulative effect of the aforementioned factors is that many adults at high risk for vaccine-preventable diseases access medical care, but only a moderate proportion undergo vaccination.

Reimbursement issues and the cost of vaccine affect who receives vaccination. Medicare covers the cost of influenza and pneumococcal vaccines, thus removing financial barriers for elderly persons. Younger adults, however, may not have insurance coverage for the vaccines they need, and some vaccines, such as hepatitis B vaccine, are relatively expensive.

Chapter Overview

Immunizations for infants, children, adolescents, and young adults through 21 years of age are discussed in Chapter 1. Immunizations specific to travelers are discussed in Chapter 20. This chapter reviews current indications and contraindications for common adult vaccinations and diseases, vaccination procedures, and strategies for increasing vaccination rates. The vaccinations discussed are listed in Table 19-2, with indications, contraindications, dosage, route of administration, and booster recommendations. A number of other vaccines are available for use in the care of adults in special circumstances. These are listed in Table 19-3 but are not discussed.

Indications for vaccination of adults are categorized as follows: *age*, recommendations for adults regardless of health status; *health*, recommendations for those with various medical conditions or who are pregnant; *occupation*, recommendations for health care workers, public safety workers, and animal handlers; *lifestyle*, such as recommendations for those at high risk because of sexual activity or use of injected drugs; and *environment*, recommendations for institutionalized adults and household contacts of persons with vaccine-preventable disease.

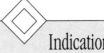

Indications for Vaccination According to Age

The substantial effect of specific vaccine-preventable diseases on mortality and morbidity, particularly among older adults, has led to recommendations for vaccination on the basis of age alone.

Influenza Vaccine

SIGNIFICANCE

Influenza is caused by one of two types of influenza virus (A and B). It is a disease of the respiratory tract characterized by abrupt onset of fever, myalgia, sore throat, and nonproductive cough. Complications include primary influenza pneumonia or secondary bacterial pneumonia. The elderly and persons with chronic health problems are at increased risk for severe disease and complications. Influenza epidemics usually occur between October and March. They increase mortality not only from influenza and pneumonia but also from cardiopulmonary and other chronic diseases.

In each of 11 recent influenza epidemics in the United States, estimated deaths related to this disease totaled more than 20,000. During some epidemics of influenza type A, as many as 172,000 hospitalizations have been attributable solely to influenza and pneumonia. The cost of a severe influenza epidemic has been estimated to be $12 billion.

The elderly, partly because they have a higher incidence of chronic medical conditions, have the highest age-specific case-fatality rate from influenza—more than 90% of deaths due to influenza and pneumonia occur among persons 65 years of age or older. Persons aged 65 years or older also undergo a high proportion of hospitalizations for influenza-like illness

(35% to 46% in recent years), although they make only 9% to 10% of office visits for such an illness. In one study involving elderly parsons, influenza vaccination resulted in a 27% to 39% reduction in hospitalizations (depending on the year studied) for acute or chronic respiratory conditions. In one year there was a 37% reduction in hospitalizations for CHF.

RECOMMENDATIONS

The American Academy of Family Physicians (AAFP) and the Advisory Committee on Immunization Practices (ACIP) recommend that beginning each September when vaccine for the upcoming influenza season becomes available, all persons 50 years of age and older who see a health care provider be offered influenza vaccine so that vaccination opportunities are not missed.

Pneumococcal Vaccine

SIGNIFICANCE

Streptococcus pneumoniae causes an estimated 3000 cases of meningitis, 50,000 cases of bacteremia, 500,000 cases of pneumonia, and 7 million cases of otitis media annually in the United States. Most cases (60% to 87%) of pneumococcal bacteremia among adults are associated with pneumonia, and the rate of bacteremia is highest among persons aged 65 years and older. *S. pneumoniae* causes 25% to 35% of the cases of community-acquired pneumonia that require hospitalization. Despite appropriate therapy, the overall case-fatality rate for pneumococcal bacteremia is 15% to 20% among adults; this climbs to approximately 30% to 40% for elderly patients. Pneumococcal polysaccharide vaccine protects against 85% to 90% of the serotypes that cause invasive pneumococcal infections, including the six serotypes that most frequently cause invasive drug-resistant pneumococcal infection.

RECOMMENDATIONS

All persons 65 years of age and older should receive one dose of pneumococcal vaccine unless they are known to have received vaccination within the past 5 years and were younger than the age of 65 years at vaccination. A prime opportunity for vaccination among this age group is hospital discharge. In one study, 61% to 62% of persons 65 years of age or older who were hospitalized with pneumonia had been discharged from a hospital within the previous 4 years.

Tetanus and Diphtheria Toxoids

Tetanus and diphtheria are discussed in Chapter 1. Both diseases are now rare in the United States.

Routine vaccination of military personnel against tetanus began in 1941, and tetanus and diphtheria toxoids were added to the childhood vaccination schedule in the late 1940s. Hence, elderly persons who did not serve in the U.S. military are unlikely to have been vaccinated during childhood and may be unprotected. Serologic surveys show that more than 48% of those 60 years of age or older have less than protective levels of antibody to tetanus, and 40% lack protective levels of antibody to diphtheria.

SIGNIFICANCE

Most of the 110 persons in the United States who contracted tetanus in 1989 and 1990 were aged 60 years or older. Only 3 (2.7%) were known to have been appropriately immunized.

In former states of the Soviet Union, where diphtheria had been well controlled for the previous 30 years, vaccination levels dropped after independence. This drop in vaccination level is held accountable for the diphtheria epidemics in these states in 1994 and 1995. Given the low levels of vaccination among older persons in the United States, it is possible that an epidemic of

Table 19-2
Common Adult Vaccines

Vaccine	Type	Series	Indications
Hepatitis A virus (HAV)	Inactivated virus	1.0 mL IM 2 doses at 0 and 6–12 months	Men who have sex with men Users of injected drugs Those who work with HAV infected primates or with HAV in a research laboratory Those with chronic liver disease Consider for those with clotting factor disorders
Hepatitis B virus (HBV)	Inactive viral antigen	1.0 mL IM at 0, 1, 6 mo or 2, 4, 6 mo Special instructions for dialysis patients	Men who have sex with men Users of injected drugs Those with multiple sex partners Household and sexual partners of HBV carriers Health care workers Public safety workers with frequent blood exposure Residents and staff of institutions for developmentally disabled Hemodialysis patients Recipients of blood clotting factors Morticians
Influenza	Inactivated virus	0.5 mL IM annually	Persons 50 yr and older Residents of nursing homes and other facilities that house persons with chronic medical conditions Those with chronic pulmonary or cardiovascular diseases, including asthma Those who need regular medical follow-up therapy for chronic metabolic diseases (including diabetes), renal disease, hemoglobinopathy or immunosuppression Children and adolescents (6 mo to 18 yr) who receive ongoing aspirin therapy (because of risk of Reye's syndrome after influenza) Women who will be in their second or third trimester of pregnancy during the influenza season Physicians, nurses, and other health care personnel

Vaccine	Type	Dose/Schedule	Indications
Mumps, measles rubella (MMR)	Live virus	0.5 mL SC Second dose, at least 1 mo after the first, for health care workers and college students	Employees of nursing homes and other long-term care facilities who have contact with residents / Providers of home care to persons at high risk / Household members of persons at high risk / Born in or after 1957 without proof of immunity
Pneumococcal	Bacterial polysaccharides	0.5 mL IM or SC Revaccination for those older than 65 yr, if first dose received more than 5 years previously at age younger than 65 yr Revaccination for immunocompromised persons and those with asplenia 5 or more years after first dose	Persons 65 yr and older / Persons 2 to 64 yr of age with chronic cardiovascular disease, chronic pulmonary disease (but not asthma), diabetes, alcoholism, chronic liver disease, cerebrospinal leaks / Persons 2 to 64 yr of age at high risk because of social or environmental conditions (Alaskan Natives or certain American Indian populations) / Persons 2 to 64 yr of age immunocompromised from disease or medical treatment
Tetanus diptheria (Td)	Inactivated toxoids	0.5 mL IM 3 doses for primary series: 2 doses 4 weeks apart, dose 3 6–12 months after dose 2 Booster every 10 yr	All adults
Varicella	Live virus	0.5 mL SC 2 doses 4 to 8 weeks apart if 13 yr or older	Those without a reliable history of disease or proof of immunity
Meningococcal	Bacterial polysaccharides	0.5 mL SC once	Consider for freshmen college students, especially those living in dormitories

Table 19-3

Immunizations for Special Circumstances

Anthrax
Bacillus of Calmette and Guérin (BCG)
Cholera
Japanese encephalitis
Lyme disease vaccine
Meningococcal
Plague
Rabies
Typhoid
Yellow fever
Haemophilus influenzae type b

diphtheria could spread to the United States from another country.

RECOMMENDATIONS

Adults who have not received a primary series of tetanus and diphtheria toxoid or whose vaccination history is unclear should have three doses of adult tetanus and diphtheria toxoid (Td). (The adult vaccine, Td, has a smaller dose of diphtheria toxoid than the pediatric vaccine, DT, used for vaccination of children younger than 7 years of age, and Td causes fewer side effects among adults.) The first two doses of Td vaccine should be given at least 4 weeks apart and the third dose 6 to 12 months after the second dose. Adults who have completed the primary vaccination series should receive a booster dose of Td vaccine every 10 years according to the ACIP. The American Academy of Family Physicians, the American College of Physicians, and the Infectious Diseases Society of America recommend Td boosters every 10 years or a single booster at 50 years of age. The U.S. Preventive Services Task Force (USPSTF) recommends periodic boosters, allowing intervals of 10 to 30 years.

Measles, Mumps, and Rubella Vaccines

The epidemiologic aspects and characteristics of measles, mumps, and rubella are discussed in Chapter 1. Persons born before 1957 can be considered immune to measles, mumps, and rubella, except for women of childbearing potential, who should be vaccinated unless they have evidence of immunity to rubella.

SIGNIFICANCE

Before introduction of a measles vaccine in 1963, approximately 3 to 4 million cases of measles and 500 deaths attributable to this disease were reported annually in the United States. After the introduction of measles vaccine, the incidence of disease dropped by more than 99%. Despite the effectiveness of measles-mumps-rubella (MMR) vaccine, outbreaks have been reported recently in the United States. A major measles epidemic (55,467 reported cases and 136 deaths) occurred in 1989 to 1991; outbreaks of rubella occurred in Massachusetts in 1993 to 1994 and in Connecticut in 1995. Persons 15 years of age or older accounted for 36% of cases of mumps in 1988 to 1993 and persons 20 years of age or older accounted for 65% of cases rubella reported from 1992 to 1994.

RECOMMENDATIONS

All adults born in 1957 or later should receive one dose of MMR vaccine unless they have documentation of at least one dose of measles-, rubella-, and mumps-containing vaccine on or after their first birthday or documentation of presumptive immunity. Documentation of immunity includes physician diagnosis of measles and mumps, but not rubella; serologic evidence; or documented vaccinations against measles, mumps, and rubella. In general, serologic screening to determine immunity is not recommended, is expensive, and can be a barrier to vaccination. All women of childbearing potential should receive rubella vaccine unless they have received at least one dose of MMR or live rubella vaccine or have serologic documentation of immunity.

Live attenuated Edmonston B measles vaccine and killed (inactivated) measles vaccine (KMV) were licensed in the United States in 1963. Persons who received KMV, which was last used in 1967, may contract an atypical form of measles characterized by fever, pneumonia, pleural effusions, edema, and an atypical rash (including maculopapules, urticaria, petechiae, and purpura). Hence, persons known to have received KMV or those vaccinated between 1963 and 1967 with a vaccine of unknown type should receive two doses of live measles vaccine separated by 1 month. Persons who received measles vaccine not known to be Edmonston B with either immune globulin or measles immune globulin should be considered susceptible to measles and should receive at least one dose of measles vaccine.

Varicella Vaccine

SIGNIFICANCE

Varicella zoster virus (VZV) infection is more likely to cause severe complications, such as pneumonia and secondary bacterial skin infections, among adults than it is among school-aged children. Almost all adults who have a history of varicella have serologic evidence of immunity. Many adults (47% to 93% depending on the study cited) who do not have a reliable history of varicella actually have seroprotection. Results of most studies suggest that most adults (71% to 93%) are protected.

RECOMMENDATIONS

Adults should be evaluated for immunity to varicella. The first thing for the clinician to do is ask whether the patient has had varicella. Those who have a reliable history of varicella are considered immune. Those who do not have a reliable history of varicella are considered susceptible. Serologic testing may be performed as a cost-effective way to determine whether vaccination is indicated. Alternatively, varicella vaccine may be administered to those without a history of varicella. Adults for whom varicella vaccination is indicated should receive two subcutaneous doses of vaccine 4 to 8 weeks apart. Varicella vaccine is recommended for the following groups:

- Susceptible persons who have close contact with persons at high risk for serious complications, such as health care workers and family contacts of immunocompromised persons. For this high-priority group, vaccination is *recommended*.
- Persons who live or work in environments in which transmission of VZV is likely (e.g., teachers of young children, day-care employees, and residents and staff in institutional settings).
- Persons who live or work in environments in which varicella transmission can easily occur (e.g., college students, inmates and staff of correctional institutions, and military personnel).
- All nonpregnant women of childbearing age without a history of varicella or other documentation of immunity should consider vaccination before pregnancy to reduce risk for congenital varicella syndrome. All women of childbearing age should be asked if they are pregnant before they are vaccinated and be advised to avoid pregnancy for 1 month after vaccination against varicella.
- Adolescents and adults living in households with children.
- International travelers. Vaccination should be offered to international travelers who do not have evidence of immunity to VZV (e.g., serologic test results), especially if the traveler

expects to have close personal contact with local populations, because varicella is endemic in most countries.

Data indicate that varicella vaccine is effective in preventing or modifying varicella infection if given within 3 days, and possibly 5 days, of exposure to mild varicella virus.

Age 50 Vaccination Check

The ACIP of the Centers for Disease Control and Prevention (CDC), U.S. Public Health Service, American College of Physicians, and American Academy of Family Physicians recommend that all adults at the age of 50 years receive a dose of Td vaccine if they have not had a booster within the last 10 years and undergone screening for high-risk conditions such as chronic pulmonary or cardiac diseases that indicate the need for administration of pneumococcal vaccines. The AAFP and ACIP recommend annual influenza vaccination beginning at the age of 50 years.

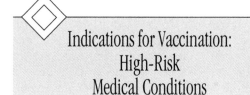

Indications for Vaccination: High-Risk Medical Conditions

There are many indications other than age for considering vaccination of older adolescents and adults against specific vaccine-preventable diseases. For example, persons who have chronic medical conditions such as chronic obstructive pulmonary disease (COPD), cardiovascular disease (CVD), and diabetes mellitus are at increased risk for death of influenza regardless of age. Influenza has a higher case-fatality rate among middle-aged persons with chronic medical conditions than among persons 65 years of age or older who are well (Table 19-4). Table 19-5 summarizes recommendations for vaccination of adults with medical conditions that place them at high risk for morbidity and mortality from vaccine-preventable diseases.

Table 19-4

Pneumonia and Influenza (P&I) Death Rates During an Influenza A Epidemic

AGE (YR) AND HIGH-RISK (HR) CONDITION STATUS[a]	NO. OF P&I DEATHS	NO. IN POPULATION	DEATHS PER 100,000
15–44 Without HR	0	134,000	0
15–44 With one HR	0	6260	0
15–44 With two or more HRs	0	260	0
45–64 Without any HR	1	43,900	2
45–64 With one HR	7	6900	100
45–64 With two or more HRs	4	1060	377
≥65 Without HR	1	11,760	9
≥65 With one HR	14	6460	217
≥65 With two or more HRs	11	1380	797

[a] Examples of high-risk conditions are rheumatic heart disease, ischemic heart disease, asthma, emphysema, nephritis, diabetes mellitus, and malignant tumors.
SOURCE: Modified from Barker WH, Mullooly JP. Pneumonia and influenza death rates during epidemics. *Arch Intern Med* 142:87, 1982. Copyright 1982, American Medical Association.

Table 19-5

Vaccine Recommendations for Adults with Various Medical Conditions

SPECIFIC ILLNESS	VACCINES TO ADMINISTER	SPECIFICS OF ADMINISTRATION
Alcoholism	Pneumococcal, influenza	Recommended
Aspirin therapy, long term	Influenza	Recommended for children and teenagers (6 mo to 18 yr of age)
Asplenia (splenic dysfunction or anatomic asplenia) including sickle cell disease and splenectomy	Hib	Consider even for adults; for elective splenectomy, give at least 2 wk before operation, if possible
	Meningococcal Pneumococcal[a]	Recommended; for elective splenectomy, give at least 2 wk before operation, if possible
Cardiac disease that alters or potentially alters hemodynamics	Influenza, pneumococcal	Recommended
Cerebrospinal fluid leak	Pneumococcal	Recommended
Cirrhosis (alcoholic)	Influenza, pneumococcal, hepatitis A	Recommended
Complement deficiency (terminal component deficiencies)	Meningococcal	Recommended
Diabetes mellitus	Influenza, pneumococcal	Recommended
Factor deficiency (hemophilia) necessitating receipt of a clotting factor concentrate	Hepatitis A	Consider[b]
	Hepatitis B	Recommended[b]
Hemoglobinopathy	Influenza	Recommended
HIV infection and AIDS	IPV (not oral poliovirus vaccine [OPV])	Household contacts also should receive IPV, not OPV, if polio vaccine is indicated
	Hepatitis B	Recommended if HIV acquired from sex between men; check titers[c]
	Hib	Recommended if child, consider if adult
	Influenza, pneumococcal	Recommended
	MMR	Recommended when otherwise indicated for susceptible HIV-infected persons who are not severely immunocompromised. HIV-infected patients with symptoms exposed to measles should receive IG[d]
	VZIG	Postexposure prophylaxis[f]

(Continued)

Table 19-5

Vaccine Recommendations for Adults with Various Medical Conditions *(Continued)*

Specific Illness	Vaccines to Administer	Specifics of Administration
Immunocompromised, severely, non-HIV-infected (congenital immuno-deficiency, leukemia, lymphoma, generalized malignant disease or therapy with alkylating agents, antimetabolites, radiation, or large amounts of corticosteroids)	IPV	OPV contraindicated, IPV if otherwise indicated for those on long-term, high-dose steroids Household contacts should receive IPV, not OPV, if polio vaccine is indicated
	Hepatitis B	Recommended when indicated using 40 μg dose[ce]
	Immunoglobulin	If exposed to measles disease[d]
	Influenza, pneumococcal[a]	Recommended[e]
Immunocompromised after solid organ transplantation, immunosuppressive therapy, or cancer chemotherapy (vaccinate >2 weeks before chemotherapy or immuno-suppressive therapy. If vaccinated during or within 2 weeks before start of immunosuppressive therapy, revaccinate ≥3 months after therapy ends)	IPV	OPV contraindicated; give IPV if indicated Household contacts should also receive IPV, not OPV, if polio vaccine indicated
	Hepatitis B	Recommended when indicated; use 40 μg dose[c]
	Hib	Recommended
	Immunoglobulin	If exposed to measles disease[d]
	Influenza, pneumococcal[a]	Recommended[e]
	VZIG	Postexposure prophylaxis[f]
Liver disease (chronic)	Hepatitis A	Recommended
Metabolic disease (chronic) that increases the likeli-hood that influenza infection will be more severe	Influenza	Recommended
Pregnant women who have medical condition that increases risk for compli-cations from influenza	Influenza	Recommended
Pregnant women in the second or third trimester during the influenza season	Influenza	Recommended

(Continued)

Table 19-5

Vaccine Recommendations for Adults with Various Medical Conditions *(Concluded)*

SPECIFIC ILLNESS	VACCINES TO ADMINISTER	SPECIFICS OF ADMINISTRATION
Pulmonary disease (chronic) including asthma and chronic obstructive pulmonary disease	Influenza, pneumococcal	Recommended
Renal disease (chronic)	Influenza, pneumococcal[a]	Recommended
Renal disease necessitating dialysis or likely to lead to dialysis or transplantation	Hepatitis B	Recommended; use 40 μg dose[c]
Varicella exposure to susceptible, immunocompetent adult	VZIG	Consider postexposure prophylaxis[f]
Varicella exposure in pregnancy	VZIG	Postexposure prophylaxis;[f] unknown if will protect fetus

[a] Pneumococcal revaccination should be considered 5 or more years after immunization if asplenia, chronic renal failure, or organ transplant occurred.

[b] Use fine needle (23-gauge or finer) and firm pressure at injection site for >2 minutes.

[c] Immunocompromised persons should received 40 μg doses of hepatitis B vaccine (special formulation of Recombivax HB7, or Engerix-B7). If Engerix-B7 is used, a 4-dose schedule is indicated. Check titers every 12 months and reimmunize if needed.

[d] Live viral vaccines are contraindicated in severely immunocompromised persons. Severely immunocompromised persons should receive IG if exposed to measles, even if they have been immunized with MMR.

[e] Vaccination ideally should occur >2 weeks before chemotherapy or immunosuppressive therapy. If vaccinated during or within 2 weeks before the start of immunosuppressive therapy, revaccinate ≥3 months after therapy ends.

[f] Before administering VZIG, determine whether (1) the patient was exposed *and* if (2) the patient is susceptible (no history of varicella and negative antibody test, if performed). Exposure includes household contact, more than 1 hour of indoor contact, prolonged direct face-to-face contact, or sharing same hospital room. Susceptibility is uncommon, only 5 to 15% of adults do not have immunity to varicella. Antibody testing may be helpful in determining susceptibility of immunocompetent persons without a history of varicella. VZIG is expensive, and supplies are limited.

ABBREVIATIONS: Hib, *Haemophilus influenzae* type b conjugated vaccine; IG, immune globulin; IPV, inactivated poliovirus vaccine; OPV, oral poliovirus vaccine; MMR, measles, mumps, rubella vaccine; VZIG, varicella zoster immune globulin.

Alcoholic Cirrhosis and Chronic Liver Disease

Alcoholism and, to a lesser degree, cirrhosis are predisposing factors for pneumonia and *S. pneumoniae* infection. Pneumococcal and annual influenza vaccinations are recommended for those with either of these conditions. Hepatitis A can be particularly severe among persons with chronic liver disease. Therefore vaccination is indicated for persons with chronic liver disease of any cause.

Asplenia

Asplenia is a risk factor for *S. pneumoniae* infection, *Neisseria meningitidis* infection, and, theoretically, *Haemophilus influenzae* type b infection. Pneumococcal and meningococcal vaccines are recommended for persons with asplenia, including those with splenic dysfunction caused by sickle cell disease. These persons also should consider *H. influenzae* type b vaccination. When splenectomy is not an emergency procedure, patients should receive vaccinations at least 2 weeks before the operation, if possible. Persons with asplenia should receive a second dose of pneumococcal vaccine 5 or more years after the first.

Chronic Cardiac and Pulmonary Conditions and Diabetes Mellitus

Chronic pulmonary disease, heart disease, and to a lesser extent, diabetes mellitus, are three of the most common predisposing factors for pneumonia, influenza, and *S. pneumoniae* infection. Patients with chronic pulmonary disease, diabetes mellitus, and heart disease with actual or potentially altered hemodynamics should receive pneumococcal vaccine and annual influenza vaccine. Asthma by itself is an indication for influenza vaccination. Annual vaccination against influenza also is indicated for household contacts of persons at high risk for complications of influenza.

Clotting Factor Deficiency

Outbreaks of hepatitis A virus (HAV) infection have occurred among persons with clotting disorders who receive factor VIII or IX concentrates. Most persons with hemophilia have serologic evidence of hepatitis B virus (HBV) infection. These persons should consider hepatitis B vaccination and hepatitis A vaccination unless they have already been infected. Because of the high HAV and HBV infection rate among those who previously received factor concentrate, testing for susceptibility to HAV and HBV is recommended before vaccination.

A fine (23-gauge or finer) needle should be used for vaccination, and after vaccination firm pressure should be applied at the injection site. Persons who have received hepatitis B vaccine should be tested for antibody to hepatitis B surface antigen (anti-HBs), ideally 1 to 2 months after vaccination, and should be revaccinated if results show an inadequate response (<10 mIU/mL).

Immunocompromising Conditions

Compromise of the immune system by high-dose or long-term use of steroids, cancer, or infection with human immunodeficiency virus (HIV) affects recommendations for and timing of administration of vaccines. Short-term (less than 2 weeks), topical, nasal, or intraarticular use of steroids generally should not be immunosuppressive and does not contraindicate use of live vaccines.

Immunosuppression increases risk for pneumonia, influenza, and *S. pneumoniae* infection. Immunocompromised persons should receive pneumococcal and annual influenza vaccination. Immunocompromised persons also should receive a second dose of pneumococcal vaccine 5 years after the first.

Use of live vaccines (oral poliovirus vaccine [OPV] and MMR) generally is contraindicated in the care of immunocompromised persons. Vaccine-associated paralytic poliomyelitis has occurred among immunocompromised persons and in one case report, a severely immunocompromised person with HIV infection contracted pneumonitis caused by measles vaccine virus after administration of MMR. Use of OPV also is contraindicated for use by household contacts of immunocompromised persons because live poliovirus can be shed in the feces and may be transmitted by the fecal-oral route to immunocompromised persons. MMR vaccination, however, is recommended for all persons with asymptomatic HIV infection who are not severely immunosuppressed and have an indication for vaccination. Use of MMR vaccine may be considered in the care of persons with symptomatic HIV infection who lack evidence of measles immunity and who are not severely immunocompromised, because measles can be severe among such persons.

Vaccines given to immunosuppressed persons may not be effective. Thus administration of immune globulin preparations may be indicated in the care of immunocompromised persons exposed to measles, varicella, or hepatitis B who have unknown or inadequate antibody titers. The CDC (1993) has published detailed recommendations for vaccination of persons with immunocompromising conditions.

Renal Disease and Hemodialysis

Chronic renal disease predisposes to pneumonia and *S. pneumoniae* infection. Persons with chronic renal disease should receive pneumococcal vaccine and be vaccinated annually against influenza. A second dose of pneumococcal vaccine is recommended 5 years after the first for persons with renal failure.

The risk for HBV infection among persons receiving hemodialysis is high. It is estimated that 15% of patients undergoing hemodialysis have serologic evidence of HBV infection, and outbreaks of HBV continue to occur in hemodialysis centers. Despite the risk for HBV infection among hemodialysis patients, many of these patients do not receive hepatitis B vaccine. Vaccinating patients before they need dialysis results in higher seroconversion rates than waiting until after hemodialysis is begun. Vaccination is recommended for patients with early-stage renal failure and for those already undergoing hemodialysis. Prevaccination testing with antibody to hepatitis B core antigen (anti-HBc) is recommended for patients who have undergone hemodialysis.

Patients undergoing hemodialysis need a higher total dosage of hepatitis B vaccine, either three doses of a special formulation (40 μg per dose) of Recombivax HB or administration at the same site of two 20 μg doses (a total of 40 μg) of Engerix-B on a four-dose schedule (0, 1, 2, and 6 months). Persons undergoing hemodialysis who have received hepatitis B vaccination appear to be immune to HBV infec-

tion only as long as the level of anti-HBs is 10 mIU/mL or more. Therefore, patients should have their anti-HBs level tested annually and should be given a booster dose of hepatitis B vaccine if the level is <10 mIU/mL.

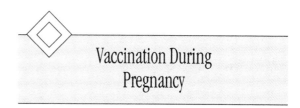

Vaccination During Pregnancy

Vaccine-related concerns for pregnancy are protection of the fetus during development, protection of the woman when lung capacity decreases, and protection of the newborn from infections at the time of delivery.

Measles-Mumps-Rubella and Varicella Vaccines

Because administering live-virus vaccines to a pregnant woman can lead to congenital infection, women of childbearing age should be asked whether they are pregnant or planning to become pregnant before receiving MMR or varicella vaccination. Nevertheless, because current data suggest little risk for congenital infection from administration of live-virus vaccine to the mother, routine pregnancy testing before MMR vaccine administration is considered unnecessary.

For women who are known to be pregnant, MMR and varicella vaccinations should be deferred until after delivery. Pregnant women who are susceptible to rubella should receive rubella vaccine in the postpartum period, preferably before discharge from the hospital or birthing center. Women should be advised to avoid pregnancy for 3 months after MMR vaccination and for 1 month after varicella vaccination.

The risk for complications of varicella is higher for women who are pregnant than for those who are not. Therefore administration of varicella zoster immune globulin should strongly be considered for pregnant women who are susceptible to and exposed to varicella. Lactating women may receive MMR, varicella, and all other vaccines.

Yellow Fever Vaccine

Yellow fever vaccine is best avoided by pregnant women unless the woman is traveling to an area where risk for yellow fever is high. In this instance the risk of vaccination is outweighed by the risk for yellow fever.

Influenza Vaccine

Data to date suggest that pregnant women with no other risk factors are at increased risk for complications of influenza, possibly because lung capacity decreases during pregnancy. It is recommended that women who will be in the second or third trimester of pregnancy during the influenza season receive influenza vaccination. Pregnant women who have high-risk medical conditions that increase the risk for complications of influenza should be vaccinated before the influenza season regardless of gestational age.

Tetanus and Diphtheria Toxoids

Pregnant women who have not received a primary series of tetanus and diphtheria toxoids (Td) should receive two doses of Td, given at least 4 weeks apart. Pregnant women who have received a primary series but have not had a booster of Td in the last 10 years should receive a booster dose.

Information about vaccine administration during pregnancy and lactation can be obtained from CDC publications (1994).

Indications for Vaccination According to Occupational Risks

Occupation is a risk factor for exposure to certain infectious diseases. For example, health care workers, public safety workers, and veterinarians and animal handlers, may be at increased risk for vaccine-preventable diseases. This has led to the development of vaccine recommendations based on occupation (Table 19-6). Persons who have served in the military can be considered to have received primary vaccinations against tetanus (vaccination began in 1941 in the military), diphtheria, measles, rubella, and polio.

Matriculation in a Post-High School Educational Program

Because outbreaks of measles have occurred on college campuses, entrants into college or other post-high school educational institutions should receive two doses of MMR before they matriculate. Entrants into college who have multiple sex partners or a history of a sexually transmitted disease (STD) also are candidates for hepatitis B vaccination. Matriculation into college is also a time to check the status of Td boosters and indications for influenza vaccination.

Entrants into medical, nursing, and other health professions schools should receive three doses of hepatitis B vaccine unless they have been vaccinated previously.

Freshmen, especially freshmen living in dormitories, are at increased risk for meningococcus disease. Although meningococcus disease is uncommon, the case-fatality rate is about 10% and another 10% have permanent sequelae. Therefore, freshmen, especially those living in dormitories, should consider meningococcal vaccination.

Table 19-6

Vaccine Recommendations in Addition to Those Recommended According to Age for Workers with Occupational Exposures

OCCUPATION	VACCINE	VACCINE INDICATIONS
Animal hide and hair (imported) workers	Anthrax	Recommended
Community service workers (teachers)	Varicella	Consider for susceptible teachers of young children and day-care[a] employees
	Influenza	Consider
Field personnel (forest rangers)	Rabies	Consider if likely to have contact with potentially rabid mammals
	Plague	Indicated if cannot avoid regular exposure to potentially plague-infected wild rodents and rabbits and their fleas
	Lyme disease	Consider if prolonged or frequent contact to tick infested habitat in areas at moderate or high-risk for Lyme disease
Health-care workers (e.g., dentists, physicians, nurses, trainees in these fields, and administrative staff)	Hepatitis B, influenza	Recommended
	Measles, mumps	For employees born in 1957 or later, one of the following is recommended: (a) 2 doses of live measles vaccine[b] and at least one dose of live mumps vaccine on or after first birthday, (b) history of physician-diagnosed disease, or (c) laboratory evidence of immunity. Consider measles vaccine for those born before 1957
	Rubella	For employees born in 1957 or later and for female employees born before 1957 who could become pregnant, one dose of vaccine on or after first birthday or laboratory evidence of immunity
	Immune globulin (for hepatitis A prevention)	Indicated when exposed to feces of infectious patients who have hepatitis A
	Varicella	For susceptible personnel.[a] Consider precautions for vaccinated personnel in whom vaccine rash develops or who are in contact with susceptible persons at high risk for complications
	VZIG, if exposed to varicella	Evaluate based on susceptibility and type of varicella exposure[c]
Staff of institutions for the developmentally disabled	Hepatitis B	Recommended for staff who work closely with clients, including staff in nonresidential day-care programs
	Varicella	Consider for susceptible staff[a]

(Continued)

Table 19-6

Vaccine Recommendations in Addition to Those Recommended According to Age for Workers with Occupational Exposures *(Concluded)*

OCCUPATION	VACCINE	VACCINE INDICATIONS
Laboratory workers	Hepatitis A	Recommended if working with hepatitis A virus in research settings
	Hepatitis B	Recommended if working around blood or other human tissues
	Anthrax, plague, rabies, typhoid, yellow fever	Recommended if working with organisms or contaminated specimens. See individual ACIP recommendations for details
	Poliovirus (IPV)	The primary series should be completed by those who anticipate close contact with specimens that may contain wild poliovirus
	Vaccinia (smallpox)	Recommended for those handling cultures or animals infected with vaccinia, recombinant vaccinia, cowpox, monkeypox, or orthopoxviruses that infect humans See CDC recommendations for details
Mortician	Hepatitis B	Recommended
Staff of nursing homes and chronic care facilities	Influenza	Recommended
Public safety workers (police, fire fighters, emergency medical service providers)	Hepatitis B	Recommended if contact with blood or blood-contaminated body fluids is anticipated
	Influenza	Consider
Sewage workers	Diphtheria and tetanus	Recommended
Staff of correctional institutions	Varicella	Consider for susceptible staff[a]
Veterinarians, animal handlers	Plague	Consider in western U.S. for veterinarians and assistants who may be exposed
	Rabies	Recommended
	Hepatitis A	Recommended if working with primates with hepatitis A virus infection

[a] Serologic screening of persons who have a negative or uncertain history of varicella is likely to be cost effective.

[b] If worker received inactivated measles vaccine, which was only available 1963–1967, or vaccine of unknown type during 1963–1967, two additional doses of MMR are needed. If worker received further attenuated vaccine (Schwarz or Moraten) simultaneously with immune globulin or measles immune globulin, consider person to be unimmunized and administer two doses of MMR. Health care facilities should consider requiring at least one dose of measles vaccine for employees born before 1957 who are at risk for occupational exposure to measles and do not have proof of immunity.

[c] Before administering VZIG, determine that worker is both (a) exposed and (b) susceptible (no history of varicella and negative antibody test, if any). Exposure includes household contact, more than 1 hour of indoor contact, prolonged direct face-to-face contact, or sharing same hospital room. Susceptibility is rare (only 5% to 15% of adults are not immune). Antibody testing may be helpful in determining susceptibility of immunocompetent persons without a history of varicella. VZIG is expensive, and supplies are limited.

Health Care Workers

Because they are more likely to come in contact with infected persons, health care workers are at increased risk for contracting certain vaccine-preventable diseases. Infectious disease in a health care worker increases risk for infection in patients, who may be chronically ill or immuno-compromised and thus have poorer outcomes if they contract infectious diseases. For example, health care workers have been known to contract and to contribute to the spread of measles within medical facilities. Vaccination of health care workers is important for their own protection and for the protection of patients.

MEASLES-MUMPS-RUBELLA VACCINATION

Health care workers are at risk for acquiring and transmitting both measles and rubella and should have documented immunity to both diseases. Those born before 1957 generally are considered to have acquired both measles and rubella and to have life-long immunity. However, some health care workers in this age group have acquired measles occupationally, so consideration should be given to administering one dose of MMR to them, especially if the health care worker is a woman with childbearing potential without serologic proof of rubella immunity.

Health care workers born in or after 1957 should have documentation of measles and rubella immunity. Documentation of measles immunity consists of one of the following: (1) two doses of measles vaccine, separated by 4 weeks, administered on or after the first birthday; (2) physician-diagnosed measles; or (3) laboratory evidence of immunity. Documentation of rubella immunity consists of one or more doses of rubella vaccine or laboratory evidence of immunity. If either measles or rubella vaccine is indicated, combined MMR is recommended. Although the CDC still accepts physician diagnosis of measles as proof of measles immunity,

it is important to realize that many clinicians today have never seen a case of measles. Therefore even with a history of physician-diagnosed measles, consideration should be given to requiring serologic evidence of immunity for those in high-risk professions.

INFLUENZA VACCINATION

Transmission of influenza from hospital staff to patients was documented in one outbreak of influenza among hospital patients. A study found that vaccination of staff in long-term care facilities reduced influenza-related morbidity and mortality among patients, even though more than 60% of patients had also received vaccination. It is therefore recommended that persons who provide health care or home care services to chronically ill patients receive influenza vaccine yearly. It is unfortunate that only about one-eighth to one-third of medical personnel are immunized each year, despite the risk their lack of immunization poses to patients.

HEPATITIS B VIRUS VACCINATION

HBV infection is a serious occupational risk for health care workers: 15 to 30% of those who have frequent exposure to blood products have serologic evidence of HBV infection. Before introduction of the hepatitis B vaccine the incidence of new HBV infections in one study was 1% per year. HBV vaccination of health care workers and their adherence to universal precautions for infection control can effectively decrease this risk, as shown by data from the CDC Viral Hepatitis Surveillance Program. The CDC found that from 1980 to 1985, 6 to 8% of cases of HBV infection occurred among health care workers, whereas after 1985, as a result of programs for HBV vaccination of health care workers and improved use of universal precautions, the proportion dropped to 3 to 4%.

The Occupational Safety and Health Administration (OSHA) requires employers to offer information about bloodborne pathogens, such as HBV, to workers at risk. OSHA defines workers at risk to be persons with "reasonably anticipated skin, eye, mucous membrane, or parenteral contact with blood or other potentially infectious materials," including semen, vaginal secretions, saliva, and any unfixed human tissue other than intact skin, "that may result from the performance of an employee's duties."

In addition to receiving vaccinations, health care workers should follow guidelines, such as those developed by the CDC, to prevent transmission of HBV and other pathogens. OSHA requires employees who have been found to be at risk for HBV exposure to attend training on universal precautions when assigned to duty and annually thereafter. The training is required to include complete information on hepatitis B vaccination. After initial training, but within 10 working days of initial assignment, the employer must offer hepatitis B vaccination at no cost to employees who are at risk for occupational exposure as defined by OSHA. Employees who decline vaccination must sign a waiver. For each employee at risk for occupational exposure to HBV, the employer must maintain a record of employee training and dates of hepatitis B vaccinations or refusal of vaccination.

Among groups with chronic HBV infection rates >2% or overall HBV infection rates >30%, prevaccination testing may be cost effective. Otherwise, prevaccination testing is not recommended. OSHA prohibits employers from requiring serologic testing before hepatitis B vaccination.

Adults at occupational risk of HBV infection should receive three doses of hepatitis B vaccine by means of intramuscular injection on a schedule of 0, 1, and 6 months. The dosage for immunocompetent adults 20 years of age and older is 10 μg Recombivax HB or 20 μg Engerix-B.

Some health care personnel have chosen not to receive hepatitis B vaccine out of concern about adverse events and possible transmission of HIV infection. However, no cases of HIV infection have ever been reported to be caused by hepatitis B vaccine, whether the vaccine was derived from plasma, as it was previously, or developed by means of recombinant technology, as is currently the case in the United States.

Postvaccination testing of an individual's anti-HBs level to determine adequacy of HBV immunization is recommended only for persons whose subsequent treatment will depend on their immunization status. Thus testing is not indicated after routine vaccination of infants, children, adolescents, or persons at low risk for exposure, such as health care workers and public safety workers who do not have contact with patients or body fluids. For those at risk for accidental needle-stick injuries or other potential exposure, postexposure treatment depends on response to immunization. Therefore workers at risk for exposure should have antibody levels to hepatitis B surface antigen (HBsAg) measured 1 to 2 months after completion of the vaccination series. An adequate antibody response to vaccination is 10 mIU/mL.

When a person has been exposed to blood products, as through accidental needle stick, the protocol outlined in Table 19-7 should be instituted as soon as possible. When indicated by this protocol, the adult dose of hepatitis B immune globulin is 0.06 mL/kg administered intramuscularly within 24 hours of exposure.

VARICELLA VACCINATION

Because nosocomial transmission of varicella is well documented, varicella vaccination is recommended for all susceptible health care workers. Serologic screening should be cost effective in identifying the need for vaccination among personnel with no history or an unclear history of varicella.

Data suggest that the benefits of administering varicella vaccine to susceptible health care workers outweigh the small potential risk for transmission of varicella organisms to patients by vaccinated workers who experience a vari-

Table 19-7

Recommendations for Hepatitis B Prophylaxis for Percutaneous or Permucosal Exposure

EXPOSED PERSON'S VACCINATION STATUS	TREATMENT WHEN SOURCE IS		
	HBsAG-POSITIVE	HBsAG-NEGATIVE	NOT TESTED OR UNKNOWN
Unvaccinated	HBIG × 1[a] and initiate hepatitis B vaccine	Initiate hepatitis B vaccine	Initiate hepatitis B vaccine
Previously vaccinated			
Known responder	No treatment	No treatment	No treatment
Known nonresponder	HBIG × 2 or HBIG × 1 and 1 dose HB vaccine	No treatment	If high-risk source, treat as if HBsAg-positive
Response unknown	Test exposed for anti-HBs: 1. If inadequate[b], give HBIG × 1 and vaccine booster 2. If adequate, no treatment	No treatment	Test exposed person for anti-HBs: 1. If inadequate, give vaccine booster 2. If adequate, no treatment

[a] HBIG dose is 0.06 mL/kg intramuscularly within 24 hours of exposure.
[b] Adequate anti-HBs level is 10 mIU/mL by radioimmunoassay or positive by enzyme immunoassay.
ABBREVIATIONS: HBsAg, Hepatitis B surface antigen; HBIG, hepatitis B immune globulin; anti-HBs, antibody to HBsAg.
SOURCE: Modified from Centers for Disease Control and Prevention. Protection against viral hepatitis: recommendation of the Immunization Practices Advisory Committee. *MMWR* 39(RR-2):1–26, 1990.

celliform rash. Nevertheless, institutions might want to consider precautions for vaccinated personnel who are in contact with patients at high risk for serious complications and for personnel who experience a rash after vaccination.

Additional vaccine recommendations for health care workers are listed in Table 19-6.

Public Safety Workers

Many public safety workers, like health care workers, are at increased risk for contact with blood or blood-contaminated body fluids and thus are at increased risk for HBV infection. It is therefore recommended that the guidelines for hepatitis B vaccination of health care workers be followed for hepatitis B vaccination of public safety workers who may be exposed to blood. Public safety workers also have extended contact with chronically ill persons who are at high risk for complications from influenza. Therefore annual influenza vaccination of these workers should be considered to prevent them from serving as a source of influenza transmission.

Veterinarians and Animal Handlers

Veterinarians and animal handlers may be at increased risk for rabies, plague, and hepatitis A.

RABIES

Veterinarians and animal handlers who have not been exposed to rabies should receive rabies vaccine, either human diploid cell vaccine (HDCV), adsorbed rabies vaccine (RVA), or purified chick embryo cell (PCEC) vaccine. Three 1.0 mL doses of one of the vaccines can be administered into the deltoid muscle on a schedule of 0, 7, and 21 or 28 days, or three 0.1 mL doses of HDCV can be given intradermally on the same schedule. Every 2 years, persons at continued occupational risk should either receive a booster dose or have their serum tested for rabies antibody and receive a booster dose if the titer is less than complete neutralization at a 1:5 serum dilution.

Recommendations for rabies postexposure prophylaxis are discussed later.

PLAGUE

Veterinarians and their assistants in the western part of the United States who may be exposed to plague should consider being vaccinated against this illness.

HEPATITIS A VIRUS

Animal handlers who work with primates infected with HAV should receive two doses of hepatitis A vaccine in the deltoid muscle. If the Havrix vaccine is used, two 1440 ELISA unit doses should be administered on a schedule of 0 and 6 to 12 months. If the Vaqta vaccine is used, two 50-unit doses should be administered on a schedule of 0 and 6 months.

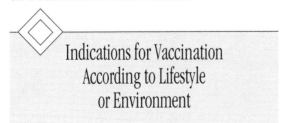

Indications for Vaccination According to Lifestyle or Environment

Lifestyle and environment are risk factors for some vaccine-preventable diseases. For exam-

ple, studies have found sexual activity (heterosexual or homosexual) to be a risk factor in 31% to 44% of cases of HBV infection and use of injected drugs to be a risk factor in 15% to 20% of cases. Recommendations for vaccination of adults on the basis of lifestyle or environment are summarized in Table 19-8 and are discussed in the following sections.

Drug Users

Outbreaks of HAV infection have occurred among users of injected drugs. For this reason, hepatitis A vaccine is recommended for users of injected drugs and users of orally or nasally administered street drugs who live in areas where epidemiologic data indicate a high incidence of hepatitis A infection. Prevaccination testing is not indicated for adolescents but may be cost effective for adults.

Outbreaks of HBV infection have occurred among users of injected drugs. The prevalence of infection among such populations ranges from 30% to 90%. Users of injected drugs should receive hepatitis B vaccine. Because more than 80% of infected users of injected drugs are infected with HBV within the first 5 years of drug use, prevaccination serologic testing is recommended.

Homosexual or Bisexual Men and Persons of Either Sex with Multiple Sex Partners

Outbreaks of HAV infection have occurred among homosexual men, and serosurveys show higher prevalence of HAV infection among homosexual men than among controls. Hepatitis A vaccination is therefore recommended for sexually active homosexual and bisexual men. Although prevaccination testing is not indicated for adolescents, it may be cost effective for adults.

Having multiple sex partners is a risk factor for HBV infection. Hepatitis B vaccination is recommended for persons who have had more than one sex partner in the previous 6 months,

Table 19-8

Vaccines for Special Environments and Lifestyle Situations in Addition to Those Recommended According to Age

SITUATION	VACCINE	VACCINE INDICATIONS
Matriculation to college, technical school, or other post–high school educational institution	Measles, mumps, rubella	For students born in or after 1957 and for women born before 1957 who could become pregnant, 2 doses of live measles vaccine[a] and ≥1 dose of rubella vaccine and of mumps vaccine on or after first birthday, or laboratory evidence of immunity or, for measles and mumps, physician-diagnosed disease
	Hepatitis B	Multiple sex partners, sexually transmitted disease or prolonged travel in endemic countries
	Meningococcal	Consider for college freshmen especially those living in dormitories
	Varicella	Consider[b]
	Influenza	Consider
Drug user	Hepatitis A	Recommended for injected-drug users and recreational users of nonprescription drugs who live in areas of high hepatitis A incidence
	Hepatitis B	Recommended for injected-drug users[c,d]
Homeless	Influenza, measles, mumps, rubella	Recommended
Homosexual or bisexual men	Hepatitis A, hepatitis B	Recommended[c,d]
Household contacts or sex partners of persons chronically infected with hepatitis B virus	Hepatitis B	Recommended[c]
Household contacts of persons at high risk for complications from influenza	Influenza	Recommended
Household contacts of persons at high risk for complications from varicella	Varicella	Recommended for susceptible contacts[b]
Household contact of typhoid carriers	Typhoid	Recommended
Outdoor activities in areas with moderate or high risk for Lyme disease	Lyme disease	Consider if frequent or prolonged exposure; not recommended if area is low risk
Residents of institutions for developmentally disabled	Hepatitis B	Recommended for new residents For current residents, screening and vaccination of susceptible residents are recommended[e]

(Continued)

Table 19-8

Vaccines for Special Environments and Lifestyle Situations in Addition to Those Recommended According to Age *(Continued)*

SITUATION	VACCINE	VACCINE INDICATIONS
	Influenza	Recommended for all residents
	Varicella	Consider for residents[b]
Native Americans	Pneumococcal	Recommended for certain Native American populations with high disease incidence
Nursing home and chronic care facility residents	Influenza	Recommended
	Pneumococcal	Recommended for persons 65 yr or older and those at increased risk for complications from pneumococcal disease due to chronic illnesses
Prison inmates (long-term correctional facility residents)	Hepatitis B	Consider[c]
	Influenza	Recommended for all inmates 50 yr and older and those with high-risk conditions, including HIV infection
	Pneumococcal	Recommended for all inmates 65 yr and older and those with high-risk conditions
	Varicella	Consider[b]
	Measles, rubella	Recommended
Sexually transmitted disease, multiple sex partners during previous 6 months, commercial sex worker (prostitute)	Hepatitis B	Recommended

[a] If person received inactivated measles vaccine, which was only available 1963–1967, or vaccine of unknown type during 1963–1967, two additional doses of MMR are needed. If person received further attenuated vaccine (Schwarz or Moraten) simultaneously with immune globulin or measles immune globulin, consider person to be unimmunized and administer two doses of MMR.

[b] Serologic screening of persons with negative or uncertain histories of varicella is likely to be cost effective.

[c] Testing for previous hepatitis B infection may be cost effective in groups with high rates of HBV infection, depending on the likelihood that persons will return for follow-up treatment.

[d] Vaccine recipients who are injected-drug users and homosexual or bisexual men and who have HIV infection should be tested for hepatitis B surface antibody, and nonrespondents should be counseled accordingly.

[e] Vaccination of clients in nonresidential day-care programs should be considered, although they are at lower risk for acquiring hepatitis B. If there is one hepatitis B carrier in a classroom, the entire class should be immunized. Staff in nonresidential day-care programs should be immunized against hepatitis B.

persons recently acquiring an STD, persons being treated in an STD clinic, homosexual or bisexual men, and persons who exchange sex for drugs or money. Some 30% to 70% of men who have unprotected sex with men become infected with HBV, particularly if they have multiple partners, have another STD, perform rectal douching, or engage in receptive anal intercourse. Because the prevalence of past or current HBV infection is high among these persons,

prevaccination serologic testing should be cost effective and is recommended.

Household Contacts of a Person with Chronic Hepatitis B Virus Infection

Hepatitis B is highly infectious, can be contracted through unapparent contamination of skin lesions, and has been transmitted within households by nonsexual means. Therefore household contacts of persons with chronic HBV infection should receive HBV vaccination.

Persons Engaged in Outdoor Activities in Locales with Lyme Disease

Persons who participate in outdoor activities in areas where Lyme disease is present may be at risk; there is marked regional variation in risk. Lyme disease is caused by *Borrelia burgdorferi*, which resides in a dormant state in the intestine of *Ixodes scapularis*, the deer tick, and *Ixodes pacificus*, the western black-legged tick. About 36 hours after a blood meal, the bacteria awaken, migrate to the salivary gland of the tick, and enter the mammal to which the tick is attached. While in the dormant state, the bacteria express outer surface protein A. Vaccines against Lyme disease induce antibodies against this protein that kill the bacteria while they are in the intestine of the tick.

Decisions about Lyme disease vaccination should be made on an individual basis. The decision process should include an assessment of risk for exposure and the risks and benefits of vaccination versus other protective measures, including early diagnosis and treatment. Vaccination is not recommended for persons who work and reside in low- or no-risk areas. In locales of high or moderate risk for the disease, one should consider the frequency of exposure to tick-infested habitat. If the exposure is frequent or prolonged, vaccination should be considered for persons 15 to 70 years of age. If the exposure is neither frequent nor prolonged, vaccination may be considered, but the benefit is uncertain. The duration of immunity from vaccination and need, if any, for repeat boosters is unknown.

Residents of Institutions for the Developmentally Disabled

HBV infection and influenza are concerns for residents of institutions for the developmentally disabled. Vaccination to prevent these infections is recommended.

HEPATITIS B VACCINE

Serosurveys show that 35% to 80% of residents of institutions for the developmentally disabled have evidence of HBV infection. Because residents and attendees in classrooms and other institutions for the developmentally disabled are at increased risk for HBV infection, particularly if one of the residents has chronic HBV infection, it is recommended that residents in such institutions receive hepatitis B vaccine. New residents ideally should be vaccinated at admission to the institution. Vaccination is particularly recommended for classmates of a person who behaves aggressively or has a medical problem such as exudative dermatitis that increases risk for exposure to blood or serous secretions. Prevaccination testing is recommended for long-term residents but not for new residents of such institutions.

INFLUENZA VACCINE

Many residents of institutions for the developmentally disabled have chronic medical conditions such as congenital heart disease that place them at risk for complications of influenza. All residents of these institutions should receive influenza vaccine annually.

Residents of Nursing Homes and Long-term Care Facilities

Influenza is extremely contagious, easily transmitted, usually by the airborne route, from person to person in semiclosed or crowded environments. Such environments include nursing homes, where influenza attack rates can approach 60% and case-fatality rates can reach 30%. Although influenza vaccine may be only 30% to 40% effective in preventing influenza among elderly persons residing in nursing homes, vaccination can be 50% to 60% effective in preventing hospitalization and pneumonia and more than 80% effective in preventing death.

Achieving a high rate of vaccination among nursing home residents can reduce the spread of infection in a facility and prevent disease through herd immunity. Institution protocols for infection control should include standing orders for vaccination of all residents of chronic-care facilities as a group. Consent for annual influenza vaccination of each resident should be obtained at the time of admission to the facility. Residents admitted during the winter but after the annual vaccination program should be vaccinated at admission.

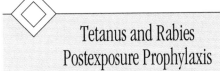

Tetanus and Rabies Postexposure Prophylaxis

In the United States during 1989 and 1990, 86 of 110 (78%) reported cases of tetanus could be attributed to an acute injury, usually of the lower extremity. Most injuries occurred outdoors, on a farm or in a garden (45%), another outdoor setting, or motor vehicle accident (21%) rather than indoors (33%). Administration of tetanus toxoid is indicated (after the wound has been cleaned, debrided if necessary, and dressed) if the patient did not complete an initial tetanus vaccination series or has not had a tetanus booster in the last 5 to 10 years. In addition, tetanus immunoglobulin (TIG) should be given if the person has not had a primary series and the wound is contaminated or complex. (See Table 19-9 for details about administration of Td and TIG.) When tetanus toxoid is indicated, administration of adult tetanus toxoid and Td is preferred. The typical dose of tetanus immune globulin (TIG) is 250 mg administered intramuscularly at a separate site from tetanus toxoid.

Any person bitten by an animal believed or proved to be rabid should begin treatment as soon as possible, preferably within 24 hours. If there is any doubt about whether treatment is

Table 19-9

Tetanus Wound Prophylaxis

| | PREVIOUS IMMUNIZATION HISTORY | | |
| | UNCERTAIN OR <3 DOSES | | 3 OR MORE DOSES |
TYPE OF WOUND	GIVE Td?	GIVE TIG?	GIVE Td?[b]
Clean, minor wound	Yes	No	No, unless <10 yr since previous dose
Wound contaminated with dirt, feces, or saliva	Yes	Yes	No, unless <5 yr since previous dose[a]
Puncture or missile wound	Yes	Yes	No, unless <5 yr since previous dose[a]
Burns, frostbite, or crush injury	Yes	Yes	No, unless <5 yr since previous dose[a]

[a] If the individual has only has three doses of the nonabsorbed (fluid) tetanus toxoid, administer a fourth dose of Td or tetanus toxoid. Nonabsorbed (fluid) vaccine is available only as single antigen tetanus toxoid; diphtheria and tetanus toxoids and pertussis vaccine (DTP), Td, and pediatric diphtheria and tetanus toxoids (DT) all use absorbed preparations.
[b] TIG not recommended.
ABBREVIATIONS: Td, adult tetanus and diphtheria toxoids; TIG, tetanus immune globulin
SOURCE: Modified from *MMWR* 1991; 40(RR-10):16.

indicated, clinicians should call their local or state health department for advice.

Postexposure treatment depends on whether those exposed have received vaccine previously. All treatment should include thorough washing of all wounds with soap and water and evaluation of the need for tetanus prophylaxis. For those previously vaccinated, no rabies immune globulin (RIG) is recommended; rabies vaccine is recommended (1.0 mL given intramuscularly) on days 0 and 3. Those not previously vaccinated should receive RIG, 20 IU/kg body weight with as much as anatomically feasible injected around the wound and the remainder given intramuscularly at a distant site. Administration of vaccine is recommended (at a different site from the RIG) on days 0, 3, 7, 14, and 28.

Vaccination Procedures

In addition to recommendations for vaccination, health care providers need to be aware of contraindications, precautions, and informational issues regarding vaccination.

Contraindications

Patient factors that may contraindicate administration of a vaccine include allergic reaction to a component of the vaccine or a serious reaction to a previous dose of the vaccine, severe febrile illness, altered immunocompetence, and pregnancy.

Anaphylactic reaction to a vaccine or components of a vaccine is a contraindication to administration of additional doses of that vaccine. Egg protein is contained in influenza and yellow fever vaccines. Persons with a history of anaphylactic allergic reactions to eggs or egg protein should avoid these vaccines. However, there are protocols for testing and desensitization for persons at high risk for complications of vaccine-preventable diseases. Contact dermatitis from neomycin is a delayed-type (cell-mediated) immune response and is a not a contraindication to vaccination. Persons who have an Arthrus type hypersensitivity reaction or a fever >39.4°C (103°F) after a dose of tetanus toxoid probably have high serum antitoxin titers and should not be given a dose of Td more often than every 10 years.

Vaccination of persons with severe febrile illnesses generally should be postponed until they have recovered from the acute phase.

Administration of live virus vaccines (measles, mumps, rubella, varicella, oral polio, yellow fever) are generally contraindicated for use by persons with immunodeficiencies or suppressed immune responses because of malignant disease or therapy with corticosteroid drugs, alkylating agents, antimetabolites, or radiation. An exception is persons with asymptomatic HIV infection, for whom MMR vaccination is recommended if the person lacks evidence of measles immunity and is not severely immunosuppressed. Severe immunocompromise among adults is defined as a CD4+ T-lymphocyte count less than 200/μL or CD4+ T lymphocytes as percentage of total lymphocytes less than 14%. MMR vaccination of persons with symptomatic HIV infection should be considered if the person lacks evidence of measles immunity and is not severely immunosuppressed. Another exception is varicella vaccine, when otherwise indicated, for persons with impaired humoral immunity (but not cellular immunodeficiencies).

Pregnancy is a contraindication to vaccination with live virus because of the theoretical risk that the live virus might affect the fetus. Women should avoid becoming pregnant within 3 months of MMR or rubella vaccination and within 1 month of mumps or varicella vaccination. Data have not shown a link between administration of live virus vaccines and fetal malformations; unintentional administration of a live-virus vaccine during pregnancy is therefore not an indication for termination of pregnancy.

Precautions

On rare occasions, administration of tetanus toxoid has been associated with the recurrence of Guillain-Barré syndrome (GBS). The benefits of any subsequent doses of tetanus toxoid should be weighed against the risks for recurrence of GBS before administration of a tetanus booster to any patient who has had GBS within 6 weeks of receiving tetanus toxoid.

Vaccine Information Statements for Patients

Patients should receive readily understandable information about the benefits and risks of immunization. Under the National Childhood Vaccine Injury Act, health care providers who administer most routine childhood vaccines are required to provide a copy of the relevant vaccine information statement (VIS) to the patient before vaccination. A VIS is available for almost all routine vaccines. When a VIS is not available, the *clinician* should provide information about the risk of the disease, the protection vaccine affords, the risk for adverse events of vaccination, and what to do if a serious adverse event occurs.

Reporting Adverse Reactions

Health care providers are required by Congress to report to the Vaccine Adverse Event Reporting System (VAERS) certain adverse events that occur after vaccine administration. Health care providers also can report other adverse reactions to the VAERS. Providers can obtain forms and instructions by calling 1-800-822-7967.

Vaccine Injury Compensation Program

The Vaccine Injury Compensation Program (VICP) is a system under which no-fault compensation can be awarded for specified injuries that are temporally related to administration of

vaccinations against measles, mumps, rubella, diphtheria, tetanus, pertussis, poliomyelitis, hepatitis B, varicella, or *H. influenzae* type b. The VICP has reduced the risk to both providers and vaccine manufacturers of litigation related to adverse events following administration of covered vaccines. Providers can obtain specific information about the adverse events covered by the VICP by calling 1-800-338-2382.

Vaccine Administration Routes

Influenza, hepatitis A, hepatitis B, and Td vaccinations are administered intramuscularly (IM) in the deltoid muscle. Pneumococcal vaccine can be administered either IM or subcutaneously (SQ). MMR, inactivated poliomyelitis vaccine, and varicella vaccine are administered.

Provider Vaccination Records

Providers administering vaccines covered by the VICP are required to record either in an office log or the recipient's permanent medical record the date of administration, manufacturer, lot number, and name, address, and title of person administering the vaccine. The ACIP recommends that providers record these data for all vaccines.

Strategies for Increasing Vaccination Rates

Many successful vaccination programs have combined elements such as education for health care workers, publicity and education targeted toward potential recipients, and efforts to remove administrative and financial barriers that prevent persons from receiving the vaccine.

Various vaccination strategies have been studied. System-oriented strategies (e.g., standing orders for nurses) have resulted in pooled vaccination rate increases of 39 and 45% for influenza and pneumococcal vaccines, respectively. Patient- or client-oriented strategies, such as postcard reminders that a dose of influenza or pneumococcal vaccine was due, resulted in vaccination rate increases of 12 and 75%, respectively. Provider-oriented strategies (e.g., chart reminders) resulted in pooled vaccination rate increases of 18 and 7.5%, respectively, for influenza and pneumococcal vaccines. Specific strategies for increasing rates of adult vaccination among target populations are as follows.

Medical Office and Clinic Patients

Several strategies have been found effective in increasing vaccination rates among patients visiting medical offices or clinics.

SYSTEM-ORIENTED STRATEGIES

Medical offices or clinics, hemodialysis centers, specialty clinics, and travel medicine clinics can use one or more system-oriented strategies to increase vaccination rates among their patients. One such strategy is to assign administration of vaccines to nursing rather than physician members of the team and to develop standing orders for vaccine administration rather than to require that a vaccination order be written for each patient individually.

For large practices or clinics, walk-in adult vaccination stations can be established in the influenza vaccine season. The stations should operate according to a written protocol and be staffed by nurses with training on recommendations and procedures for vaccination.

PATIENT-ORIENTED STRATEGIES

Patient-oriented strategies to increase adult vaccination rates include providing informa-

tional pamphlets on adult vaccines and displaying informational posters in patient waiting areas. Individual candidates for vaccination can be found by means of checking computerized billing records for vaccination indications, which include patient age, diagnosis code (for a high-risk medical condition), and receipt of influenza vaccine at an office visit the previous year. These persons can be reminded personally of their need for vaccination through a postcard or telephone call, perhaps with an autodialing machine to decrease staff time spent on this task.

PROVIDER-ORIENTED STRATEGIES

At least three patient surveys have shown that persons who receive vaccinations are more likely to report that their provider recommended vaccination than are those who do not receive vaccinations. In two of these surveys, the most powerful factor in whether patients were vaccinated appears to have been provider advice.

Strategies to ascertain who is a candidate for vaccination and to remind providers to recommend vaccination include: (1) developing protocols for office staff to identify candidates for vaccination based on age or diagnoses, (2) developing protocols for nursing personnel to assess vaccination status when they obtain vital signs, or (3) using computer-generated prompts, when available. Computerized systems have been instrumental in the ability of health maintenance organizations to increase use of preventive services. The need to recommend vaccination can be communicated among office or clinic personnel by marking the patient's chart with a colored sticker or stamp or including a checklist or questionnaire about preventive services. Placing such reminders on patient charts has been reported to increase vaccination rates. For pneumococcal vaccine in particular, meta-analysis of data from several studies of moderate to high quality showed vaccination rate increases of 7 to 37% with use of such reminders in clinic and hospital settings.

Another provider-oriented strategy for increasing vaccination rates is to offer financial incentives to providers for achieving vaccination rate targets. In one such study, influenza vaccination rates were 56% for the control group and 73% for the financial incentive group.

To improve vaccination rates among patients of a medical office or clinic, the most important steps are: (1) assessment of the practice's vaccination rates, (2) identification of target populations for vaccination, (3) formulation of a specific vaccination goal (percentage of target population to be immunized), (4) development of a plan of action, and (5) provision of ongoing feedback to individual clinicians about vaccination rates among their own patients. Clinician feedback is especially important.

Residents of Nursing Homes and Other Long-term Care Facilities

Standing orders should be written for adult vaccinations to be provided to all residents of long-term care facilities. Consent for vaccination should be obtained from the resident or a family member at admission to the facility. For influenza vaccine, all residents should be vaccinated ideally at one time, immediately before the influenza season.

Patients Discharged from Hospitals

Many (39 to 45%) of those who die from influenza and pneumonia have been hospitalized within the preceding year, which suggests that hospitalization is an indicator of increased risk for a serious influenza infection. Persons discharged from the hospital between September and March should be offered influenza vaccine. Hospital-based influenza vaccination programs carried out according to a specific protocol by nurses and ward secretaries can be effective in enhancing influenza immunization rates.

Hospital-based vaccination programs also work for pneumococcal vaccine. In one study, infection-control nurses who ascertained whether a patient was a candidate for pneumococcal vaccination and administration of vaccine according to a standing order resulted in a 78% increase in vaccination rates. In another study, patients hospitalized in acute-care wards who were offered pamphlets describing the recommendations for pneumococcal vaccination or pamphlets plus follow-up discussion had a 75% higher rate of vaccination than those on the same units who were not offered either intervention.

Women of Childbearing Age

MMR should be offered routinely to women of childbearing age as part of routine or contraceptive-related care. Women who have just given birth should be immunized before hospital discharge if they lack proof immunization to rubella.

Health Care Workers

Administrators of all health care facilities should arrange for influenza vaccine to be offered to all personnel before the influenza season. Particular emphasis should be placed on vaccination of persons who care for members of high-risk groups (e.g., staff of intensive care units and employees of nursing homes). Practical approaches include using a mobile cart to provide vaccination on hospital wards or at other work sites and offering vaccination on evening, night, and weekend work shifts in addition to weekday shifts.

Other Adult Populations

Other adult populations who should be offered vaccination on site include residents of retirement communities, those who attend adult recreation centers, patients of acute care or urgent care centers, clients of facilities that provide outpatient care for high-risk conditions (e.g., dialysis centers), clients of visiting nurses, and those visiting travel clinics.

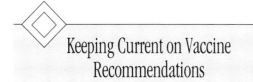

Keeping Current on Vaccine Recommendations

Vaccine recommendations change frequently. It is difficult for practicing clinicians to stay up to date in this field. One of the best sources of information is the *MMWR Morbidity and Mortality Weekly Report* published weekly by the CDC. The MMWR contains regular updates on the ACIP vaccine recommendations and is available on the Internet at www2.cdc.gov/mmwr. Information is also available at websites of professional academies (e.g., www.aafp.org).

This chapter is adapted from a continuing medical education (CME) article written as a component of the Teaching Immunization for Medical Education (TIME) project, a collaborative effort of the CDC, the Association of Teachers of Preventive Medicine (ATPM), and the University of Pittsburgh School of Medicine. Information about CME modules on vaccine-preventable diseases and case-based materials designed for medical students and residents can be obtained from ATPM at 800-789-6737 or www.atpm.org. Some of the CME modules are available on line at www.upmc.edu/CCEHS/cme.

Bibliography

American Academy of Family Physicians: *Summary of Policy Recommendations for Periodic Health Examination*, AAFP Policy Action. American Academy of Family Physicians, Leawood, KS, 1996, pp 2–14.

American College of Physicians Task Force on Adult Immunization and Infectious Diseases Society of America: *Guide for Adult Immunization*, 3rd ed. Philadelphia: American College of Physicians, 1994.

Bloom BS, Hillman AL, Fendrick AM, et al: A reappraisal of hepatitis B virus vaccination strategies using cost effectiveness analysis. *Ann Intern Med* 118:298–306, 1993.

Centers for Disease Control and Prevention: Yellow fever vaccine: Recommendations of the Immunization Practices Advisory Committee (ACIP). *MMWR Morb Mortal Wkly Rep* 39(RR-6):1–6, 1990.

Centers for Disease Control and Prevention: Rubella prevention: Recommendations of the Immunization Practices Advisory Committee (ACIP). *MMWR Morb Mortal Wkly Rep* 39(RR-15):1–18, 1990.

Centers for Disease Control and Prevention: Vaccinia (smallpox) vaccine: Recommendations of the Immunization Practices Advisory Committee (ACIP) [published erratum appears in *MMWR Morb Mortal Wkly Rep* 1992;41:31]. *MMWR Morb Mortal Wkly Rep* 40(RR-14):1–10, 1991.

Centers for Disease Control and Prevention: Tetanus surveillance—United States, 1989–1991. *MMWR Morb Mortal Wkly Rep* 41(SS-8):1–9, 1992.

Centers for Disease Control and Prevention: Recommendations of the Advisory Committee on Immunization Practices (ACIP): Use of vaccines and immune globulins in persons with altered immunocompetence. *MMWR Morb Mortal Wkly Rep* 42(RR-4):1–18, 1993.

Centers for Disease Control and Prevention: General Recommendations on immunization: Recommendations of the Advisory Committee on Immunization Practices (ACIP). *MMWR Morb Mortal Wkly Rep* 43(RR-1):1–38, 1994.

Centers for Disease Control and Prevention: Assessing adult vaccination status at age 50 years. *MMWR Morb Mortal Wkly Rep* 44:561–563, 1995.

Centers for Disease Control and Prevention: Mumps surveillance—United States, 1988–1993. *MMWR Morb Mortal Wkly Rep* 44(SS-3):1–14, 1995.

Centers for Disease Control and Prevention: Update: Diphtheria epidemic—New independent states of the former Soviet Union, January 1995–March 1996. *MMWR Morb Mortal Wkly Rep* 45:693, 1996.

Centers for Disease Control and Prevention: Outbreaks of hepatitis B virus infection among hemodialysis patients—California, Nebraska, and Texas, 1994. *MMWR Morb Mortal Wkly Rep* 45:285–209, 1996.

Centers for Disease Control and Prevention: Measles pneumonitis following measles-mumps-rubella vaccination of a patient with HIV infection, 1993. *MMWR Morb Mortal Wkly Rep* 45:603–606, 1996.

Centers for Disease Control and Prevention: Prevention of varicella: Recommendations of the Advisory Committee on Immunization Practices (ACIP). *MMWR Morb Mortal Wkly Rep* 45(RR-11):1–36, 1996.

Centers for Disease Control and Prevention: Update: Vaccine side effects, adverse reactions, contraindications, and precautions—Recommendations of the Advisory Committee on Immunization Practices (ACIP). *MMWR Morb Mortal Wkly Rep* 45(RR-12):1–35, 1996.

Centers for Disease Control and Prevention: Prevention of hepatitis A through active or passive immunization: Recommendations of the Advisory Committee on Immunization Practices (ACIP). *MMWR Morb Mortal Wkly Rep* 45(No. RR-15):1–30, 1996.

Centers for Disease Control and Prevention: *Information for International Travel 1996–1997*. Atlanta, Department of Health and Human Services, 1996–1997.

Centers for Disease Control and Prevention: Immunization of health care workers: Recommendations of the Advisory Committee on Immunization Practices (ACIP) and the Hospital Infection Control Practices Advisory Committee (HICPAC). *MMWR Morb Mortal Wkly Rep* 46:1–42, 1997.

Centers for Disease Control and Prevention: Poliomyelitis prevention in the United States: Introduction of a sequential vaccination schedule of inactivated poliovirus vaccine followed by oral poliovirus vaccine: Recommendations of the Advisory Committee on Immunization Practices (ACIP). *MMWR Morb Mortal Wkly Rep* 46(RR-3):1–25, 1997.

Centers for Disease Control and Prevention: Prevention of pneumococcal disease: Recommendations of the Advisory Committee on Immunization Practices (ACIP). *MMWR Morb Mortal Wkly Rep* 46(RR-8):1–24, 1997.

Centers for Disease Control and Prevention: Prevention and control of influenza: Recommendations of the Advisory Committee on Immunization Practices (ACIP). *MMWR Morb Mortal Wkly Rep* 47:1–26, 1998.

Centers for Disease Control and Prevention: Influenza and pneumococcal vaccination levels among adults aged >65 years—United States, 1997. *MMWR Morb Mortal Wkly Rep* 47:797–802, 1998.

Centers for Disease Control and Prevention: Measles, mumps, and rubella—vaccine use and strategies for elimination of measles, rubella and congenital rubella syndrome and control of mumps: Recommendations of the Advisory Committee on Immunization Practices (ACIP). *MMWR Morb Mortal Wkly Rep* 47(RR-8):1–57, 1998.

Centers for Disease Control and Prevention: *Epidemiology and Prevention of Vaccine-Preventable Diseases*, 5th ed. Atlanta: Centers for Disease Control and Prevention, 1999.

Centers for Disease Control and Prevention: Hepatitis B virus infection: A comprehensive immunization strategy to eliminate transmission in the United States—Recommendations of the Advisory Committee on Immunization Practices (ACIP). *MMWR Morb Mortal Wkly Rep* (in press).

Jernigan DB, Cetron MS, Breiman RF: Minimizing the impact of the drug-resistant *Streptococcus pneumoniae* (DRSP): A strategy from the DRSP working group. *JAMA* 275:206–209, 1996.

Kent JH, Chapman LE, Schmeltz LM, et al: Influenza surveillance—United States, 1991–1992. *MMWR Morb Mortal Wkly Rep* 41:35–43, 1992.

Kouides RW, Lewis B, Bennett NM, et al: A performance-based incentive program for influenza immunization in the elderly. *Am J Prev Med* 9:250–255, 1993.

LeBaron CW, Birkhead GS, Parsons P, et al: Measles vaccination levels of children enrolled in WIC during the 1991 measles epidemic in New York City. *Am J Public Health* 86:1551–1556, 1996.

Nichol KL: Long-term success with the national health objective for influenza vaccination: An institution-wide model. *J Gen Intern* Med 7:595–600, 1992.

Nichol KL, Margolis KL, Wuorenma J, Von Sternberg T: The efficacy and cost effectiveness of vaccination against influenza among elderly persons living in the community. *N Engl J Med* 331:778–784, 1994.

Occupational Safety and Health Administration: *Bloodborne Pathogens and Acute Care Facilities*, 1995 rev. ed. Washington, DC: U.S. Department of Labor, Occupational Safety and Health Administration, 1995.

Sisk JE, Moskowitz AJ, Whang W: Cost effectiveness of vaccination against pneumococcal bacteremia among elderly people. *JAMA* 278:1333, 1997.

Thompson RS: What have HMOs learned about clinical prevention services? An examination of the experience at Group Health Cooperative of Puget Sound. *Milbank Q* 74:469–509, 1996.

US Preventive Services Task Force: *Guide to Clinical Preventive Services*, 2nd ed. Baltimore, Williams & Wilkins, 1996.

Randa M. Kutob
Ron E. Pust

Chapter
20

The Traveler

How Common Is International Travel?

College students, business executives, medical missionaries, government officials—these are some of the faces of the international traveler today. Travel around the globe is easier and accessible to more people than it has ever been, most destinations being attainable in little over a day's travel. It is estimated that more than 500 million international tourists embark annually, but this number does not include undocumented and involuntary travel often related to poor social conditions and political unrest. The relative distribution of documented travelers is shown in Figure 20-1. Each global region presents some unique and some ubiquitous health risks. These combined with the relative ease of travel and short incubation period of many infectious diseases pose considerable health threats for individual travelers and a challenge for disease control programs. Primary care clinicians are in a front-line position to help minimize these risks with a pretravel risk assessment

and posttravel follow-up evaluation. Clinician and patient can work together to develop specific disease prevention strategies.

These strategies, consisting of immunizations, screening tests, counseling, and chemoprophylaxis, are influenced by the destination of the planned trip and by specific itineraries between and within nations, such as travel in a rural or urban area. Prevention strategies have to be tailored to the individual patient's needs. Increasingly today travelers are not only vacationers. Travelers now include persons working or studying abroad, such as military personnel, college students, health care professionals, and undocumented migrant workers. Each person has specific risks based on age, sex, and general health status that must be taken into account when prevention strategies are designed.

Travel medicine is an exciting and constantly changing field. At the end of the chapter (Table 20-1) is a comprehensive list of resources for up-to-the-minute information. The Centers for Disease Control and Prevention (CDC) web site at http://www.cdc.gov/travel/index.htm is an excellent source of information with weekly updates. More specific information may also be obtained by calling the CDC hotline at 888-232-

Figure 20-1

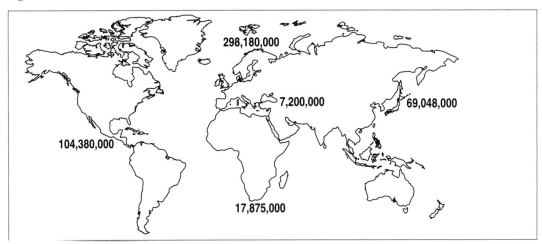

International tourist arrivals by region. (Reproduced with permission from SM Ostroff, P Kozarsky, *Infect Dis Clin North Am* 12:232, 1998.)

3228. We strongly recommend both of these as a supplement to the material presented in this chapter.

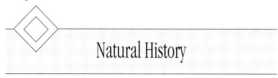

Natural History

One-third of travelers have travel-related illness. One study of travelers to eastern Europe and developing countries found diarrhea and upper respiratory illness to be the most common disor-

ders. Figure 20-2 further delineates travel-acquired illnesses reported by travelers to tropical areas. Infectious diseases account for most reported health problems.

Traveler's Diarrhea

Traveler's diarrhea is the bane of 20% to 50% of persons traveling to the developing world. Although rarely life threatening, traveler's diarrhea takes a toll in terms of work and vacation days lost. Enterotoxigenic and other pathogenic

Figure 20-2

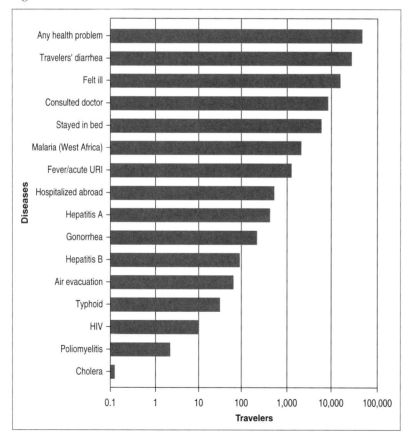

Estimated monthly prevalence of health problems per 100,000 travelers to tropical areas. (Reproduced with permission from L Dick, Travel medicine: Helping patients prepare for trips abroad. *Am Fam Phys* 58:385, 1998.)

strains of *Escherichia coli* are the most commonly identified organisms, accounting for 50% of cases. Other bacterial agents such as *Salmonella* and *Shigella* organisms, *Campylobacter jejuni*, and *Vibrio parahaemolyticus* have been identified. The role of viruses is less easy to document, but rotaviruses and hepatitis A are highly prevalent. Parasites, such as *Giardia, Entamoeba,* and *Cryptosporidium* organisms, are less common causes of traveler's diarrhea, but with the longer incubation periods of such parasites, clinical symptoms may begin weeks after the traveler has returned home.

Typhoid Fever

Typhoid fever, caused by *Salmonella typhi,* is endemic in the developing world. It is spread by feces-contaminated food and water and is characterized by bloody diarrhea and high fever. The incidence of typhoid fever is low among U.S. travelers (an estimated 58 to 174 cases per 1 million travelers). Mexico, Peru, Pakistan, and India are countries with higher transmission rates. Immunizations of moderate (70%) efficacy do exist and may be indicated for travelers who will be living in rural areas under less than sanitary conditions.

Hepatitis A

Hepatitis A is a viral disease characterized by nausea, vomiting, malaise, jaundice, and diarrhea. The incubation period of the virus is 15 to 50 days, so symptoms can appear long after the trip is over. Although it is endemic in developing nations, hepatitis A also is of low endemicity in developed nations. Risk for acquiring hepatitis A increases with duration of travel. In one study it was found that hepatitis A affected 5 of every 1000 short-term travelers and 2 of every 100 long-term travelers. It is the most common travel-related disease that can be prevented with vaccination.

Malaria

In 1997, the World Health Organization (WHO) estimated that high risk for malaria existed in 100 countries and territories. Every year travelers die of malaria. It is of utmost importance to consider the diagnosis of malaria in every returning traveler who has a fever. Between 300 and 500 million people worldwide are infected with one of the four species of malaria, *Plasmodium falciparum, P. vivax, P. malaria,* and *P. ovale.* Each year 25 to 30 million persons from nontropical countries visit malaria-endemic countries. As many as 30,000 North American and European travelers contract malaria annually. One does not have to travel far away or even out of his or her country of origin to be exposed. Outbreaks occurring near major airports have been dubbed "airport" or "runway" malaria. Cases have even been documented among travelers who never left the plane while at a stopover in a malaria-endemic area. It seems mosquitoes have joined the world of the frequent flyer!

Malaria causes between 1.5 and 2.7 million deaths annually. These deaths are almost exclusively caused by *P. falciparum* malaria. Most deaths occur in sub-Saharan Africa among children younger than 5 years of age, who have a higher case-fatality rate because they have not yet developed immunity. Travelers, because they also have not developed immunity, are at higher risk for death from *P. falciparum* malaria. Complicating the situation is the problem of *P. falciparum* drug resistance and resistance of the *Anopheles* mosquito vector to insecticides. Because of these two factors, malaria is reemerging in many parts of the world where it had previously been considered controlled.

Dengue Fever

Arboviral infections, especially dengue fever, are on the increase. Again, insecticide resistance of the insect vector, the *Aedes* mosquito, is a major reason. Approximately 100 million cases of dengue fever occur annually worldwide. Most of the reported cases among travelers occur among those returning from the Caribbean, Mexico, and Central and South America. Dengue causes high fevers and severe myalgia, thus earning its colloquial name, "break-bone fever." In its most severe forms, dengue hemorrhagic fever and dengue septic shock, this illness can lead to sepsis and death. An outbreak in Cuba in 1981 affected 344,203 persons, resulting in 116,000 hospitalizations and 158 deaths. There is currently no available vaccine or therapy for dengue. Persons who have had dengue and are later reinfected actually are more likely to suffer from severe forms of the disease. Immunization may therefore actually increase morbidity and mortality through unknown mechanisms of immune system activation. Avoidance of the mosquito vector is the principal means of prevention.

Yellow Fever

Yellow fever is another arboviral disease transmitted by *Aedes* mosquitoes. An estimated 200,000 cases occur annually, most in sub-Saharan Africa. This number has been increasing over the last decade. The case-fatality rate can be as high as 60% among persons who are not immune. Yellow fever is not a common disease among travelers, but fatal cases have occurred among unvaccinated tourists visiting rural areas within the yellow fever endemic areas of Africa and South America. Several countries require proof of vaccination before entry, especially for those arriving from endemic areas.

Cardiovascular Disease and Traumatic Injury

Although much of the focus of travel medicine is on infectious diseases, most travel-associated mortality among expatriates is caused by cardiovascular disease and motor vehicle crashes. Cardiovascular disease accounts for one-half of the deaths among U.S. travelers, and motor vehicle crashes are responsible for one-fourth. Each year 25,000 U.S. travelers are injured and 750 are killed in motor vehicles. Complicating this situation is a blood supply in many countries contaminated with HIV, hepatitis B virus, and hepatitis C virus, leading to an increased risk for acquisition of these infections if blood transfusions are performed after a traumatic injury.

Summary

Simple preventive measures can greatly reduce risk for acquisition of the aforementioned. Vaccines exist for several of the infectious diseases, chemoprophylaxis prevents malaria, and education focused on risk-reduction behavior minimizes the traveler's exposure to infectious and noninfectious diseases and trauma. Travelers also can be instructed that if prevention fails, self-initiation of treatment, especially for the diarrheal diseases and in some isolated settings, malaria, at the first sign of symptoms, can be effective. The clinician's first step is to identify travel-related risks.

Pretravel Risk Assessment

No two travelers are alike. Each has different travel-associated risks. Patients ideally should visit their clinician 6 to 8 weeks before anticipated travel. This allows ample time for vaccine administration and initiation of chemoprophylactic medication. The pretravel risk assessment may be aided by development of a questionnaire the patient completes before meeting with the physician. The focus of questions for the assessment of travel risk should be epidemiologic, that is, based on place and time period of desired travel and the person's general health status.

Place and Time

Risk varies greatly with itinerary. It is important to know whether the patient is planning a trip to an urban or a rural area. Knowledge of accommodations (e.g., a four-star hotel versus camping in the wilderness) also is important. How many days, weeks, or months will the patient be traveling? Many tropically acquired illnesses (e.g., trypanosomiasis, schistosomiasis) rarely are acquired by travelers making brief trips to urban centers. Such diseases are more common among medical missionaries and others who stay in rural areas for prolonged periods.

Person

Age and sex are important factors to consider in the pretravel risk assessment. The very old and very young have higher case-fatality rates for most infectious diseases. Especially for these groups, routine vaccination status should be reviewed to make sure they are current. Pregnancy or the presence of a chronic disease also influences prevention planning.

THE PREGNANT TRAVELER

Women who are pregnant or planning pregnancy deserve special attention, not only to routine preventive measures such as prenatal vitamins containing folate, which may not be available in some countries, but also to unique travel-associated risks. They should not receive live-virus vaccines, and no safety data exist for many of the inactivated vaccines. Therefore the clinician must discuss specific travel risks in relation to the planned itinerary. The risks and benefits of specific vaccinations must be care

fully weighed with the patient. Certain chemo-prophylaxis and treatment agents such as doxy-cycline for malaria or ciprofloxacin for traveler's diarrhea are unsafe during pregnancy. Alternative medicines that are safe in pregnancy should be offered.

Travel in the third trimester should be discussed. In some instances, patient and clinician may want to postpone travel until after delivery, if possible. Most airlines restrict the travel of pregnant women after 36 weeks' gestation. Women anticipating delivery in another country should be informed of the level of obstetric and neonatal care facilities available and the safety of blood products should transfusion be necessary. Pregnant patients should be aware that many insurance plans do not cover deliveries outside a designated area.

PERSONS WITH CHRONIC DISEASE

Patients with chronic conditions such as diabetes and asthma pose unique challenges. Persons with diabetes, especially those who need insulin, should be aware that travel and time zone changes may affect blood glucose level. Regular eating intervals should be maintained as much as possible in spite of time zone changes. Increased blood glucose monitoring may be appropriate. The patient should be educated to alter insulin dosing according to blood glucose values.

Exposure to upper respiratory illnesses or secondhand smoke during prolonged airplane trips may make exacerbations of asthma likely. High altitudes, temperature variations, and dust also may trigger asthma. Patients should be instructed in appropriate use of an inhaler and may want to consider regular use of an inhaled steroid while traveling. For reliable patients, the clinician may consider giving a limited supply of oral steroids so that the patient may initiate treatment if standard medical care is difficult to reach in a timely manner.

PERSONS WITH IMMUNOCOMPROMISE OR HIV INFECTION

Immunocompromised persons or those with HIV infection may be at increased risk for acquiring opportunistic infections when traveling. The use of prophylactic antibiotics by travelers with HIV infection has not been well studied, but empirical therapy for traveler's diarrhea is recommended. In general, BCG (Bacille Calmette-Guérin) and live virus vaccines, such as oral polio, oral typhoid, varicella, and yellow fever should be avoided. Inactivated vaccines are available for several of these diseases and are discussed later. There are conflicting recommendations regarding measles vaccine, but 1998 CDC guidelines do support the use of measles vaccine in the care of persons with HIV infection. Persons with HIV infection who are planning extended stays (e.g., those involved in study-abroad programs) should be aware that many nations will not issue visas without documentation of a negative result of an HIV test.

Immunizations

Although immunizations are not the only reason to visit a clinician before embarking on a trip, vaccines are an important part of disease prevention. Vaccines can be thought of in two categories—required and recommended. The recommended vaccines can be further classified into those that are routinely given in the United States but that may require a booster (e.g., tetanus-diphtheria toxoid [Td], polio), and special vaccinations (e.g., typhoid, hepatitis A) unique to travel.

Required Immunizations

YELLOW FEVER

Yellow fever vaccine is the only vaccine still required by some countries. Under the international health regulations adopted by the WHO, certificates of vaccination are necessary and must be shown to port-of-entry officials in the countries listed in Table 20-2. The CDC recommends the vaccine to travelers anticipating stays in areas where yellow fever is endemic, especially for travel to rural areas, even if not required by those nations (sub-Saharan Africa and parts of South America; Figure 20-3). Current information on countries requiring proof of vaccination and those for which vaccination is recommended can be obtained through the blue sheet on the CDC web site (http://www.cdc.gov/travel/index.htm) or by calling the 24-hour telephone line at 888-232-3228.

Table 20-2

Countries That Require Yellow Fever Vaccination Certificate for Direct Travel from the United States

Benin	French Guiana	Niger
Burkina Faso	Gabon	Rwanda
Cameroon	Ghana	Sao Tome and Principe
Central African Republic	Liberia	Togo
Congo	Mali	Zaire
Côe d'Ivoire	Mauritania (for stay >2 wk)	

For travel to and between other countries, check the individual country requirements.
SOURCE: Centers for Disease Control and Prevention, 1996–1997.

Figure 20-3a

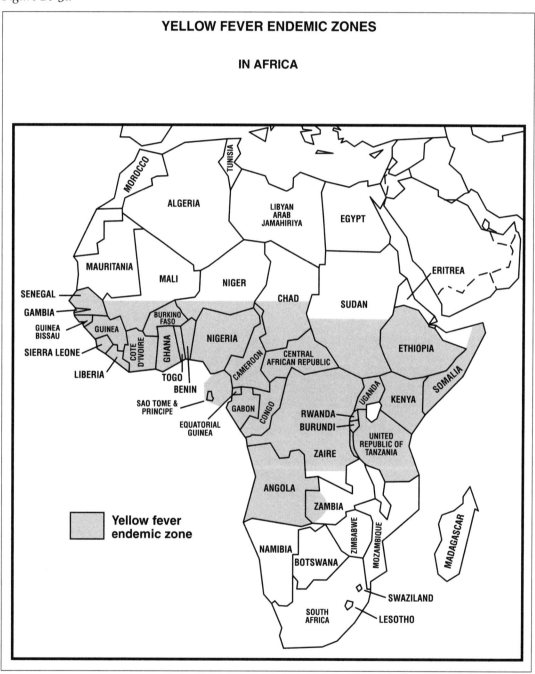

Yellow fever endemic zones. (Reproduced from Centers for Disease Control and Prevention, 1996–1997.)

Figure 20-3b

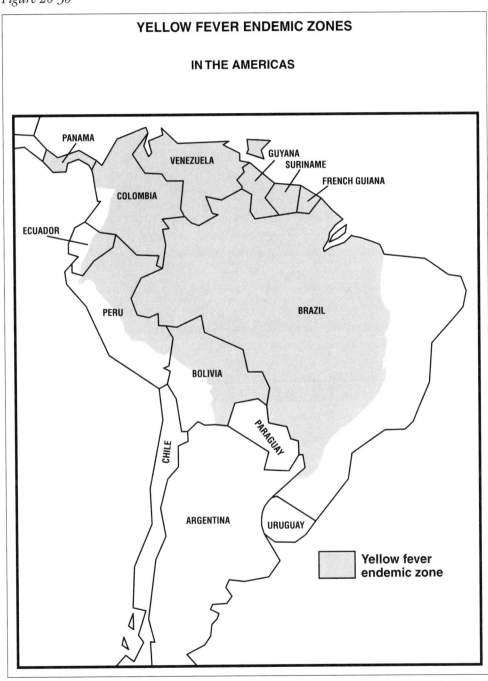

Yellow fever endemic zones. (Reproduced from Centers for Disease Control and Prevention, 1996–1997.)

Yellow fever vaccine is highly effective. It is an attenuated, live-virus vaccine and is produced by several manufacturers worldwide, which must be approved by WHO. The vaccine must be administered at an approved yellow fever vaccination center. Information on approved centers and how to obtain approval can be obtained from the local health department. The vaccine is administered in a 0.5 mL subcutaneous dose at least 10 days before entry into the endemic area. A booster is recommended every 10 years (Table 20-3).

Yellow fever vaccine is absolutely contraindicated for infants younger than 4 months of age because of a number of reported cases of vaccine-induced encephalitis among this age group. For infants 4 to 9 months of age yellow fever vaccine may be considered if travel is planned to an endemic area, but the risk for vaccine-induced encephalitis remains. After 9 months of age the vaccine is considered safe. Because it is a live-virus vaccine, use of yellow fever vaccine is generally contraindicated for use in pregnant women or immunocompromised persons. However, if a patient is traveling to an endemic area where the potential for infection is high, vaccination may be considered. The CDC recommends that clinicians discuss with their patients the risks and benefits in these special circumstances.

Recommended Immunizations

ROUTINE IMMUNIZATIONS

Booster doses of all the standard vaccinations given in the United States are recommended for travelers. Persons who have not completed the primary series should do so before travel. These vaccines, including primary series, accelerated series, and booster doses, are discussed in Chapters 1 and 19. A summary follows.

DIPHTHERIA-TETANUS-PERTUSSIS   Diphtheria, tetanus, and pertussis are common in many countries where routine immunization is not available. Pertussis outbreaks also have been reported in several areas in the United States. All children should therefore receive the primary series, which may be given according to the accelerated schedule. A Td booster is recommended for adults every 10 years. This booster dose can be given in pregnancy and to immunocompromised individuals.

HAEMOPHILUS INFLUENZAE TYPE B   All children younger than 5 years of age should receive vaccination against *Haemophilus influenzae.* This vaccine is not indicated in the care of persons 5 years of age and older unless an immunocompromising condition exists. The vaccine may be given to persons with HIV infection, but the immune response may vary depending on the stage of HIV infection.

HEPATITIS B   Hepatitis B is a disease of low endemicity in the United States but is highly endemic in southeast Asia, China, Africa, the Middle East, the Amazon Basin, the Dominican Republic, and Haiti (see Figure 20-4). In the United States the vaccine is recommended for children, adolescents, and occupational groups at high risk for exposure to blood products. Travelers to areas of high or intermediate endemicity who are planning a stay of more than 6 months should receive the vaccine. Health care workers or travelers anticipating sexual contact with local populations also should receive the vaccine. Hepatitis B vaccine may be administered to immunocompromised persons. Pregnancy is not a contraindication to vaccination.

INFLUENZA   During fall and winter (October to March in the northern hemisphere and April to September in the southern hemisphere) travelers should be encouraged to receive vaccination against influenza. Travelers to the tropics should consider the vaccine regardless of the time of year. This vaccine may be used by pregnant women after 14 weeks' gestation and by children older than 6 months of age. The vaccine should be offered to persons with HIV infection and those with immunocompromising conditions.

MEASLES-MUMPS-RUBELLA   All persons born in or after 1957 who have not had two documented doses of MMR vaccine should receive a booster. This vaccine is contraindicated in the care of women who are pregnant or are planning to become pregnant within 3 months of vaccination. In general, the MMR vaccine should not be given to immunocompromised persons. Those infected with HIV, however, may receive the vaccine because limited studies have shown no adverse effects. The CDC therefore does recommend that the MMR vaccine be offered to all adult travelers who have HIV infection who are not severely immunocompromised. If immune globulin (rather than the vaccine) is used to prevent hepatitis A, MMR vaccine should be administered at least 14 days before immunoglobulin. MMR and yellow fever vaccination may be administered at the same time, but if not given concomitantly, should be separated by a 1-month interval.

PNEUMOCOCCAL INFECTION   Pneumococcal vaccine should be offered to all adults older than 65 years of age. Persons with asplenia or those with chronic diseases, including HIV infection or immunocompromise, should receive the vaccine. The vaccine should not be given to children younger than 2 years of age. Although it is an inactivated bacterial vaccine and not contraindicated in pregnancy, pneumococcal vaccine need not be given to pregnant women unless the risk for acquiring pneumococcal disease is great.

POLIOMYELITIS   A polio booster is recommended for travelers to countries in which wild poliovirus is endemic or epidemic, that is, most developing countries (except in Latin America) and eastern Europe. Adults who need a booster should receive inactivated polio vaccine (IPV).

Use of oral polio vaccine (OPV) is contraindicated in the care of immunocompromised persons; IPV is preferred. In general, OPV and IPV should be avoided by pregnant women. According to WHO, however, OPV may be administered to pregnant women when the risk for acquiring disease is considered great.

VARICELLA   Any person who has never had chickenpox should be offered the varicella vaccine. Use of this vaccine is contraindicated in the care of pregnant women or those planning pregnancy within 3 months of receiving the vaccine. It also is contraindicated in the care of persons with HIV infection and immunocompromise.

SPECIAL IMMUNIZATIONS

CHOLERA   Cholera vaccination is neither required nor recommended by WHO for international travelers, because their risk for acquiring cholera is very low. Although no country officially requires proof of immunization, according to anecdotal information from travelers, local authorities do occasionally demand this before granting entry. The CDC recommends cholera immunization for those who will be living and working for an extended time in endemic areas with unsanitary conditions without access to medical care. Routine travelers to endemic areas still need to follow food and beverage precautions (discussed later).

Cholera vaccine is an inactivated-bacteria vaccine. It is 50% effective against the El Tor strain, *V. cholerae* 01, but is not effective against *V. cholerae* 0139, the so-called Bengal strain which was identified in south Asia in 1992. A new oral vaccine is available in Switzerland and Canada and may become available in the United States. It, however, also is not effective against the Bengal strain.

The primary adult series for the injectable cholera vaccine consists of two 0.5 mL doses administered subcutaneously or intramuscularly

Table 20-3
Travel-related Vaccinations

Vaccine	Vaccine Type	Adult Primary Series	Time Interval Between Last Dose and Expected Travel	Booster	Contraindications[a]	Interactions
Yellow fever	Attenuated, live virus	0.5 mL SC, one time dose	10 d	Every 10 yr	Children <4 mo, *Children 4–9 mo, pregnancy, immunocompromise, HIV*	Cholera, (separate by 3 wk) MMR (give at same time or 1 mo apart)
Cholera	Inactivated bacteria	0.5 mL SC, IM, or 0.2 mL ID, 2 doses, 1 wk apart	6 d	Every 6 mo	*Pregnancy* Children <6 mo	Yellow fever (separate by 3 wk)
Hepatitis A	Inactivated virus	1 mL IM	4 wk	6–12 mo after first dose, (unclear how long immunity lasts)	Children <2 yr *Pregnancy*	Immune globulin (give at different site)
Hepatitis A immune globulin	Serum globulin	0.02 mL/kg IM (length of stay <3 months) 0.06 mL/kg (length of stay >3 months)	2 d	Every 6 mo	—	Hepatitis A (give at different site) measles vaccine (give 14 d before or 3 mo after immune globulin)
Japanese B encephalitis	Inactivated virus	1.0 mL SC dose on days 0, 7, and 30	10 d	Every 3 yr (unclear how long immunity lasts)	Children <1 yr *Pregnancy*	—

Disease	Vaccine	Dose			Contraindications	Comments
Meningococcal disease	Polysaccharide, inactivated bacteria sero groups A/C/Y/W-135	0.5 mL SC single dose	1–2 wk	3–5 yr	Children <2, *Pregnancy*	—
Rabies	Inactivated virus	HDCV, RVA, PCEC 1.0 mL IM deltoid muscle or 0.1 mL HDCV ID days 0, 7, 21 or 28	30 d	2 yr	*Pregnancy*	Antimalarials with HDVC given ID (use IM if doses cannot be completed before start of antimalarials)
Typhoid	Typhoid V_1, polysaccharide	0.5 mL IM 1 dose	2 wk	Every 2 yr	*Pregnancy*	
	Ty21a, attenuated bacteria	1 capsule days 0, 2, 4, 6	1 wk	Every 5 yr	*Pregnancy*, HIV, immuno-compromise	Mefloquine
	Typhoid, heat phenol inactivated	0.5 mL SQ 2 doses 4 wks apart	2 wk	Every 3 yr	*Pregnancy*	

[a] Italics indicate relative contraindication.

ABBREVIATIONS: HDCV, human diploid cell vaccine; RVA, rabies vaccine, absorbed; PCEC, purified chick embryo cell vaccine.

Figure 20-4

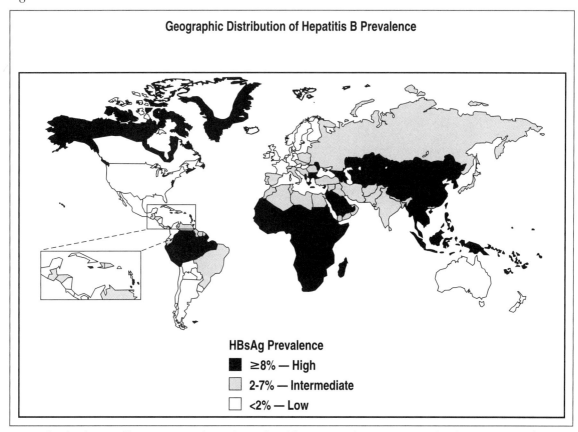

Geographic distribution of hepatitis B prevalence. (Reproduced from Centers for Disease Control and Prevention, 1996–1997.)

1 week apart. The vaccine also can be given intradermally in a 0.2 mL dose. A single dose 6 days before entry should be enough to satisfy countries with unofficial vaccination requirements. The vaccine is effective for only 3 to 6 months, so a booster at 6 months is indicated. The vaccine, if time permits, should be given 3 weeks before or after yellow fever vaccine, because decreased efficacy of both has been documented with concomitant administration. Although the injectable vaccine is inactivated, no data exist regarding its efficacy and safety in pregnancy. Given the low risk for acquiring cholera for most travelers, it would rarely be

indicated for pregnant women. Persons with HIV infection also would rarely need vaccination, but the vaccine is not contraindicated for them.

HEPATITIS A Hepatitis A vaccine is recommended for travelers to countries where the infection is highly or intermediately endemic (Figure 20-5). The two vaccines are inactivated-virus vaccines and are highly efficacious. The first dose (adult dose is 1 mL given intramuscularly) should be administered at least 4 weeks before travel. A booster dose may be given 6 to 12 months after the first. It is unclear how long

Figure 20-5

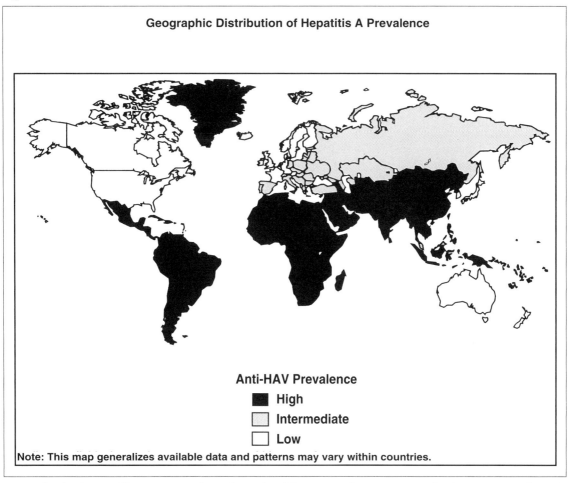

Geographic distribution of hepatitis A prevalence. (Reproduced from Centers for Disease Control and Prevention, 1996–1997.)

immunity lasts, because currently available vaccines have been evaluated only over a 5-year period.

Hepatitis A vaccine should not be given to children younger than 2 years of age. No data exist concerning safety in pregnancy. Therefore clinician and patient should discuss risks and benefits. The vaccine may be used in the care of immunocompromised individuals.

HEPATITIS A IMMUNOGLOBULIN (IMMUNE SERUM GLOB-ULIN) Immune globulin until relatively recently was the only option for hepatitis A protection. Now the vaccine is preferred because of its higher efficacy and longer duration of action. Travelers, however, who will depart in less than 4 weeks still may benefit from immune globulin in addition to hepatitis A vaccine. Immune globulin is safe for children younger than 2 years of age. It is 60% to 70% efficacious. A single intra-muscular injection of 0.02 mL/kg should be administered for persons planning a 3-month stay or less. A dose of 0.06 ml/kg is needed for stays longer than 3 months and is effective for up to 6 months. Immune globulin may be given at the same time as hepatitis A vaccine, but it should be given at a different site and may decrease antibody production. Immune globulin may be given in pregnancy and can be given to immunocompromised persons. No bloodborne infections have been traced to immune globulin produced in the United States.

JAPANESE B ENCEPHALITIS Japanese B encephalitis vaccination is recommended for travelers to China, Korea, the Indian subcontinent, and southeast Asia who are planning a trip longer than 1 month's duration or who will be spending time in rural areas where exposure to the Culex mosquito vector is highest. Because the risk for acquiring Japanese B encephalitis varies with season, consultation with the CDC web site (see earlier) is recommended. Transmission rates are highest between May and September.

The Japanese B encephalitis vaccine is composed of inactivated virus. The primary series for those 3 years of age and older is 1.0 mL given subcutaneously in three doses on days 0, 7, and 30. The last dose should be given at least 10 days before travel. This schedule may be shortened with the last dose administered on day 14 if travel plans do not allow the preferred schedule. Two doses 1 week apart may be given but will confer only short-term immunity among 80% of persons vaccinated. For children 1 to 3 years of age the same schedule is followed, but 0.5 mL is given. A booster dose may be given after 3 years, but duration of immunity is unknown. The vaccine is not recommended for children aged younger than 1 year and has not been tested in pregnancy. It should therefore be given in pregnancy only if the risk for acquiring disease is high. Japanese B encephalitis vaccination is not contraindicated for persons with HIV infection or immunocompromise.

MENINGOCOCCAL DISEASE Vaccination against meningococcus is recommended for travelers to the so-called meningococcus belt, consisting mostly of countries in sub-Saharan Africa (see Figure 20-6). Although the disease is rare among U.S. travelers, the vaccination is advised by the CDC especially for those planning extended stays in this area. The CDC has rescinded its recommendations for countries outside the belt, namely Burundi, Tanzania, Kenya, Mongolia, Nepal, and northern India. Travelers to these countries no longer need to be vaccinated. The vaccine is still required by the Saudi Arabian government for travelers making the annual *hajj*.

The meningococcus vaccine is a polysaccharide, inactivated-bacteria vaccine. It is 80% to 95% effective against serogroups A, C, Y, and W-135 but not against B. The B serogroup is responsible for one-half of cases of meningitis in the United States and recently has caused several epidemics in Brazil and Chile. The vaccine is administered in a 0.5 mL subcutaneous dose 1 to 2 weeks before departure. A booster dose every 3 to 5 years is recommended.

Although no adverse effects have been found among pregnant patients, the vaccine is not recommended for pregnant women unless the risk for acquiring disease is very high. Meningococcal vaccine should not be given to children younger than 2 years of age. The vaccine may be given to immunocompromised persons.

RABIES Travelers planning trips longer than 30 days to areas in which a high prevalence of dog rabies exists should consider rabies vaccination. The vaccine also is recommended for spelunkers (cave explorers) and those working with animals. Postexposure prophylaxis also is highly efficacious, but may not be available in some areas.

The preexposure rabies series consists of one of three inactivated-virus vaccines: human diploid cell vaccine (HDCV); rabies vaccine, adsorbed (RVA); and purified, chick embryo cell

Figure 20-6

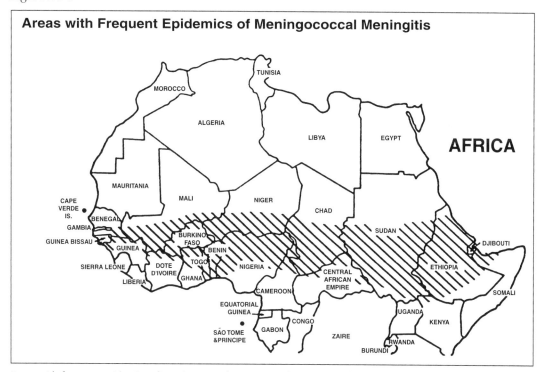

Areas with Frequent Epidemics of Meningococcal Meningitis

Areas with frequent epidemics of meningococcal meningitis. (Reproduced from Centers for Disease Control and Prevention, 1996–1997.)

vaccine (PCEC). A dose of 1.0 mL is given into the deltoid muscle on days 0, 7, and 21 or 28. To decrease cost, the HDCV vaccine also may be given as 0.1 mL intradermally on the same schedule. However, vaccination should be completed before the administration of antimalarial agents because antimalarials have been shown to interfere with the development of immunity when HDCV is given intradermally.

All travelers should be advised to immediately cleanse all wounds with soap and water and to seek medical attention after any animal bite or scratch so that rabies immunoglobulin (if preexposure vaccination has not been administered) and postexposure prophylaxis may be given.

Neither pregnancy nor immunocompromise is a contraindication to postexposure prophylaxis. Preexposure vaccination of pregnant women is recommended only if the risk for exposure to disease is high.

TYPHOID Typhoid vaccine is recommended by the CDC for persons traveling in endemic areas for longer than 3 weeks. Three bacteria-derived vaccine options are: (1) a new, injectable, polysaccharide vaccine (Typhim Vi), (2) an oral, live-attenuated vaccine (Ty21a), and (3) the old, heat-phenol inactivated vaccine (typhoid vaccine). Efficacy is in the 50% to 80% range for all three. Dosing and administration vary (Table 20-3). Depending on the vaccine, the primary series should be completed 1 to 2 weeks before travel.

The Typhim Vi and Ty21a vaccines are preferred because of their lower side-effect profiles; however, the oral vaccine should not be given to immunocompromised travelers. The oral vaccine also should not be given with mefloquine, because coadministration can diminish the effectiveness of the vaccine. No data exist about use of any of the vaccines during pregnancy, but theoretical risks to the fetus exist with use of the live-attenuated, Ty21a vaccine and the often fever-inducing typhoid vaccine.

Screening

Tuberculosis

There is no efficacious vaccine against tuberculosis. BCG vaccine is not recommended for travelers because of its low efficacy.

The purified protein derivative (PPD) skin test remains the most sensitive and specific screening test for early detection of *Mycobacterium tuberculosis*. Early detection of asymptomatic infection allows for treatment with isoniazid to prevent development of active disease.

Skin testing before travel is recommended for persons planning to live and work in close, crowded conditions in countries where rates of tuberculosis are high. Testing should be repeated when the traveler returns and 3 months after potential exposure. The PPD test should not be administered immediately after vaccination with live-virus because of risk for a false-negative result. The PPD test should be begun the same day or 4 to 6 weeks after live-virus vaccines are administered. A PPD result is measured according to amount of induration not of erythema. The size of reaction considered a positive result varies with age and risk (Table 20-4).

Table 20-4

Classification of Tuberculosis Skin Test

≥5 MM IS POSITIVE
Persons known or believed to have HIV infection
Close contacts of a person with infectious tuberculosis (TB)
Those with a chest radiograph suggestive of TB
Persons who inject drugs if their HIV status is unknown

≥10 MM IS POSITIVE
Persons with the following medical conditions 　Diabetes 　Silicosis 　Cancer of the head and neck 　Hematologic and reticuloendothelial diseases 　End-stage renal disease 　Intestinal bypass or gastrectomy 　Chronic malabsorption 　Prolonged corticosteroid therapy 　Other immunosuppressive therapy
Persons who inject drugs if HIV negative
Foreign-born persons from areas with high TB rates
Medically underserved, low-income populations
Residents of long-term care facilities
Children younger than 4 yr of age
Locally identified high-risk groups

≥15 MM POSITIVE
All persons with no known risk factors for TB

For adult travelers who have not undergone a tuberculosis skin test in several years, a two-step test is recommended. Delayed-type hypersensitivity to tuberculin can wane over the years. This can cause a negative reaction among those tested years after infection. A skin test can boost immunity, causing a positive reaction to subsequent tests. This boosted reaction may be misinterpreted as recent infection or skin test conversion. To avoid this, two-step testing is recommended. If the first test reaction is negative, a second skin test is performed 1 to 3 weeks later. A positive reaction to the second skin test represents a positive test result and is most likely a boosted reaction, indicating past infection.

Differentiating a boosted reaction from true skin test conversion is important because isoniazid might be or might not be recommended to a traveler whose pretrip skin test result is positive. Determining factors are age, history of exposure, and likely time since infection. Isoniazid is recommended for a returned traveler whose skin test reaction indicates recent infection, unless a contraindication to prophylaxis exists.

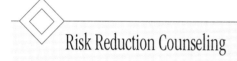

Risk Reduction Counseling

Although immunizations and screening are important, risk reduction counseling is an effective means to ensure that patients have a safe, healthy travel experience. Counseling should be aimed at accident prevention, insect avoidance, and prevention of traveler's diarrhea and sexually transmitted diseases.

Injuries and Blood Transfusions

Because trauma (motor vehicle crashes, in particular) is one of the leading causes of travel-related death, travelers should be instructed to use seat belts. Night travel should be restricted because many countries lack adequate street lighting. This in addition to the presence of animals and livestock on the road makes evening travel in rural areas especially hazardous.

Travelers should be advised to use the same common-sense approaches to risk reduction recommended in the United States, such as use of seat belts and shoulder harnesses, driving vehicles that are in good condition and equipped with airbags and antilock brakes, avoiding driving when impaired by alcohol or drugs, not riding with an impaired driver, and using protective head gear when riding a motorcycle or bicycle.

Travelers visiting countries where cars travel on the left side of the road should be advised to be cautious and look in both directions before crossing streets. The potential to be a victim of violence can be minimized by seeking and heeding advice from local residents and tour guides about areas and situations to avoid.

In the event of a serious accident in another country, travelers need to be advised of their options regarding blood transfusion. All blood products should be screened for HIV, hepatitis B virus, hepatitis C virus, and *Plasmodium* organisms before being administered. If a nonemergency surgical procedure is planned, the patient should be informed of the option of donations from known donors, such as family members or coworkers who have consented to blood product testing.

Insect-borne Infectious Diseases

Avoidance is by far the most effective strategy for dealing with most of the infectious diseases for which vaccines do not exist. For mosquito-borne or other insect-borne illnesses, travelers should be advised to wear protective clothing, such as long-sleeved shirts tucked into long pants or full-length skirts. Because many insects are most active in the early morning and early evening hours, travelers should limit their exposure at these times by staying indoors, ideally in a screened environment. They also should be instructed to use insect repellents containing diethyltoluamide (DEET) which is highly efficacious. DEET is toxic in high concentrations, and concentrations vary markedly among products. Rare cases of toxic encephalopathy have occurred among children exposed to DEET. To minimize this risk, a maximum of 10% DEET should be used on children and 30% on adults. Travelers should be advised to apply these products sparingly to exposed skin and avoid contact with eyes or mucous membranes. Repellents used correctly provide hours of effective relief and protection. They should be washed off as soon as possible after risk for exposure has passed.

Sleeping under permethrin-coated bed nets also effectively reduces risk for exposure to insect-borne diseases not only for travelers but also for local populations. Bed nets or small-net tents may be purchased from camping stores in the United States and from WHO. These nets may then be dipped in or sprayed with permethrin.

Traveler's Diarrhea

Travelers should eat only properly cooked foods (e.g., no salads or fresh fruit that is not peeled.) They should be warned against eating raw or partially cooked meat and consuming unpasteurized milk and milk products, such as cheese. The potential for ciguatera fish poisoning exists with many types of sea fish and is unpredictable, especially in the tropics and subtropics. Sea fish should probably be avoided.

Water should never be obtained from the tap unless the water supply is known to be safe. Finding reliable information on the safety of local water supplies can be a challenge. If there are times when the water system does not work, this indicates that water pressure is not being maintained. Because constant water pressure is necessary to maintain purity, this is an indicator of an unsafe system. Constant pressure, however, does not guarantee safe water.

Bottled water and other bottled, carbonated drinks may be safely consumed, but water on the outside of the container and on the container opening should be wiped off with a clean cloth. Travelers often forget and therefore need to be reminded that tooth brushing should be performed with bottled, not tap, water. Ice

cubes also should be avoided because freezing does not effectively kill the pathogens responsible for traveler's diarrhea.

If bottled water is not available, water can be purified by means of boiling, iodine treatment, or filtration. Water should be boiled for 1 minute. At high altitudes (>2 km [6562 ft]), water should be boiled for 3 minutes. Iodine treatment can be done with tincture of iodine or iodine-containing tablets, which can be purchased from sporting goods or camping stores. The manufacturer's instructions should be followed. Filtration has not been as well studied as the other two methods, and efficacy may vary depending on the features of the specific filter. These devices may be purchased from sporting goods or camping stores.

Sexually Transmitted Diseases

All travelers should also be educated about safe sex practices (e.g., appropriate condom use) before travel. Abstinence is the safest strategy.

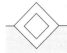

Chemoprophylaxis

Malaria

Travelers to areas where malaria is endemic should be given chemoprophylaxis with appropriate instructions. Clinicians should contact the CDC hotline to obtain the most up to date recommendations, which vary with season and itinerary. Whether chloroquine-resistant *P. falciparum* (CRPF) is present in an area can be learned through the CDC hotline. This vital information helps one determine optimum regimens for chemoprophylaxis. At present CRPF is widespread wherever malaria is present, except in the Dominican Republic, Haiti, Central America west of the Panama Canal Zone, Egypt, and most countries of the Middle East (Figure 20-7).

Figure 20-7

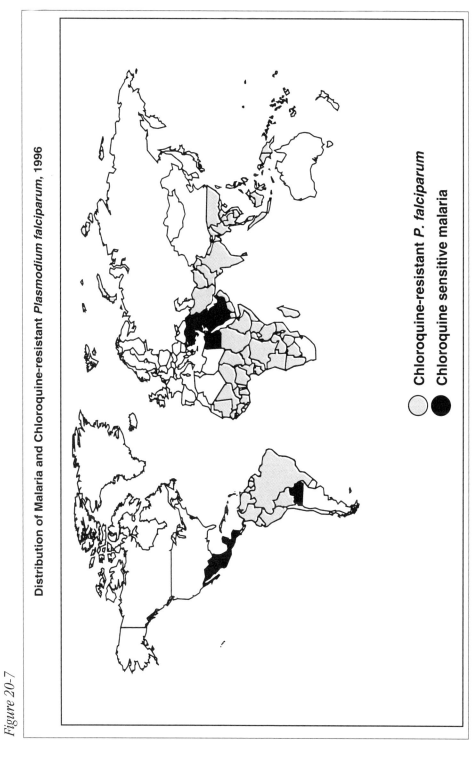

Distribution of malaria and chloroquine-resistant *P. falciparum*, 1996. Source: Health Information for the International Traveler. U.S. Department of Health and Human Services, Center for Disease Control, Atlanta, Georgia, 1996–1997.

The CDC recommends mefloquine for the prevention of CRPF (Table 20-5). It should be initiated 2 weeks before travel and taken in a dose of 250 mg a week. This dosage should be continued for 4 weeks after return from an area where malaria is endemic. Patients need to be warned of possible side effects of mefloquine, including gastrointestinal upset, insomnia, dizziness, and in rare instances psychosis and convulsions. Mefloquine therefore is contraindicated for use by those with psychiatric or seizure disorders. It also is contraindicated for patients with cardiac arrhythmias.

Daily doxycycline is an effective alternative to mefloquine (except for pregnant women and children younger than 8 years). It should be taken in a dose of 100 mg daily started 2 days before departure and continued for 4 weeks

Table 20-5

Drugs Used in the Prophylaxis of Malaria

DRUG	ADULT DOSE	PEDIATRIC DOSAGE
Mefloquine	228 mg base (250 mg salt) orally once a week	<15 kg: 4.6 mg/kg (base); 5 mg/kg (salt) 15–19 kg: ¼ tab/wk 20–30 kg: ½ tab/wk 31–45 kg: ¾ tab/wk >45 kg: 1 tab/wk
Doxycycline	100 mg orally once a day	>8 yr: 2 mg/kg body weight orally once a day up to adult dose of 100 mg/day
Chloroquine phosphate	300 mg base (500 mg salt) orally once a week	5 mg/kg base (8.3 mg/kg salt) orally once a week up to maximum adult dose of 300 mg base
Hydroxychloroquine sulfate	310 mg base (400 mg salt) orally once a week	5 mg/kg base (6.5 mg/kg salt) orally once a week up to maximum adult dose
Proguanil	200 mg orally once a day in combination with weekly chloroquine	<2 years: 50 mg/day 2–6 years: 100 mg/day 7–10 years: 150 mg/day >10 years: 200 mg/day
Primaquine	15 mg base (26.3 mg salt) orally once a day for 14 days	0.3 mg/kg base (0.5 mg/kg salt) orally once a day for 14 days
For Presumptive treatment pyrimethamine sulfadoxine (Fansidar)	3 tablets (75 mg pyrimethamine and 1500 mg sulfadoxine) orally as a single dose	5–10 kg : ½ tablet 11–20 : 1 tablet 21–30 : 1½ tablet 31–45 : 2 tablets >45 : 3 tablets

SOURCE. Centers for Disease Control and Prevention, 1996–1997.

after return. Side effects include gastrointestinal upset and photosensitivity. It is the drug of choice for those traveling to Thailand, where mefloquine resistance has been well documented.

Chloroquine in combination with proguanil is a third, much less effective option for patients with contraindications to both mefloquine and doxycycline. Studies have found increased efficacy of chloroquine taken with proguanil for prophylaxis of CRPF compared with use of chloroquine alone. This is true for travelers to Africa but not those who travel to Thailand. Travelers who use chloroquine with proguanil also may be given a treatment dose of pyrimethamine-sulfadoxine. In the event of high fever, the traveler can take three pyrimethamine-sulfadoxine tablets by mouth as a one-time dose and seek prompt medical attention. Table 20-4 shows pediatric dosages. Persons with an allergy to sulfa-containing drugs should not take pyrimethamine-sulfadoxine.

For patients traveling to those rapidly diminishing areas of the world in which there exists no documented chloroquine resistance, chloroquine remains a reasonable option. The dose is 500 mg of the salt or 300 mg of the base taken once a week. Doses should start 2 weeks before departure and continue for 4 weeks on return. Side effects can include gastrointestinal upset, headaches, dizziness, blurred vision, and pruritis.

After completing travel to an area where *P. vivax* or *P. ovale* is heavily endemic, it also is of vital importance to take primaquine in a dose of 26.3 mg of the salt once a day for 2 weeks. This is the only drug known to be efficacious in managing the hepatic forms or hypnozoites of these two species, which can remain dormant in the liver for years. (*P. falciparum* and *P. malariae* do not have hepatic forms.) This drug should not be used by persons with glucose-6-phosphate dehydrogenase deficiency, because hemolytic anemia can occur. It also is contraindicated during pregnancy.

Women who are pregnant or planning pregnancy may take chloroquine, which should be combined with daily doses of proguanil as described for those planning travel in CRPF areas. On returning from areas where P. ovale or P. vivax is endemic, pregnant patients can continue weekly chloroquine during the remainder of the pregnancy followed by 2 weeks of primaquine dosage after delivery.

Traveler's Diarrhea

For prevention of traveler's diarrhea, avoidance is by far the best option. Although several agents have been evaluated, controversy remains in regard to their role in chemoprophylaxis. Diphenoxylate and other antiperistaltic agents have not been shown to prevent traveler's diarrhea; use of diphenoxylate actually may increase the likelihood of occurrence. Drugs such as halogenated hydroxyquinoline derivatives (e.g., clioquinil, iodoquinil, MexaForm, Intestospan, and Enterovioform) have not been demonstrated to be effective and have serious side effects.

Bismuth subsalicylate found in brand name Pepto-Bismol has been shown to decrease the incidence of traveler's diarrhea by as much as 60% when taken in high doses (2 tablets or 2 oz. [60 mL] four times a day). However, side effects caused by and contraindications owing to the salicylate content (e.g., potential for Reye's syndrome among children) call into question routine use of this medicine. The CDC states that bismuth subsalicylate may be effective but is not recommended for more than 3 weeks' use.

The CDC does not recommend use of any antimicrobial agent for prophylaxis of traveler's diarrhea. Several studies have shown 52% to 95% efficacy of these agents, but varying resistance patterns and serious potential side effects make routine use unattractive. No studies have demonstrated a benefit to use of these agents by immunocompromised persons.

A traveler who contracts a diarrheal illness while traveling can be advised to take medicines for symptom control or treatment. Activated charcoal is ineffective at producing symptom relief, as are kaolin and pectin preparations, although the latter two might improve stool consistency. Lactobacillus-containing preparations have not been well studied. Bismuth subsalicylate (1 oz. [30 mL] every 30 minutes for 8 doses) has been shown to decrease stooling and shorten the duration of illness. However, patients with aspirin allergy or other contraindications should be advised not to use this medicine. Antimotility agents (e.g., opiates, diphenoxylate, and loperamide) can provide temporary symptomatic relief but should not be used in the presence of high fever, bloody stools, or symptoms that persist more than 48 hours.

Antimicrobial agents, such as ciprofloxacin in a dose of 500 mg two a day for 3 days, are effective treatment and may be prescribed before travel for use if diarrhea occurs. Ciprofloxacin is not recommended for pregnant women or children, but trimethoprim-sulfamethoxazole is a reasonable alternative for children and pregnant women between 12 and 36 weeks' gestation. It should be used twice a day for 3 days.

Hydration is crucial, ideally with a balanced electrolyte solution. Such a solution can be prepared with relatively simple ingredients—salt, sugar, and baking powder. WHO oral rehydration packs are readily available at stores and pharmacies in many developing countries.

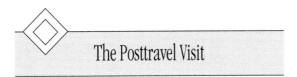

The Posttravel Visit

After the journey is completed, the clinician and patient have an opportunity not only to share experiences but also to reassess travel-related health risks. To have the most effect, this post-

travel visit should be scheduled for approximately 1 month after the traveler has returned home. Arrangements for this appointment can be made at the pretravel visit. The posttravel assessment provides an important opportunity to review the traveler's itinerary and to use this as a basis to discuss additional screening, counseling, or diagnostic testing. If potential exposure to tuberculosis occurred during travel, a repeat PPD test should be performed. Patients should be advised to seek medical attention immediately in the event of fever or persistent diarrhea, and to inform evaluating clinicians of their recent travel history. If the patient has symptoms, appropriate diagnostic tests (stool culture and stool for ova and parasites) can be performed. This also is an important opportunity to confirm completion of 4 weeks of posttravel malaria chemoprophylaxis and to assess the need for primaquine, which often is forgotten as soon as the traveler returns home.

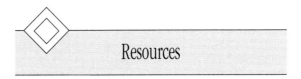

Resources

One of the challenges of travel medicine is keeping up with the diseases themselves. As with malaria, geographic and seasonal variations within countries rapidly change disease patterns. We therefore strongly recommend consultation with the web sites listed in Table 20-1 when considering each traveler's itinerary and exposure risks.

Health insurance in the event of illness during travel also is an important consideration. Many health insurers provide limited travel coverage. This often comes with a price of higher deductibles or copayments. Patients should be advised to check with their insurers before departure and to obtain specific information on what to do and where to go if illness occurs during travel. Many credit card companies and

Table 20-1

Travel Medicine On-Line Resources

CDC Home Travel Information Page	http://www.cdc.gov/travel/index.htm
World Health Organization (WHO)	http://www.who.ch/
American Journal of Tropical Medicine and Hygiene	http://www.astmh.org/journal.html
Journal of Travel Medicine	http://www.istm.org/jtm.html
U.S. State Department Consular Information and Travel Advisories	http://travel.state.gov/travel_warnings.html
Shoreland's Travel Health On-Line	http://www.tripprep.com

life insurance agencies offer short-term travel insurance.

Common Errors

Probably the most common error in preparing for travel is not allowing enough time before departure to receive the recommended vaccines at the recommended intervals and sequence. Careful planning is needed.

Risk reduction counseling often does not cover the potential for trauma from motor vehicle crashes. Advice to avoid ice and tooth brushing with tap water also is frequently neglected.

The potential for sexual encounters with residents of other countries often is overlooked and not asked about. Advice about safe sex practices and vaccine for hepatitis B should not be avoided simply because the future traveler does not admit to plans for sexual contact.

It is also common for advice about malaria prophylaxis not to include consideration of primaquine.

Finally, the posttravel visit and assessment sometimes are overlooked, and the travel history and likelihood of exposure to infectious disease are not considered when travel-related diseases manifest themselves after return.

Emerging Trends

New or evolving infectious diseases have received much attention from the news media and among the medical community. These changing disease patterns present a challenge to clinicians assessing patients' travel-related risks and offering prevention advice. Ready access to accurate and dependable sources of information is important.

Vaccines will likely be available against some serious travel-related health risks such as malaria and some of the causes of traveler's diarrhea. If it becomes a reality, an HIV vaccine would change risks associated with receipt of blood products and sexual encounters.

Computer-related technology has changed and will continue to change travel medicine. Web sites worldwide can provide advice even to remote areas by means of satellites. Medical records can be carried on computer disks, as can treatment recommendations. Advances in computer technology, telemedicine, and satellite communication will be used to make medical information more readily available worldwide.

Travel often provides patients with life-changing insights. With appropriate pretravel prevention and posttravel follow-up care, most trips abroad can be completed without being marred by serious illness. The clinician is in a unique position to share in this experience. As participants in the process, clinicians can reinforce health behaviors that apply not only to the travel at hand but also that last a lifetime.

Bibliography

Bruni M, Steffen R: Impact of travel related health impairments. *J Travel Med* 4:61–64, 1997.

Centers for Disease Control and Prevention: *Health Information for the International Traveler.* Atlanta: US Department of Health and Human Services, 1996–1997.

Centers for Disease Control and Prevention: *Blue Sheet.* Atlanta, U.S. Department of Health and Human Services, November 20, 1998.

Cohen J: Cholera and typhoid vaccine. *Aust Fam Phys* 26:943–946, 1997.

Conlon CP, Berendt AR, Dawson K, et al: Runway malaria. *Lancet* 335:472, 1990.

Dick L: Travel medicine: Helping patients prepare for trips abroad. *Am Fam Phys* 58:383–398, 1998.

Freedman DO: Keeping current: Travel medicine resources available on the Internet. *Infect Dis Clin North Am* 12:543–547, 1998.

Hans LO, Kozarsky PE: Update on prevention of malaria for travelers. *JAMA* 278:1767–1771, 1997.

Hargarten SW, Baker TD, Guptill K: Oversees fatalities of US citizen travelers: An analysis of deaths related to international travel. *Ann Emerg Med* 20: 622–626, 1991.

Kouri G, Guzman MG, Bravo J: Hemorrhagic dengue in Cuba: History of an epidemic. *Bull Pan Am Health Organ* 20:24–30, 1986.

Kroeger A, Mancheno M, Alarcon J, et al: Insecticide-impregnated bed nets for malaria control: varying experiences from Ecuador, Colombia, and Peru concerning acceptability and effectiveness. *Am J Trop Med Hyg* 53:313–323, 1995.

Lange WR, Beall B, Denny SC: Dengue fever: A resurgent risk for the international traveler. *Am Fam Phys* 45:1161–1168, 1992.

Mileno MD, Bia FJ: The compromised traveler. *Infect Dis Clin North Am* 12:369–412, 1998.

Osmitz TG, Murphy JV: Neurological effects associated with use of the insect repellent N,N-diethyl-m-toluamide (DEET). *J Toxicol Clin Toxicol* 35: 435–441, 1997.

Ostroff SM, Kozarsky P: Emerging infectious diseases and travel medicine. *Infect Dis Clin North Am* 12: 231–241, 1998.

Pust RE, Campos-Outcalt D, Cordes DH: International travel: Preparing your patient. *Prim Care* 18:213–240, 1991.

Pust RE, Peate WF, Cordes, DH: Comprehensive care of travelers. *J Fam Pract* 23:572–579, 1986.

Robertson SE, Hull BP, Tomori O, et al: Yellow fever: A decade of reemergence. *JAMA* 276:1157–1162, 1996.

Samuel BU, Barry M: The pregnant traveler. *Infect Dis Clin North Am* 12:325–355, 1998.

Steffen, R, Kane MA, Shapiro CN, et al: Epidemiology of hepatitis A in travelers. *JAMA* 272:885–889, 1994.

Thanassi WT: Immunizations for international travelers. *West J Med* 168:197–202, 1998.

Thompson R: *Travel and Routine Immunizations: A Practical Guide for the Medical Office.* Milwaukee: Shoreland, 1998.

Welsby PD: Highlights from the Fifth International Conference on travel medicine held in Geneva, Switzerland, on 24–27 March 1997. *Postgrad Med J* 74:61–62, 1998.

Wolfe MS: hepatitis A and the American traveler. *J Infect Dis* 171(Suppl 1):S29–S32, 1995.

World Health Organization: *The World Health Report 1997.* Geneva, World Health Organization, 1997.

Index

Page numbers followed by the letters *f* and *t* indicate figures and tables, respectively.

ISBN 0-07-012044-7

90000